Impact of COVID-19 on the Dental Community

Impact of COVID-19 on the Dental Community

Editors

Hans-Peter Howaldt
Sameh Attia

MDPI

Basel • Beijing • Wuhan • Barcelona • Belgrade • Novi Sad • Cluj • Manchester

Editors

Hans-Peter Howaldt
Justus-Liebig University Giessen
Giessen
Germany

Sameh Attia
Justus-Liebig University Giessen
Giessen
Germany

Editorial Office
MDPI
St. Alban-Anlage 66
4052 Basel, Switzerland

This is a reprint of articles from the Topical Collection published online in the open access journal *Journal of Clinical Medicine* (ISSN 2077-0383) (available at: https://www.mdpi.com/journal/jcm/topical_collections/Impact_Covid-19_Dental_Community).

For citation purposes, cite each article independently as indicated on the article page online and as indicated below:

Lastname, A.A.; Lastname, B.B. Article Title. *Journal Name* **Year**, *Volume Number*, Page Range.

ISBN 978-3-0365-9002-8 (Hbk)
ISBN 978-3-0365-9003-5 (PDF)
doi.org/10.3390/books978-3-0365-9003-5

Contents

About the Editors . . . . **vii**

Sameh Attia and Hans-Peter Howaldt
Impact of COVID-19 on the Dental Community: Part I before Vaccine (BV)
Reprinted from: *J. Clin. Med.* **2021**, *10*, 288, doi:10.3390/jcm10020288 . . . . **1**

Adi Kasem, Idan Redenski, Daniel Oren, Adeeb Zoabi, Samer Srouji and Fares Kablan
Decline in Maxillofacial Injuries during the Pandemic: The Hidden Face of COVID-19
Reprinted from: *J. Clin. Med.* **2023**, *12*, 128, doi:10.3390/jcm12010128 . . . . **3**

Nada O. Binmadi, Suad R. Aljohani, Maha T. Alsharif, Soulafa A. Almazrooa and Amal M. Sindi
Oral Manifestations of COVID-19: A Cross-Sectional Study of Their Prevalence and Association with Disease Severity
Reprinted from: *J. Clin. Med.* **2022**, *11*, 4461, doi:10.3390/jcm11154461 . . . . **11**

Balazs Feher, Cordelia Wieser, Theresa Lukes, Christian Ulm, Reinhard Gruber and Ulrike Kuchler
The Effect of the COVID-19 Pandemic on Patient Selection, Surgical Procedures, and Postoperative Complications in a Specialized Dental Implant Clinic
Reprinted from: *J. Clin. Med.* **2022**, *11*, 855, doi:10.3390/jcm11030855 . . . . **23**

Karin Christine Huth, Leonard von Bronk, Maximilian Kollmuss, Stefanie Lindner, Jürgen Durner, Reinhard Hickel and Miriam Esther Draenert
Special Teaching Formats during the COVID-19 Pandemic—A Survey with Implications for a Crisis-Proof Education
Reprinted from: *J. Clin. Med.* **2021**, *10*, 5099, doi:10.3390/jcm10215099 . . . . **31**

Magdalena Sycinska-Dziarnowska, Marzia Maglitto, Krzysztof Woźniak and Gianrico Spagnuolo
Oral Health and Teledentistry Interest during the COVID-19 Pandemic
Reprinted from: *J. Clin. Med.* **2021**, *10*, 3532, doi:10.3390/jcm10163532 . . . . **43**

Nima Farshidfar, Dana Jafarpour, Shahram Hamedani, Arkadiusz Dziedzic and Marta Tanasiewicz
Proposal for Tier-Based Resumption of Dental Practice Determined by COVID-19 Rate, Testing and COVID-19 Vaccination: A Narrative Perspective
Reprinted from: *J. Clin. Med.* **2021**, *10*, 2116, doi:10.3390/jcm10102116 . . . . **55**

Abanoub Riad, Andrea Pokorná, Sameh Attia, Jitka Klugarová, Michal Koščík and Miloslav Klugar
Prevalence of COVID-19 Vaccine Side Effects among Healthcare Workers in the Czech Republic
Reprinted from: *J. Clin. Med.* **2021**, *10*, 1428, doi:10.3390/jcm10071428 . . . . **73**

Sajjad Shirazi, Clark M. Stanford and Lyndon F. Cooper
Characteristics and Detection Rate of SARS-CoV-2 in Alternative Sites and Specimens Pertaining to Dental Practice: An Evidence Summary
Reprinted from: *J. Clin. Med.* **2021**, *10*, 1158, doi:10.3390/jcm10061158 . . . . **91**

Mohamed Mekhemar, Sameh Attia, Christof Dörfer and Jonas Conrad
The Psychological Impact of the COVID-19 Pandemic on Dentists in Germany
Reprinted from: *J. Clin. Med.* **2021**, *10*, 1008, doi:10.3390/jcm10051008 . . . . **103**

Stéphane Derruau, Jérôme Bouchet, Ali Nassif, Alexandre Baudet, Kazutoyo Yasukawa, Sandrine Lorimier, et al.
COVID-19 and Dentistry in 72 Questions: An Overview of the Literature
Reprinted from: *J. Clin. Med.* **2021**, *10*, 779, doi:10.3390/jcm10040779 . . . . **121**

Barbora Hocková, Abanoub Riad, Jozef Valky, Zuzana Šulajová, Adam Stebel, Rastislav Slávik, et al.
Oral Complications of ICU Patients with COVID-19: Case-Series and Review of Two Hundred Ten Cases
Reprinted from: *J. Clin. Med.* **2021**, *10*, 581, doi:10.3390/jcm10040581 . . . . **167**

Christopher J. Coke, Brandon Davison, Niariah Fields, Jared Fletcher, Joseph Rollings, Leilani Roberson, et al.
SARS-CoV-2 Infection and Oral Health: Therapeutic Opportunities and Challenges
Reprinted from: *J. Clin. Med.* **2021**, *10*, 156, doi:10.3390/jcm10010156 . . . . **181**

Andrea Butera, Carolina Maiorani, Valentino Natoli, Ambra Bruni, Carmen Coscione, Gaia Magliano, et al.
Bio-Inspired Systems in Nonsurgical Periodontal Therapy to Reduce Contaminated Aerosol during COVID-19: A Comprehensive and Bibliometric Review
Reprinted from: *J. Clin. Med.* **2020**, *9*, 3914, doi:10.3390/jcm9123914 . . . . **201**

Dorota Pylińska-Dąbrowska, Anna Starzyńska, Wiesław Jerzy Cubała, Karolina Ragin, Daniela Alterio and Barbara Alicja Jereczek-Fossa
Psychological Functioning of Patients Undergoing Oral Surgery Procedures during the Regime Related with SARS-CoV-2 Pandemic
Reprinted from: *J. Clin. Med.* **2020**, *9*, 3344, doi:10.3390/jcm9103344 . . . . **231**

Alona Emodi-Perlman, Ilana Eli, Joanna Smardz, Nir Uziel, Gniewko Wieckiewicz, Efrat Gilon, et al.
Temporomandibular Disorders and Bruxism Outbreak as a Possible Factor of Orofacial Pain Worsening during the COVID-19 Pandemic—Concomitant Research in Two Countries
Reprinted from: *J. Clin. Med.* **2020**, *9*, 3250, doi:10.3390/jcm9103250 . . . . **243**

Bruna Sinjari, Damiano D'Ardes, Manlio Santilli, Imena Rexhepi, Gianmaria D'Addazio, Piero Di Carlo, et al.
SARS-CoV-2 and Oral Manifestation: An Observational, Human Study
Reprinted from: *J. Clin. Med.* **2020**, *9*, 3218, doi:10.3390/jcm9103218 . . . . **259**

Sunita Manuballa, Marym Abdelmaseh, Nirmala Tasgaonkar, Vladimir Frias, Michael Hess, Heidi Crow, et al.
Managing the Oral Health of Cancer Patients during the COVID-19 Pandemic: Perspective of a Dental Clinic in a Cancer Center
Reprinted from: *J. Clin. Med.* **2020**, *9*, 3138, doi:10.3390/jcm9103138 . . . . **273**

Aneta Olszewska and Piotr Rzymski
Children's Dental Anxiety during the COVID-19 Pandemic: Polish Experience
Reprinted from: *J. Clin. Med.* **2020**, *9*, 2751, doi:10.3390/jcm9092751 . . . . **283**

Cinzia Maspero, Andrea Abate, Davide Cavagnetto, Mohamed El Morsi, Andrea Fama and Marco Farronato
Available Technologies, Applications and Benefits of Teleorthodontics. A Literature Review and Possible Applications during the COVID-19 Pandemic
Reprinted from: *J. Clin. Med.* **2020**, *9*, 1891, doi:10.3390/jcm9061891 . . . . **295**

About the Editors

Hans-Peter Howaldt

Prof. Howaldt, Dr. med. Dr. med. dent., is well known in the field of maxillofacial surgery. He began his journey in 1997 when he was appointed as a full professor at the University Hospital in Gießen. Prof. Howaldt's dedication is evident through his involvement as a member and former executive of both the German Society for Oral and Maxillofacial Surgery (DGMKG) and the European Association for Cranio-Maxillo-Facial Surgery (EACMFS). He also serves as the head of the ethical committee of the medical university in Gießen. His expertise and leadership have made a lasting impact on maxillofacial surgery, inspiring many aspiring surgeons to follow in his footsteps. Prof. Howaldt is widely respected in the medical community for his contributions and commitment to his profession.

Sameh Attia

PD Dr. med. dent. Sameh Attia, M.Sc., is a dentist, oral surgeon, and part of the scientific staff at the Clinic and Polyclinic for Oral and Maxillofacial Surgery at the University Hospital Giessen in Germany. He is also serving as a senior physician at the same hospital and is the head of the Dental Polyclinic and Initial Admission Clinic and Polyclinic for Oral and Maxillofacial Surgery. Additionally, he is responsible for the dental emergency service.

Dr. Attia obtained his Doctorate in Dentistry from Justus Liebig University Giessen and a Master of Science in International Master of Applied Scientific Dental/Medical Education and Research from Christian-Albrechts University Kiel. He has also achieved Habilitation (Venia legendi) in Dentistry, Oral and Maxillofacial Surgery from the Faculty of Medicine at Justus Liebig University Giessen. Currently, he is serving as a Visiting Professor at the Faculty of Medicine at Masaryk University in Brno, Czech Republic.

Journal of
Clinical Medicine

MDPI

Editorial

Impact of COVID-19 on the Dental Community: Part I before Vaccine (BV)

Sameh Attia * and Hans-Peter Howaldt

Department of Oral and Maxillofacial Surgery, Justus-Liebig University of Giessen, Klinikstr. 33, 35392 Giessen, Germany; HP.Howaldt@uniklinikum-giessen.de
* Correspondence: sameh.attia@dentist.med.uni-giessen.de

One year has passed with the COVID-19 pandemic and its impact is still evident everywhere on the globe and in all fields and domains. It was very clear that we all were not prepared for such a situation which was completely new for the living generation. However, the light of optimism has been shed with the onset of vaccination.

From beginning of the pandemic, authors realized the imminent impact on the dental field. The route of transmission via contact with droplets and aerosols puts dentists at high risk of infection. Dental treatment became a challenge during the outbreak. Initially, the publications dealing with the COVID-19 and the dental field were limited; then, we had a stream of papers with different quality grades. With this Special Issue, we aim to act as a scientific meeting point for all kinds of high-quality research dealing with the management of the COVID-19 crisis within the dental community. However, the main problem faced by scientific groups in multiple countries has been that health authorities were hesitant to approve clinical investigations for research purposes on COVID-19 patients to reduce the spread of infection.

To date, we have been able to publish eight high-quality research and review papers which significantly added knowledge to the scientific community and the recognized progress of the pandemic. With the beginning of vaccination, a very important milestone was achieved, and we recommend dividing the pandemic time into: before vaccine (BV) and after vaccine (AV). This classification allows a better understanding of the research circumstances, psychologies, and perspectives.

In the first pandemic phase (BV), most non-essential dentist visits were canceled or postponed to avoid the spread of infection. Tele-dentistry arose as a promising field, allowing to maintain recall visits without physical contact [1]. This technology can be also used post-COVID especially in some dental disciplines and when clinical or radiological investigations are not required. However, dental emergency treatment is still available and requires a physical visit to the dental office. While dental anxiety of children under pandemic circumstances did not show any increase, as it was tested in a specific group [2] another study presented an enhancement of dental anxiety among patients undergoing oral surgery procedures [3]. Providing treatment for oral cancer patients can be considered as an urgent treatment that has to be maintained during the pandemic. This goal can be achieved with an adequate treatment protocol to protect immunocompromised patients and involved health care professional workers [4]. Other protocols using bio-inspired systems in nonsurgical periodontal treatment led to a reduction in aerosol generation and therefore limited the spreading of COVID-19 infection [5]. Over time, it became clear that the SARS-CoV-2 virus directly affected the oral cavity with several signs and symptoms such as xerostomia, impaired taste, burning sensation, and difficulty in swallowing [6,7]. An indirect impact of Coronavirus was detected in patients in two countries who had worsening bruxism and temporomandibular dysfunction (TMD) symptoms [8].

It can be concluded from the present editorial which contains a summary of the published papers usque ad diem, that we learned a lot about the pandemic in its first

Citation: Attia, S.; Howaldt, H.-P. Impact of COVID-19 on the Dental Community: Part I before Vaccine (BV). *J. Clin. Med.* **2021**, *10*, 288. https://doi.org/10.3390/jcm10020288

Received: 7 January 2021
Accepted: 13 January 2021
Published: 14 January 2021

phase (BV). There remains a lot of work to do in the next phase of the pandemic (AV). All scientific works and well-conducted clinical reviews regarding the COVID-19 outbreak and its effects on the dental field are more than welcome and of great importance in the second pandemic phase.

Funding: This research received no external funding.

Acknowledgments: The guest editors acknowledge their respect to all distinguished authors who conducted clinical studies and reviews which were published in this special issue.

Conflicts of Interest: The authors declare no conflict of interest.

References

1. Maspero, C.; Abate, A.; Cavagnetto, D.; El Morsi, M.; Fama, A.; Farronato, M. Available technologies, applications and benefits of teleorthodontics. A literature review and possible applications during the COVID-19 Pandemic. *J. Clin. Med.* **2020**, *9*, 1891. [CrossRef] [PubMed]
2. Olszewska, A.; Rzymski, P. Children's Dental Anxiety during the COVID-19 Pandemic: Polish Experience. *J. Clin. Med.* **2020**, *9*, 2751. [CrossRef]
3. Pylińska-Dąbrowska, D.; Starzyńska, A.; Cubała, W.J.; Ragin, K.; Alterio, D.; Jereczek-Fossa, B.A. Psychological Functioning of Patients Undergoing Oral Surgery Procedures during the Regime Related with SARS-CoV-2 Pandemic. *J. Clin. Med.* **2020**, *9*, 3344. [CrossRef] [PubMed]
4. Manuballa, S.; Abdelmaseh, M.; Tasgaonkar, N.; Frias, V.; Hess, M.; Crow, H.; Andreana, S.; Gupta, V.; Wooten, K.E.; Markiewicz, M.R. Managing the Oral Health of Cancer Patients During the COVID-19 Pandemic: Perspective of a Dental Clinic in a Cancer Center. *J. Clin. Med.* **2020**, *9*, 3138. [CrossRef] [PubMed]
5. Butera, A.; Maiorani, C.; Natoli, V.; Bruni, A.; Coscione, C.; Magliano, G.; Giacobbo, G.; Morelli, A.; Moressa, S.; Scribante, A. Bio-Inspired Systems in Nonsurgical Periodontal Therapy to Reduce Contaminated Aerosol during COVID-19: A Comprehensive and Bibliometric Review. *J. Clin. Med.* **2020**, *9*, 3914. [CrossRef] [PubMed]
6. Sinjari, B.; D'Ardes, D.; Santilli, M.; Rexhepi, I.; D'Addazio, G.; Di Carlo, P.; Chiacchiaretta, P.; Caputi, S.; Cipollone, F. SARS-CoV-2 and Oral Manifestation: An Observational, Human Study. *J. Clin. Med.* **2020**, *9*, 3218. [CrossRef]
7. Coke, C.J.D.B.; Fields, N.; Fletcher, J.; Rollings, J.; Roberson, L.; Challagundla, K.B.; Sampath, C.; Cade, J.; Farmer-Dixon, C.; Gangula, P.R. SARS-CoV-2 Infection and Oral Health: Therapeutic Opportunities and Challenges. *J. Clin. Med.* **2021**, *10*, 20. [CrossRef]
8. Emodi-Perlman, A.; Eli, I.; Smardz, J.; Uziel, N.; Wieckiewicz, G.; Gilon, E.; Grychowska, N.; Wieckiewicz, M. Temporomandibular Disorders and Bruxism Outbreak as a Possible Factor of Orofacial Pain Worsening during the COVID-19 Pandemic—Concomitant Research in Two Countries. *J. Clin. Med.* **2020**, *9*, 3250. [CrossRef] [PubMed]

Journal of
Clinical Medicine

Article

Decline in Maxillofacial Injuries during the Pandemic: The Hidden Face of COVID-19

Adi Kasem [1,†], Idan Redenski [1,†], Daniel Oren [1], Adeeb Zoabi [1], Samer Srouji [1,2,*] and Fares Kablan [1]

1 Department of Oral and Maxillofacial Surgery, Galilee College of Dental Sciences, Galilee Medical Center, Nahariya 2210001, Israel
2 The Azrieli Faculty of Medicine, Bar-Ilan University, Safed 1311502, Israel
* Correspondence: dr.samersrouji@gmail.com
† These authors contributed equally to this work.

Abstract: Maxillofacial injuries result from a variety of daily activities. Traffic accidents, interpersonal violence, and falls represent some of the most common etiological factors behind maxillofacial fractures. During the COVID-19 outbreak, the social distancing measures imposed by healthcare authorities aimed at abolishing the spread of the viral infection. This study aimed to evaluate the effect of social distancing measures on the incidence of maxillofacial injuries. Methods: Data were retrieved from the medical file registry at the Galilee Medical Center, Nahariya, Israel. Incidence, gender, age, etiology, and cost of hospitalization during the COVID-19 lockdown and the previous periods were retrieved. Results: A decrease in maxillofacial fractures was registered during the 2020 lockdown; younger patients had the largest share of maxillofacial traumas during this period. The midface was the most involved facial region in both periods, and a reduction of 62.3% in the cost of OMF fracture treatment was observed during the COVID-19 era. Conclusions: The occurrence, etiology, and cost of treatment of maxillofacial injuries during the COVID-19 period were different from those in the corresponding period in the pre-COVID-19 era. These results can provide a guide to help design programs for the prevention of OMF trauma.

Keywords: maxillofacial injuries; facial bone fractures; COVID-19

Citation: Kasem, A.; Redenski, I.; Oren, D.; Zoabi, A.; Srouji, S.; Kablan, F. Decline in Maxillofacial Injuries during the Pandemic: The Hidden Face of COVID-19. *J. Clin. Med.* **2023**, *12*, 128. https://doi.org/10.3390/jcm12010128

Academic Editors: Hans-Peter Howaldt and Sameh Attia

Received: 8 November 2022
Revised: 19 December 2022
Accepted: 20 December 2022
Published: 24 December 2022

1. Introduction

Maxillofacial injuries are among the most common injuries and are usually combined with fractures of facial bones. Facial bone fractures may include the zygomatic complex and the malar bones, the maxilla and the mandible, the orbital walls, the alveoli and the teeth, and the nasal and frontal sinus bones [1,2]. Different traumatic events may affect the maxillofacial region, e.g., road accidents, falls (falls from heights, falls due to systemic illness), interpersonal violence, work accidents, sport, and other injuries [3–5]. Israeli government organizations have been investing resources and facilities in an attempt to control and decrease those leading causes, all without improvement. In the past three years, there was an average of approximately 190,000 road accidents in Israel annually. In 2019, 81,000 people were injured, and 343 were killed there. The economic cost of road accidents in Israel is ca. 4.9 billion US dollars a year, which is about 1.3% of the national product [6].

COVID-19 is an infectious disease that was first reported in December 2019 in Wuhan, China, and has since spread globally, resulting in the ongoing coronavirus pandemic fueled by human-to-human transmission [7]. One of the essential ways to control it that has been utilized worldwide is decreasing interpersonal contact. In Israel, the first case was described in February 2020. Since March 2020, the whole country has been on lockdown to slow down the spread of the infection. In addition, there was a shutdown of public transport, road transport and trains, educational institutions, business centers, parks, and other social interaction points.

The GMC is considered a high-level trauma center localized in the north of Israel, and the Department of Maxillofacial Surgery is an essential part of this center. In our hospital, there was a significant reduction in the rate of admission of patients suffering from traumatic injuries during March and April 2020 (COVID-19 era). The aim of this study is to evaluate the occurrence of maxillofacial injuries in our hospital in the period of COVID-19 and compare it to the corresponding pre-COVID-19 era (2017, 2018, and 2019).

2. Materials and Methods

This retrospective study was approved by the GMC Helsinki committee. Medical files of all the maxillofacial trauma patients who were admitted to the GMC during the year 2019, as well as of the patients admitted for trauma during March and April 2020 (COVID-19 lockdown) and the corresponding periods prior to the COVID-19 lockdown, i.e., March–April for 2017 and 2018 (termed "pre-COVID periods") were reviewed. Only patients who had sustained an injury with subsequent facial bone fractures were included in the study. Etiology of injury, age, gender, treatment, site of injury, operative time, number of plates and screws, and duration of hospitalization were all included in the analysis. The patients were divided into five groups according to the period they were admitted to the GMC trauma center. The first group included OMF fractures admitted to the hospital during the year 2019. The second, third, and fourth groups belonged to the pre-COVID-19 era and included the patients who were admitted to the hospital during March and April of each year from 2017 to 2019. The fifth group included the trauma patients admitted during March–April 2020, which corresponded to the COVID-19 lockdown.

Statistical analysis was performed using IBM SPSS statistics software version 27.0. Continuous data were described using the means and range. Categorical data were presented by frequencies and percentages. For the calculation of maxillofacial injuries incidence and odds ratios, the general population used for analysis included the entire population in the region of Acre in Western Galilee, served by the hospital during the corresponding years.

Continuous variables were analyzed using the Mann–Whitney test. Categorical variables (gender, etiological factors, trauma site, etc.) for different years were compared and analyzed using Pearson's chi-squared test, Fisher–Freeman–Halton exact test (if expectancy < 5), and univariate logistic regression analysis (the results were reported as odds ratios (OR) and each year from the pre-COVID era was compared to the COVID-19 lockdown period in 2020); the differences were considered significant at $p < 0.05$. Two-sided p-values were presented unless otherwise noted.

3. Results

3.1. Incidence of OMF Admissions

One hundred five maxillofacial trauma patients were admitted to the GMC emergency department in 2019. The peak in OMF fractures was registered in March and April of that year (Figure 1).

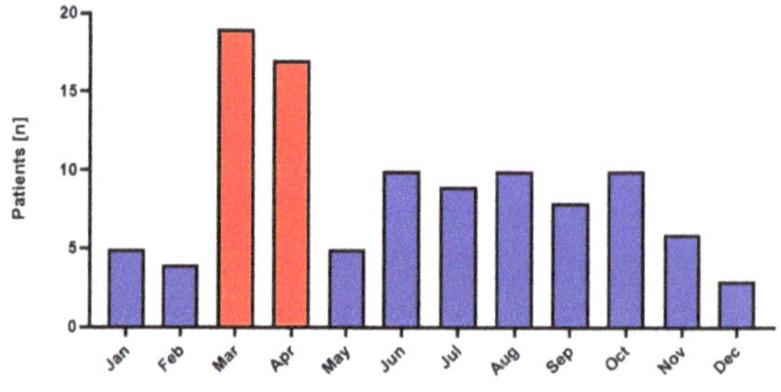

Figure 1. Trauma patients admitted to the Galilee Medical Center in 2019.

The patients admitted during March and April before the COVID-19 outbreak included a total of 89 maxillofacial fractures (Figure 2). The average number of monthly admissions in these periods was 12 patients, and the average age of the trauma patients admitted was 45.6 years. During the COVID-19 lockdown in 2020, seven patients were admitted to the hospital with an average age of 28.7 years upon admission.

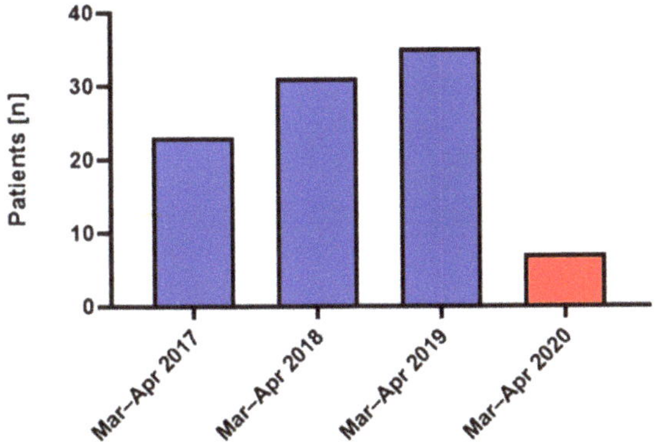

Year	*P* value	OR	95% CI for OR	
			Lower	Upper
2017	0.004	3.4	1.5	8.0
2018	<0.001	4.5	2.0	10.3
2019	<0.001	5.1	2.2	11.4

Figure 2. Trauma patients admitted to the Galilee Medical Center during March and April of 2017, 2018, and 2019 compared to the same period in 2020 corresponding to the COVID–19 lockdown, presented with univariate logistic regression analysis.

While during the COVID-19 lockdown, the cases of facial trauma were 1.07 cases per 100,000 residents. In the previous years, 2017, 2018, and 2019, the incidence of facial trauma was 3.65, 4.86, and 5.4 cases per 100,000 residents, respectively. Logistic regression indicated significant differences compared to the 2020 COVID-19 period, being 3.4, 4.5, and 5.1 higher in 2017, 2018, and 2019, respectively (Figure 2).

Both in the COVID-19 and the corresponding pre-COVID-19 periods, the admission rate of male patients was higher than that of female patients (a total of 74 male patients compared to 22 females), a ratio of 3.36/1. For males, a significantly higher occurrence of maxillofacial injuries was registered in the years 2017, 2018, and 2019, being 3.3, 3.6, and 4.7 times higher compared to the COVID-19 lockdown in 2020 (Figure 3, *p*-values = 0.011, 0.006, and 0.001, respectively). The same trend regarding the occurrence of maxillofacial injuries was registered for female patients, being 4.216, 10.27, and 7.09 higher in the years 2017, 2018, and 2019 compared to the COVID-19 lockdown in 2020 (Figure 3, *p*-values = 0.067, 0.026, and 0.202, respectively).

3.2. *Age and Etiology*

Age ranged from 5 to 89 years, with an average age of 44 ± 23 years upon admission. In 2017, 2018, and 2019, the corresponding periods showed a clear trend, with the majority of OMF trauma patients being older than 29 years of age (52.17%, 74.19%, and 71.42%, respectively). However, while the involvement of age groups varied across the periods under investigation, one trend seemed consistent. The lockdown period (March–April 2020) showed a distinct increase in trauma patients aged 20–29 years compared to the same period in 2017, 2018, and 2019 (an increase of 31.06%, 40.46%, and 42.86% compared to 2020, respectively), reaching a total of 57.14% of the patients as described in Figure 4. While age differences were not found to be significantly different between 2017 and the year 2020, a significant difference was found via a one-sided hypothesis for 2018 and 2019 (p-values = 0.039 and 0.05, respectively).

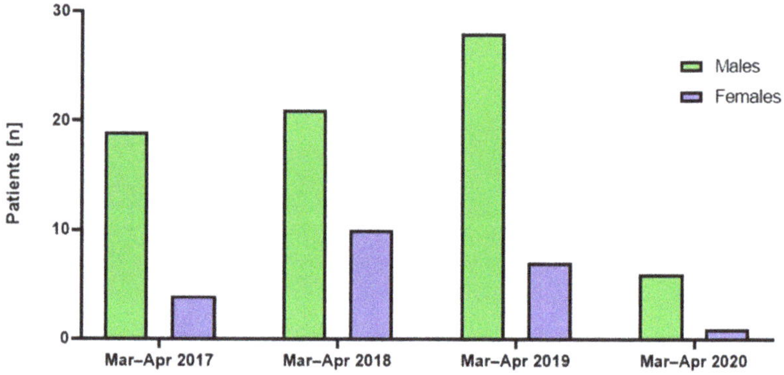

Figure 3. Trauma patients (males and females) admitted during March and April to the GMC trauma center in the years 2017–2020.

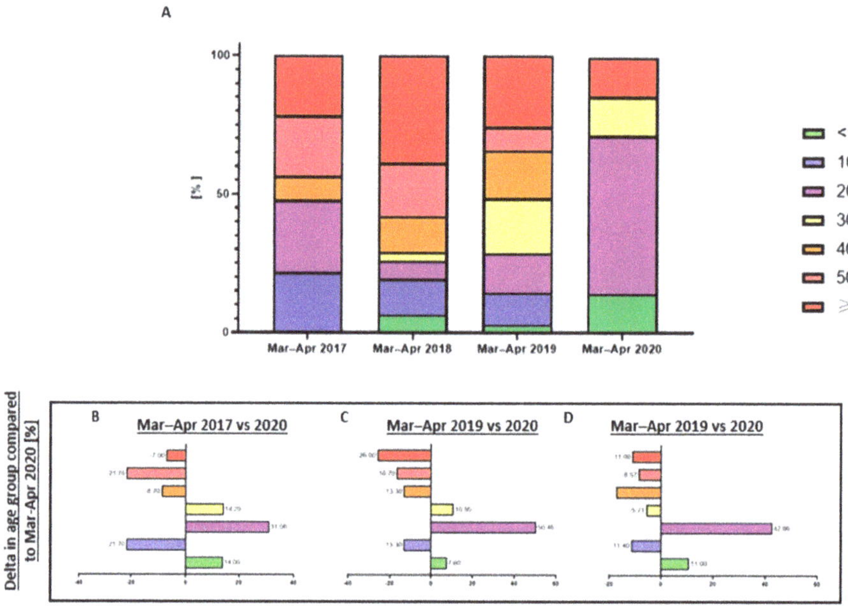

Figure 4. Age distribution across the trauma patients admitted during March and April to the GMC trauma center in the years 2017–2020. (**A**) Admissions as the percentage of the total admissions during March and April of each year. (**B–D**) Change in each age group admitted during 2017, 2018, and 2019 compared to the period corresponding to the COVID–19 lockdown.

The leading cause of traumatic maxillofacial fractures in the patients admitted during the COVID-19 lockdown and the corresponding periods in 2017, 2018, and 2019 were falls, followed by road accidents. Together, these etiologies comprised well over 50% of the hospital admissions during March and April in 2017, 2018, 2019, and 2020 (69.56%, 87.09%, 68.57%, and 57.15%, respectively, Figure 5). Etiological factors did not show statistically significant changes before and during the COVID-19 lockdown, possibly due to the low number of facial trauma admissions during the 2020 COVID-19 lockdown.

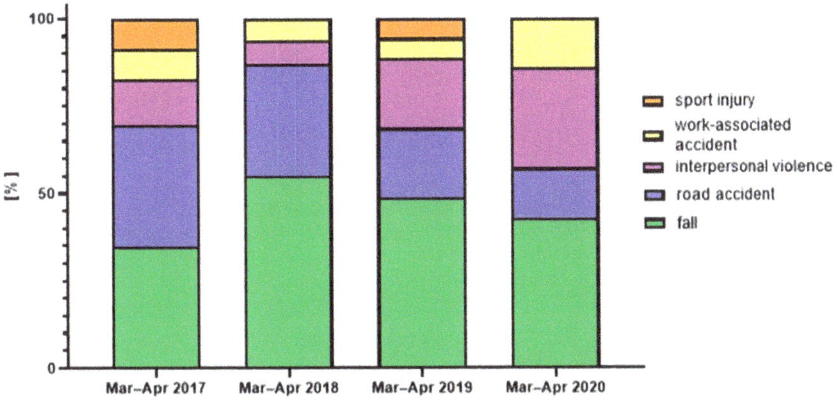

Figure 5. Etiology of OMF fractures admitted to the GMC trauma center during March and April in the years 2017–2020.

3.3. Injury Site and Costs

The majority of facial fractures across the periods involved both the mandible and the midface, with a cumulative occurrence of over 60% across the periods analyzed (Figure 5). Interestingly, injuries involving the upper third of the facial skeleton were not registered at all during the lockdown (Figure 6).

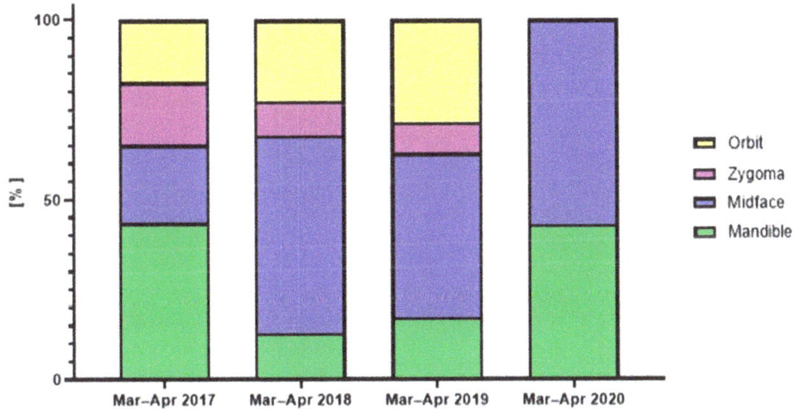

Figure 6. OMF fractures according to the site of injury in the patients admitted to the GMC trauma center during March and April in the years 2017–2020.

As for the total treatment cost during March and April in the pre-COVID-19 period as well as the corresponding COVID-19 lockdown, a reduction of 62.3% in the total cost of OMF fractures was registered (Figure 7). The average treatment cost per month during the pre-COVID-19 era was 52,874 USD, while during the COVID-19 lockdown, the treatment expenses decreased substantially, reaching as low as 19,945 USD.

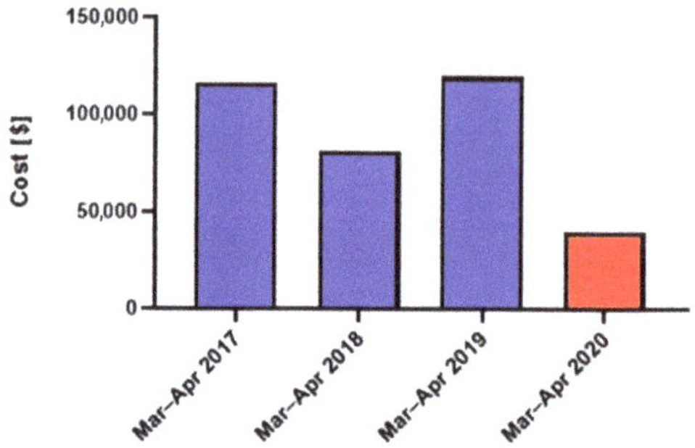

Figure 7. Total costs associated with maxillofacial fractures in the patients admitted during the COVID era and the corresponding periods in 2017–2019.

4. Discussion

The outbreak of the COVID-19 virus was a challenge for the world community. Despite all scientific progress nowadays, social distancing and personal hygiene were the most effective tools to prevent the spread of the virus. Most countries had imposed lockdowns and social distancing, with Israel being amongst the countries that adopted a strict social distancing policy, imposing a lockdown on all amenities of life, specifically during the period between March and April 2020 [8] with the intention of slowing down the spread of the COVID-19 infection. Thus, a total shutdown of all public transportation and gathering areas was in effect and included trains, major roads closure, and shutdown of educational institutions, business centers, cultural centers, and public parks [9].

Generally, when winter ends, and spring begins, most Israeli citizens are on holiday, spending more time outdoors and having face-to-face interactions. This period usually correlates with a rise in traumatic injuries, including OMF injuries [10]. During 2019, one hundred and five patients were admitted to our department suffering from different OMF fractures, with the average number of patients per month being 8.33 patients. Specifically, during the months of March and April in the same year, the average number of patients admitted was 17.5, more than a fourfold rise in admissions of patients with OMF injuries compared to the previous months in 2019. These results were in accordance with other studies where the peak in the incidence of OMF injuries was registered in March and April [11,12].

In the pre-COVID period, during March and April, the monthly average number of patients was 14.83, with traffic accidents being the main etiological factor for OMF fractures admission. This trend corresponds with previous reports that described traffic accidents as the leading cause of OMF fractures [10–12]. However, during the COVID-19 lockdown, a dramatic reduction in admissions of patients with maxillofacial fractures was registered, with an average of 3.5 patients per month. The lowered admission rates were in line with reports from other healthcare centers during the pandemic [13]. The average age upon admission during the COVID-19 lockdown was 28.7 years, compared to 45.6 years during the corresponding periods in the pre-COVID era. The fact that younger patients were more involved in injuries resulting from outdoor and interpersonal activities correlates with reports regarding the perceived importance of quarantine measures amongst younger people. Among respondents on the perceived importance of social distancing measures and self-isolation guidelines, younger respondents reported lower adherence to full self-isolation periods and less compliance with social distancing measures [14]. Moreover, almost no compliance was reported among people of lower age, in children and adolescents, who were also admitted to the GMC during the pandemic [15]. Thus, the change in age distribution between the pre-COVID era and the COVID-19 outbreak corresponded to the perceived importance of safety measures amongst younger patients during these times.

A major result of the lower admissions rate during the pandemic was a reduction of 62.3% in the total cost of OMF fractures treatment at the GMC trauma center. This trend correlated with the reduced admission rate during the pandemic. However, while the cost of trauma-related therapy was reduced, it was outweighed by the cost of treatment of infected COVID-19 patients, accompanied by the dramatic reduction in elective services [16,17].

5. Conclusions

Treatment of trauma injuries worldwide has seen a dramatic change during the COVID-19 pandemic. These changes were also observed in Israel, with a massive reduction in admissions due to OMF fractures. Thus, the social distancing and "stay-at-home" policy had a clear positive effect on the incidence of facial injuries.

Author Contributions: Conceptualization, S.S. and F.K.; Methodology, D.O. and A.Z.; Formal analysis, I.R.; Investigation, A.K., D.O. and F.K.; Resources, S.S.; Data curation, A.K. and I.R.; Writing—original draft, A.K. and I.R.; Writing—review & editing, S.S. and F.K.; Project administration, S.S. All authors have read and agreed to the published version of the manuscript.

Funding: This research received no external funding.

Institutional Review Board Statement: The study was conducted in accordance with the Declaration of Helsinki and approved by the Institutional Ethics Committee of The Galilee Medical Center (protocol 0156-20-NHR, approved 5 August 2020).

Conflicts of Interest: The authors declare no conflict of interest.

References

1. Iida, S.; Kogo, M.; Sugiura, T.; Mima, T.; Matsuya, T. Retrospective Analysis of 1502 Patients with Facial Fractures. *Int. J. Oral Maxillofac. Surg.* **2001**, *30*, 286–290. [CrossRef] [PubMed]
2. Ellis, E.; El-Attar, A.; Moos, K.F. An Analysis of 2,067 Cases of Zygomatico-Orbital Fracture. *J. Oral Maxillofac. Surg.* **1985**, *43*, 417–428. [CrossRef] [PubMed]
3. Gassner, R.; Tuli, T.; Hächl, O.; Rudisch, A.; Ulmer, H. Cranio-Maxillofacial Trauma: A 10 Year Review of 9543 Cases with 21 067 Injuries. J. *Cranio Maxillofac. Surg.* **2003**, *31*, 51–61. [CrossRef]
4. Subhashraj, K.; Nandakumar, N.; Ravindran, C. Review of Maxillofacial Injuries in Chennai, India: A Study of 2748 Cases. *Br. J. Oral Maxillofac. Surg.* **2007**, *45*, 637–639. [CrossRef] [PubMed]
5. Ruslin, M.; Wolff, J.; Forouzanfar, T.; Boffano, P. Maxillofacial Fractures Associated with Motor Vehicle Accidents: A Review of the Current Literature. *J. Oral Maxillofac. Surg. Med. Pathol.* **2015**, *27*, 303–307. [CrossRef]
6. Hertzog, C.; Azulai, E.; Ziggel, A.; Gutsman, E. Traffic Accident Costs for the National Economy. Available online: https://www.gov.il/he/departments/publications/reports/2020_cost_accidents_israel (accessed on 19 March 2022).
7. Yang, C.L.; Qiu, X.; Zeng, Y.K.; Jiang, M.; Fan, H.R.; Zhang, Z.M. Coronavirus Disease 2019: A Clinical Review. *Eur. Rev. Med. Pharmacol. Sci.* **2020**, *24*, 4585–4596. [CrossRef]
8. Leshem, E.; Afek, A.; Kreiss, Y. Buying Time with COVID-19 Outbreak Response, Israel. *Emerg. Infect. Dis.* **2020**, *26*, 2251–2253. [CrossRef]
9. Esquivel-Gómez, J.D.J.; Barajas-Ramírez, J.G. Efficiency of Quarantine and Self-Protection Processes in Epidemic Spreading Control on Scale-Free Networks. *Chaos* **2018**, *28*, 013119. [CrossRef]
10. Agarwal, P.; Mehrotra, D.; Agarwal, R.; Kumar, S.; Pandey, R. Patterns of Maxillofacial Fractures in Uttar Pradesh, India. Craniomaxillofac. *Trauma Reconstr.* **2017**, *10*, 48–55. [CrossRef]
11. Boffano, P.; Kommers, S.C.; Karagozoglu, K.H.; Forouzanfar, T. Aetiology of Maxillofacial Fractures: A Review of Published Studies during the Last 30 Years. *Br. J. Oral Maxillofac. Surg.* **2014**, *52*, 901–906. [CrossRef] [PubMed]
12. Van Hout, W.M.M.T.; Van Cann, E.M.; Abbink, J.H.; Koole, R. An Epidemiological Study of Maxillofacial Fractures Requiring Surgical Treatment at a Tertiary Trauma Centre between 2005 and 2010. *Br. J. Oral Maxillofac. Surg.* **2013**, *51*, 416–420. [CrossRef] [PubMed]
13. Kamine, T.H.; Rembisz, A.; Barron, R.J.; Baldwin, C.; Kromer, M. Decrease in Trauma Admissions with COVID-19 Pandemic. *West. J. Emerg. Med.* **2020**, *21*, 819–822. [CrossRef] [PubMed]
14. Zhao, S.Z.; Wong, J.Y.H.; Wu, Y.; Choi, E.P.H.; Wang, M.P.; Lam, T.H. Social Distancing Compliance under COVID-19 Pandemic and Mental Health Impacts: A Population-Based Study. *Int. J. Environ. Res. Public Health* **2020**, *17*, 6692. [CrossRef] [PubMed]
15. Saurabh, K.; Ranjan, S. Compliance and Psychological Impact of Quarantine in Children and Adolescents Due to COVID-19 Pandemic. *Indian J. Pediatr.* **2020**, *87*, 532–536. [CrossRef] [PubMed]

16. Ellison, A. Hospitals Face Financial Fallout from COVID-19: 6 Things to Know. Available online: https://www.beckershospitalreview.com/finance/hospitals-face-financial-fallout-from-covid-19-6-things-to-know.html (accessed on 24 April 2022).
17. Haut, E.R.; Leeds, I.L.; Livingston, D.H. The Effect on Trauma Care Secondary to the COVID-19 Pandemic: Collateral Damage From Diversion of Resources. *Ann. Surg.* **2020**, *272*, e204–e207. [CrossRef] [PubMed]

Journal of
Clinical Medicine

MDPI

Article

Oral Manifestations of COVID-19: A Cross-Sectional Study of Their Prevalence and Association with Disease Severity

Nada O. Binmadi *, Suad Aljohani, Maha T. Alsharif, Soulafa A. Almazrooa and Amal M. Sindi

Department of Oral Diagnostic Sciences, King Abdulaziz University Faculty of Dentistry, Jeddah 21589, Saudi Arabia; sraljohani@kau.edu.sa (S.A.); mtyalsharif@kau.edu.sa (M.T.A.); salmazrooa@kau.edu.sa (S.A.A.); amsindi@kau.edu.sa (A.M.S.)
* Correspondence: nmadi@kau.edu.sa

Abstract: Background: COVID-19, caused by SARS-CoV-2, has impacted the world in an unprecedented way since December 2019. SARS-CoV-2 was found in the saliva of patients, and entry points for the virus may have been through the numerous angiotensin-converting enzyme 2 receptors in the oral cavity. Oral manifestations of COVID-19 could contribute to the burden of oral disease. Objective: To determine the prevalence of oral manifestations of COVID-19 in patients and their association with disease severity. Methods: Interviews were conducted with adult participants diagnosed with COVID-19 between October 2021 and March 2022 to document their demographic and health status data, symptoms, and the presence of oral manifestations of COVID-19. Chi-square and the Fisher's exact test were used to compare data on the presence or absence of oral manifestations of COVID-19. Results: Of 195 participants interviewed, 33% were 18 to 24 years old, 33% were 25 to 34 years old, and 75% were female. A total of 57 (29%) had oral manifestations; the most common were taste disorders (60%), xerostomia (42%), and oral ulcers (11%). There was no relationship between the severity of COVID-19 and the presence of the oral manifestations. Conclusion: Oral manifestations of COVID-19 were common among female patients and linked to certain general COVID-19 symptoms regarding frequency and extent.

Keywords: COVID-19; cross-sectional study; oral manifestations; oral cavity; SARS-CoV-2; taste disorders; xerostomia

Citation: Binmadi, N.O.; Aljohani, S.; Alsharif, M.T.; Almazrooa, S.A.; Sindi, A.M. Oral Manifestations of COVID-19: A Cross-Sectional Study of Their Prevalence and Association with Disease Severity. *J. Clin. Med.* **2022**, *11*, 4461. https://doi.org/10.3390/jcm11154461

Academic Editors: Hans-Peter Howaldt and Sameh Attia

Received: 3 July 2022
Accepted: 28 July 2022
Published: 30 July 2022

1. Introduction

In December 2019 in Wuhan, Hubei Province, China, a cluster of patients were seen who had shortness of breath, fever, and pneumonia. On 7 January 2020, the Chinese government identified the cause of this pneumonia as a newly isolated coronavirus of 2019 (and the disease was named COVID-19). The virus quickly spread, and by 11 March 2020, more than 136 countries were affected by the disease. The World Health Organization (WHO) then declared the disease a global pandemic [1]. By 31 May 2022, COVID-19 had infected 528,816,317 individuals and resulted in 6,294,969 deaths globally [2]. Saudi Arabia reported its first case in March of 2020, and by 31 May 2022, the country had reported 768,648 cases of and 9149 deaths from the disease [3].

SARS-CoV-2, the agent of COVID-19, is a member of the family Coronaviridae. It belongs to the Betacoronavirus subfamily, together with two other highly pathogenic viruses, SARS-CoV and MERS-CoV. It is a positive-sense single-stranded RNA (+ssRNA) virus with envelope-anchored spike protein receptors that facilitate its entry into host cells [4,5]. Angiotensin-converting enzyme 2 (ACE2) is the main receptor involved in COVID-19 pathogenesis [5]. It is abundantly present on the ciliated cells of the airway epithelium, or alveolar type 2 cells, which are the primary sites attacked by the virus. Direct contact with patients and their respiratory droplets is a well-known mode of transmission [4].

The most common symptoms reported by patients with COVID-19 are fever; respiratory symptoms, such as a cough or shortness of breath; and general fatigue. Other less common symptoms include headache, taste distortion, anosmia, and sore throat. Additionally, some patients present with gastrointestinal symptoms, such as diarrhea, nausea, or vomiting. The severity of these symptoms depends on many factors, such as the time of exposure to the virus and the patient's age and gender, as well as the presence of coexisting diseases. Investigators found that patients with autoimmune diseases were more prone to the infection [6].

At the beginning of the pandemic, it was assumed that the disease did not affect the oral cavity, and this was considered a factor that distinguished COVID-19 from other viral exanthemas. Later, however, SARS-CoV-2 was detected in the saliva of patients with COVID-19. The reverse transcriptase–polymerase chain reaction (RT-PCR) test of saliva was found to be more sensitive than a routine nasopharyngeal test in detecting the virus [6]. ACE2 receptors are distributed all over the oral cavity and especially on the dorsum of the tongue and in the salivary glands; these locations make these sites potential entry points for the virus. Therefore, COVID-19 could contribute to the burden of oral disease [6–8]. The most commonly reported affected sites were the tongue (38%), labial mucosa (26%), and palate (22%). Oral lesions were symptomatic in 68% of the cases [6,8,9].

Many researchers reported that oral manifestations were associated with COVID-19. The types of manifestations varied significantly. Taste disorder was the first and most common oral symptom [8]. Other oral manifestations were aphthous-like lesions, herpetiform lesions, periodontitis, candidiasis, mucormycosis and oral lesions of Kawasaki-like disease, pustules, a fissured or depapillated tongue, macules, papules, plaques, abnormal pigmentation, halitosis, whitish areas, hemorrhagic crusts, necrosis, petechiae, swelling, erythema, and spontaneous bleeding [5,7,9,10]. The risk of some of these manifestations can be reduced by taking probiotics, as proposed by Butera et al. [11]. Little is known about the prevalence of these oral manifestations in adults. It also has not been affirmed whether the oral symptoms are a direct manifestation of the infection or merely a consequence of the immune response to it. We aimed in the present study to determine the prevalence of the oral manifestations of COVID-19 in patients and their association with disease severity and general symptoms.

2. Materials and Methods

2.1. Study Design and Setting

A cross-sectional survey was carried out at the King Abdulaziz University Faculty of Dentistry (KAUFD), Department of Oral Diagnostic Sciences, Jeddah, Saudi Arabia, between October of 2021 and March of 2022 to determine the prevalence of oral manifestations in patients diagnosed with COVID-19 and their association with disease severity and to describe the patterns of the oral manifestations. Ethical approval to conduct the study was granted by the Research Ethics Committee at KAUFD (study approval number: 204-01-21). Potential participants were informed that their participation was voluntary and that they were free to decline to participate in the study or to halt participation at any point during the study. All participants provided written informed consent. All data were anonymized and stored on secure servers that could only be accessed by authorized healthcare professionals from the Department of Oral Diagnostic Sciences, Faculty of Dentistry, King Abdulaziz University.

2.2. Study Population

Participants were 18 years of age or older, had been diagnosed with COVID-19 between March of 2020 and March of 2022, could read and write in English/Arabic, and could provide informed consent. We included participants who stated that they had confirmed COVID-19 disease based on a test performed at a government center or a private hospital/laboratory or on a self-test [12].

2.3. Sample Size Calculation

We used the sample size for cross-sectional studies [13], in which published systematic reviews reported a prevalence of 45% of taste disorders in COVID-19 patients (95% confidence interval [CI], 34% to 55%) (taste disorders were the commonest oral manifestation of COVID-19) [14]. We used a z-value from the standard normal distribution that reflected a 95% CI (e.g., $z = 1.96$ for 95%) and a margin of error of 7% [15]. This yielded a sample size of 185. A random sampling technique was used to recruit participants.

2.4. Study Procedures

Invitations were sent randomly via email, WhatsApp, or SMS to recruit eligible candidates. A reminder was sent 2 weeks and 1 month after the first invitation was sent. If we received an acceptance, we invited the participant to an interview with researchers via Zoom, Facetime, or a phone call or to an in-person interview. A standardized web-based survey (http://www.surveymonkey.com (accessed on 3 March 2021)) was used by the researchers when they interviewed the participants. We restricted multiple responses from the participants by using unique identification codes for each interviewer and participant. Before we interviewed participants, a face validity test was carried out by experts in the field of oral pathology or oral medicine to check if the survey covered all the needed questions and was appropriately written. Additionally, a pilot test of the questionnaire on 20 participants was performed to study the questions' clarity and verify reliability. We revised the survey and collection tool based on the outcomes of the pretesting procedures.

2.5. Data Collection

A total of 208 persons accepted our invitation and agreed to be interviewed and answer the survey, which took 10 min to complete. Survey questions asked about participants' demographic data and health status, their history of exposure to COVID-19, symptoms of COVID-19, and oral manifestations of COVID-19. We inquired about the presence of the following general symptoms of COVID-19: fever, cough, fatigue, myalgia/arthralgia, dyspnea, headache, sore throat, nausea/vomiting, diarrhea, nasal obstruction, or loss of smell. Individuals were also free to document any other symptoms. We also obtained information on the severity of COVID-19 (i.e., mild, moderate, severe, or critical) based on the guidelines in the document titled WHO COVID-19: Clinical Management, Interim Guidelines [16]. Information on the severity of each general symptom of COVID-19, whether mild, moderate, or severe, was assessed using the subjective Visual Analogue Scale (VAS), with 0 indicating no symptom and 10 the most severe symptom [17]. We assessed the duration of each symptom (i.e., 1 to 2 days, 3 to 4 days, or 5+ days), frequency of each symptom (i.e., occurred once, occurred intermittently, or occurred constantly), whether hospitalization was needed due to COVID-19, the reason for hospitalization, and the duration of hospitalization.

To determine the prevalence of oral manifestations of COVID-19, the participants were asked about their history of xerostomia, oral ulcerations, gingivitis, necrotizing periodontal disease, candidiasis, distortion of taste, vesiculobullous lesions, erythema migrans, geographic tongue, petechiae, and leukoplakia. Participants were also free to document any other symptoms. The severity, duration, frequency, location, and outcome of the oral manifestations were documented.

2.6. Data Analysis

Data were downloaded from the web-based tool Survey Monkey and imported into SAS version 9.2 for analysis. Continuous variables were expressed as the mean and standard deviation if they were normally distributed or as the median and range if they were skewed. Categorical variables were expressed as frequencies and proportions. Chi-square statistics or the Fisher's exact test was used to compare the findings and determine the proportions of participants with the findings, which were the overall severity of COVID-19, the presence or absence of oral manifestations of COVID-19, the general symptoms of COVID-19 with the presence or absence of oral manifestations of COVID-19, and the oral manifestations of COVID-19 by severity, duration, and frequency with the overall severity of COVID-19. Additionally, participants with different oral manifestations and the timing of the oral manifestations were described.

3. Results

3.1. Participant Selection

An invitation to participate in a survey was randomly sent out, and 208 individuals accepted the invitation. A total of 201 were eligible and consented to an interview by the research team. After individuals with incomplete documentation (n = 6) were excluded, 195 were deemed acceptable for inclusion in the final analysis.

3.2. Participant Characteristics, COVID-19 Disease Severity, and COVID-19 Exposure

Participants who had been previously diagnosed with COVID-19 rated their status at the time of diagnosis as asymptomatic or having mild symptoms (21%), moderate symptoms (59%), or severe and critical symptoms (20%). Of the patients, 33% were 18 to 24 years old and 33% were 25 to 34 years old. Most participants were female (75%). Approximately 33% were current or previous smokers, 18% were taking medications, and 9% had been hospitalized due to COVID-19. There was a significantly high proportion of participants older than 55 years with mild COVID-19 symptoms compared with other age groups (p = 0.0175). There was a significantly high proportion of moderate and severe COVID-19 symptoms in patients who were hospitalized compared with those with mild disease (p = 0.0002). Participants did not differ in COVID-19 severity based on gender, smoking history, or medication status (Table 1).

Table 1. Participant characteristics of COVID-19 with and without oral manifestations.

Participant Characteristics	All Participants (N = 195) n/N	COVID-19 Severity			p-Value **	Oral Manifestations of COVID-19		p-Value **
		Mild 41 (21%)	Moderate 115 (59%)	Severe and Critical ** 39 (20%)		Had Oral Manifestations of COVID-19 (n = 57; 29%)	Did Not Have Oral Manifestations of COVID-19 (n = 138; 71%)	
Age group:								
18–24 years	64 (33%)	15 (23%)	41 (64%)	8 (13%)	**0.0175**	18 (28%)	46 (72%)	0.3166
25–34 years	64 (33%)	7 (11%)	43 (67%)	14 (22%)		18 (285)	46 (72%)	
35–44 years	41 (21%)	12 (29%)	22 (54%)	7 (17%)		9 (22%)	32 (78%)	
45–54 years	13 (7%)	2 (15%)	5 (39%)	6 (46%)		6 (46%)	7 (54%)	
55+ years	13 (5%)	5 (38%)	4 (31%)	4 (31%)		6 (46%)	7 (54%)	
Sex:								
Female	147 (75%)	27 (18%)	88 (60%)	32 (22%)	0.2208	49 (33%)	98 (67%)	**0.0275**
Male	48 (25%)	14 (29%)	27 (56%)	7 (15%)		8 (17%)	40 (83%)	
Smoking history (current and previous smoker)	65 (33%)	9 (14%)	39 (60%)	17 (26%)	0.1192	16 (25%)	43 (75%)	0.3163
Taking medication €	36 (18%)	9 (25%)	21 (58%)	9 (17%)	0.7482	49 (33%)	98 (67%)	0.0275
Positive history of hospitalization due to COVID-19	17 (9%)	0 (0%)	7 (41%)	10 (59%)	**0.0002**	4 (24%)	13 (76%)	0.7819

** Chi = square statistics or Fisher's exact test. € These categories were not mutually exclusive.

Patients taking medications (n = 36; 18%) were taking antihypertensives (7), antihistamines (8), thyroid medication (7), antidiabetics (5), antiasthmatics (3), proton pump inhibitors (2), nutritional supplements (2), antiepileptics (2), antidepressants (1), osteoarthritis medication (1), benign prostatic hyperplasia medication (1), hormone replacements (1), or laxatives (1). These categories were not mutually exclusive (data not shown).

Although most had strictly followed the recommended COVID-19 preventive measures (73%), had not travelled abroad during the pandemic (86%), and were not healthcare providers (76%), the majority had been in contact with a person with COVID-19 (82%) and half had been in crowded places or attended a group gathering (50%) (data not shown).

3.3. COVID-19 General Symptoms, Severity, and Hospitalization Due to COVID-19

The general COVID-19 symptoms among all participants were fever (95%, n = 140), headache (65%, n = 127), fatigue (65%, n = 126), cough (63%, n = 122), myalgia/arthralgia (53%, n = 104), loss of smell (53%, n = 102), sore throat (50%, n = 97), shortness of breath or dyspnea (40%, n = 78), nausea or vomiting (21%, n = 41), and diarrhea (15%, n = 30). These categories were not mutually exclusive; a participant could report more than one symptom. The highest proportion of patients with severe symptoms had loss of smell; this symptom lasted 5+ days and was constant throughout that entire time (Table 2). Seventeen patients (9%) were hospitalized due to COVID-19 for 1 to 21 days, 10 for 1 to 7 days, 2 for 7 to 14 days, and 2 for 15 to 21 days; the duration for three participants was not documented. The reasons for hospitalization for the 11 participants who responded to this question varied; these were allergy (one participant), precautionary (one), back pain (one), chest pain (two), difficulty in breathing (two), fever (two), diarrhea and intravenous medication (one), and headache and fever (one).

Table 2. Relationships between general symptoms of COVID-19 in terms of severity, duration, and the frequency and presence of oral manifestations of COVID-19.

Symptom	Total 195	Severity of Specific COVID-19 Symptom				Duration of Specific COVID-19 Symptom				Frequency of Specific COVID-19 Symptom			
		Mild	Moderate	Severe	*p*-Value	1–2 Days	3–4 Days	5+ Days	*p*-Value	Once	Intermittent	Constant	*p*-Value
Fever	140 (72%)	34 (24%)	81 (58%)	25 (18%)		47 (35%)	46 (35%)	40 (30%)		13 (11%)	65 (53%)	45 (36%)	
Oral manifestations +	43 (31%)	9 (26%)	30 (37%)	4(16%)	0.8751	15 (32%)	13 (28%)	14 (35%)	0.7971	5 (39%)	22 (34%)	11 (24%)	0.4745
Oral manifestations −	97 (69%)	25 (74%)	51 (68%)	21 (84%)		32 (68%)	33 (72%)	26 (65%)		8 (62%)	43 (66%)	34 (76%)	
Headache	127 (65%)	33 (24%)	42 (33%)	52 (41%)		25 (22%)	29 (25%)	61 (53%)		10 (9%)	55 (49%)	47 (42%)	
Oral manifestations +	38 (29%)	11 (33%)	12 (29%)	15 (28%)	0.8832	6 (24%)	9 (31%)	20 (33%)	0.7214	0 (0%)	22 (40%)	22 (40%)	0.0336
Oral manifestations −	89 (71%)	22 (67%)	30 (71%)	37 (72%)		19 (76%)	20 (69%)	41 (67%)		10 (100%)	33 (60%)	34 (72%)	
Fatigue	126 (65%)	33 (26%)	48 (38%)	45 (36%)		19 (16%)	36 (31%)	61 (53%)		3 (3%)	37 (34%)	69 (63%)	
Oral manifestations +	40 (32%)	13 (39%)	17 (35%)	10 (22%)	0.2151	2 (11%)	7 (19%)	30 (49%)	0.0007	0 (0%)	13 (35%)	22 (32%)	0.4548
Oral manifestations −	86 (68%)	20 (61%)	31 (65%)	35 (78%)		17 (89%)	29 (82%)	31 (51%)		3 (100%)	24 (65%)	47 (68%)	
Cough	122 (63%)	41 (34%)	49 (40%)	32 (26%)		19 (17%)	29 (25%)	66 (58%)		5 (5%)	56 (55%)	41 (40%)	
Oral manifestations +	39 (32%)	17 (42%)	16 (33%)	6 (19%)	0.1176	3 (16%)	12 (41%)	23 (35%)	0.1669	2 (40%)	21 (38%)	11 (27%)	0.5188
Oral manifestations −	83 (68%)	24 (58%)	33 (67%)	26 (81%)		16 (84%)	17 (59%)	43 (65%)		3 (60%)	35 (62%)	30 (73%)	
Myalgia/arthralgia	104 (53%)	26 (25%)	37 (36%)	41 (39%)		18 (19%)	24 (26%)	52 (55%)		6 (54%)	36 (40%)	49 (6%)	
Oral manifestations +	32 (31%)	11 (42%)	13 (35%)	8 (20%)	0.1111	3 (17%)	8 (33%)	20 (38%)	0.2375	0 (0%)	16 (44%)	15 (31%)	0.0736
Oral manifestations −	72 (69%)	15 (58%)	24 (65%)	33 (80%)		15 (83%)	16 (67%)	32 (62%)		6 (100%)	20 (56%)	34 (69%)	
Loss of smell	102 (53%)	9 (9%)	19 (19%)	74 (72%)		5 (5%)	8 (9%)	80 (86%)		1 (1%)	4 (5%)	78 (94%)	
Oral manifestations +	40 (39%)	5 (55%)	10 (53%)	25 (34%)	0.1865	1 (20%)	7 (88%)	31 (39%)	0.0122	0 (0%)	2 (50%)	33 (42%)	1.0000

Table 2. *Cont.*

Symptom	Total 195	Severity of Specific COVID-19 Symptom				Duration of Specific COVID-19 Symptom				Frequency of Specific COVID-19 Symptom			
		Mild	Moderate	Severe	*p*-Value	1–2 Days	3–4 Days	5+ Days	*p*-Value	Once	Intermittent	Constant	*p*-Value
Oral manifestations −	62 (61%)	4 (44%)	9 (47%)	49 (66%)		4 (80%)	1 (12%)	49 (61%)		1 (100%)	2 (50%)	45 (58%)	
Sore throat	97 (50%)	33 (34%)	38 (39%)	26 (27%)		18 (20%)	39 (44%)	32 (36%)		9 (11%)	27 (33%)	47 (56%)	
Oral manifestations +	34 (35%)	14 (42%)	10 (26%)	10 (38%)	0.3338	5 (28%)	15 (38%)	12 (38%)	0.7181	2 (22%)	11 (41%)	17 (36%)	0.6056
Oral manifestations −	63 (65%)	19 (58%)	28 (74%)	16 (62%)		13 (72%)	24 (62%)	20 (62%)		7 (78%)	26 (59%)	30 (64%)	
Dyspnea	78 (40%)	22 (28%)	24 (31%)	32 (41%)		10 (15%)	22 (32%)	36 (53%)		8 (12%)	35 (54%)	22 (34%)	
Oral manifestations +	22 (28%)	8 (36%)	7 (29%)	7(22%)	0.5048	2 (20%)	8 (36%)	11 (31%)	0.6485	2 (25%)	13 (37%)	5 (23%)	0.4818
Oral manifestations −	56 (72%)	14 (64%)	17 (71%)	25 (78%)		8 (80%)	14 (64%)	25 (69%)		6 (75%)	22 (67%)	17 (77%)	
Nausea/vomiting	41 (21%)	20 (49%)	15 (36%)	6 (15%)		11 (34%)	7 (22%)	14 (44%)		5 (13%)	22 (71%)	4 (16%)	
Oral manifestations +	11 (27%)	5 (25%)	5 (33%)	1 (17%)	0.7991	1 (9%)	3 (43%)	5 (36%)	0.2099	2 (40%)	6 (27%)	1 (25%)	0.8367
Oral manifestations −	30 (73%)	15 (75%)	10 (67%)	5 (83%)		10 (91%)	4 (57%)	9 (64%)		3 (60%)	16 (73%)	3 (75%)	
Diarrhea	30 (15%)	19 (63%)	8 (27%)	3 (10%)		13 (57%)	4 (17%)	6 (26%)		6 (29%)	11 (52%)	4 (19%)	
Oral manifestations +	11 (37%)	7 (37%)	4 (50%)	0 (0%)	0.3861	6 (46%)	1 (25%)	2 (33%)	0.7085	4 (67%)	3 (27%)	1 (25%)	0.2329
Oral manifestations −	19 (63%)	12 (63%)	4 (50%)	3 (100%)		7 (54%)	3 (75%)	4 (67%)		2 (33%)	8 (73%)	3 (75%)	

Oral manifestations +: Patient(s) developed oral manifestations of COVID-19 simultaneously with having the general symptom listed just above it. Oral manifestations −: Patient(s) did not have oral manifestations of COVID-19 simultaneously with the general symptom listed above it.

3.4. Oral Manifestations of COVID-19

A total of 57 participants (29%) had oral manifestations of COVID-19. The majority were age 45 to 54 years and 55+ years. There was a significantly higher proportion of females than males with oral manifestations (33% vs. 17%, $p = 0.0275$). Approximately 25% of current or previous smokers, 33% of those taking medications, and 24% of those who had been hospitalized due to COVID-19 developed oral manifestations. Thirteen participants with oral manifestations were taking medications (Table 1).

Of patients who had oral manifestations ($n = 57$, 29%), thirty-four (60%) had distortion of taste, twenty-four (42%) had xerostomia, six (11%) had oral ulcerations, three (6%) had gingivitis, three (6%) had petechiae, three (6%) had candidiasis, two (4%) had necrotizing periodontal disease, two (4%) had vesiculobullous lesions, two (4%) had erythema migrans, and two (4%) had a geographic tongue. These categories were not mutually exclusive; a participant could report more than one oral manifestation (Table 3).

Table 3. Characteristics of patients with oral manifestations of COVID-19.

Participant Characteristics	All Participants with Oral Manifestations of COVID-19 N = 57 n/N	Oral Manifestation of COVID-19 among 195 Participants									
		Dysgeusia (n = 34; 60%)	Xerostomia (n = 24; 42%)	Oral Ulceration (n = 6; 11%)	Gingivitis (n = 3; 6%)	Petechiae (n = 3; 6%)	Candidiasis (n = 3; 6%)	Necrotizing Periodontal Disease (n = 2; 4%)	Vesiculobullous Lesions (n = 2; 4%)	Erythema Migrans (n = 2; 4%)	Geographic Tongue (n = 2; 4%)
Age group											
18–24 years	18 (32%)	11 (32%)	5 (21%)	4 (67%)	1 (33%)	1 (33%)	1 (50%)	1 (50%)	1 (50%)	1 (50%)	1 (50%)
25–34 years	18 (32%)	13 (38%)	8 (33%)	1 (17%)	1 (33%)	2 (67%)	0 (0%)	1 (50%)	1 (50%)	1 (505)	1 (50%)
35–44 years	9 (16%)	6 (18%)	5 (13%)	0 (0%)	0 (0%)	0 (0%)	1 (50%)	0 (0%)	0 (0%)	0 (0%)	0 (0%)
45–54 years	6 (10%)	3 (95%)	5 (21%)	1 (17%)	0 (0%)	0 (0%)	0 (0%)	0 (0%)	0 (0%)	0 (0%)	0 (0%)
55+ years	6 (10%)	1 (3%)	3 (12%)	0 (0%)	1 (33%)	0 (0%)	1 (6%)	0 (0%)	0 (0%)	0 (0%)	0 (0%)
Sex (female)	49 (86%)	30 (88%)	21 (87%)	5 (83%)	2 (67%)	2 (67%)	2 (67%)	1 (50%)	1 (50%)	1 (50%)	1 (50%)
Smoking history (current or previous smoker)	16 (28%)	9 (27%)	7 (29%)	3 (50%)	1 (33%)	2 (67%)	0 (0%)	1 (50%)	1 (50%)	1 (50%)	1 (50%)
Taking medication €	13 (23%)	7 (21%)	4 (17%)	0 (0%)	1 (33%)	0 (0%)	2 (15%)	0 (0%)	0 (0%)	0 (0%)	0 (0%)
Positive history of hospitalization	4 (7%)	1 (3%)	1 (4%)	1 (17%)	0 (0%)	0 (0%)	1 (33%)	0 (0%)	0 (0%)	0 (0%)	0 (0%)

€ These categories are not mutually exclusive.

3.5. Relationship between Oral Manifestations of COVID-19 and Overall Severity of COVID-19

Of participants with mild, moderate, severe, or critical COVID-19, 27%, 30%, 29%, and 25% of participants, respectively, developed oral manifestations. The following symptoms were described as moderate or severe and lasting 3 to 4 or 5+ days before resolution: distortion of taste, xerostomia, and oral ulcerations. Candidiasis was most often described as mild and lasting for 1 to 2 days. There was no statistically significant association between the severity, duration, and frequency of each oral manifestation of COVID-19 and the overall severity of COVID-19 symptoms (Supplementary Table S1).

3.6. Relationship between Oral Manifestations of COVID-19 and Specific General COVID-19 Symptoms in Terms of Severity, Duration, and Frequency

There was no relationship between the severity of specific general COVID-19 symptoms and the presence of oral manifestations. However, patients with fatigue lasting more than 5 days were more likely to develop oral manifestations ($p < 0.0007$). Patients with loss of smell for 3 to 4 days were more likely to develop oral manifestations, and the most common one was a taste disorder ($p = 0.0122$) [12]. Patients with headaches that were constant or intermittent were more likely to develop oral manifestations ($p = 0.0336$) (Table 2).

3.7. Timing of Oral Manifestations of COVID-19 Relative to General Symptoms of and Therapy for COVID-19

Fifty-three of the fifty-seven participants with oral manifestations could recall the time of appearance of the oral manifestations in relation to the general symptoms and therapy they received. The oral manifestations developed concurrently with the general symptoms in 47%, after the general symptoms occurred in 43%, and before the general symptoms occurred in 9%. Patients with mild disease developed oral manifestations before the appearance of general symptoms, whereas those with moderate or severe disease developed oral manifestations concurrently with or after the appearance of general symptoms (Table 4).

Table 4. Temporal relationship of oral manifestations of and general symptoms of COVID-19 in 53 of the 57 participants with oral manifestations of COVID-19.

COVID-19 Severity	Total ± 57 n/N	Timing of Oral Manifestations Relative to COVID-19 General Symptoms		
		Before COVID-19 General Symptoms (n = 5; 9%)	Concurrent with COVID-19 General Symptoms (n = 25; 47%)	After COVID-19 General Symptoms (n = 23; 43%)
Mild	11 (19%)	3 (60%)	4 (16%)	4 (17%)
Moderate	35 (61%)	2 (40%)	15 (60%)	15 (65%)
Severe or critical	11 (19%)	1 (20%)	6 (24%)	4 (17%)

± Three patients with distortion of taste did not give information on the timing of oral manifestations relative to COVID-19 general symptoms.

4. Discussion

COVID-19 patients presented with different symptoms and manifestations in different body systems, such as the cutaneous, gastrointestinal, and respiratory systems [8,18,19]. In this study, we aimed to determine the prevalence of oral manifestations of patients diagnosed with COVID-19 and their association with disease severity. The prevalence of oral manifestations among all participants was 29%. These patients were predominantly female, 45 to 54 years of age or older than 55 years, and nonsmokers; were not taking any medications; and had never been hospitalized for COVID-19. Patients with the oral manifestations of COVID-19 were more likely to have moderate or severe COVID-19. The most common oral manifestations of COVID-19 reported in our cohort were distortion of taste, xerostomia, and oral ulceration, which is congruent with what has been reported in the literature [9,14,20]. Martín Carreras-Presas et al. were the first to report oral ulcerations as an oral manifestation associated with COVID-19 [21]. Several reports followed a heterogeneous group of lesions in suspected and confirmed cases of COVID-19, with, as reported in the current study, altered taste and oral ulcerations being the most common symptoms [20]. The development of oral lesions in a setting of COVID-19 infection may be explained by the affinity of the coronavirus for ACE2 receptors, which are highly expressed in the respiratory and oral epithelium. The binding of the virus to these receptors may disrupt the epithelial lining and the functioning of keratinocytes [7]. However, the cause-and-effect relationship of the development of oral manifestations in confirmed cases of COVID-19 is still unclear. Whether it is a direct effect of the virus on the oral mucosal tissue or a consequence of an impaired immune response or concurrent infection needs to be investigated.

Moreover, the exacerbated vigor and activity of innate immune response mechanisms [22] and hormonal modulations in females may be responsible for the higher prevalence of oral manifestations among female participants [23], as previously reported [14,24,25]. A higher proportion of elderly patients developed oral manifestations, as in the study by Iranmanesh et al. [8]. Immune suppression due to advances in age may be responsible for a higher prevalence of oral manifestations in this age group.

Patients with oral manifestations tended to have moderate or severe COVID-19. It was observed that patients of older age and a higher degree of severity of COVID-19 suffered from more severe episodes of oral lesions [6,8,10]. Oral manifestations developed regardless of the severity of COVID-19. However, some studies found that most of the oral manifestations were linked to severe COVID-19 [26,27]. This could be attributed to the hyperinflammatory response to COVID-19 [8]. Nonetheless, we were able to establish a link between the presence of oral manifestations and the presence of specific general symptoms of COVID-19. Similar to other cohorts studied in Saudi Arabia, most of the participants in our study described the general symptom of a chemosensory disorder, such as the loss of smell and taste, as being severe and extending for more than 5 days [28]. Loss of taste along with anosmia was concurrent and attributed to edema of the respiratory system [6]. This lends credence to the theory that olfactory and gustatory dysfunctions are potential indications of COVID-19. Xerostomia was the second most common manifestation (41%; $n = 24$) in the current study in patients who were nonsmokers and were not taking medications; it appeared concurrently with general symptoms and was associated with moderate severity of COVID-19. Another study showed that xerostomia was the most common oral manifestation in COVID-19 patients [23], indicating that salivary gland symptoms and disorders are highly prevalent among these patients. However, further case–control studies are suggested to confirm this observation.

Patients with mild disease developed oral manifestations prior to the onset of general symptoms, whereas those with more severe disease developed oral manifestations at the same time or after the appearance of general symptoms. Oral symptoms could have developed secondarily to the use of medications or to adverse reactions to medications such as corticosteroids with increased severity of the disease. Other studies reported the appearance of oral lesions after the onset of COVID-19 regardless of the severity of disease [24].

There are some limitations in the current study, which was conducted to be descriptive only, without multivariant analysis. It was not possible to analyze the oral manifestations for some patients because the data regarding duration and frequency of their self-reported symptoms were incomplete. Because the study relied on participants' self-reporting, the prevalence of some symptoms may have been overestimated or underestimated. Moreover, the current study cannot be generalized, because the validity of the self-reported symptoms was not corroborated by objective measures, and therefore reporting bias could not be prevented. We excluded patients under age 18 years, so our study did not provide data for this population. To our knowledge, our study was the first study that addressed the relationship between oral manifestations of COVID-19 and specific general symptoms of COVID-19 in terms of severity, duration, and frequency. This study reported the oral manifestations associated with COVID-19 in patients with symptoms ranging from mild to severe. We found that taste distortion could increase the clinical suspicion for COVID-19 and could be a potential indicator for patient screening.

Oral manifestations of COVID-19 were common in female patients and were linked to specific general COVID-19 symptoms. Taste distortion, xerostomia, and oral ulcerations were the most reported oral manifestations. Future studies should be undertaken to elucidate the controversial link between oral lesions and COVID-19 infection using validated measurement tools. Dentists and other health practitioners should be careful during dental examinations because oral manifestations of COVID-19 may emerge before the onset of general symptoms of COVID-19, as they did in this study population. Dental professionals may also promote awareness of the common oral manifestations of COVID-19, which may persist for long durations, and provide the proper management and medical attention for them.

Supplementary Materials: The following supporting information can be downloaded at: https://www.mdpi.com/article/10.3390/jcm11154461/s1, Table S1: Frequency, severity, and duration of oral manifestations of COVID-19.

Author Contributions: Conceptualization, N.O.B. and S.A.A.; methodology, N.O.B., S.A., S.A.A. and M.T.A.; software, N.O.B.; validation, S.A., S.A.A. and M.T.A.; formal analysis, N.O.B. and S.A.; data curation, N.O.B., M.T.A., S.A., S.A.A. and A.M.S.; writing, N.O.B. and M.T.A.; writing review and editing, S.A., S.A.A. and A.M.S.; visualization, A.M.S.; project administration, N.O.B.; funding acquisition, N.O.B. All authors have read and agreed to the published version of the manuscript.

Funding: This research was funded by the Deputyship for Research & Innovation, Ministry of Education in Saudi Arabia, through project number IFPHI-093-165-2020 and King Abdulaziz University, DSR, Jeddah, Saudi Arabia.

Institutional Review Board Statement: The study was conducted in accordance with the Declaration of Helsinki and approved by the Research Ethics Committee at King Abdulaziz University Faculty of Dentistry (Approval No. 204-01-21; approved on 26 September 2021).

Informed Consent Statement: Informed consent was obtained from all subjects involved in the study.

Data Availability Statement: The data presented in this study are available on request from the corresponding author.

Acknowledgments: The authors extend their appreciation to the Deputyship for Research & Innovation, Ministry of Education, in Saudi Arabia for funding this research work through project number IFPHI-093-165-2020 and King Abdulaziz University, DSR, Jeddah, Saudi Arabia.

Conflicts of Interest: The authors declare no conflict of interest.

References

1. Centers for Disease Control and Prevention. CDC Museum COVID-19 Timeline. Available online: https://www.cdc.gov/museum/timeline/covid19.html (accessed on 22 March 2022).
2. World Health Organization. WHO Coronavirus (COVID-19) Dashboard. Available online: https://covid19.who.int/ (accessed on 3 June 2022).
3. World Health Organization. Saudi Arabia Situation. Available online: https://covid19.who.int/region/emro/country/sa (accessed on 18 July 2022).
4. Harapan, H.; Itoh, N.; Yufika, A.; Winardi, W.; Keam, S.; Te, H.; Megawati, D.; Hayati, Z.; Wagner, A.L.; Mudatsir, M. Coronavirus disease 2019 (COVID-19): A literature review. *J. Infect. Public Health* **2020**, *13*, 667–673. [CrossRef] [PubMed]
5. Wan, Y.; Shang, J.; Graham, R.; Baric, R.S.; Li, F. Receptor Recognition by the Novel Coronavirus from Wuhan: An Analysis Based on Decade-Long Structural Studies of SARS Coronavirus. *J. Virol.* **2020**, *94*, e00127-20. [CrossRef] [PubMed]
6. Paradowska-Stolarz, A.M. Oral manifestations of COVID-19: Brief review. *Dent. Med. Probl.* **2021**, *58*, 123–126. [CrossRef] [PubMed]
7. Brandão, T.B.; Gueiros, L.A.; Melo, T.S.; Prado-Ribeiro, A.C.; Nesrallah, A.C.F.A.; Prado, G.V.B.; Santos-Silva, A.R.; Migliorati, C.A. Oral lesions in patients with SARS-CoV-2 infection: Could the oral cavity be a target organ? *Oral Surg. Oral Med. Oral Pathol. Oral Radiol.* **2021**, *131*, e45–e51. [CrossRef]
8. Iranmanesh, B.; Khalili, M.; Amiri, R.; Zartab, H.; Aflatoonian, M. Oral manifestations of COVID-19 disease: A review article. *Dermatol. Ther.* **2021**, *34*, e14578. [CrossRef]
9. Erbaş, G.S.; Botsali, A.; Erden, N.; Arı, C.; Taşkın, B.; Alper, S.; Vural, S. COVID-19-related oral mucosa lesions among confirmed SARS-CoV-2 patients: A systematic review. *Int. J. Dermatol.* **2022**, *61*, 20–32. [CrossRef]
10. Jimenez-Cauhe, J.; Ortega-Quijano, D.; de Perosanz-Lobo, D.; Burgos-Blasco, P.; Vañó-Galván, S.; Fernandez-Guarino, M.; Fernandez-Nieto, D. Enanthem in Patients With COVID-19 and Skin Rash. *JAMA Dermatol.* **2020**, *156*, 1134–1136. [CrossRef]
11. Butera, A.; Maiorani, C.; Natoli, V.; Bruni, A.; Coscione, C.; Magliano, G.; Giacobbo, G.; Morelli, A.; Moressa, S.; Scribante, A. Bio-Inspired Systems in Nonsurgical Periodontal Therapy to Reduce Contaminated Aerosol during COVID-19: A Comprehensive and Bibliometric Review. *J. Clin. Med.* **2020**, *9*, 3914. [CrossRef]
12. Centers for Disease Control and Prevention. Self-Testing at Home or Anywhere: For Doing Rapid COVID-19 Tests Anywhere. Available online: https://www.cdc.gov/coronavirus/2019-ncov/testing/self-testing.html (accessed on 3 June 2022).
13. Pourhoseingholi, M.A.; Vahedi, M.; Rahimzadeh, M. Sample size calculation in medical studies. *Gastroenterol. Hepatol. Bed Bench* **2013**, *6*, 14–17.
14. Dos Santos, J.A.; Normando, A.G.; Da Silva, R.L.C.; Acevedo, A.C.; Canto, G.D.L.; Sugaya, N.; Santos-Silva, A.R.; Guerra, E.N.S. Oral Manifestations in Patients with COVID-19: A Living Systematic Review. *J. Dent. Res.* **2020**, *100*, 141–154. [CrossRef]
15. Taherdoost, H. Determining sample size: How to calculate survey sample size. *Int. J. Econ. Manag. Syst.* **2017**, *2*, 237–239.
16. World Health Organization. Clinical Management of COVID-19: Interim Guidance. Available online: https://apps.who.int/iris/handle/10665/332196 (accessed on 3 March 2022).
17. Salepci, E.; Turk, B.; Ozcan, S.N.; Bektas, M.E.; Aybal, A.; Dokmetas, I.; Turgut, S. Symptomatology of COVID-19 from the otorhinolaryngology perspective: A survey of 223 SARS-CoV-2 RNA-positive patients. *Eur. Arch. Otorhinolaryngol.* **2021**, *278*, 525–535. [CrossRef]
18. Galván Casas, C.; Català, A.; Carretero Hernández, G.; Rodríguez-Jiménez, P.; Fernández-Nieto, D.; Rodríguez-Villa Lario, A.; Navarro Fernández, I.; Ruiz-Villaverde, R.; Falkenhain-López, D.; Llamas Velasco, M.; et al. Classification of the Cutaneous Manifestations of COVID-19: A Rapid Prospective Nationwide Consensus Study in Spain with 375 Cases. *Br. J. Dermatol.* **2020**, *183*, 71–77. [CrossRef]
19. Patel, K.P.; Patel, P.A.; Vunnam, R.R.; Hewlett, A.T.; Jain, R.; Jing, R.; Vunnam, S.R. Gastrointestinal, hepatobiliary, and pancreatic manifestations of COVID-19. *J. Clin. Virol.* **2020**, *128*, 104386. [CrossRef]
20. Farid, H.; Khan, M.; Jamal, S.; Ghafoor, R. Oral manifestations of Covid-19-A literature review. *Rev. Med. Virol.* **2022**, *32*, e2248. [CrossRef]
21. Martín Carreras-Presas, C.; Amaro Sánchez, J.; López-Sánchez, A.F.; Jané-Salas, E.; Somacarrera Pérez, M.L. Oral vesiculobullous lesions associated with SARS-CoV-2 infection. *Oral Dis.* **2021**, *27* (Suppl. S3), 710–712. [CrossRef]
22. Oertelt-Prigione, S. The influence of sex and gender on the immune response. *Autoimmun. Rev.* **2012**, *11*, A479–A485. [CrossRef]

23. Taneja, V. Sex Hormones Determine Immune Response. *Front. Immunol.* **2018**, *9*, 1931. [CrossRef]
24. Dos Santos, J.A.; Normando, A.G.C.; da Silva, R.L.C.; Acevedo, A.C.; Canto, G.D.L.; Sugaya, N.; Santos-Silva, A.R.; Guerra, E.N.S. Oral Manifestations in Patients with COVID-19: A 6-Month Update. *J. Dent. Res.* **2021**, *100*, 1321–1329. [CrossRef]
25. Aragoneses, J.; Suárez, A.; Algar, J.; Rodríguez, C.; López-Valverde, N.; Aragoneses, J.M. Oral Manifestations of COVID-19: Updated Systematic Review with Meta-Analysis. *Front. Med.* **2021**, *8*, 726753. [CrossRef]
26. Ganesan, A.; Kumar, S.; Kaur, A.; Chaudhry, K.; Kumar, P.; Dutt, N.; Nag, V.L.; Garg, M.K. Oral Manifestations of COVID-19 Infection: An Analytical Cross-Sectional Study. *J. Maxillofac. Oral Surg.* **2022**, 1–10. [CrossRef] [PubMed]
27. Sharma, P.; Malik, S.; Wadhwan, V.; Palakshappa, S.G.; Singh, R. Prevalence of oral manifestations in COVID-19: A systematic review. *Rev. Med. Virol.* **2022**, e2345. [CrossRef] [PubMed]
28. Natto, Z.S.; Afeef, M.; Khalil, D.; Kutubaldin, D.; Dehaithem, M.; Alzahrani, A.; Ashi, H. Characteristics of Oral Manifestations in Symptomatic Non-Hospitalized COVID-19 Patients: A Cross-Sectional Study on a Sample of the Saudi Population. *Int. J. Gen. Med.* **2021**, *14*, 9547–9553. [CrossRef] [PubMed]

Journal of
Clinical Medicine

MDPI

Article

The Effect of the COVID-19 Pandemic on Patient Selection, Surgical Procedures, and Postoperative Complications in a Specialized Dental Implant Clinic

Balazs Feher [1,2,*], Cordelia Wieser [3], Theresa Lukes [3], Christian Ulm [1], Reinhard Gruber [2,4,5] and Ulrike Kuchler [1]

[1] Department of Oral Surgery, University Clinic of Dentistry, Medical University of Vienna, 1090 Vienna, Austria; christian.ulm@meduniwien.ac.at (C.U.); ulrike.kuchler@meduniwien.ac.at (U.K.)
[2] Department of Oral Biology, University Clinic of Dentistry, Medical University of Vienna, 1090 Vienna, Austria; reinhard.gruber@meduniwien.ac.at
[3] Department of Dental Training, University Clinic of Dentistry, Medical University of Vienna, 1090 Vienna, Austria; n1445032@students.meduniwien.ac.at (C.W.); n1242565@students.meduniwien.ac.at (T.L.)
[4] Austrian Cluster for Tissue Regeneration, Ludwig Boltzmann Institute for Experimental and Clinical Traumatology, 1200 Vienna, Austria
[5] Department of Periodontology, School of Dental Medicine, University of Bern, 3012 Bern, Switzerland
* Correspondence: balazs.feher@meduniwien.ac.at; Tel.: +43-1-40070-2623

Abstract: During the coronavirus disease 2019 (COVID-19) pandemic, aerosol-generating procedures, including dental implant treatments, are considered high-risk. With dental implant treatment mostly an elective procedure, we aimed to assess whether the pandemic influenced patient selection, surgical procedures, and postoperative complications. We compared dental implant treatments during (March to December 2020) and before (December 2018 to February 2020) the COVID-19 pandemic based on patient and implant parameters, as well as postoperative complications. For analysis, we used the Chi-squared test with the Holm–Sidak correction for multiple comparisons. The number of implants placed during the COVID-19 pandemic (696 implants in 406 patients, 70 implants per month) was comparable to pre-pandemic levels (1204 implants in 616 patients, 80 implants per month). Regarding patient parameters, there were no significant differences in respiratory ($p = 0.69$) and cardiovascular conditions ($p = 0.06$), diabetes ($p = 0.69$), and smoking ($p = 0.68$). Regarding implant parameters, there was a significant difference in the distribution of augmentative procedures (no augmentation, guided bone regeneration, and sinus floor elevation, $p = 0.01$), but no significant differences in the types of edentulous spaces ($p = 0.19$) and the timing of implant placement ($p = 0.52$). Regarding complications, there were significantly fewer minor complications ($p < 0.001$) and early (i.e., before loading) implant failures ($p = 0.02$) compared with pre-pandemic levels. Our results suggest that the COVID-19 pandemic had no effect on patient selection and only a slight effect on the surgical procedures. However, postoperative complications, including early failures, were significantly less prevalent during the pandemic.

Keywords: dentistry; surgery; oral; dental implantation; retrospective studies; population characteristics

Citation: Feher, B.; Wieser, C.; Lukes, T.; Ulm, C.; Gruber, R.; Kuchler, U. The Effect of the COVID-19 Pandemic on Patient Selection, Surgical Procedures, and Postoperative Complications in a Specialized Dental Implant Clinic. *J. Clin. Med.* **2022**, *11*, 855. https://doi.org/10.3390/jcm11030855

Academic Editors: Hans-Peter Howaldt, Sameh Attia and Mark A. Reynolds

Received: 10 December 2021
Accepted: 2 February 2022
Published: 6 February 2022

1. Introduction

The airborne transmission of severe acute respiratory syndrome coronavirus 2 (SARS-CoV-2), the RNA virus that causes coronavirus disease 2019 (COVID-19), poses a considerable challenge in the dental setting, where patients are unable to wear masks or other facial barriers while in close contact to the personnel providing care [1]. Furthermore, aerosol-generating procedures, including dental implant placement, are generally considered high-risk as they can produce and spread contaminated droplets [2–5]. Surface contamination through these droplets is substantial at close proximity and still detectable at a maximum distance of 4 m from the source [6]. Consequently, multiple guidelines have recommended prioritizing no-aerosol over aerosol-generating procedures (e.g., using manual over rotary or ultrasonic instruments [1]) or postponing aerosol-generating procedures of potentially infectious patients or patients at an increased risk for COVID-19 entirely, especially if these procedures are elective [7–10].

In general, dental implant treatment is an elective procedure. Nevertheless, implant placement cannot be postponed indefinitely, as edentulous bone is subject to catabolic dimensional changes over time [11]. In addition, there is a highly important quality-of-life aspect to dental implant treatment [12,13]. Thus, the clinical decision-making process during the COVID-19 pandemic must balance this increase in quality of life against a potentially increased risk of SARS-CoV-2 transmission. This could affect both patient selection and surgical procedures. Patients with relevant comorbidities (e.g., respiratory and cardiovascular conditions [14], diabetes [15]) might choose to—or be advised to—postpone their dental implant treatment until such time that they are at no increased risk for SARS-CoV-2 transmission. In addition, oral surgeons might choose to limit the number and complexity of procedures (e.g., restricting augmentative procedures to where indisputably necessary) to minimize the patients' and their own risk of transmission.

Previous work has focused on various guidelines, preventive measures, as well as the epidemiological aspect of dental treatments during the COVID-19 pandemic [8]. However, the effect of the pandemic on the treatments themselves remains elusive. The aim of this study was therefore to retrospectively assess whether the COVID-19 pandemic had an effect on patient selection, surgical procedures, and postoperative complications.

2. Materials and Methods

This is a retrospective study designed and conducted in accordance with the Declaration of Helsinki and its subsequent revisions [16]. The study protocol was approved by the institutional review board of the Medical University of Vienna (No. 1282/2021). We reviewed and extracted data from the electronic patient records (Medfolio, Nexus, Donaueschingen, Germany) of our clinic. We included patients that received at least one dental implant at our clinic between 1 December 2018 and 1 December 2020. Data were extracted into a standardized patient–feature matrix by two researchers (CW, TL) and subsequently error-proofed by two different researchers (BF, UK) in an independent manner. Only complete data were used in this study. Results are reported in accordance with STROBE criteria for observational studies [17]; the complete checklist is available as a Supplementary File.

Patient parameters included demographic data and medical history. They comprised age, sex, smoking status, comorbidities (e.g., respiratory conditions, cardiovascular conditions, diabetes mellitus), implant location, and type of edentulous space (single-tooth gap, extended gap, distal extension, edentulous jaw). We considered the following implant parameters: length, diameter, bone augmentation (guided bone regeneration or sinus floor elevation), and timing of implant placement (immediate, early, or late [18]). In addition, we assessed minor postoperative complications (e.g., bleeding, suppuration, swelling, local infection, hematoma, temporary neurosensory disturbance), as well as early implant failure (i.e., before loading [19]).

The sample for the statistical analysis included every patient who received a dental implant between 1 December 2018 and 1 December 2020, for which complete data were available in the electronic patient records. We first collected all data and checked them for possible errors. The dataset was then split into a sample before the pandemic (control sample, December 2018 to February 2020) and a sample during the pandemic (test sample, March 2020 to December 2020). We analyzed all parameters in a descriptive manner. We further compared the prevalence and distributions of smoking, respiratory conditions, cardiovascular conditions, types of gaps, bone augmentation, timing of implant placement, minor postoperative complications, as well as early implant failures using the Chi-squared test. To correct for multiple comparisons, we used the Holm–Bonferroni correction with the Sidak modification. We set the level of significance at $\alpha < 0.05$. Statistical analysis was performed by one researcher (BF) using Prism 9.2.0 (GraphPad Software, La Jolla, CA, USA).

3. Results

3.1. Sample Characteristics

The sample during the pandemic included 406 patients (median age at first implantation: 54.0 years, interquartile range: 41.9–62.2, 56% female, 16% smokers) and 696 implants (70 implants per month, 54% maxilla). The number of implants per patient ranged from 1 (n = 236) to 10 (n = 1), with an average of 1.7 implants per patient. The mean implant diameter was 4.1 ± 0.5 mm (standard deviation). The mean implant length was 11.0 ± 1.3 mm.

The sample before the pandemic included 616 patients (median age at first implantation: 54.0 years, interquartile range: 42.5–63.5, 53% female, 19% smokers) and 1204 implants (80 implants per month, 47% maxilla). The number of implants per patient ranged from 1 (n = 320) to 11 (n = 2), with an average of 2.0 implants per patient. The mean implant diameter was 4.1 ± 0.5 mm. The mean implant length was 11.0 ± 1.2 mm. A detailed description of the samples is shown in Table 1, and age distributions are shown in Figure 1.

Table 1. Subject and implant characteristics.

	Before the Pandemic		During the Pandemic	
Patient Parameters	**Patients, n (%)**	**Implants, n (%)**	**Patients, n (%)**	**Implants, n (%)**
Sex				
Female	324 (53)	646 (54)	227 (56)	382 (55)
Male	292 (47)	558 (46)	179 (44)	314 (45)
Smoking				
Non-smoker	493 (80)	941 (78)	339 (84)	583 (84)
Light smoker (<10 d^{-1})	46 (7)	88 (7)	24 (6)	32 (5)
Heavy smoker (≥10 d^{-1})	76 (12)	175 (15)	41 (10)	81 (12)
Comorbidities				
Respiratory conditions [1]	37 (6)	68 (6)	21 (5)	51 (7)
Cardiovasc. Conditions [2]	137 (22)	312 (26)	64 (16)	106 (15)
Diabetes	22 (4)	50 (4)	11 (3)	25 (4)
Implant Parameters		**Implants, n (%)**		**Implants, n (%)**
Treatment indication				
Single implant		556 (46)		348 (50)
Extended gap		198 (16)		121 (17)
Distal extension		225 (19)		132 (19)
Empty jaw		225 (19)		95 (14)
Timing				
Immediate		41 (3)		34 (5)
Early		10 (1)		9 (1)
Late		1153 (96)		653 (94)
Augmentation technique				
GBR [3]		213 (18)		82 (12)
Sinus floor elevation		208 (17)		145 (21)
None		783 (35)		469 (67)

[1] Positive if patient history included asthma (International Classification of Diseases [ICD] 11 code CA23), chronic obstructive pulmonary disease (CA22), or pulmonary embolism (BB00). [2] Positive if patient history included hypertension (BA00), hypotension (BA2Z), arrythmia (BC80, BC81), thrombosis/thromboembolism (BD71, BD72), or cardiac/vascular transplants/grafts (QB50). [3] Guided bone regeneration.

3.2. Patient Parameters

First, we compared patient parameters between the samples. There were 339 non-smokers (84%), 24 light smokers (fewer than 10 cigarettes per day, 6%), and 41 heavy smokers (at least 10 cigarettes per day, 10%) during the pandemic, compared to 493 non-smokers (80%), 46 light smokers (7%), and 76 heavy smokers (12%) before the pandemic (p = 0.68) (Figure 2a). Respiratory conditions were reported by 21 patients (5%) during the pandemic, compared to 37 patients (6%) before the pandemic (p = 0.69) (Figure 2b). Cardiovascular conditions were reported by 64 patients (16%) during the pandemic, compared to 137 patients (22%) before the pandemic (p = 0.06) (Figure 2c). Diabetes was reported by 11 patients (3%) during the pandemic, compared to 22 patients (4%) before the pandemic (p = 0.69) (Figure 2d). Taken together, the data suggest that the populations treated during and before the pandemic were largely comparable. While there were fewer cardiovascular conditions reported during the pandemic, this difference was not significant.

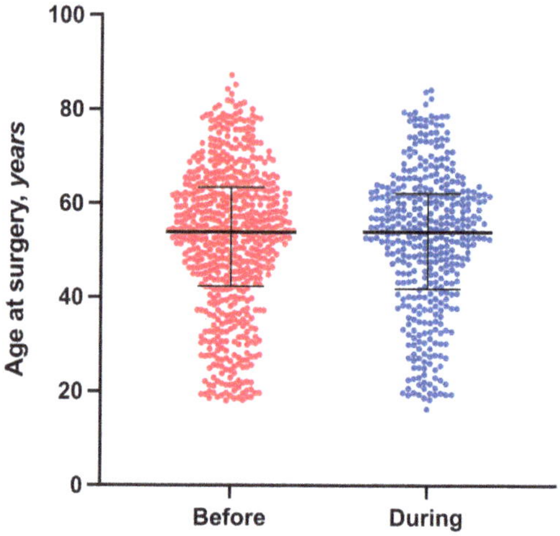

Figure 1. Age distribution. Bars represent medians and interquartile ranges.

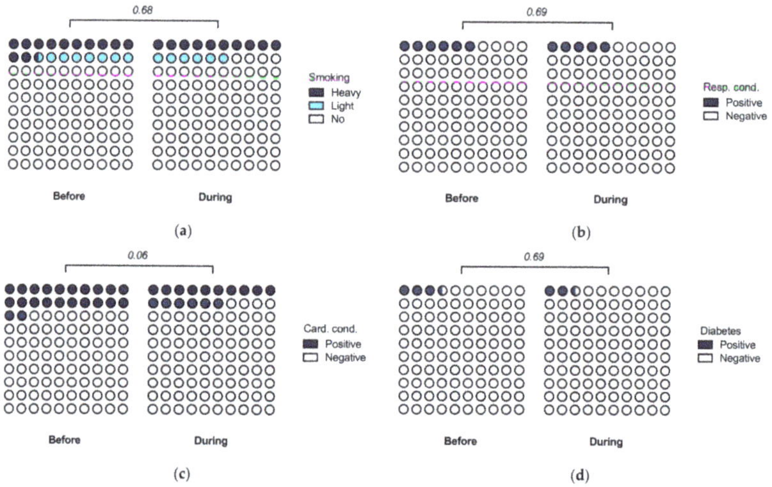

Figure 2. Patient parameters. (**a**) Smoking. Patients were considered light smokers if they smoked fewer than 10 cigarettes per day. (**b**) Respiratory conditions. Positive if patient history included asthma (International Classification of Diseases [ICD] 11 code CA23), chronic obstructive pulmonary disease (CA22), or pulmonary embolism (BB00). (**c**) Cardiovascular conditions. Positive if patient history included hypertension (BA00), hypotension (BA2Z), arrythmia (BC80, BC81), thrombosis/thromboembolism (BD71, BD72), or cardiac/vascular transplants/grafts (QB50). (**d**) Diabetes (5A14). All p-values using the Chi-squared test with the Holm–Sidak correction for multiple testing.

3.3. Implant Parameters

Next, we compared implant parameters between the samples. There were 348 single implants (50%), 121 implants placed in extended edentulous gaps (17%), 132 implants placed as distal extensions (19%), and 95 implants placed in empty jaws (14%) during the pandemic, compared to 556 single implants (46%), 198 implants placed in extended edentulous gaps (16%), 225 implants placed as distal extensions (19%), and 225 implants placed in empty jaws (19%) before the pandemic ($p = 0.19$) (Figure 3a). There were 34 immediate implants (5%), 9 implants placed early (1%), and 653 implants placed late (94%) during the pandemic, compared to 41 immediate implants (3%), 10 implants placed early (1%), and 1153 implants placed late (96%) before the pandemic ($p = 0.52$) (Figure 3b).

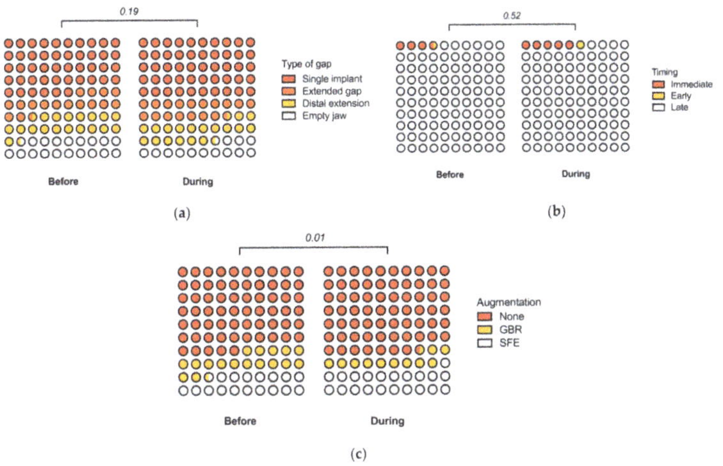

Figure 3. Implant parameters. (**a**) Type of edentulous space. (**b**) Timing of implant placement. Immediate implant placement took place in the same surgery as tooth extraction. Early implant placement took place no later than 8 weeks following tooth extraction. (**c**) Bone augmentation. *GBR*—guided bone regeneration; *SFE*—sinus floor elevation. All *p*-values using the Chi-squared test with the Holm-Sidak correction for multiple testing.

There were 469 implants placed without bone augmentation (67%), 82 implants placed with guided bone regeneration (12%), and 145 implants placed with sinus floor elevation (21%) during the pandemic, compared with 783 implants placed without bone augmentation (35%), 213 implants placed with guided bone regeneration (18%), and 208 implants placed with sinus floor elevation (17%) before the pandemic ($p = 0.01$) (Figure 3c). Taken together, the data suggest a significant difference in the use of bone augmentation, but no differences were found between the types of edentulous spaces as well as the timing of implant placements performed during and before the pandemic.

3.4. Postoperative Complications

Finally, we compared postoperative complications between the sample. Minor complications included bleeding or suppuration, swelling, local infection, hematoma, as well as temporary neurosensory disturbance. These occurred in 23 patients (6%) and affected 42 (6%) of the implants during the pandemic, compared to 133 patients (22%) and 261 implants (22%) before the pandemic ($p < 0.001$ at the patient level) (Figure 4a). A total of 3 implants failed before loading (<1%) during the pandemic, compared to 26 implants (2%) before the pandemic ($p = 0.02$) (Figure 4b). Taken together, the data suggest a significantly lower prevalence of postoperative complications, including early implant failure, between treatments during and before the pandemic.

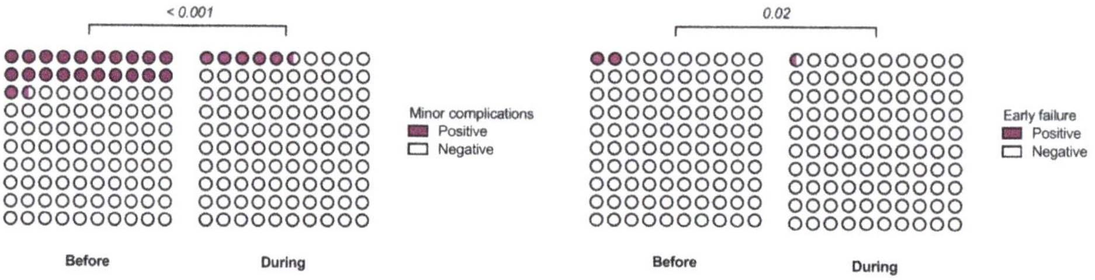

(a) (b)

Figure 4. Postoperative complications. (**a**) Minor complications. Positive if patient bleeding, suppuration, swelling, local infection, hematoma, or temporary neurosensory disturbance was either reported by the patient or observed during a follow-up visit. (**b**) Early (i.e., before loading) implant failures. All p-values using the Chi-squared test with the Holm–Sidak correction for multiple testing.

4. Discussion

We studied dental implant treatments during the COVID-19 pandemic and compared them to a pre-pandemic control population with regards to patient and implant factors as well as postoperative complications. First, we found that the patient populations treated during and before the pandemic were largely comparable. While there were fewer cardiovascular conditions reported during the pandemic, this difference was not significant. Second, our data suggested a significant difference in the use of bone augmentation but no differences between the types of edentulous spaces as well as timing of implant placements performed during and before the pandemic. Third, we observed significantly fewer postoperative complications, including early implant failure, between treatments during and before the pandemic. Overall, the data show that the COVID-19 pandemic had virtually no effect on most aspects of dental implant treatment. Nonetheless, both minor postoperative complications and early implant failures were significantly less prevalent during the pandemic.

Our findings with regards to patient selection and surgical procedures relate well to others who found that after mostly restricting their work to emergency care in the initial phase of the pandemic, dental health care professionals resumed elective care [5]. Notably, the consideration to return to elective surgery soon after the first wave of the pandemic can also be observed in other surgical fields (e.g., cardiac [20], orthopedic [21,22], and plastic [23] surgery). Notably, ours is among the first studies to provide a retrospective analysis reporting on a large patient cohort treated during the pandemic. Importantly, with very strict measures in place to prevent transmission of SARS-CoV-2, there have been to date no clusters among patients or providers. This is also in line with recent work from other surgical fields showing no increased number of infections following elective surgery [24,25].

The clinical relevance of our findings is threefold. First, the data suggest that with adequate preventive measures in place, the benefits of dental implant treatment for patients outweighed their risk of SARS-CoV-2 transmission. It appears that postponing their dental implant treatment had too high an opportunity cost for patients. This is an important finding with regards to the quality-of-life increase patients expect from a dental implant treatment. Second, the data suggest much fewer postoperative complications and early implant failures. We believe the findings with regards to postoperative complications should be interpreted with caution. While all pre-pandemic dental implants had already been placed under sterile conditions, additional personal protective equipment (e.g., filtering face pieces) might have played a beneficial role in preventing surgical site infections. It is further possible that patients wanted to minimize the number of visits to our clinic during the pandemic and therefore chose to not report minor complications. While patients might have decided to undergo dental implant surgery notwithstanding the risk of SARS-CoV-2 transmission, they might not have made the same decision for a postoperative check-up visit. In comparison, early implant failure is not a subjective complication. Notably, 3 out of 696 implants failed before loading during the pandemic, compared with 26 out of 1204 implants before the pandemic, making the early failure rate 75% lower during the pandemic. While it is difficult to explain this finding, we believe its clinical relevance is unquestionable. One possible explanation is the overall lower prevalence of comorbidities and extensive augmentative procedures, albeit these differences were not significant in this study. Nonetheless, it should be noted that in our previous work using a dataset of over 2400 implants in over 1100 patients, neither comorbidities nor surgical procedures could accurately predict early implant failure [26]. Third, the data suggest that datasets containing dental implant treatments during the pandemic are comparable to pre-pandemic datasets, allowing their use for training or validation of statistical models. Prior to our study, this would not have been possible as we could not know whether the patient population can be considered homogenous.

The main limitation of our study is its potentially limited generalizability due to its sample being from a single institute in one location, focusing on a subset of oral surgical procedures using endosseous implants. It remains to be assessed whether other specialized implant clinics observed similarly unchanged tendencies with regards to patient selection and surgical procedures, especially clinics offering different implant types (e.g., zygomatic or subperiostal implants). It further remains to be assessed whether our findings are relatable to dental procedures, especially elective treatments, where the time component is not as relevant as in dental implant treatment (i.e., cosmetic dentistry). Further research should consider collating large datasets from different sources and including other dental treatments. However, the inclusion of new features must be balanced against maintaining a high quality of the patient–feature matrix to not compromise the analysis.

5. Conclusions

Within the limitations of this study, the results suggest that the COVID-19 pandemic had no effect on patient selection and only a slight effect on the surgical procedures. Nonetheless, postoperative complications, including early implant failure, were significantly less prevalent during the pandemic.

Supplementary Materials: The following supporting information can be downloaded at: https://www.mdpi.com/article/10.3390/jcm11030855/s1.

Author Contributions: Conceptualization, B.F., C.W., T.L. and U.K.; methodology, B.F.; formal analysis, C.W. and T.L.; resources, C.U.; data curation, B.F.; writing—original draft preparation, B.F. and R.G.; writing—review and editing, C.U. and U.K.; visualization, B.F.; supervision, C.U., R.G. and U.K.; project administration, B.F., C.U. and U.K. All authors have read and agreed to the published version of the manuscript.

Funding: This research received no external funding.

Institutional Review Board Statement: The study was conducted according to the guidelines of the Declaration of Helsinki and approved by the Institutional Review Board of the Medical University of Vienna (protocol No. 1282/2021).

Informed Consent Statement: Not applicable.

Data Availability Statement: Data supporting the reported findings are available from the corresponding author upon reasonable request.

Acknowledgments: The authors thank Stefan Lettner for his advice on the statistical analyses.

Conflicts of Interest: The authors declare no conflict of interest.

References

1. Banakar, M.; Lankarani, K.B.; Jafarpour, D.; Moayedi, S.; Banakar, M.H.; MohammadSadeghi, A. COVID-19 transmission risk and protective protocols in dentistry: A systematic review. *BMC Oral Health* **2020**, *20*, 1–12. [CrossRef] [PubMed]
2. Epstein, J.B.; Chow, K.; Mathias, R. Dental procedure aerosols and COVID-19. *Lancet Infect. Dis.* **2020**, *21*, e73. [CrossRef]

3. Izzetti, R.; Nisi, M.; Gabriele, M.; Graziani, F. COVID-19 Transmission in Dental Practice: Brief Review of Preventive Measures in Italy. *J. Dent. Res.* **2020**, *99*, 1030–1038. [CrossRef] [PubMed]
4. Nulty, A.; Lefkaditis, C.; Zachrisson, P.; Van Tonder, Q.; Yar, R. A clinical study measuring dental aerosols with and without a high-volume extraction device. *Br. Dent. J.* **2020**, 1–8. [CrossRef]
5. Brunello, G.; Gurzawska-Comis, K.; Becker, K.; Becker, J.; Sivolella, S.; Schwarz, F.; Klinge, B. Dental care during COVID-19 pandemic: Follow-up survey of experts' opinion. *Clin. Oral Implant. Res.* **2021**, *32*, 342–352. [CrossRef]
6. Allison, J.R.; Currie, C.C.; Edwards, D.C.; Bowes, C.; Coulter, J.; Pickering, K.; Kozhevnikova, E.; Durham, J.; Nile, C.J.; Jakubovics, N.; et al. Evaluating aerosol and splatter following dental procedures: Addressing new challenges for oral health care and rehabilitation. *J. Oral Rehabil.* **2020**, *48*, 61–72. [CrossRef]
7. Coulthard, P. Dentistry and coronavirus (COVID-19)—Moral decision-making. *Br. Dent. J.* **2020**, *228*, 503–505. [CrossRef]
8. Becker, K.; Gurzawska-Comis, K.; Brunello, G.; Klinge, B. Summary of European guidelines on infection control and prevention during COVID-19 pandemic. *Clin. Oral Implant. Res.* **2021**, *32*, 353–381. [CrossRef]
9. Luo, W.; Lee, G.H.; Nalabothu, P.; Kumar, H. Paediatric dental care during and post-COVID-19 era: Changes and challenges ahead. *Pediatr. Dent. J.* **2021**, *31*, 33–42. [CrossRef]
10. Gurzawska-Comis, K.; Becker, K.; Brunello, G.; Gurzawska, A.; Schwarz, F. Recommendations for Dental Care during COVID-19 Pandemic. *J. Clin. Med.* **2020**, *9*, 1833. [CrossRef]
11. Rutkowski, J.L.; Camm, D.P.; El Chaar, E. AAID White Paper: Management of the Dental Implant Patient During the COVID-19 Pandemic and Beyond. *J. Oral Implant.* **2020**, *46*, 454–466. [CrossRef] [PubMed]
12. Reissmann, D.R.; Dard, M.; Lamprecht, R.; Struppek, J.; Heydecke, G. Oral health-related quality of life in subjects with implant-supported prostheses: A systematic review. *J. Dent.* **2017**, *65*, 22–40. [CrossRef]
13. Ali, Z.; Baker, S.; Shahrbaf, S.; Martin, N.; Vettore, M.V. Oral health-related quality of life after prosthodontic treatment for patients with partial edentulism: A systematic review and meta-analysis. *J. Prosthet. Dent.* **2018**, *121*, 59–68.e3. [CrossRef]
14. Gao, Y.D.; Ding, M.; Dong, X.; Zhang, J.J.; Azkur, A.K.; Azkur, D.; Gan, H.; Sun, Y.L.; Fu, W.; Li, W.; et al. Risk factors for severe and critically ill COVID-19 patients: A review. *Allergy* **2021**, *76*, 428–455. [CrossRef] [PubMed]
15. Hill, M.A.; Mantzoros, C.; Sowers, J.R. Commentary: COVID-19 in patients with diabetes. *Metabolism* **2020**, *107*, 154217. [CrossRef] [PubMed]
16. World Medical Association. World Medical Association Declaration of Helsinki: Ethical principles for medical research involving human subjects. *JAMA* **2013**, *310*, 2191–2194. [CrossRef] [PubMed]
17. Von Elm, E.; Altman, D.G.; Egger, M.; Pocock, S.J.; Gøtzsche, P.C.; Vandenbroucke, J.P. The Strengthening the Reporting of Observational Studies in Epidemiology (STROBE) statement: Guidelines for reporting observational studies. *J. Clin. Epidemiol.* **2008**, *61*, 344–349. [CrossRef]
18. Hämmerle, C.H.; Chen, S.T.; Wilson, T.G., Jr. Consensus statements and recommended clinical procedures regarding the placement of implants in extraction sockets. *Int. J. Oral Maxillofac. Implant.* **2004**, *19*, 26–28.
19. Esposito, M.; Hirsch, J.M.; Lekholm, U.; Thomsen, P. Biological factors contributing to failures of osseointegrated oral implants. (I). Success criteria and epidemiology. *Eur. J. Oral. Sci.* **1998**, *106*, 527–551. [CrossRef]
20. Shehata, I.M.; Elhassan, A.; Jung, J.W.; Urits, I.; Viswanath, O.; Kaye, A.D. Elective cardiac surgery during the COVID-19 pandemic: Proceed or postpone? *Best Pr. Res. Clin. Anaesthesiol.* **2020**, *34*, 643–650. [CrossRef]
21. Anoushiravani, A.A.; Barnes, C.L.; Bosco, J.A., 3rd; Bozic, K.J.; Huddleston, J.I.; Kang, J.D.; Ready, J.E.; Tornetta, P., 3rd; Iorio, R. Reemergence of Multispecialty Inpatient Elective Orthopaedic Surgery During the COVID-19 Pandemic: Guidelines for a New Normal. *J. Bone Jt. Surg. Am.* **2020**, *102*, e79. [CrossRef] [PubMed]
22. O'Connor, C.M.; Anoushiravani, A.A.; DiCaprio, M.R.; Healy, W.L.; Iorio, R. Economic Recovery After the COVID-19 Pandemic: Resuming Elective Orthopedic Surgery and Total Joint Arthroplasty. *J. Arthroplast.* **2020**, *35*, S32–S36. [CrossRef]
23. Kaye, K.; Paprottka, F.; Escudero, R.; Casabona, G.; Montes, J.; Fakin, R.; Moke, L.; Stasch, T.; Richter, D.; Benito-Ruiz, J. Elective, Non-urgent Procedures and Aesthetic Surgery in the Wake of SARS-COVID-19: Considerations Regarding Safety, Feasibility and Impact on Clinical Management. *Aesthetic Plast. Surg.* **2020**, *44*, 1014–1042. [CrossRef] [PubMed]
24. Kamal, A.; Widodo, W.; Kuncoro, M.; Karda, I.; Prabowo, Y.; Singh, G.; Liastuti, L.; Trimartani; Hutagalung, E.; Saleh, I.; et al. Does elective orthopaedic surgery in pandemic era increase risk of developing COVID-19? A combined analysis of retrospective and prospective study at Cipto Mangunkusumo Hospital, Jakarta, Indonesia. *Ann. Med. Surg.* **2020**, *60*, 87–91. [CrossRef] [PubMed]
25. Ji, C.; Singh, K.; Luther, A.Z.; Agrawal, A. Is Elective Cancer Surgery Safe During the COVID-19 Pandemic? *World J. Surg.* **2020**, *44*, 3207–3211. [CrossRef] [PubMed]
26. Feher, B.; Lettner, S.; Heinze, G.; Karg, F.; Ulm, C.; Gruber, R.; Kuchler, U. An advanced prediction model for postoperative complications and early implant failure. *Clin. Oral Implant. Res.* **2020**, *31*, 928–935. [CrossRef]

Journal of
Clinical Medicine

MDPI

Article

Special Teaching Formats during the COVID-19 Pandemic—A Survey with Implications for a Crisis-Proof Education

Karin Christine Huth *, Leonard von Bronk, Maximilian Kollmuss, Stefanie Lindner, Jürgen Durner, Reinhard Hickel and Miriam Esther Draenert

Department of Conservative Dentistry and Periodontology, University Hospital, LMU Munich, Goethestrasse 70, 80336 Munich, Germany; lvonbron@dent.med.uni-muenchen.de (L.v.B.); kollmuss@dent.med.uni-muenchen.de (M.K.); stlindne@dent.med.uni-muenchen.de (S.L.); juergen.durner@med.uni-muenchen.de (J.D.); hickel@dent.med.uni-muenchen.de (R.H.); mdraener@dent.med.uni-muenchen.de (M.E.D.)

* Correspondence: khuth@dent.med.uni-muenchen.de

Abstract: Modern teaching formats have not been considered necessary during the COVID-19 pandemic with uncertain acceptance by students. The study's aim was to describe and evaluate all measures undertaken for theoretical and practical knowledge/skill transfer, which included objective structured practical examinations (OSPEs) covering a communication skills training. The students' performance in the OSPE as well as the theoretical knowledge level were assessed, of which the latter was compared with previous terms. In conservative dentistry and periodontology (4th and 5th year courses), theoretical teaching formats were provided online and completed by a multiple-choice test. Practical education continued without patients in small groups using the phantom-head, 3D printed teeth, and objective structured practical examinations (OSPEs) including communication skills training. Formats were evaluated by a questionnaire. The organization was rated as very good/good (88.6%), besides poor Internet connection (22.8%) and Zoom® (14.2%) causing problems. Lectures with audio were best approved (1.48), followed by practical videos (1.54), live stream lectures (1.81), treatment checklists (1.81), and virtual problem-based learning (2.1). Lectures such as .pdf files without audio, articles, or scripts were rated worse (2.15–2.30). Phantom-heads were considered the best substitute for patient treatment (59.5%), while additional methodical efforts for more realistic settings led to increased appraisal. However, students performed significantly worse in the multiple-choice test compared to the previous terms ($p < 0.0001$) and the OSPEs revealed deficits in the students' communication skills. In the future, permanent available lectures with audio and efforts toward realistic treatment settings in the case of suspended patient treatment will be pursued.

Keywords: dental education; COVID-19; OSPE; communications skills; remote

Citation: Huth, K.C.; von Bronk, L.; Kollmuss, M.; Lindner, S.; Durner, J.; Hickel, R.; Draenert, M.E. Special Teaching Formats during the COVID-19 Pandemic—A Survey with Implications for a Crisis-Proof Education. *J. Clin. Med.* **2021**, *10*, 5099. https://doi.org/10.3390/jcm10215099

Academic Editors: Hans-Peter Howaldt, Sameh Attia and Emmanuel Andrès

Received: 14 September 2021
Accepted: 28 October 2021
Published: 30 October 2021

1. Introduction

On 12 March 2020, the World Health Organization announced that the Coronavirus disease-19 (COVID-19) was considered as a global pandemic [1], affecting all areas of life around the world. This includes all fields of dentistry [2,3], from dental care [4] to education. Dentists are known to have a high risk of infection due to possible transmission via aerosols and droplets [5,6], which are unavoidable for many dental procedures as well as close proximity to many patients. As a result, increased hygienic demands and requirements for social distancing were implemented within the already high hygiene standards in dentistry [7]. Dental students face the same potential risks as dental health care staff within the patients' treatment and chairside education. In particular, chairside dental education creates a high proximity between the patient, the student with assistance, and the teacher. Therefore, students and professionals across the globe [8–11] were faced with the challenge of adapting dental education in a crisis-proof manner [12]. The current literature stresses the demand for an international exchange of measures to address this new challenge [13].

Furthermore, a huge portfolio of different teaching approaches has been described. The scope ranges from recorded lectures, live stream lectures, and online conferences using various platforms (e.g., Microsoft Teams, Blackboard, or Zoom) [11,14–16] to final examinations in the form of MEQs (modified essay questions), MCQs (multiple choice questions), OSCEs, and online interviews [17]. Most formats have been compared to face-to-face teaching, mainly in terms of student's attitude rather than objective assessment of knowledge level. During the first lockdown in early 2020, and in part ongoing throughout 2020 and 2021, measures have been undertaken to minimize the risk of infection for the students, the staff, and the patients [18,19]. Different measures have been reported internationally to reduce the contact between staff and patients, most importantly, personal protection equipment (PPE), entrance checkpoints with temperature measurements, and contact history questionnaires as well as workforce shift schedules [20]. Aside from the increased hygienic measures, the education of undergraduate dental students was switched from face-to-face education to online lecturing and practical teaching without patients. To compensate for the resulting lack of patient communication, a new OSPE (objective structured practical examination) was additionally performed and evaluated.

The objective structured practical examination (OSPE) is an examination format primarily in medical school that is designed to assess clinical competence. This examination format consists of a course with different stations in which practical skills, theoretical knowledge, and communication skills are tested [21,22]. Problem-based learning (PBL) is an educational learning model in which a clinical problem serves as an impetus for active learning. Participants work together in small groups to define their own learning objectives and gain a comprehensive understanding of a problem. Here, the aim of PBL is to develop strategies to solve a complex dental patient case. It also helps to develop clinical reasoning, teamwork, and communication skills [23].

The aim of this study was to describe all measures and special formats of theoretical and practical knowledge/skills transfer within the undergraduate clinical dental education in the field of conservative dentistry and periodontology during the COVID-19 summer term in 2020. Furthermore, the students' attitude toward this alternative teaching concept was surveyed by an electronic questionnaire. In addition, the theoretical knowledge level was assessed and compared with previous terms. We explored the following questions: Is teaching without practical patient contact as efficient as teaching with patients? Do additional digital teaching formats support knowledge transfer? In light of the present literature, the added value of this study may derive from issuing not only a theoretical, but also practical and communication skills training without patients such as a training and assessment OSPE in periodontology followed by structured feedback.

From the results, conclusions can be drawn, of which the alternative education formats should be maintained in the future for a contemporary, crisis-proof, and sustainable dental education.

2. Materials and Methods

2.1. Setting and Participants

The special teaching formats and their evaluation involved 4th and 5th year undergraduate students (n = 86) attending the first and second clinical course in the Department of Conservative Dentistry and Periodontology, Ludwig-Maximilians University, Munich, from April until August 2020 (approval of the ethics committee no. 20-547 KB, 15.06.2020). The participants (69% female, 31% male; mean age 26.5 years) were motivated to participate in the evaluation after completing the OSPE. The questionnaire contained different parts: (1) General (two questions); (2) Digital setting (five questions), (3) Theoretical teaching (20 questions); and (4) Practical teaching (10 questions). The 5th year students also evaluated the OSPE (eight questions). The questions regarding teaching formats were rated as either very good, good, satisfactory, bad, and very bad. In terms of using the Likert scale, we considered the answer choices of fully agree, rather agree, partially agree, disagree, and fully disagree. A detailed explanation of the increased hygienic measures for clinical as well as educational settings at our department can be found in Diegritz et al. [7]. Furthermore, separate entrances for students were installed, two groups were formed to diminish the number of students simultaneously present in the building, and one-way walking markings were set up in the course rooms as well as distance lines in waiting areas (e.g., in front of the students' stock issue).

2.2. Theoretical Education

Within a regular term, the face-to-face lectures are available afterward as .pdf files on Moodle® (Modular Object-Oriented Dynamic Learning Environment, West Perth WA 6872, Australia) together with scripts, checklists, videos, and virtual problem-based learning seminars (VHB).

In the Corona summer term of 2020, the theoretical education began with a systematic six-week theory module, while the practical education was postponed to avoid any social contact. The majority of lectures were either prerecorded with an audio file or broadcast as a live-stream with online chat and recorded, which were both available on Moodle® throughout the entire term. Most of them were also available as .pdf files. Six additional videos regarding organizational procedures, hygiene briefing, and rules of conduct were generated, while videos showing specific treatment sequences were increased up to 64. Table 1 shows the change in the theoretical education elements from the regular semester to the 2020 Corona summer term in detail.

Table 1. Theoretical and practical dental education in the 2020 Corona summer term in comparison to a regular term (4th and 5th year courses, Department of Conservative Dentistry and Periodontology).

	Teaching Format	Regular Term	Corona Summer Term 2020
Theoretical Education	Lectures with audio (*n*)	None	41 33 additionally as .pdf files 8 exclusively as lectures with audio
	Live stream lectures (*n*)	None	10 8 additionally as .pdf files 2 exclusively as live stream lectures
	Practical instructional videos (*n*)	62	64
	Introducing videos (e.g., hygiene briefing) (*n*)	None	6
	Treatment checklists (*n*)	7	7
	Lectures (only .pdf file) (*n*)	41	43 33 additionally as lectures with audio 10 exclusively available as .pdf files)
	Virtual problem-based learning (VHB) (*n*)	6	6
	Scripts (*n*)	2	2
	Scientific articles/recommended literature (*n*)	None	6
	Case presentation (endodontology) (*n*)	None	1
	Tutorial periodontology (*n*)	None	1
Practical education	Restorative Dentistry	Regular patient treatment	Phantom head treatment, add on in clinical difficulty (veneers)
	Endodontology	Regular patient treatment	Phantom head treatment, Problem based Learning (PBL) case presentations, root canal treatment using 3D printed teeth
	Periodontology	Regular patient treatment	Phantom head treatment, Tutorial (PBL) followed by virtual presentations OSPE including communication training with simulated patients

In pediatric dentistry, the new digital competences of staff and students were valued to offer an international webinar on thee "oral pathology in children" by an Australian specialist via Zoom® (Zoom video communications, San Jose, CA 95113, USA).

2.3. Practical Education

Normally, students are trained in practical and communication skills by treating patients supervised by Assistant Professors according to the National Competency Based Catalogue of Dental Education (NKLZ) [24]. In the 2020 Corona summer term, the educational challenge was to create, even without patients, an add on in practical skills training and clinical context compared with the phantom course in the first clinical term. Next to a realistic phantom head positioning without the possibility of tooth replacement accompanied by realistic hygiene procedures, each field has found its own approach to accomplish this task. In the field of restorative dentistry, the fabrication of ceramic partial crowns and inlays (4th year) and veneers (5th year) is required. In endodontology, students of both courses receive problem-based learning (PBL) [21,23] seminars followed by realistic and comparative training in root canal treatment using 3D printed teeth based on patient DVT data [25].

In periodontology, the 5th year students solely received practical training at the phantom head, while the 4th year students first ran through a PBL tutorial. Each student received an exemplary patient case, which should be planned from anamnesis and diagnosis up to prognosis and treatment planning. They had to virtually present and discuss their cases in small supervised groups via Zoom®. In the following, an individual objective structured practical examination (OSPE) [22,26] was implemented covering practical skills (34 achievable points) and theoretical knowledge (34 points) as well as communication skills training (32 points). The latter was accomplished by a fellow student acting as a patient based on a prewritten script regarding anamnesis facts and oral health complaints together with respective X-rays, while the assessment was based on the Calgary Cambridge Observation Guide (CCOG) [27]. The OSPE was followed by structured feedback [22,28], and upon agreement, the student could watch the recorded session to ensure self-reflection and competence development [29,30].

Regarding the difference between the 4th and 5th year courses, the 5th year students had to undertake 33.3% more practical work than the 4th year students, while the education methods were the same for both courses except in periodontology.

2.4. Final Examination

At the end of the 2020 summer term, theoretical examinations took place for both courses, each consisting of 30 "Pick N Type" multiple-choice (MC) questions with four answer choices [31,32]. The results were compared to the mean of the grades of the four previous terms (2018 summer term up to the 2019/2020 winter term).

2.5. Questionnaire

A questionnaire (Table 2) was developed and electronically provided via Moodle®, which anonymously evaluated the students' acceptance regarding organization, technical requirements, and the different theoretical and practical teaching formats. It was addressed through the student's identification number for both the 4th and 5th year students, whereby the 4th year questionnaire contained additional questions about the OSPE in periodontology.

In addition to site-specific questions, literature research was conducted with the search terms e-learning, remote learning, students' acceptance of dental education, evaluation/assessment of new teaching forms in dentistry, COVID-19 dental education, and digitalization within the dental curriculum, which resulted in a pool of 143 questions after the elimination of redundancies. Based on the nominal group technique (NGT) [33,34], a prioritization of the questions was carried out by the authors assigning 1–3 points to each question according to its subjective importance, yielding a descending list according to the sum of points awarded. To ensure a feasible time to complete the questionnaire of around 15 min, the list was cut from the end to a total of 62 questions followed by a content related arrangement. The answer options were mostly based on modified Likert scales [35–37], while multiple answer options or free text were also included.

Table 2. Two exemplary questions regarding the evaluation of the different teaching formats in the summer term 2020 together with answer options.

How do you rate your personal learning success with regard to the individual theoretical teaching forms in the summer term 2020?					
Lectures with audio	☐ Very good	☐ Good	☐ Satisfactory	☐ Bad	☐ Very bad
Live Stream lectures	☐ Very good	☐ Good	☐ Satisfactory	☐ Bad	☐ Very bad
Lectures (only .pdf files)	☐ Very good	☐ Good	☐ Satisfactory	☐ Bad	☐ Very bad
Scripts	☐ Very good	☐ Good	☐ Satisfactory	☐ Bad	☐ Very bad
Scientific articles	☐ Very good	☐ Good	☐ Satisfactory	☐ Bad	☐ Very bad
Virtual problem-based learning (VHB)	☐ Very good	☐ Good	☐ Satisfactory	☐ Bad	☐ Very bad
In the future I would like to have "Lectures with audio" permanently available	☐ Fully agree	☐ Rather agree	☐ Partially agree	☐ Disagree	☐ Disagree at all

2.6. Statistics

Data were analyzed descriptively and given graphically (Microsoft Excel, version 16.43, Redmond, WA, USA; GraphPad Prism, San Diego, CA, USA). Theoretical examination scores, separately for the 4th and 5th year courses, were statistically compared (Mann–Whitney U-test) between groups (2020summer term versus pooled previous four terms) after testing the normal distribution of the data (Shapiro–Wilk test). Alpha level was set at ≤ 0.05. The power as well as the effect size *d* were also given for the comparisons (GPower 3.1).

3. Results

The response rate of the questionnaire was 91% (4th year 42/45 students, 5th year 37/42 students, total 79/87, female 55 (69.6%), male 24 (30.4%)).

3.1. Evaluation of the General Learning Conditions

The organization was rated as "very good" (44.3%) or "good" (44.3%) (together 88.6%) by the majority of students (satisfactory 10.1%, bad 1.3%, very bad 0%). While most participants did not experience any technical problems (63.3%), the most frequent complaints were a poor Internet connection (22.8%) and problems with Zoom® (14.2%).

3.2. Evaluation of Theoretical Teaching Formats

Using grades from 1 (very good) to 5 (poor), lectures with audio were rated best with an average grade of 1.48 (Figure 1), followed by videos (1.54), live stream lectures including the webinar in pediatric dentistry (1.81), treatment checklists (1.81), and virtual problem-based learning (VHB) (2.1). Lectures only available as .pdf files (2.15), scientific articles (2.29), and scripts (2.30) were at the end. The aforementioned pediatric webinar (38 participating students) was particularly highlighted among the free-text responses, due to the promoting of English terminology, and the interaction with an international lecturer.

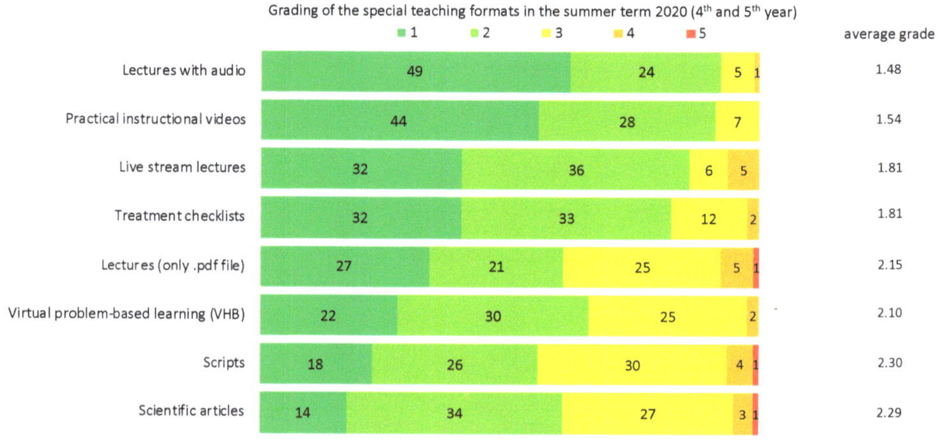

Figure 1. Students' ($n = 79$ out of 86) overall assessment of different teaching formats in grades. Evaluation was conducted using school grades: 1 = very good, 2 = good, 3 = satisfactory, 4 = bad, 5 = very bad. Given are the different teaching formats (left), the absolute number of different grades per teaching form (middle), and the average grade (right).

Regarding the students' wish to maintain the newly developed theoretical teaching formats in the future, lectures with audio were mostly named (91% "fully agree" and "partially agree"), followed by the videos (85%), live stream lectures (67%), and lectures provided solely as .pdf files at the end (32.91%) (Figure 2).

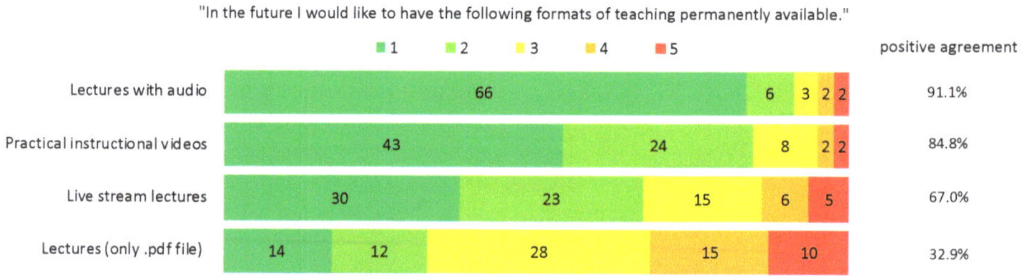

Figure 2. Evaluation of different teaching formats regarding the students' wish for maintenance. Rating was conducted using a modified Likert scale, 1 = fully agree, 2 = rather agree, 3 = partially agree, 4 = rather disagree, 5 = disagree at all. Given are the newly developed teaching formats (left), and the absolute number of given answers (middle). In addition, ratings 1 and 2 are given together as positive agreement (right).

Furthermore, the students were asked to compare the virtual theoretical teaching formats with the traditional face-to-face teaching regarding their efficacy of knowledge transfer (Figure 3). The ratings "distinctly better" and "better" were taken together and considered as "superior perception". This was the case in 78.5% for the lectures with audio, 39.2% for the live stream lectures, 30.4% for the virtual problem-based learning (VHB), and only 16.5% for the lectures solely given as .pdf files.

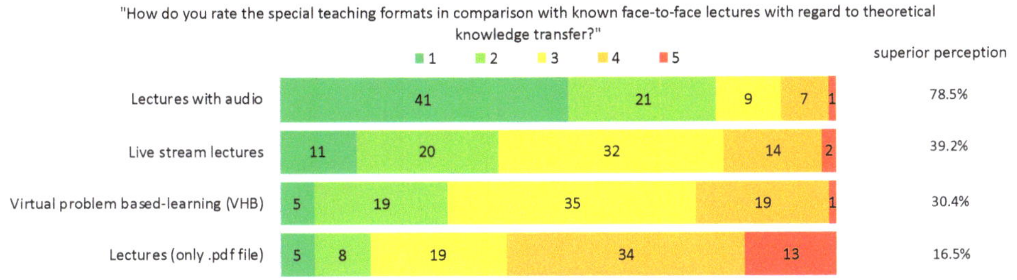

Figure 3. Assessment of the virtual theoretical teaching formats in comparison with traditional theoretical face-to-face teaching. Evaluation was conducted using a modified Likert scale, 1 = distinctly better, 2 = better, 3 = similar, 4 = worse, 5 = distinctly worse. Given are the different theoretical teaching formats (left), and the absolute number of given ratings (middle). In addition, ratings 1 and 2.

3.3. Evaluation of the Practical Training

Most students fully or rather agreed that the phantom head was the best possible replacement for treatment of a patient (59.5%). However, 69.4% of the students indicated, that they did not have the same respect toward the phantom head. Only 30.4% of the students stated they would appreciate additional training opportunities at the phantom head in the future. As advantages, the students primarily mentioned a relaxed working atmosphere (64.6%), equal conditions for all students (55.7%), gaining practical routine by working without complications (no saliva, no tongue; 54.4%), and no risk of infection (54.4%). As disadvantages, the lack of specific treatment parts, for example, injection (96.2%), anatomical individuality (96.2%), patient feedback such as pain perception (93.7%), and lack of communication (87.3%) were named.

The practical teaching in restorative dentistry was rated as "very good" or "good" by 85.7% of the 4th year and 81.0% of the 5th year students. In endodontology, it was rated as "very good" or "good" by 83.3% (4th year) and even by 91.1% of the 5th year students. In periodontology, it was graded as "very good" or "good" by 78.6% (4th year students), however, by only 27.0% of the 5th year students. The 4th year students rated the combination of tutorial and OSPE to be more realistic due to the simulated communication (69.0%), and appreciated it as further training of the complex periodontal diagnostic process, and would welcome its maintenance in the future (71.4%). Analyzing the students' performance within the OSPE, they achieved 79.8 ± 9.6% (mean ± SD) of the possible points (theoretical part 77.8 ± 3.6%, practical part 91.9 ±3.2%, communication skills 67.2 ± 1.0%).

Taking the theoretical and practical education together, 95% of the students rated their progress in theoretical knowledge and practical skills equal to that in a regular term.

3.4. Final Examination

In the 2020 summer term, the 4th year students achieved 40.4 ± 5.3 points, and the 5th year students 44.4 ± 3.6 points (mean ± SD) (maximum score 60 points, pass mark 36 points). This was significantly less than in the pooled examinations of the last four terms (4th year 45.9 ± 5.2 points, and 5th year 48.8 ± 5.4 points (mean ± SD) ($p < 0.0001$) (Figure 4). The comparison within the 4th year and 5th year students before and during Corona showed a power of 99.98 and an effect size d of 1.04 as well as 99.88 and 0.95, respectively.

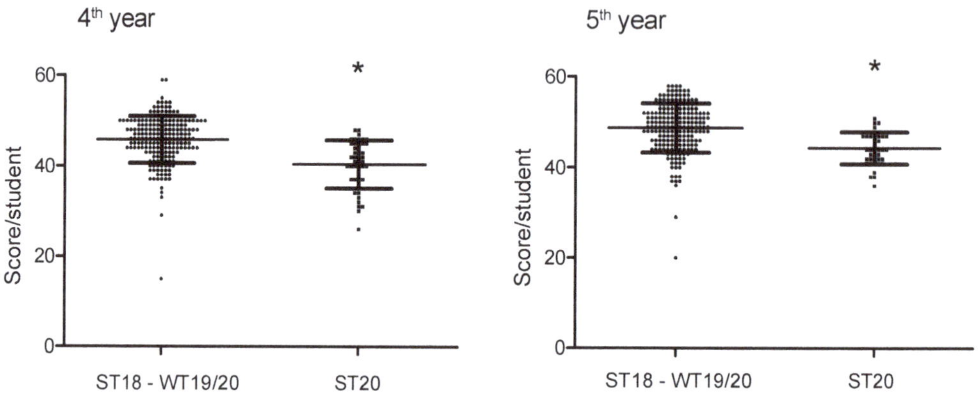

Figure 4. Evaluation of final examinations under regular and Corona conditions. Given are the 4th (**left**) and 5th year (**right**) students' scores in the final theoretical examination; each graph contrasts the results from the 2018 summer term to the 2019/2020 winter term (ST18-WT19/20), the results of the 2020 Corona summer term (ST20) (each dot represents one student, the bars depict mean ± SD, Mann–Whitney U-Test, * $p < 0.0001$).

4. Discussion

4.1. Theoretical Education

Regarding theoretical education, several approaches toward online availability were developed such as lectures with audio, live stream lectures, practical instructional videos, and introducing videos, which replaced hygienic or equipment briefings on site. The newly acquired online skills were also used for international exchange (webinar in pediatric dentistry). According to the questionnaire, lectures with audio were rated best among these approaches and should be maintained in the future, according to the opinion of most of the students. They especially emphasized the availability at any time and place via the Internet, and the possibility to repeat and pause sequences. These features would create a highly efficient and individual learning, which can be adapted to their own pace and daily routines. Interestingly, formats such as scripts, scientific articles, and lectures given solely as .pdf files without audio were rated worse, which may underline the importance of embedding content into an explaining frame. Besides, although not counted in particular, lecturers had the feeling of a higher number of attendees during their online lectures than their past face-to-face lectures. In contrast, it became clear from the free text comments within the survey that the students missed the communication between each other and the staff to eliminate uncertainties. Furthermore, they disapproved the lack of a clear separation of life and work, which would have a negative impact on their learning motivation. The mentioned findings are in accordance with recent studies from all over the world (e.g., Germany, Italy, and Jordan), which also evaluated the online learning possibilities during the COVID-19 pandemic [11,15,16,38,39].

However, the presented study revealed no hints that students would feel insufficiently qualified for patient treatment after the 2020 summer term, as this was critically mentioned by various studies [11,39] nor did the presented study point to an increased burnout risk, which was brought up as a concern in the case of sustained teaching without attendance [40,41]. In contrast, 95% of our students rated their progress in theoretical knowledge and practical skills equal to that in a regular term, although their theoretical test results were worse compared to the previous terms. Most of the recent studies assessed the students' subjective attitude toward the different teaching formats rather than their effectiveness in terms of knowledge gain. Instead, we tried to objectively evaluate their knowledge level based on end of term examinations. In this way, the success of the corona term in its entirety was evaluated and not solely the effect of specific formats.

4.2. Practical Education

To substitute the suspended patient treatment in the 2020 summer term, several approaches were offered to fulfill the practical education in this crisis situation, which ranged from demanding preparations at the phantom head, PBL presentations in combination with root canal treatments in 3D-printed teeth [25] to tutorials and OSPEs including communication skills training with acting patients. Although the students' treatment using phantom heads were only a surrogate for real patient treatment, the participants highly appreciated the provided efforts. However, this positive response should be viewed critically, since the newly offered formats could appear subjectively interesting and tended to be evaluated more positively. As disadvantages, the lack of typical treatment attributes such as salivation, tongue movements, patient feedback, anatomical individuality, and communication were named.

Interestingly, 4th year students rated the education in periodontology better than the 5th year students. The difference was that the 4th year course was provided with a tutorial and an OSPE including communication training with an acting patient in addition to the practical skills training at the phantom head. The 5th year course trained solely at the phantom head. Therefore, one could conclude that the more patient-centered simulation of periodontal treatment covering different aspects such as in this case, anamnesis, diagnosis, and treatment planning, taking the information of a simulated patient into account in combination with communication, found more acceptance by the students. Another aspect might have been, that the 5th year students had already treated patients in their 4th year course and therefore felt the difference to the phantom head and the associated loss of the mentioned attributes possibly even more. Communication was deemed important as a key process within the patient–doctor relationship as stressed already in the literature [27,42–44]. This is consistent with well-known learning theories that emphasize the need for teaching methods with social interaction. This is not only evident with a view to Miller's pyramid of competencies [45], but also according to Kolb [46], who, following the concept of "experiential learning", describes learning as a social process supported by experiences, educational moments, and a safe environment. In the 2020 summer term, the OSPE format was not primarily used for assessment but rather an excellent teaching tool seeking a higher level of competency [26]. According to Miller´s pyramid of competence [45], we could reach level 3a "shows how" (i.e., performance based on simulated patients). This requires the knowledge regarding cognitive levels 1 "know" and 2 "knows how", which was taught in the tutorials and at the phantom head.

As a welcome side effect when looking at the free text comments, the participants highlighted the better supervision relation between students and staff. Interestingly, the new approbation regulation for dentists, which becomes effective as of 2021, will provide a better relation of 1:3 for treatments of patients and of 1:6 for teaching at the patient [47].

5. Conclusions

Regarding the theoretical education, the study especially suggests maintaining digital lectures with audio on demand in future education accompanied by Q&A sessions with staff. A stable Internet connection is a prerequisite of utmost importance. While nothing can really replace patient treatment in practical education, for a crisis proof practical training/assessment without patients, approaches toward a higher level of competence such as OSPEs should be applied including as many aspects of patient treatment as possible. Special attention should also be paid to the training of communication skills. Nevertheless, a limitation of this study is that only students from a single dental school participated in this study. Therefore, especially, in view of the high relevance of this subject, review articles are necessary to gain a comprehensive overview of the measures undertaken worldwide.

Author Contributions: Conceptualization K.C.H., M.E.D., L.v.B.; methodology, K.C.H., M.E.D., L.v.B.; formal analysis and investigation K.C.H., M.E.D., L.v.B., M.K., S.L.; writing—original draft preparation, K.C.H., M.E.D., L.v.B.; writing—review and editing, K.C.H., M.E.D., L.v.B., R.H., J.D.; visualization, L.v.B.; supervision, K.C.H., M.E.D., R.H. All authors have read and agreed to the published version of the manuscript.

Funding: This research received no external funding.

Institutional Review Board Statement: The study was conducted according to the guidelines of the Declaration of Helsinki, and approved by the medical faculty's ethics committee of the Ludwig Maximilians University, Munich (No. 20-547 KB; Datum).

Informed Consent Statement: Formal consent was not required.

Data Availability Statement: The data can be made available upon reasonable request from the corresponding author.

Conflicts of Interest: The authors declare no conflict of interest.

References

1. WHO Europe's Standing Committee. WHO Declares COVID 19 Outbreak a Pandemic. Available online: https://www.euro.who.int/de/health-topics/health-emergencies/coronavirus-covid-19/news/news/2020/3/who-announces-covid-19-outbreak-a-pandemic (accessed on 13 April 2020).
2. Peng, X.; Xu, X.; Li, Y.; Cheng, L.; Zhou, X.; Ren, B. Transmission routes of 2019-nCoV and controls in dental practice. *Int. J. Oral Sci.* **2020**, *12*, 9. [CrossRef]
3. Meng, L.; Hua, F.; Bian, Z. Coronavirus disease 2019 (COVID-19): Emerging and future challenges for dental and oral medicine. *J. Dent. Res.* **2020**, *99*, 481–487. [CrossRef] [PubMed]
4. Walter, E.; von Bronk, L.; Hickel, R.; Huth, K.C. Impact of COVID-19 on Dental Care during a National Lockdown: A Retrospective Observational Study. *Int. J. Environ. Res. Public Health* **2021**, *18*, 7963. [CrossRef] [PubMed]
5. Van Doremalen, N.; Bushmaker, T.; Morris, D.H.; Holbrook, M.G.; Gamble, A.; Williamson, B.N.; Tamin, A.; Harcourt, J.L.; Thornburg, N.J.; Gerber, S.I. Aerosol and surface stability of SARS-CoV-2 as compared with SARS-CoV-1. *N. Engl. J. Med.* **2020**, *382*, 1564–1567. [CrossRef] [PubMed]
6. Herrera, D.; Serrano, J.; Roldán, S.; Sanz, M. Is the oral cavity relevant in SARS-CoV-2 pandemic? *Clin. Oral Investig.* **2020**, *24*, 2925–2930. [CrossRef]
7. Diegritz, C.; Manhart, J.; Bücher, K.; Grabein, B.; Schuierer, G.; Kühnisch, J.; Kunzelmann, K.-H.; Hickel, R.; Fotiadou, C. A detailed report on the measures taken in the Department of Conservative Dentistry and Periodontology in Munich at the beginning of the COVID-19 outbreak. *Clin. Oral Investig.* **2020**, *24*, 2931–2941. [CrossRef]
8. Chang, T.-Y.; Hong, G.; Paganelli, C.; Phantumvanit, P.; Chang, W.-J.; Shieh, Y.-S.; Hsu, M.-L. Innovation of dental education during COVID-19 pandemic. *J. Dent. Sci.* **2020**, *16*, 15–20. [CrossRef]
9. Desai, B.K. Clinical implications of the COVID-19 pandemic on dental education. *J. Dent. Educ.* **2020**, *84*, 512. [CrossRef]
10. Iyer, P.; Aziz, K.; Ojcius, D.M. Impact of COVID-19 on dental education in the United States. *J. Dent. Educ.* **2020**, *84*, 718–722. [CrossRef]
11. Schlenz, M.A.; Schmidt, A.; Wöstmann, B.; Krämer, N.; Schulz-Weidner, N. Students' and lecturers' perspective on the implementation of online learning in dental education due to SARS-CoV-2 (COVID-19): A cross-sectional study. *BMC Med. Educ.* **2020**, *20*, 1–7. [CrossRef]
12. Machado, R.A.; Bonan, P.R.F.; Perez, D.E.d.C.; Martelli JÚnior, H. COVID-19 pandemic and the impact on dental education: Discussing current and future perspectives. *Braz. Oral Res.* **2020**, *34*, e083. [CrossRef] [PubMed]
13. Quinn, B.; Field, J.; Gorter, R.; Akota, I.; Manzanares, M.; Paganelli, C.; Davies, J.; Dixon, J.; Gabor, G.; Amaral Mendes, R. COVID-19: The immediate response of european academic dental institutions and future implications for dental education. *Eur. J. Dent. Educ.* **2020**, *24*, 811–814. [CrossRef] [PubMed]
14. Goob, J.; Erdelt, K.; Güth, J.F.; Liebermann, A. Dental education during the pandemic: Cross-sectional evaluation of four different teaching concepts. *J. Dent. Educ.* **2021**, *85*, 1574–1587. [CrossRef] [PubMed]
15. Varvara, G.; Bernardi, S.; Bianchi, S.; Sinjari, B.; Piattelli, M. Dental Education Challenges during the COVID-19 Pandemic Period in Italy: Undergraduate Student Feedback, Future Perspectives, and the Needs of Teaching Strategies for Professional Development. *Healthcare* **2021**, *9*, 454. [CrossRef]
16. Hattar, S.; AlHadidi, A.; Sawair, F.A.; Abd Alraheam, I.; El-Ma'aita, A.; Wahab, F.K. Impact of COVID-19 pandemic on dental education: Online experience and practice expectations among dental students at the University of Jordan. *BMC Med. Educ.* **2021**, *21*, 1–10. [CrossRef] [PubMed]
17. Khalaf, K.; El-Kishawi, M.; Moufti, M.A.; Al Kawas, S. Introducing a comprehensive high-stake online exam to final-year dental students during the COVID-19 pandemic and evaluation of its effectiveness. *Med. Educ. Online* **2020**, *25*, 1826861. [CrossRef] [PubMed]

18. Universität Bayern e.V.; Bayerische Universitätenkonferenz. Richtlinien zum Vollzug der Bayerischen Infektionsschutzmaßnahmenverordnung an den Bayerischen Universitäten. Available online: https://www.mathematik-informatik-statistik.uni-muenchen.de/e-mails-corona/corona-update-_30_4_20-21_30_.pdf (accessed on 6 July 2020).
19. Ludwig-Maximilians Universität. Ergänzende Regelungen der LMU zu den Richtlinien des Universität Bayern e.V. *zum Vollzug der Bayerischen Infektionsschutzmaßnahmenverordnung an den bayerischen Universitäten*. Available online: https://www.studium.geowissenschaften.uni-muenchen.de/aktuelles/20-06-30-lmu-ergaenzende-regelungen-infektionsschutz.pdf (accessed on 10 July 2020).
20. Al Kawas, S.; Al-Rawi, N.; Talaat, W.; Hamdoon, Z.; Salman, B.; Al Bayatti, S.; Jerjes, W.; Samsudin, A.R. Post COVID-19 lockdown: Measures and practices for dental institutes. *BMC Oral Health* **2020**, *20*, 1–7. [CrossRef]
21. Rohlin, M.; Petersson, K.; Svensäter, G. The Malmö model: A problem-based learning curriculum in undergraduate dental education. *Eur. J. Dent. Educ.* **1998**, *2*, 103–114. [CrossRef]
22. Larsen, T.; Jeppe-Jensen, D. The introduction and perception of an OSCE with an element of self-and peer-assessment. *Eur. J. Dent. Educ.* **2008**, *12*, 2–7. [CrossRef]
23. Bassir, S.H.; Sadr-Eshkevari, P.; Amirikhorheh, S.; Karimbux, N.Y. Problem–Based Learning in Dental Education: A Systematic Review of the Literature. *J. Dent. Educ.* **2014**, *78*, 98–109. [CrossRef]
24. Fischer, M.R.; Bauer, D.; Karin Mohn, N. Finally finished! National competence based catalogues of learning objectives for undergraduate medical education (NKLM) and dental education (NKLZ) ready for trial. *GMS Z. Für Med. Ausbild.* **2015**, *32*, Doc35.
25. Reymus, M.; Fotiadou, C.; Kessler, A.; Heck, K.; Hickel, R.; Diegritz, C. 3D printed replicas for endodontic education. *Int. Endod. J.* **2019**, *52*, 123–130. [CrossRef] [PubMed]
26. Gerhard-Szep, S.; Guentsch, A.; Pospiech, P.; Söhnel, A.; Scheutzel, P.; Wassmann, T.; Zahn, T. Assessment formats in dental medicine: An overview. *GMS J. Med. Educ.* **2016**, *33*, 6–8. [CrossRef]
27. Kurtz, S.; Silverman, J. The Calgary—Cambridge Referenced Observation Guides: An aid to defining the curriculum and organizing the teaching in communication training programmes. *Med. Educ.* **1996**, *30*, 83–89. [CrossRef] [PubMed]
28. Kollewe, T.; Sennekamp, M.; Ochsendorf, F. *Medizindidaktik*; Springer: Berlin/Heidelberg, Germany, 2018.
29. McGaghie, W.C.; Issenberg, S.B.; Petrusa, E.R.; Scalese, R.J. A critical review of simulation-based medical education research: 2003–2009. *Med Educ.* **2010**, *44*, 50–63. [CrossRef]
30. Kurtz, S.; Draper, J.; Silverman, J. *Teaching and Learning Communication Skills in Medicine*; CRC Press: Boca Raton, FL, USA, 2017.
31. Haladyna, T.M. *Developing and Validating Multiple-Choice Test Items*; Routledge: New York, NY, USA, 2004.
32. Bauer, D.; Holzer, M.; Kopp, V.; Fischer, M.R. Pick-N multiple choice-exams: A comparison of scoring algorithms. *Adv. Health Sci. Educ.* **2011**, *16*, 211–221. [CrossRef]
33. Carney, O.; McIntosh, J.; Worth, A. The use of the nominal group technique in research with community nurses. *J. Adv. Nurs.* **1996**, *23*, 1024–1029. [CrossRef]
34. Gallagher, M.; Hares, T.; Spencer, J.; Bradshaw, C.; Webb, I. The nominal group technique: A research tool for general practice? *Fam. Pract.* **1993**, *10*, 76–81. [CrossRef]
35. Norman, G. Likert scales, levels of measurement and the "laws" of statistics. *Adv. Health Sci. Educ.* **2010**, *15*, 625–632. [CrossRef]
36. Likert, R. A technique for the measurement of attitudes. *Arch. Psychol.* **1932**, *140*, 1–55.
37. Sullivan, G.M.; Artino, A.R., Jr. Analyzing and interpreting data from Likert-type scales. *J. Grad. Med Educ.* **2013**, *5*, 541. [CrossRef]
38. Mukhtar, K.; Javed, K.; Arooj, M.; Sethi, A. Advantages, Limitations and Recommendations for online learning during COVID-19 pandemic era. *Pak. J. Med Sci.* **2020**, *36*, S27. [CrossRef]
39. Abbasi, S.; Ayoob, T.; Malik, A.; Memon, S.I. Perceptions of students regarding E-learning during Covid-19 at a private medical college. *Pak. J. Med Sci.* **2020**, *36*, S57. [CrossRef]
40. Chen, E.; Kaczmarek, K.; Ohyama, H. Student perceptions of distance learning strategies during COVID-19. *J. Dent. Educ.* **2020**, *85*, 1190–1191. [CrossRef]
41. De Oliveira Araújo, F.J.; de Lima, L.S.A.; Cidade, P.I.M.; Nobre, C.B.; Neto, M.L.R. Impact of Sars-Cov-2 and its reverberation in global higher education and mental health. *Psychiatry Res.* **2020**, *288*, 112977. [CrossRef]
42. Silverman, J.; Kurtz, S.; Draper, J. *Skills for Communicating with Patients*; CRC Press: Boca Raton, FL, USA, 2016.
43. Field, J.; Cowpe, J.; Walmsley, A. The graduating European dentist: A new undergraduate curriculum framework. *Eur. J. Dent. Educ.* **2017**, *21*, 2–10. [CrossRef] [PubMed]
44. Cowpe, J.; Plasschaert, A.; Harzer, W.; Vinkka-Puhakka, H.; Walmsley, A.D. Profile and competences for the graduating European dentist–update 2009. *Eur. J. Dent. Educ.* **2010**, *14*, 193–202. [CrossRef]
45. Miller, G.E. The assessment of clinical skills/competence/performance. *Acad. Med.* **1990**, *65*, S63–S67. [CrossRef] [PubMed]
46. Kolb, D.A. Experience as the source of learning and development. *Up. Sadle River Prentice Hall* **1984**, *2*, 31–49.
47. Bundesgesundheitsministerium. Approbationsordnung für Zahnärzte und Zahnärztinnen (ZApprO). 2019. Available online: https://www.buzer.de/ZApprO.htm (accessed on 4 January 2020).

Journal of
Clinical Medicine

MDPI

Article

Oral Health and Teledentistry Interest during the COVID-19 Pandemic

Magdalena Sycinska-Dziarnowska [1], Marzia Maglitto [2], Krzysztof Woźniak [1] and Gianrico Spagnuolo [2,3,*]

1 Department of Orthodontics, Pomeranian Medical University in Szczecin, Powstańców Wielkopolskich Street 72, 70111 Szczecin, Poland; magdadziarnowska@gmail.com (M.S.-D.); krzysztof.wozniak@pum.edu.pl (K.W.)
2 Department of Neurosciences, Reproductive and Odontostomatological Sciences, University of Naples "Federico II", 80131 Napoli, Italy; mar.maglitto@gmail.com
3 Institute of Dentistry, I. M. Sechenov First Moscow State Medical University, 119435 Moscow, Russia
* Correspondence: gspagnuo@unina.it

Abstract: Background: The COVID-19 pandemic outbreak has significantly changed access to dental treatments. Methods: The data related to oral health and teledentistry topics were collected from the open database Google Trends. The analyzed material was collected from 19 June 2016 to 6 June 2021 among anonymous search engine users. The following expressions were analyzed: "dental care", "emergency dental care", "oral health", "periodontitis", "teledentistry", "is it safe to go to the dentist", and "COVID-19" and "PPE dentist". Results: During the first lockdown in 2020, a significant increase in "emergency dental care" phrase queries was detected, with a simultaneous decrease in regular "dental care" questions, as well as a peak in the queries for "periodontitis" preceded by lower interest in "oral health." The number of searches stated for "teledentistry" increased during the time of the pandemic 5 times and for and "PPE dentist" 30 times. The risk of visiting the dental studio was seen in almost 40 times increase in the query "is it safe to go to the dentist." Conclusions: The COVID-19 imprinted a stigma on oral health care. In this difficult epidemiological situation, teledentistry might become a helpful solution.

Keywords: oral health; teledentistry; Google Trends; COVID-19 pandemic

Citation: Sycinska-Dziarnowska, M.; Maglitto, M.; Woźniak, K.; Spagnuolo, G. Oral Health and Teledentistry Interest during the COVID-19 Pandemic. *J. Clin. Med.* **2021**, *10*, 3532. https://doi.org/10.3390/jcm10163532

Academic Editors: Hans-Peter Howaldt and Sameh Attia

Received: 22 July 2021
Accepted: 10 August 2021
Published: 11 August 2021

1. Introduction

In late June 2021, about 182 million COVID-19 cases were reported globally, with almost 4 million people deaths [1]. It seems very likely that the COVID-19 pandemic had an impact on oral health-related behaviors. The stringent measures undertaken to limit the spread of COVID-19 disease with social distancing rules made access to dental offices more troublesome. The risk of contagion can be reduced by introducing teledentistry [2]. Teleconsultation, which begins with an online triage, was a compromise that limited patient access but also ensured effective treatment and relief from symptoms [3]

According to some studies, routine dental care and emergency dental care have been immensely influenced by the waves of COVID-19 [4–7]. The large impact of the COVID-19 pandemic on dentistry was shown in the study conducted by Soltani et al., in which as many as 659 articles published by dental journals were found in PubMed regarding implications of the COVID-19 pandemic in dentistry [8]. Moreover, many people did not want to visit the dental studios due to the fear of virus transmission. Moreover, as proved in many studies in pre-pandemic time, the prolonged lack of regular oral health check-ups may lead to periodontitis [9,10]. Another unprecedented situation happened during the COVID-19 pandemic. Greater demand for personal protective equipment (PPE) was detected globally and led to a shortage in masks, gloves, and almost all PPE [11]. Difficult access to PPE was significant and obvious in the early phase of the COVID-19 pandemic. In order to minimize the viral spread risk during the current COVID-19 pandemic and post-pandemic times, the global project to define the best organization of dental offices was conducted [12].

Rapid changes in the epidemiological situation might be easily and strongly visible in the surveillance of the more widely used search engines, for example, the Google search engine, the most used engine with the vast majority of the market share, as much as 92.26% [13].

The aim of this study was to analyze the impact of the COVID-19 pandemic on oral health and the interest in teledentistry.

2. Materials and Methods

The data for the study were collected from the open database—Google Trends (GT) service among anonymous search engine users related to oral health and teledentistry subjects [14,15]. Each data record represents a weekly worldwide number of queries processed by Google engine and available according to the selected time period. In the study, the analyzed material was collected from 19 June 2016 to 6 June 2021. All data imported from GT represent queries were normalized to the time and location. The resulting numbers are scaled on a range of 0 to 100, where 100 is the maximum number of searches in a stated period of time. The following expressions were analyzed: "dental care", "emergency dental care", "oral health", "periodontitis", "COVID-19" and "PPE dentist", as well as the phrases "teledentistry" and "is it safe to go to the dentist", were investigated to check the interest for online consultations.

The data analysis was divided into two sections. The first section provides the detailed level description of data, its structure, and main samples characteristics needed in order to perform further calculations. In the second section, the pairwise correlation between data series was analyzed. For each time series data, the trend, cyclical, and random fluctuations analyses were performed. The purposes of this section were as follows:

- To present pairwise time series visualizations;
- To perform time series decompositions indicating the trend, cyclical, and random fluctuations;
- To analyze the cross-correlation between chosen time series pairs with statistically significant estimation;
- To evaluate a pairwise of mutual influence (where possible).

To estimate the dynamics rate (hereinafter), the comparisons of two mean rates for two periods were made: first one for the period before the 22–23 January 2020, when the World Health Organization (WHO) Director gathered an Emergency Committee to discuss whether the new virus outbreak determined a public health emergency of worldwide concern [16] (that refers to dates from 19 June 2016 to 19 January 2020 in our weekly split data set) and the second one from 19 January 2020 to 6 June 2021. For simplicity, we further refer to those periods as before and during the pandemic. In the study, we aimed to check the time before the official pandemic onset, as the search engines may have shown some interest in the subject before official regulations were made.

For the qualitative and quantitative analysis of the correlation, the time series collections were divided into the following 4 pairs:

- "Dental care"–"emergency dental";
- "Oral health"–"periodontitis";
- "Teledentistry"–"is it safe to go to the dentist";
- "COVID-19"–"PPE-dentist".

All statistical estimations with data visualizations were programmed by the "R" programming language [17] with "R studio" version 1.4.1106 open-source software for data science, scientific research, and technical communication [18].

3. Results

3.1. Time Series Visualizations

A graphical illustration of time series was presented by a paired graph of the dynamics of requests in the study period. For the purposes of analyzing the trend, cyclical, and random fluctuations, the time series were decomposed for each collection separately.

The pairwise time series visualization of "dental care"–"emergency dental care" is presented in Figure 1a. The plot clearly shows a high proportion of uncertainty in demand for dental services at the very beginning of 2020. This is evidenced by a sharp decline in demand for planned dental procedures with a simultaneous sharp increase in demand for emergency ones. However, this phase had a short-term character, and during the next 1–2 months, the structure of demand returned to its normal state.

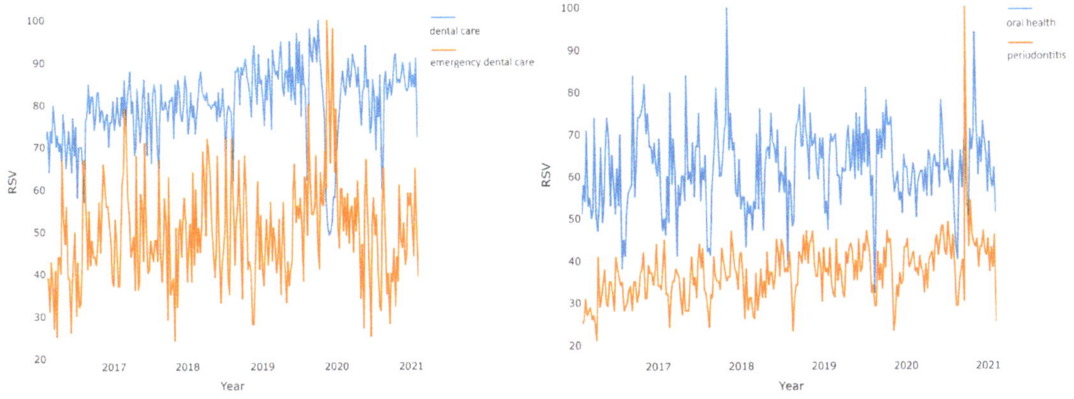

(a) (b)

Figure 1. Pairwise comparison of weekly requests during 2016–2021: (**a**) "dental care"–"emergency dental care"; (**b**) "oral health"–"periodontitis".

The pairwise, time series visualization of "oral health"–"periodontitis" is presented in Figure 1b. The plot shows large interest growth when regarding "periodontitis" with the peak at the beginning of the year 2020 with stable and slight growth in the number of questions asked during the analyzed period. The number of queries for "oral health" is more stable. A peak in "periodontitis" queries was detected after the hard lockdown and the lower interest in the "oral health" subject.

Furthermore, the pairwise, time series visualization of "teledentistry"–"is it safe to go to the dentist" is presented in Figure 2a. Both terms under consideration rarely occurred in the pre-pandemic time. Only at the beginning of 2020 did these concepts become widespread. The plot clearly shows a peak when the request for both terms reaches its maximum. The demand for the "teledentistry" term then begins to decline exponentially until the end of the period under review, reaching levels preceding the pandemic, and the expression "is it safe to go to the dentist" is characterized by steady demand throughout almost all of 2020, reaching local highs during periods of lockdowns and exacerbations of restrictions. However, at the end of the period under review, requests for this term also reached a minimum, slightly exceeding pre-pandemic levels.

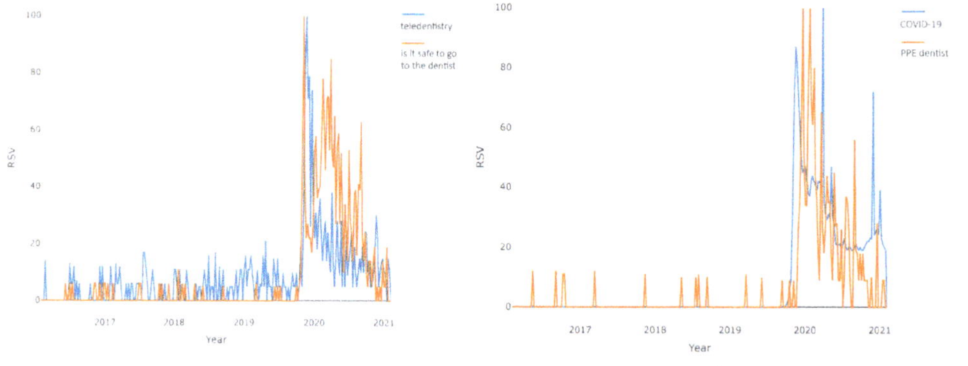

(**a**) (**b**)

Figure 2. Pairwise comparison of weekly requests during 2016–2021: (**a**) "teledentistry"–"is it safe to go to the dentist"; (**b**) "COVID-19"–"PPE dentist".

The pairwise, time series visualization of "COVID-19"–"PPE dentist" is presented in Figure 2b. Both expressions came into use immediately with the onset of the pandemic. The demand curve for "COVID-19" is characterized by the presence of three global highs that occurred at the junction of 2019–2020, in the first quarter of 2020, and at the junction of 2020/2021, which corresponds to the time of global pandemic waves. The topic "PPE dentist" standing for personal protective equipment was characterized by the greatest demand at the beginning of the pandemic; over the next 1.5 years, the level of interest dropped exponentially, until the end of the period under review, where it again reached the pre-pandemic level.

3.2. Trends Analysis

Regarding the "dental care" time series, during the period under consideration, there are two periods of trend growth Figure 3a: the first (more pronounced) from the beginning of 2018 to the beginning of 2019, and the second (more smoothed) from the beginning of 2020. There was no downtrend during the pandemic period. Regarding the "emergency dental care" time series (Figure 3b), the direction is multidirectional (with local ups and downs) with a general upward trend. After reaching the minimum in 2018 through mid-2020, there was a significant increase, followed by a short-term moderate decline (probably during the general lockdown). An upward trend was observed since the second half of 2020, which reached its maximum values at the end of the period under review.

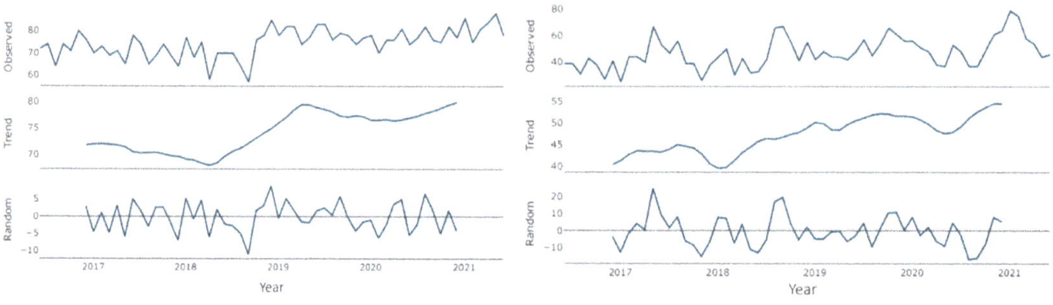

(**a**) (**b**)

Figure 3. Decomposition of time series (month granularity): (**a**) "dental care"; (**b**) "emergency dental care".

Regarding the "oral health" time series, during the period under consideration, there are two periods of trend growth Figure 4a: the first (minor one) from the beginning of 2017 to the beginning of 2018, and the second (a pronounced one) from mid-2018 to early 2020. Periods of growth are followed by periods of decline with similar severity and duration. Since the beginning of the pandemic, a negative trend was recorded with small periods of stabilization with a tendency to smooth out. There were no upward trends. In mid-2021, the level of demand is close to the minimum values for the period under review. Furthermore, regarding the "periodontitis" time series (Figure 4b), for most of the period under review, the trend was characterized as moderately growing with small corrections and short declines. Since the beginning of 2019, there has been protracted growth, which reached its maximum during the pandemic. At the end of the period under review, there is a slight decrease in the trend, which, however, exceeds the demand levels of the pre-pandemic period.

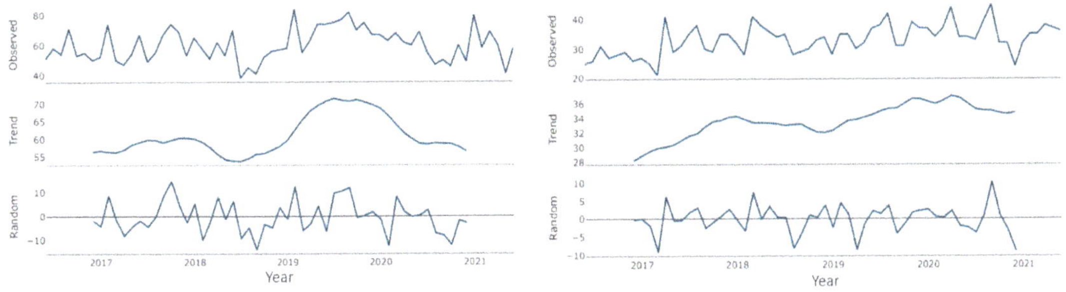

(a) (b)

Figure 4. Decomposition of time series (month granularity): (**a**) "oral health"; (**b**) "periodontitis".

Regarding the "teledentistry" time series (Figure 5a), until the second half of 2019, the trend was an almost flat curve, with a barely noticeable increase, which is replaced by a sharp growth phase lasting about a year. The growth for the specified period was about 20 points. Then, the growth phase was replaced by a moderate decline phase, which continued until the end of the period under review. Similarly, in the "is it safe to go to the dentist" time series (Figure 5b), until the second half of 2019, the trend was a flat line with a zero value, which was replaced by a phase of sharp growth that lasted for about a year. The growth for the indicated period was about 40 points. Then, the growth phase gave way to a moderate decline phase, which lasted until the end of the period under review.

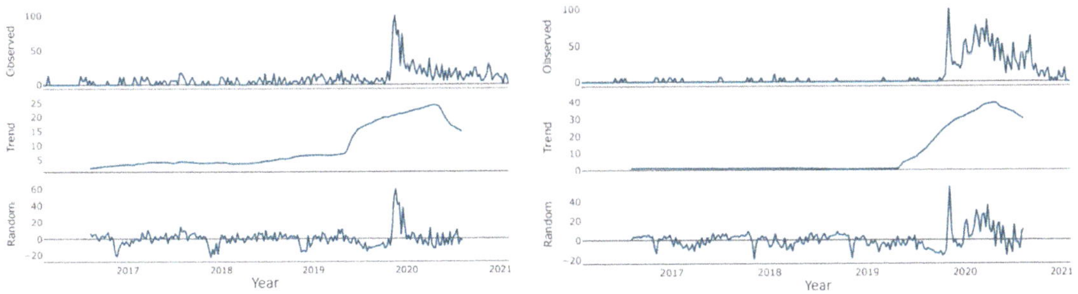

(a) (b)

Figure 5. Decomposition of time series (week granularity): (**a**) for "teledentistry"; (**b**) for "is it safe to go to the dentist".

The trend line for both expressions in Figure 6a,b—"COVID-19" and "PPE dentist"—repeats the pattern of the previous pair. Until mid-2019, a horizontal line at the 0 level is observed, after which the annual growth phase with a maximum increase of up to 30 points is observed. The growth phase is replaced by a moderate decline phase, which continues until the end of the period under consideration (the volume of decline for "COVID-19"—5 points, for "PPE dentist"—10 points).

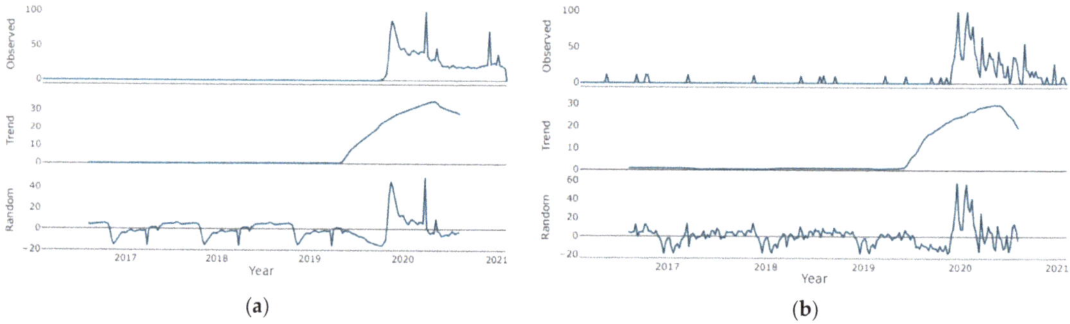

Figure 6. Decomposition of time series (week granularity): (**a**) for "COVID-19"; (**b**) for "dentist PPE".

3.3. Cyclical and Random Fluctuations Indications Analysis

In the "dental care" time series (Figure 3a), there is a single negative peak of average severity in the second half of 2018. There were no positive peaks in the similar intensity. When regarding the "emergency dental care" time series Figure 3b, there are two peaks: the most pronounced at the beginning of the period (breaking through the 20 marks) and slightly less pronounced in the second half of 2018 (approaching the 20 marks). Negative peaks of similar intensity were not observed.

Regarding the "oral health" time series (Figure 4a), there are several cycles of low severity breaking through the 10-point mark in both directions. Moreover, in the "periodontitis" time series (Figure 4b), there are several peaks of average severity approaching the 10-point mark in both directions. The most pronounced is the positive cycle at the end of the period under consideration.

In the "teledentistry" time series (Figure 5a), there is one pronounced cycle with an increase in the parameter of about 60 points, and there is one pronounced cycle with an increase in the parameter of more than 40 points when describing the "is it safe to go to the dentist" time series (Figure 5b).

Two pronounced cycles are clearly visible in the "COVID-19" time series in Figure 6a—at the junction of 2019/2020 and in the first half of 2020, with an increase of about 35 points. No pronounced negative peaks are observed. A series of peaks regarding the expression "PPE dentist" at the junction of 2019/2020 with gains of more than 50 points is clearly visible. No pronounced negative peaks were recorded (Figure 6b).

3.4. Changes in Request Average during COVID-19 Pandemic

The mean of "dental care" time series request rate in the pre-pandemic period has a rate of 79.9; during the pandemic, the mean rate was increased to 80.2. Thus, from the pandemic onset to the present, the "dental care" requests mean rate has remained particularly unchanged (the increasing rate is about 0.4%). Moreover, the mean of the "emergency dental care" time series request rate in the pre-pandemic period has a rate of 48.73, and during the pandemic, the mean rate increased to 52.6. Thus, from the pandemic onset to the present, the main rate of "emergency dental care" increased by 7.9%. The mean of the "oral health" time series request rate in the pre-pandemic period has a rate of 62.0; during the pandemic, the mean rate changed to 61.8. Thus, from the pandemic onset to the present, the "oral health" requests mean rate remained particularly unchanged (the decreasing rate is about 0.3%). The mean of the "periodontitis" request rate in the pre-pandemic period has a rate of 35.7; during the pandemic, the mean rate changed to 41.1. Thus, from the pandemic onset to the present, the main rate of "periodontitis" increased by 15.1%. Moreover, the mean of the "teledentistry" time series request rate in the pre-pandemic period has a rate of 4.3; during the pandemic, the mean rate changed to 21.4. Thus, from the pandemic onset to the present, the "teledentistry" requests mean rate characterized by a 5 times increase. The mean of the request rate for the "is it safe to go to the dentist" time series in the pre-pandemic period has a rate of 0.8; during the pandemic, the mean rate changed to 31.9. Thus, from the pandemic onset to the present, the requests mean rate is characterized by an increase of almost 40 times. The mean of the "PPE dentist" request rate in the pre-pandemic period has a rate of 0.8; during the pandemic, the mean rate changed to 24.0. Thus, from the pandemic onset to the present, the "PPE dentist" request mean rate is characterized by an increase of 30 times. When regarding the "COVID-19" time series, this expression did not exist before the pandemic.

3.5. Cross-Correlation

The time series pair "dental care"–"emergency dental" cross-correlation function plot is shown in Figure 7a. There are a number of significant correlations on both sides of 0. All significant correlations are positive, from which it follows, an increase in one parameter leads to an increase in another. There is no significant correlation at h = 0. Furthermore, the time series pair "oral health"–"periodontitis" cross-correlation function plot is shown in Figure 7b. The correlation magnitude and the number of significant correlations are greater on the left side of 0. The most dominant cross-correlation occurs at h = −2. The correlation is positive, indicating that an above-average value of "oral health" is likely to lead to an above-average value of "periodontitis" about 2 months later. Additionally, a below-average value of "oral health" is associated with a likely below-average "periodontitis" value about 2 months later. Moreover, the time series pair "teledentistry"–"is it safe to go to the dentist" cross-correlation function plot is shown in Figure 7c. There are a number of significant correlations only on the right side of 0. All significant correlations are positive. Finally, the time series pair "COVID-19"–"PPE dentist" cross-correlation function plot is shown in Figure 7d. There are a number of significant correlations on both sides of 0. There is also a significant correlation at h = 0. All significant correlations are positive, from which it follows, an increase in one parameter leads to an increase in another. An above-average value of "COVID-19" is highly likely to lead to an above-average value of "PPE dentist" about 4 weeks later. Since both expressions existed in GT searches for less than 2 years, the use of month granularity was impossible, which is why, in this case, a week granularity was used.

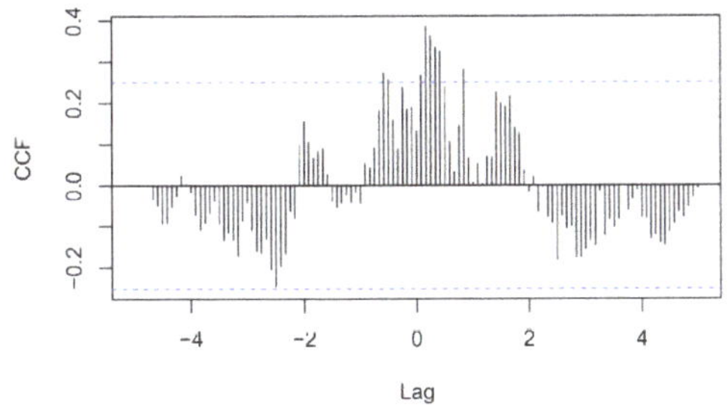

(a)

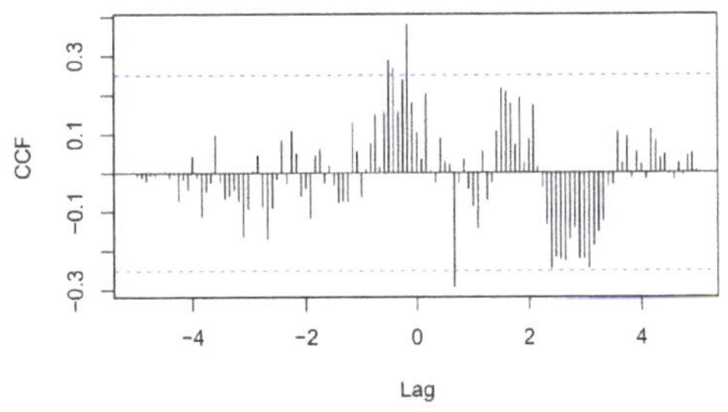

(b)

Figure 7. *Cont.*

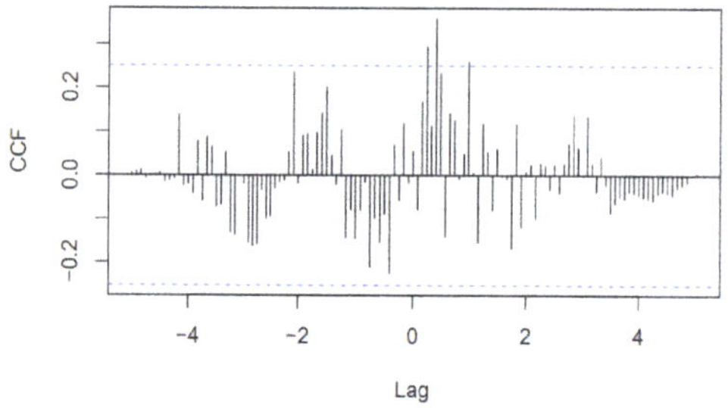

(c)

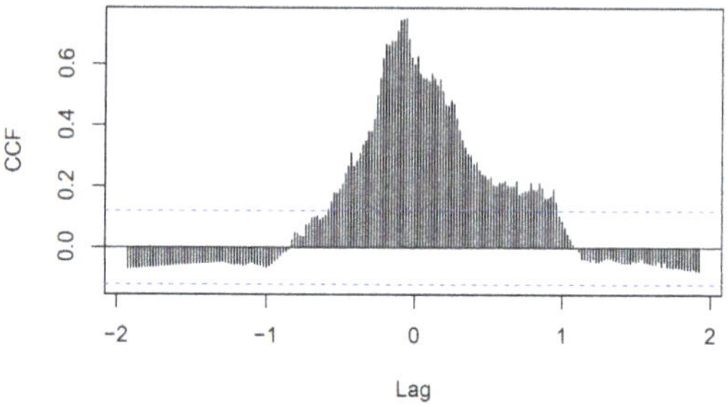

(d)

Figure 7. Cross-correlation plots: (**a**) "dental care"–"emergency dental" (granularity: month); (**b**) "oral health"–"periodontitis" (granularity: month); (**c**) "teledentistry"–"is it safe to go to the dentist" (granularity: month); (**d**) "COVID-19"–"PPE dentist" (granularity: week).

4. Discussion

The aim of the study was to investigate the impact of the COVID-19 pandemic on oral health and teledentistry subjects. To the best of our knowledge, this is one of the few studies [19,20] tracing the GT expressions connected with oral health during the COVID-19 pandemic. The first noticeable outcome of the research was a large increase in emergency dental care questions asked during the spring lockdown in 2020 with a simultaneous decrease in regular dental care queries. Our results strongly show that the COVID-19 pandemic had significantly influenced dental-care-seeking behavior. According to the recommendations and because of the fear surrounding the epidemic, people were averse to be outside and less willing to visit dental studios. Moreover, dental care was not widely available during the early phase of the pandemic, with a large number of patients expected to seek emergency dental service only when urgent care was needed [5]. In line with our study, the outcomes of the study conducted by Faccini et al. indicate that during the hard lockdown, 64.6% of dentists carried out only emergency treatments, with 26.1% of dentists still maintaining the routine planned appointments, and with 9.3% of dental offices closed for the duration of the lockdown. An increase in urgent dental procedures was noted by 44.1% of the dentists. It occurred most often due to the lower availability for a longer period of time for regular dental care. The main causes of emergency appointments were toothache, dental trauma, or broken restorations [21]. Similarly, a study conducted in Beijing, China, with 2537 patients involved in the study, indicated that at the beginning of the COVID-19 pandemic, 38% fewer patients sought dental emergency care than before. Dental problems and oral infection increased from 51.0% in the pre-pandemic period to 71.9% during the COVID-19 pandemic period [5]. A finding in line with our study is that the COVID-19 pandemic outbreak had strongly influenced the emergency dental services. The large influence of COVID-19 disease on oral cavity was shown in the study conducted by Gherlone et al., as 83.6% of patients reported anomalies of the oral cavity, such as dry mouth or salivary gland ectasia, that lasted even up to 3 months after hospitalization due to COVID-19 [22].

According to recent studies, people with serious medical conditions such as diabetes, heart diseases, lung or kidney chronic disease, and older persons were at high risk for developing more severe COVID-19 infection. On the other hand, poor oral health and hygiene may increase the risk of developing the abovementioned medical problems. Therefore, improving oral health among the whole population may lead to a lower risk of developing systemic diseases and, in this way, reduce the morbidity due to COVID-19 [9,23]. In the study among a group of 568 patients, the higher risk of intensive care unit admission with the need for assisted ventilation and worse disease outcomes, leading even to the death of COVID-19 patients, was associated with periodontitis. Similarly, COVID-19 patients with periodontitis had significantly higher blood levels of D-dimer and C-reactive protein and white blood cells [24]. After a lower level of interest in oral health was detected in the number of queries asked in GT during the hard lockdown, in the conducted study, we detected a peak in periodontitis questions and about a 15% interest growth in the subject.

During the pandemic, telemedicine represented an opportunity to improve accessibility to medical treatments. According to some studies, teledentistry could be comparable to face-to-face visits for oral screening, especially in areas with limited access to oral health care. In fact, the identification of oral pathologies via teleconsultations is widely possible and valid [25]. The online examination using intraoral scans may become helpful in detecting dental problems. The remote assessment of intraoral scans can allow an efficient screening and the correct triage of patients. Improved intraoral scans can provide even three-dimensional images with true colors [26]. Nowadays, to minimize contact with the patient and to ensure patient safety clinicians may follow up with patients online, for example, through video calls. In the present study, a 5-time increase in query rates for teledentistry during the COVID-19 pandemic was detected because of the anxiety to visit the dentist. The query "is it safe to go to the dentist" increased the question rate during the pandemic almost 40 times. It may indicate the usefulness of such a digital tool during epidemiological threats. The screening for other chronic viral infections was previously conducted in dental offices, for example, for HCV virus [27]; such easy, free-of-charge prevention campaigns may use teleconsultation in the post-pandemic time.

In addition, specific recommendations and lots of preventive measures against COVID-19 were undertaken in dental offices with infection control strategies. The urgent need for dental emergency care required fast delivery of the appropriate PPE. The initial shortage and distribution challenges of PPE was seen globally [11,28], as well as the large interest in PPE connected with dentists was observed in our study, with a 30-time increase of requests mean rate. The patient management protocols were applied to reduce the risk of infection and to prevent the spread of the cross-infection, for example, clinical triage for patient screening with a questionnaire on recent disease symptoms, body temperature measurement, avoiding crowding in the waiting room, a hand sanitizer available to patients before entering the operating rooms, and the use of PPEs and oral rinses with hydrogen peroxide before the dental treatment [29–32]. The WHO recommended the use of FFP3 masks according to the European terminology or N100, according to the United States nomenclature [33]. Members of the oral healthcare team should be acquainted with the COVID-19 transmission and preventive measures, as the oral cavity is an important site for COVID-19 infection and a potential route of virus transmission [34]. Cross-infection control measures should be applied to all patients because asymptomatic COVID-19 persons may also need emergency dental treatment [35].

This study has some limitations. Firstly, the analyzed data were collected from one search engine; nevertheless, Google engine has nearly four billion users worldwide and covers more than 90% of all queries on the internet, with near 7 billion queries per day. With 4.39 billion internet users worldwide, the number of Google users is globally nearly four billion [36]. In our study, the GT request sample size for 5 years period is about big data collections. Thus, the nature of the data and sample size is appropriate for the purpose and nature of the study. Moreover, when considering the overlapping of expressions meaning, in a small sample, it might be discussed as a limitation; however, the sample of expressions gathered in the presented study is huge, the time of observation is long, and therefore, it should not induce significant changes in results. Secondly, the study was carried out globally, in order not to add too much manual categorization, by providing expressions in different languages. When adding queries in many languages across countries, it becomes more difficult to choose the best fitting expression used in a specific country. Finally, there are no strict rules on how to analyze the GT in health care research [37]; on the other hand, the GT data are recognized by the scientific community as a reliable source on the basis of which scientific papers in various fields are published [38,39]. Because of the anonymized approach of data collection, GT enables the analysis and forecasting of sensitive topics especially in medicine [37,40–43]. Because of using the revealed and not stated users' preferences, it is possible to obtain information that would be otherwise impossible to collect. Moreover, GT offers a substantial promise for the global monitoring of diseases in countries that lack clinical surveillance but have sufficient internet coverage to allow for surveillance via digital epidemiology [44].

5. Conclusions

1. Firstly, according to the search queries analysis from GT, the COVID-19 pandemic had a large impact on oral health problems;
2. Moreover, emergency dental care became more required during the onset of pandemic and hard lockdown than regular dental care;
3. Finally, teledentistry gained in popularity during the lockdowns according to globally asked questions in GT service.

Author Contributions: Conceptualization, M.S.-D. and G.S.; methodology, M.S.-D.; software, M.S.-D.; validation, M.S.-D. and M.M.; formal analysis, M.S.-D.; investigation, M.S.-D.; resources, M.S.-D.; data curation, M.S.-D.; writing—original draft preparation, M.S.-D.; writing—review and editing, M.S.-D., K.W., M.M., and G.S.; visualization, M.S.-D. and M.M.; supervision, G.S. All authors have read and agreed to the published version of the manuscript.

Funding: This research received no external funding.

Institutional Review Board Statement: Not applicable.

Informed Consent Statement: Not applicable.

Data Availability Statement: The data presented in this study are available on request from the corresponding author.

Conflicts of Interest: The authors declare no conflict of interest.

References

1. Worldometer—COVID-19 Coronavirus Pandemic. Available online: https://www.worldometers.info/coronavirus/?utm_campaign=homeAdvegas1 (accessed on 28 June 2021).
2. Barca, I.; Novembre, D.; Giofrè, E.; Caruso, D.; Cordaro, R.; Kallaverja, E.; Ferragina, F.; Cristofaro, M.G. Telemedicine in Oral and Maxillo-Facial Surgery: An Effective Alternative in Post COVID-19 Pandemic. *Int. J. Environ. Res. Public Health* **2020**, *17*, 7365. [CrossRef]
3. Beauquis, J.; Petit, A.; Michaux, V.; Sagué, V.; Henrard, S.; Leprince, J. Dental Emergencies Management in COVID-19 Pandemic Peak: A Cohort Study. *J. Dent. Res.* **2021**, *100*, 352–360. [CrossRef]
4. Cagetti, M.G.; Balian, A.; Camoni, N. Guglielmo Campus Influence of the COVID-19 Pandemic on Dental Emergency Admissions in an Urgent Dental Care Service in North Italy. *Int. J. Environ. Res. Public Health* **2021**, *18*, 1812. [CrossRef]
5. Guo, H.; Zhou, Y.; Liu, X.; Tan, J. The impact of the COVID-19 epidemic on the utilization of emergency dental services. *J. Dent. Sci.* **2020**, *15*, 564–567. [CrossRef]
6. Yu, J.; Zhang, T.; Zhao, D.; Haapasalo, M.; Shen, Y. Characteristics of Endodontic Emergencies during Coronavirus Disease 2019 Outbreak in Wuhan. *J. Endod.* **2020**, *46*, 730–735. [CrossRef] [PubMed]
7. Chakraborty, T.; Jamal, R.; Battineni, G.; Teja, K.; Marto, C.; Spagnuolo, G. A Review of Prolonged Post-COVID-19 Symptoms and Their Implications on Dental Management. *Int. J. Environ. Res. Public Health* **2021**, *18*, 5131. [CrossRef] [PubMed]
8. Soltani, P.; Baghaei, K.; Tafti, K.T.; Spagnuolo, G. Science Mapping Analysis of COVID-19 Articles Published in Dental Journals. *Int. J. Environ. Res. Public Health* **2021**, *18*, 2110. [CrossRef] [PubMed]
9. Campisi, G.; Bizzoca, M.E.; Muzio, L.L. COVID-19 and periodontitis: Reflecting on a possible association. *Head Face Med.* **2021**, *17*, 1–6. [CrossRef] [PubMed]
10. Echeverría, J.J.; Echeverría, A.; Caffesse, R.G. Adherence to supportive periodontal treatment. *Periodontology* **2019**, *79*, 200–209. [CrossRef]
11. Mandrola, J. COVID-19 e dispositivi di protezione individuale: Qualcuno di noi morirà per la loro carenza. *Recent. Prog. Med.* **2020**. [CrossRef]
12. Campus, G.; Diaz-Betancourt, M.; Cagetti, M.G.; Carvalho, J.C.; Carvalho, T.S.; Cortés-Martinicorena, J.F.; Deschner, J.; Douglas, G.V.; Giacaman, R.A.; Machiulskiene, V.; et al. Study Protocol for an Online Questionnaire Survey on Symptoms/Signs, Protective Measures, Level of Awareness and Perception Regarding COVID-19 Outbreak among Dentists. A Global Survey. *Int. J. Environ. Res. Public Health* **2020**, *17*, 5598. [CrossRef]
13. Top 10 Search Engines In The World (2021 Update). Available online: https://www.reliablesoft.net/top-10-search-engines-in-the-world/ (accessed on 11 May 2021).
14. Google Trends. Available online: https://trends.google.com/trends (accessed on 20 August 2020).

15. Wikipedia Google Trends. Available online: https://en.wikipedia.org/wiki/Google_Trends (accessed on 20 August 2020).
16. Archived: WHO Timeline—COVID-19. Available online: https://www.who.int/news/item/27-04-2020-who-timeline---covid-19 (accessed on 15 May 2021).
17. R Core Team. R: A Language and Environment for Statistical Computing. Available online: https://www.r-project.org/ (accessed on 11 August 2021).
18. RStudio | Open Source & Professional Software for Data Science Teams—RStudio. Available online: https://www.rstudio.com/ (accessed on 17 April 2021).
19. Sycinska-Dziarnowska, M.; Paradowska-Stankiewicz, I. Dental Challenges and the Needs of the Population during the COVID-19 Pandemic Period. Real-Time Surveillance Using Google Trends. *Int. J. Environ. Res. Public Health* **2020**, *17*, 8999. [CrossRef]
20. Sofi-Mahmudi, A.; Shamsoddin, E.; Ghasemi, P.; Bahar, A.M.; Azad, M.S.; Sadeghi, G. Association of COVID-19-imposed lockdown and online searches for toothache in Iran. *BMC Oral Health* **2021**, *21*, 1–7. [CrossRef]
21. Faccini, M.; Ferruzzi, F.; Mori, A.A.; Santin, G.C.; Oliveira, R.C.; De Oliveira, R.C.G.; Queiroz, P.M.; Salmeron, S.; Pini, N.I.P.; Sundfeld, D.; et al. Dental Care during COVID-19 Outbreak: A Web-Based Survey. *Eur. J. Dent.* **2020**, *14*, S14–S19. [CrossRef]
22. Gherlone, E.; Polizzi, E.; Tetè, G.; De Lorenzo, R.; Magnaghi, C.; Querini, P.R.; Ciceri, F. Frequent and Persistent Salivary Gland Ectasia and Oral Disease After COVID-19. *J. Dent. Res.* **2021**, *100*, 464–471. [CrossRef] [PubMed]
23. Botros, N.; Iyer, P.; Ojcius, D.M. Is there an association between oral health and severity of COVID-19 complications? *Biomed. J.* **2020**, *43*, 325–327. [CrossRef]
24. Marouf, N.; Cai, W.; Said, K.N.; Daas, H.; Diab, H.; Chinta, V.R.; Hssain, A.A.; Nicolau, B.; Sanz, M.; Tamimi, F. Association between periodontitis and severity of COVID-19 infection: A case–control study. *J. Clin. Periodontol.* **2021**, *48*, 483–491. [CrossRef] [PubMed]
25. Alabdullah, J.H.; Daniel, S.J. A Systematic Review on the Validity of Teledentistry. *Telemed. e-Health* **2018**, *24*, 639–648. [CrossRef] [PubMed]
26. Steinmeier, S.; Wiedemeier, D.; Hämmerle, C.H.F.; Mühlemann, S. Accuracy of remote diagnoses using intraoral scans captured in approximate true color: A pilot and validation study in teledentistry. *BMC Oral Health* **2020**, *20*, 1–8. [CrossRef] [PubMed]
27. Tecco, S.; Parisi, M.R.; Gastaldi, G.; Polizzi, E.; D'Amicantonio, T.; Zilocchi, I.; Gardini, I.; Gherlone, E.; Lazzarin, A.; Capparè, P. Point-of-care testing for hepatitis C virus infection at an Italian dental clinic: Portrait of the pilot study population. *New Microbiol.* **2019**, *42*, 133–138. [PubMed]
28. Dave, M.; Seoudi, N.; Coulthard, P. Urgent dental care for patients during the COVID-19 pandemic. *Lancet* **2020**, *395*, 1257. [CrossRef]
29. Ather, A.; Patel, B.; Ruparel, N.B.; Diogenes, A.; Hargreaves, K.M. Coronavirus Disease 19 (COVID-19): Implications for Clinical Dental Care. *J. Endod.* **2020**, *46*, 584–595. [CrossRef]
30. Villani, F.A.; Aiuto, R.; Paglia, L.; Re, D. COVID-19 and Dentistry: Prevention in Dental Practice, a Literature Review. *Int. J. Environ. Res. Public Health* **2020**, *17*, 4609. [CrossRef] [PubMed]
31. Giudice, R.L.; Giudice, R.L. The Severe Acute Respiratory Syndrome Coronavirus-2 (SARS-CoV-2) in Dentistry. Management of Biological Risk in Dental Practice. *Int. J. Environ. Res. Public Health* **2020**, *17*, 3067. [CrossRef]
32. Gherlone, E.; Polizzi, E.; Tetè, G.; Capparè, P. Dentistry and COVID-19 Pandemic: Operative Indications Post-Lockdown. *New Microbiol* **2021**, *44*, 1–11.
33. World Health Organization. Infection Prevention and Control of Epidemic- and Pandemic-Prone Acute Respiratory Infections in Health Care. Available online: https://apps.who.int/iris/bitstream/handle/10665/112656/9789241507134_eng.pdf (accessed on 5 May 2021).
34. NIH COVID-19 Autopsy Consortium; HCA Oral and Craniofacial Biological Network; Huang, N.; Pérez, P.; Kato, T.; Mikami, Y.; Okuda, K.; Gilmore, R.C.; Conde, C.D.; Gasmi, B.; et al. SARS-CoV-2 infection of the oral cavity and saliva. *Nat. Med.* **2021**, *27*, 892–903. [CrossRef] [PubMed]
35. Odeh, N.D.; Babkair, H.; Abu-Hammad, S.; Borzangy, S.; Abu-Hammad, A.; Abu-Hammad, O. COVID-19: Present and Future Challenges for Dental Practice. *Int. J. Environ. Res. Public Health* **2020**, *17*, 3151. [CrossRef] [PubMed]
36. Revealing Google Statistics and Facts to Know in 2020. Available online: https://review42.com/resources/google-statistics-and-facts/ (accessed on 13 July 2021).
37. Nuti, S.V.; Wayda, B.; Ranasinghe, I.; Wang, S.; Dreyer, R.P.; Chen, S.I.; Murugiah, K. The Use of Google Trends in Health Care Research: A Systematic Review. *PLoS ONE* **2014**, *9*, e109583. [CrossRef] [PubMed]
38. Mavragani, A.; Ochoa, G. Google Trends in Infodemiology and Infoveillance: Methodology Framework. *JMIR Public Health Surveill.* **2019**, *5*, e13439. [CrossRef]
39. Fabbian, F.; Rodríguez-Muñoz, P.; López-Carrasco, J.; Cappadona, R.; Rodríguez-Borrego, M.; López-Soto, P. Google Trends on Obesity, Smoking and Alcoholism: Global and Country-Specific Interest. *Healthcare* **2021**, *9*, 190. [CrossRef] [PubMed]
40. Liu, M.; Caputi, T.L.; Dredze, M.; Kesselheim, A.S.; Ayers, J.W. Internet Searches for Unproven COVID-19 Therapies in the United States. *JAMA Intern. Med.* **2020**, *180*, 1116–1118. [CrossRef] [PubMed]
41. Pelat, C.; Turbelin, C.; Bar-Hen, A.; Flahault, A.; Valleron, A.J. More Diseases Tracked by Using Google Trends. *Emerg. Infect. Dis.* **2009**, *15*, 1327–1328. [CrossRef] [PubMed]

42. Barros, J.M.; Melia, R.; Francis, K.; Bogue, J.; O'Sullivan, M.; Young, K.; Bernert, R.A.; Rebholz-Schuhmann, D.; Duggan, J. The Validity of Google Trends Search Volumes for Behavioral Forecasting of National Suicide Rates in Ireland. *Int. J. Environ. Res. Public Health* **2019**, *16*, 3201. [CrossRef]
43. Anastasiou, M.; Pantavou, K.; Yiallourou, A.; Bonovas, S.; Nikolopoulos, G.K. Trends of Online Search of COVID-19 Related Terms in Cyprus. *Epidemiologia* **2021**, *2*, 36–45. [CrossRef]
44. Bakker, K.M.; Martinez-Bakker, M.E.; Helm, B.; Stevenson, T.J. Digital epidemiology reveals global childhood disease seasonality and the effects of immunization. *Proc. Natl. Acad. Sci. USA* **2016**, *113*, 6689–6694. [CrossRef]

Journal of
Clinical Medicine

MDPI

Perspective

Proposal for Tier-Based Resumption of Dental Practice Determined by COVID-19 Rate, Testing and COVID-19 Vaccination: A Narrative Perspective

Nima Farshidfar [1,*,†], Dana Jafarpour [2,†], Shahram Hamedani [3], Arkadiusz Dziedzic [4,*] and Marta Tanasiewicz [4]

1 Student Research Committee, Shiraz University of Medical Sciences, Shiraz 71348-14336, Iran
2 Faculty of Dentistry, McGill University, Montreal, QC H3A 1G1, Canada; dana.jafarpour@mail.mcgill.ca
3 Oral and Dental Disease Research Center, School of Dentistry, Shiraz University of Medical Sciences, Shiraz 71956-15878, Iran; shahramhamedani@yahoo.com
4 Department of Restorative Dentistry with Endodontics, Medical University of Silesia, 40-055 Katowice, Poland; martatanasiewicz@sum.edu.pl
* Correspondence: n.farshidfar@icloud.com (N.F.); adziedzic@sum.edu.pl (A.D.)
† These authors contributed equally to this work.

Abstract: Since the emergence of the new coronavirus disease (COVID-19), profound alterations in general and specialist dental practice have been imposed to provide safe dental care. The guidelines introduced in response to the COVID-19 pandemic to mitigate healthcare disruption are inconsistent regarding the dental practice re-installation, particularly during a transitional time. Despite the successful mass vaccination campaigns rolled out in 2021, the presence of more than 80 genotypes of COVID-19, rapid neutralisation of antibodies within a short period of seropositivity, and the likelihood of recurrent infection raise some doubts on whether vaccination alone will provide long-term immunity against COVID-19 and its variants. Here, from this perspective, we aim to provide an initial proposal for dental services reinstallation, easily applicable in various care settings. We discuss the potential options for the transition of dental services, as well as challenges and opportunities to adapt to new circumstances after mass COVID-19 vaccination. The proposal of the universal three-tier system of dental services resumption, determined by regional COVID-19 rates, testing accessibility, and vaccination rollout has been presented. Following herd COVID-19 immunity enhancement, it would be prudent to confer various preventative measures until virus spread naturally diminishes or becomes less virulent. Based on modelling data, dental practices may not return to normal, routine operation even after global vaccination as there would still be a significant risk of outbreaks of infection. Variable, multi-level measures will still be required, depending on the local COVID-19 cases rate, to secure safe dental care provision, despite predicted success of vaccination agendas. This approach can be implemented by achievable, practical means as a part of risk assessment, altered work pattern, and re-arrange of dental surgery facilities. The adequate standard operating procedure, with the support of rapid point-of-care testing at workplace, would vastly intensify the uninterrupted recovery of the dental care sector.

Keywords: COVID-19; SARS-CoV-2; coronavirus; dental care; resumption; mitigating measures; vaccination; rapid testing

Citation: Farshidfar, N.; Jafarpour, D.; Hamedani, S.; Dziedzic, A.; Tanasiewicz, M. Proposal for Tier-Based Resumption of Dental Practice Determined by COVID-19 Rate, Testing and COVID-19 Vaccination: A Narrative Perspective. *J. Clin. Med.* **2021**, *10*, 2116. https://doi.org/10.3390/jcm10102116

Academic Editors: Paul R. Cooper, Gianrico Spagnuolo, Hans-Peter Howaldt and Sameh Attia

Received: 4 April 2021
Accepted: 11 May 2021
Published: 14 May 2021

1. Introduction

The new coronavirus disease (COVID-19) pandemic has dramatically changed the main aspects of healthcare systems globally, including dental care provision on all levels of primary and secondary care [1,2]. This unprecedented phenomenon has triggered inevitable major workplace changes, global vaccination, as well as rapid testing innovations [3,4]. The consequences of severe acute respiratory syndrome coronavirus 2 (SARS-CoV-2) threat have given an impetus for innovative trends and technologies, as often happens when humanity faces a global challenge [5]. Besides its obvious negative impact, the COVID-19 pandemic has also created opportunities for the dental care sector (Figure 1). It is predicted that dental practice will survive the pandemic as altered as the rest of the healthcare sectors. Disruptive pandemic events can give sudden, overall positive impetus for acceleration of organizational changes.

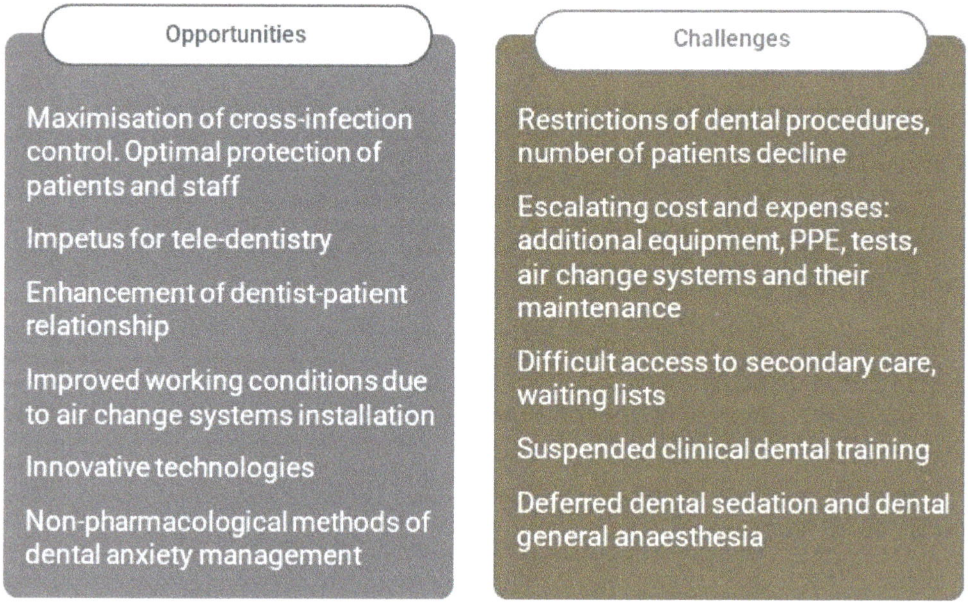
Opportunities
Maximisation of cross-infection control. Optimal protection of patients and staff
Impetus for tele-dentistry
Enhancement of dentist-patient relationship
Improved working conditions due to air change systems installation
Innovative technologies
Non-pharmacological methods of dental anxiety management
Challenges
Restrictions of dental procedures, number of patients decline
Escalating cost and expenses: additional equipment, PPE, tests, air change systems and their maintenance
Difficult access to secondary care, waiting lists
Suspended clinical dental training
Deferred dental sedation and dental general anaesthesia

Figure 1. The impact of COVID-19 on the dental care sector. Potential opportunities and negative consequences.

Globally, the authorities have released safety protocols and guidelines to decrease the risk of SARS-CoV-2 transmission and help dental care providers control the spread of the virus during the first wave of the pandemic and the health services re-installation phase [4,6]. Accordingly, these heterogeneous recommendations constantly evolve, supporting medical and dental workforce by ensuring safe working conditions and subsequently, putting in place locally implemented measures, adequate to any dental settings. In particular, dental care workers (DCWs) who perform their duties in the proximity of upper respiratory tract and are usually exposed to air-borne infectious bio-aerosols, have to rely on specific protective measures and guidelines to minimise the risk of being infected [6]. They face a high risk of contracting COVID-19 because of exposure to potentially contaminated saliva and microdroplets during aerosol-generating dental procedures (AGPs) [2].

This perspective aims to broaden the outlook of dental practice management following immense COVID-19 vaccination campaigns and puts forward constructive suggestions for routine dental service resumption after vaccination has been implemented on a global scale. To date, relatively few proposals of structured reinstallation of dental care provision have been presented during the transitional period, in the light of subsequent pandemic waves. This is surprising, considering mass inoculation and recently developed modern modalities to contain COVID-19 in the form of rapid testing. Undoubtedly, the response to immunization and prevention of virus transmission is not only largely driven by vaccine distribution, but also by the emergence of new SARS-CoV-2 variants. To the best of our knowledge, this is the first report of the universal tiers-based proposal for dental services reinstallation after COVID-19 emergence.

2. Primary Measure: The Adequate Standard Operating Procedures (SOP) Comprising Vaccination Status

Health authorities such as the World Health Organization (WHO) [7], Centers for Disease Control and Prevention (CDC) [8], the American Dental Association (ADA) [9] and the United Kingdom National Health Service (UK NHS) [10] have introduced essential guidelines for dental practice during the COVID-19 outbreak. These rigorous region-specific or national mitigating measures have been proposed to protect the staff and patients simultaneously, and to decrease the spread of COVID-19 by offering a consistent and scientifically proven series of steps. However, the concern remains whether professionals will disregard proposed guidelines after widespread vaccination programs have been completed, and also if the dental practice could then return to the way it had been operating before the pandemic.

Considering the prospect of COVID-19 vaccination, there is ongoing dispute regarding how dental practice would change if population-wide immunity against COVID-19 is achieved. Currently, limited recommendations from regulatory bodies exist regarding the safe resumption of routine dental care services during recovery period in 2021 [7–10]. It is predicted that the shift from strict Standard Operating Procedure (SOP) for dental management and the use of enhanced personal protective equipment (PPE) towards a more routine approach will occur, based on vaccination success and available rapid testing. The specifically adjusted SOP in dentistry aims to provide uninterrupted and efficient safe working environment while reducing the risk of COVID-19 infection. It highlights various crucial aspects to secure health and safety in the workplace.

The timeframe for the reinstallation of dental care since the pandemic outbreak is yet unpredictable, depending on potential new COVID-19 waves, virus variants, access to extended vaccination, cohorts' immune response, and 'self-adjustment' of the dental sector to the new clinical reality. The fluctuating COVID-19 rates are predicted to escalate the conundrum of dentistry re-establishment across the world. Therefore, rolling out rapid in vitro diagnostics for DCWs at the workplace on a larger scale appears to be a viable option to detect asymptomatic cases and subsequently amplify the service recovery. It might be, however, challenging and compromised by logistic and/or financial constraints (Figure 2). It is predicted that dental services based in the university hospitals, community clinics or dental schools, and multi-unit dental corporate bodies would face a quicker adaptation and 're-invention' of the new reality, compared to small general dental practices.

Even though evidence from studies regarding mass vaccination campaigns is promising [11], the presence of more than 80 genotypes of the COVID-19 coronavirus, neutralising antibodies with a short period of seropositivity, and the likelihood of re-infection have raised doubts whether vaccination will lead to long-term immunity [12]. A recent study demonstrated that the newly emerged SARS-CoV-2 variants B.1.1.7 (UK), B.1.351 (South Africa), and P.1 (Brazil) can escape immune response induced by vaccination or infection, with serious implications for pandemic mitigation [13]. Predominantly, it has been shown that the serological levels of immunoglobulin do not accurately correlate with the shedding of virus particles and the risk of transmissibility [12]. The homogeneity of infected populations in a particular timeframe might not be achieved due to the short-term immunity against the virus. Consequently, there might be no long-term, continuous herd immunity due to the possibility of re-infection, which might take place even with the existence of neutralising immunoglobulins [14]. Individuals need to be reminded to attend for the second vaccine dose, as missing this could lead to spreading, mutating of the virus, and potentially to becoming vaccine-resistant [15].

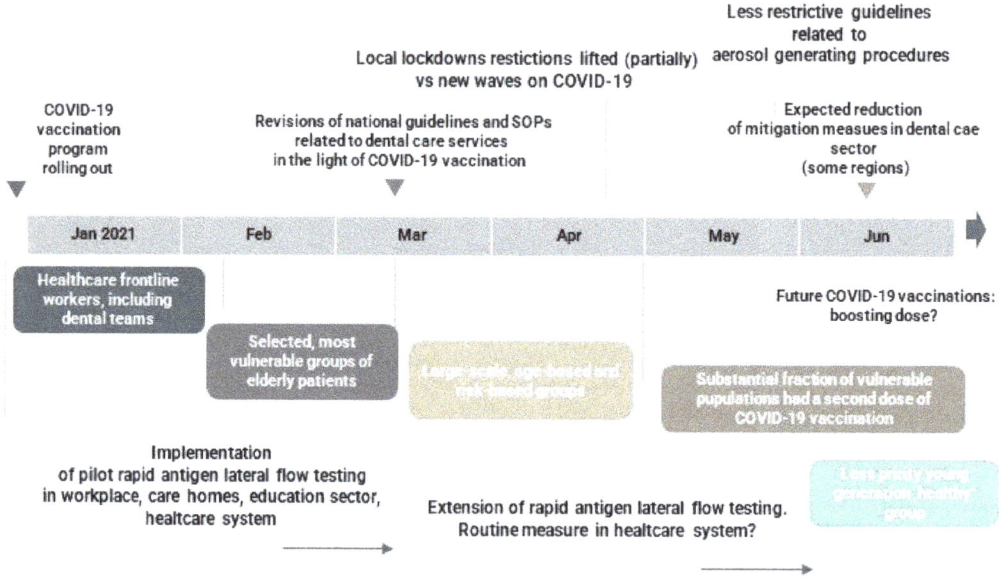

Figure 2. The predicted timescale of staged de-escalation and reinstallation of dental care services in 2021. Sequelae determined by COVID-19 mass vaccination.

A concern regarding the firstly introduced COVID-19 vaccines is the necessity of administering two doses. Moreover, as new vaccines begin to emerge, this challenge persists and may particularly hinder the sufficient supply to less developed countries [12,14]. The obvious inequalities associated with the access to COVID-19 vaccine, and its disproportionate distribution across the world (for various reasons) may considerably compromise combating COVID-19. These factors are likely to increase the equity gap between countries and delay the eradication pandemic. Hence, the continuation of basic preventive measures for DCWs should be maintained until further evidence related to the virulence rate and its pathogenicity is revealed [14]. Prevention is particularly important in dentistry, where mutual contact between the DCWs and patients is unavoidable.

3. Optimizing Risk-Reduction: Teleconsultations and Chair-Side Tests Following Immunity Enhancement

Since 2020, remote teleconsultations have become a standard part of the SOP protocol to assess, diagnose, and protect DCWs, as well as to detect COVID-19 cases. It underpins the efforts to restore the normal pattern of clinical work. In fact, the COVID-19 pandemic may lead to a permanent re-organisation in dentistry with further development of new software for multi-purpose teledentistry [16,17]. Reduction of the risk of infection and protection of staff have been the main reasons for developing teledentistry. Virtual appointments, online consultations, and follow-ups, as well as the application of artificial intelligence to support clinical diagnosis have now been rendered practical through tele-dentistry [18]. In terms of risk mitigation and given the reduced risk of viral transmission using teledentistry, it is expected to become a pivotal, routine aspect of patient' management following rapid testing to find out whether patients are infected or not [17]. A recent survey study has shown significant patient satisfaction towards using virtual consultations via teledentistry [19].

Hence, dental providers are encouraged to adopt telehealth as an optimal mode of consultation, initial examination and triaging during recovery time. It should be widely incorporated as a COVID-19 outbreak response, including specific SOP [20] and subsequently as a pillar of restored services. Moreover, consultations with the orthodontist during the orthodontic treatments and follow-up procedures can be easily performed via teledentistry. Recent studies have proposed a new concept of dental monitoring which integrates teledentistry with artificial intelligence in order to monitor orthodontic treatments in a semi-automatic manner [21]. Due to these substantial advantages of tele-dentistry in data collection, risk-assessment, saving of time, and providing better access to oral healthcare, this modern modality can eventually become an essential adjunct to the traditional approaches in dental practice [20]. Due to the 'nature' of dental profession, obviously they cannot substitute restorative or surgical services in people with active dental diseases and substantial needs of complex dental care.

Until now, although results have been promising as regards effective vaccination, it has been suggested that individuals should continue to aim for prevention and diagnosis of COVID-19 until a worldwide introduction of effective vaccine programs is in place (Figure 3). Given these circumstances, and taking into account the risk of asymptomatic carriers, it is rational to assume that 'conventional' dental practice might continue to expose DCWs to the risk of infection [22]. Therefore, fit-for-purpose SOP constitutes the core aspect of dental practice management to secure safe work environment for staff and patients.

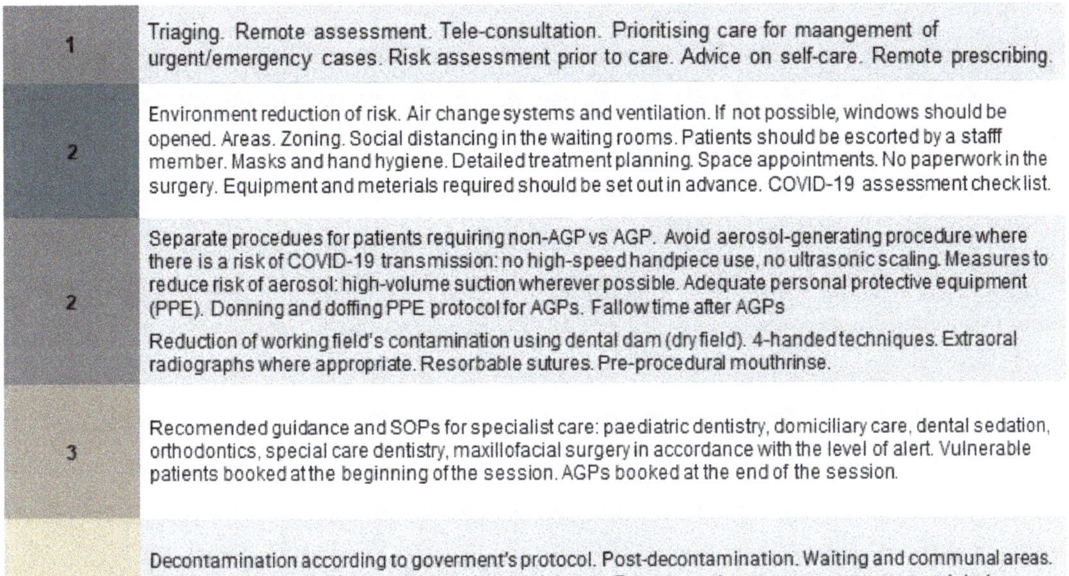

Figure 3. The essential elements of standard operating procedures applicable for the dental service.

Rapid Antigen Tests: A Gamechanger?

Although teleconsultation and triaging may support the detection of symptomatic cases in the medical and dental sectors, reverse transcription-quantitative PCR (RT-qPCR) tests are the gold standard to diagnose COVID-19 [23,24]. Yet, the application of these laboratory tests is not feasible in dental clinics due to long waiting times for test results and lack of RT-qPCR testing facilities. Many rapid antigen qualitative tests such as commercial lateral flow assays have been developed for initial triage and rapid qualitative assessment of SARS-CoV-2 antigens [25]. These rapid lateral flow antigen tests (LFATs) can provide valid results within 10 to 20 min with sensitivity and specificity similar to quantitative immunoassays [26]. The opportunity to perform LFATs as rapid point-of-care tests (POCTs) outside the clinical laboratory is of great assistance, particularly in the clinical contexts where triaging patients is required. In general, LFATs mainly based on colloidal gold immunochromatography assay are intended for the qualitative detection of nucleocapsid antigens from human nasal and throat swabs, as well as sputum samples [26,27].

Considering the core priorities to combat a pandemic, it has been proposed that performing reliable and validated POCTs with acceptable sensitivity and specificity could potentially become a crucial element for triaging/screening all patients attending dental appointments. Particularly, chair-side LFATs can become a game changer on global scale. Rapid testing seems especially justified in the multi-unit clinical settings, i.e., hospital-based community medical/dental services, university hospitals and clinics. Besides standard nasal/pharyngeal swabs—because saliva is a relevant specimen for COVID-19 diagnosis and its collection is inexpensive, non-invasive, fast, and safe—accurate saliva-based POCT can help dental teams take the leading position in COVID-19 diagnosis, even in the post-vaccination era [24,28,29]. Employing more advanced diagnostics such as smartphone-based microfluidic systems could pave the way for straightforward pre-treatment diagnosis of other viruses in the dental setting [24].

Apart from key and obvious benefits, such as its simple use in clinical settings and its rapid results, LFATs have some disadvantages, including lower sensitivity compared to RT-qPCR and—as a result—potentially more false-negative results if SARS-CoV-2 antigen load in a sample is low [25–27]. However, the advantages of applying LFATs as an additional measure to protect DCWs while resuming the routine dental care prevail over their limitations (Table 1).

Table 1. The main advantages and disadvantages of rapid lateral flow antigen tests.

Advantages	Disadvantages	Limitations
Simplified use and performance in outpatients' clinic. Suitable to be used at the workplace, including dental surgery.	Suboptimal relative sensitivity (wide range 74–94%), false-negative results if low viral antigen load in a sample. A negative result does not eliminate the possibility of SARS-CoV-2 infection	Positive results do not rule out co-infections with other pathogens
Short reaction time, rapid results within 5–20 min.	Test's sensitivity depends on the active phase of viral infection	Specimens collected after five days of illness are more likely to be negative compared to RT-PCR assay
A small amount of sampling material required	Positive results need to be verified by molecular RT-PCR testing	Negative results are not intended to rule out other viral or bacterial infections
High specificity about 100%. High accuracy 98–99%	Results may not correlate with the clinical history and other diagnostic methods performed on the same specimen	The amount of antigen in a sample may decrease as the duration of illness increases
Can detect both viable and non-viable material	Cost	
To be used for the qualitative detection of SARS-CoV-2 antigens from nasal swabs, throat swabs or sputum samples only		
Equally sensitive for different SARS-CoC-2 variants		

What is more, the positive 'psychological effect' of rapid COVID-19 testing in dental settings cannot be underestimated, enabling reassurance, and strengthening patients'/staff confidence [30]. As a result, this approach, although costly and logistically challenging in resource-limited areas, would improve the patient attendance rate and reduce the employee's absence rate [30]. Most importantly, regular rapid LFATs are recommended as a routine protocol for staff members who provide special care dentistry for medically compromised individuals, persons with special needs (intellectual or developmental disabilities), and frail care home residents, to limit the treatment-related risk of SARS-CoV-2 infection [31].

Rapid testing in dentistry also depends on sufficient expertise, perception and attitude of managers/dental practice owners', which account for their decisions. Primarily, LFATs constitute a particularly viable option to increase service capacity and decrease access inequalities in special care dentistry, as its provision was significantly reduced due to the pandemic [32]. Considering supply limits, rapid LFATs allow for more personalized care, prioritizing groups of patients with unmet healthcare needs. As persons with special needs present with generally poorer oral health, they are likely to require urgent dental care, and also are susceptible to COVID-19 contraction due to the high prevalence of infections in care institutions. This propagation of LFATs in dental and/or any other primary care settings, would considerably support public health 'surveillance' policy to monitor the trends of SARS-CoV-2 rate in asymptomatic local communities.

In the United Kingdom, LFATs have been already incorporated in primary care and care homes for staff and residents since the end of 2020 [31,33]. Moreover, LFATs are recommended for other occupational groups with increased risk of mass-spreading infection, e.g., in education sector. Recently, Conwey et al. [34] demonstrated feasibility of implementation a rapid screening and testing protocol in asymptomatic patients presented in dental surgery as response to the pandemic.

4. Will the COVID-19 Vaccines Modify PPE Use for High-Risk Procedures?

After the commencement of the mass vaccination campaigns in December 2020, an important issue could be the continued use of conventional vs. enhanced PPE in dental practice. Scientists predict that SARS-CoV-2 virus, which causes COVID-19, may outsmart immunity stimulation and it will eventually become an endemic strain, despite successful global vaccination in the future [35]. A recent modelling study [36] concluded that the vaccination for COVID-19 alone is unlikely to prevent further spread of the infection, to enable achievement of herd immunity, and to fully control the virus. The above-mentioned study predicts that the indicative R number will be still high, around 1.58 in the United Kingdom, even if the vaccine prevents a vast proportion of new infections [36]. Thus, even with mass-scale immunisation, the protective measures for routine clinical practice that were used pre-pandemic might not be sufficient, particularly during dental treatment involving aerosol-generating procedures (AGPs) creating potentially infectious aerosol [37]. This requires further scientific evidence regarding the virus pathogenicity, transferability, and rate of spreading.

To protect DCWs, it is imperative to choose suitable PPE according to the level of exposure to risk. Predominantly, the main concerns are costs, impact on the environment (waste), and physical discomfort, which reduce the necessary versatility, comfort, and vision needed for precise dental work [38]. Despite the intrinsic drawbacks of using traditional PPE (heat stress, lack of mobility, fall hazard, physiological effects, and anxiety), PPE has recently benefitted from high-tech developments [38], protecting DCWs adequately without compromising their comfort and capacity to perform clinical tasks.

Due to the anticipated reduction of AGPs in general, it is predicted that some dental specialities will introduce 'AGPs-limited' protocols. This may involve more common use of Hall (stainless steel crowns) and atraumatic restorative technique in paediatric dentistry, the usage of 3D intraoral technology instead of conventional impressions in prosthodontics and orthodontics, pre-procedural mouth rinse, disinfection of dentures and removable orthodontic appliances during their adjustment [39,40]. What is more, broader utilization of conscious dental sedation, instead of treatment under general anaesthesia in patients with special needs [40], as well as digital procedures in orthodontics [41] would become common standards in clinical practice.

Recent studies demonstrated that the materials used in PPE, especially soft surfaces, might act as carriers for the acquisition and transfer of pathogens after having been contaminated with them [38]. Additionally, the survival of infectious pathogens on PPE can expose DCWs and patients, particularly when PPE get damp or when protein-enriched biological waste is present on them [38]. Kasloff et al. [42] found significant variations in virus stability after drying SARS-CoV-2 over 21 days on the surfaces of commonly used PPE items and surfaces found in healthcare facilities. The viability of SARS-CoV-2 on non-porous and porous surfaces was between 4 (gloves) and 21 days (plastic, N-95, and N-100 masks) [42]. As SARS-CoV-2 has been found to persist on the surfaces of various types of PPE for several days [42], the use of superior textile materials, particularly in dental health care settings, should be considered an alternative to overcome the previously stated drawbacks of conventional PPE. These materials should also have both fluid-resistant and antimicrobial properties to reduce the probability of contamination, growth, and transmission of contagious pathogens on their surfaces [38]. Therefore, the reduction of additional, enhanced PPE use following inoculation and POC testing during and after the reinstallation phase appears paramount. This approach which is based on safety checks, will also have a positive impact on reduction of global carbon footprint.

Without widely applied and easy-to-be used rapid testing, the acquired herd immunity against COVID-19 acquired via vaccinated cohorts would allow the gradual transition to the reduced use of enhanced PPE only in some circumstances, when dental patients belong to the low-risk category (Table 2), with expected COVID-19 negative status and mainly in the areas with low, steadily declining COVID-19 rates. At the end of 2020, All Wales Clinical Dental Leads COVID-19 Group prepared a report for the Welsh Government, recommending Standard Operating Procedure (SOP) for dental services as part of de-escalating the COVID-19 response, which includes COVID-19 risk categories of patients [43].

Table 2. COVID-19 risk categories of patients.

Low Risk	Medium Risk	High Risk
Triaged or clinically assessed patients with no symptoms, with known recent COVID-19 status, or patients who recently have self-isolated, shielded.	Triaged or clinically assessed patients with no symptoms, with no known recent COVID-19 contact	Untriaged persons present for assessment or treatment (status and symptoms unknown)
Persons who have recovered from COVID-19 recently and had few days without any symptoms	Asymptomatic persons with unknown infectious status	Symptomatic or suspected COVID-19 persons
Patients who had a negative COVID-19 PCR test within 72 h of treatment and had been self-isolating from the test date	Asymptomatic persons who declined testing	History of contact with COVID-19 individual, they are waiting for test results

Traffic light' system, adapted and modified, Standard Operating Procedure for the Dental Management of Non-COVID-19 Patients in Wales, v.1.01, Wales, UK.

5. The Inevitably Altered and Adjusted Dental Facilities

According to the Occupational Safety and Health Administration (OSHA) professional hazard pyramid for COVID-19, DCWs are placed in the 'remarkably high exposure risk' category during AGP. Therefore, the attempt to reduce bio-aerosol microdroplets will be likely to remain a top priority for the dental profession even after widespread COVID-19 vaccination [44]. Apart from a standard recommendation, such as routine use of high-volume suction, installing fit-for-purpose air change ventilation systems (AVSs), with negative pressure operating rooms (NPRs) and airborne infection isolation rooms is deemed imperative for dentists to be able to treat patients safely during the pandemic. However, most health authorities across the world have declared this to be an arbitrary requirement if the patient history and physical examination results suggest an asymptomatic patient [44]. Based on the existing data and taking into account the practicability of proposed alterations in dental surgeries, we believe that AVSs and NPRs will become the main element of COVID-19 adjustments to curb the risk of infection and shall allow full re-installation of routine dentistry.

The instant removal of microparticles and microdroplets by incorporating AVSs during AGP is equally paramount and cost-effective; therefore, it should be considered mandatory, or at least a highly recommended option in the future. According to the regulatory bodies, it is recommended that treatment rooms, including dental surgeries, should provide minimum ten air changes per hour as inadequate ventilation in the clinical setting increases the risk of SARS-CoV-2 transmission [45]. The number of air changes per hour per surgery affects the decontamination time following AGP and estimation of this number estimation has to be done for each individual surgery. High-efficiency particulate arrestor (HEPA) filters, which can eliminate 99.97% of 0.3 μm particles could be also used to filter the contaminated air in the treatment zone during the pandemic [45] as an alternative option when the installation of AVSs cannot be carried out. However, there a possibility that HEPA filters become a source of microorganisms if there is microbe proliferation in the air filter, also they are difficult to clean and expensive to replace [45]. Therefore, imposing isolation and negative pressure operating rooms should be considered an optimal scenario following widespread vaccination for COVID-19. Predicting future changes, AVSs and NPRs may become mandatory requirements for any AGPs in clinical settings.

The suggested proposal of the decision–action plan for dental providers, based on the presence of in-surgery air changing systems, known COVID-19 vaccination status, and access to LFATs is presented in Figure 4. These different approaches can be practically implemented in a situation when the COVID-19 cases rate fluctuates (new waves), based on the combined AVS's, COVID-19 rapid testing and vaccine status during the transition phase.

The potential three different pathways with accompanying SOP measures can be executed as part of staged resumption of the dental services. These meaningful scenarios as a response to COVID-19 depend upon economic and social aspects, reflecting specific policies and regulations imposed globally. If broadly utilized, they will alleviate the existing local inequalities in using more advanced anti-COVID-19 measures and shall vastly improve access to routine primary and specialist dental interventions, predominantly in community or hospital services. Considering the advantages of these realistic approaches, dental providers have evidence-based options to support them in restoring activities, although a locally specific fine-tuning would be required.

The knowledge of aerosol-generating mechanisms and way of COVID-19 spread has contributed to the subsequent correction of the mishaps occurring in daily dental practice [46]. It has been acknowledged that there is urgent need for change in the current architecture of dental clinics. A recent study [47] has suggested a modification in clinics' design, clearly separating the treatment areas (where patients are in direct contact with the dentist) from non-treatment areas (waiting areas, reception, lavatory, rest rooms, and office space). Preferably, dental laboratories and X-ray rooms should be located in the proximity of the treatment areas, while the reception area and consultation/waiting rooms should be near the main entrance [47]. Similarly, short-treatment units, e.g., in dental schools, should be designed next to the consultation rooms, whereas units used to provide lengthy procedures should be located far from the main clinical hub space. In both cases, the treatment areas are required to be large enough and equipped with sufficient ventilation and efficient air change systems to prevent exposed surfaces from contamination during AGPs [47].

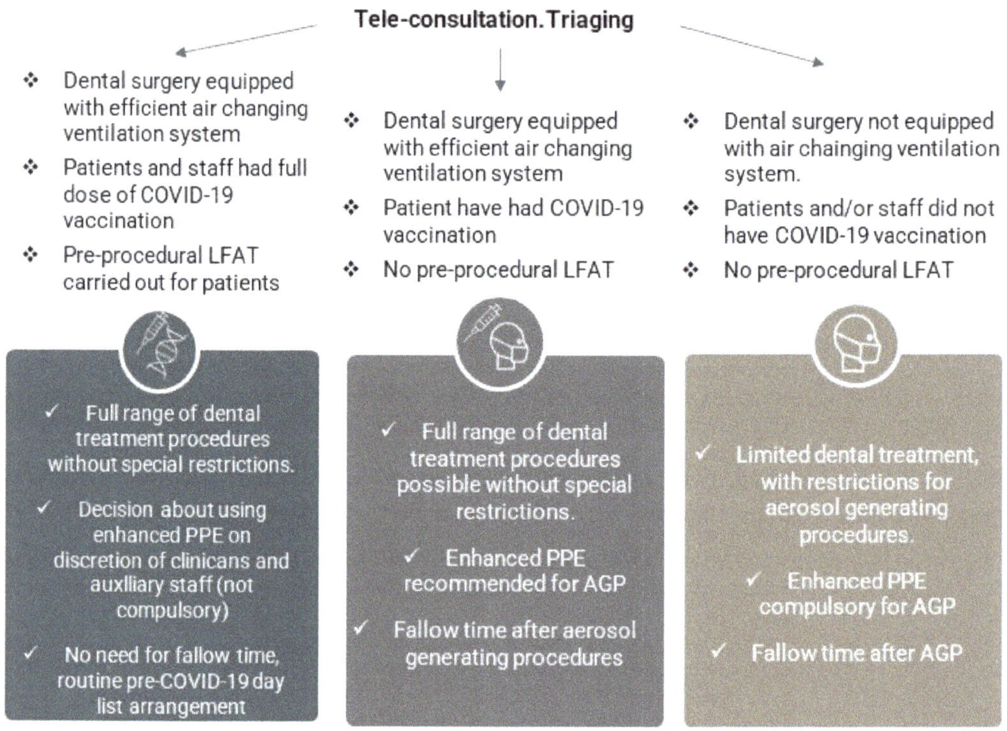
Tele-consultation.Triaging
Dental surgery equipped with efficient air changing ventilation system
Patients and staff had full dose of COVID-19 vaccination
Pre-procedural LFAT carried out for patients
Dental surgery equipped with efficient air changing ventilation system
Patient have had COVID-19 vaccination
No pre-procedural LFAT
Dental surgery not equipped with air chainging ventilation system.
Patients and/or staff did not have COVID-19 vaccination
No pre-procedural LFAT
Full range of dental treatment procedures without special restrictions.
Decision about using enhanced PPE on discretion of clinicans and auxlliary staff (not compulsory)
No need for fallow time, routine pre-COVID-19 day list arrangement
Full range of dental treatment procedures possible without special restrictions.
Enhanced PPE recommended for AGP
Fallow time after aerosol generating procedures
Limited dental treatment, with restrictions for aerosol generating procedures.
Enhanced PPE compulsory for AGP
Fallow time after AGP

Figure 4. Optimal plan for dental care service resumption subject to adequate SOP, adapted facilities, COVID-19 diagnostics, and immunity status. Regions with fluctuating and unpredictable COVID-19 rate.

In addition to current rigorous infection control measures, a broad implementation of negative pressure dental operating rooms seems to be a priority, regardless of the level of dental care (primary vs. secondary) or geographical location. This can be combined with the modification of the design, and materials used for contact surfaces in dental clinics should also be re-considered. The incorporation of 'smart', bioactive materials, metal and/or metal oxide nanoparticles into surfaces could be considered as part of the new measures since they effectively reduce contamination of the environment [46]. In relation to the specifics of dental treatments, decontamination of removable prosthodontic or orthodontic appliance should also be taken into account since they are demonstrated to be a source of intra-oral microbiota transmission [39]. As a result, dental clinics set up will need to undergo essential modifications and adjustments shortly, in order to protect dental teams and patients more effectively.

6. The Predicament; Combined SOP/COVID-19 Test/Vaccine Approach

Substantial reduction to limit the risk of exposure to both DCWs and patients is paramount. While the proposed actions would involve increased costs and levels of complexity for DCWs, they impose a serious task for management [48]. Treatment would become more time-consuming and costly. Subsequently, the number of daily treatments to be performed would be limited [48]. These major disruptions to dental healthcare should be perceived as a red flag, indicating a need to change the way we manage patients. Challenges around the development and implementation of new measures, along with practical solutions, can be efficiently managed with the support of policymakers, dental healthcare commissioners, and agenda for constructive changes (Figure 5). Therefore, the adequate and updated SOP, a gradual relaxation of special measures, high vaccine uptake with effective protection, and rapid testing are essential to restore dental care provision, by minimising future outbreaks.

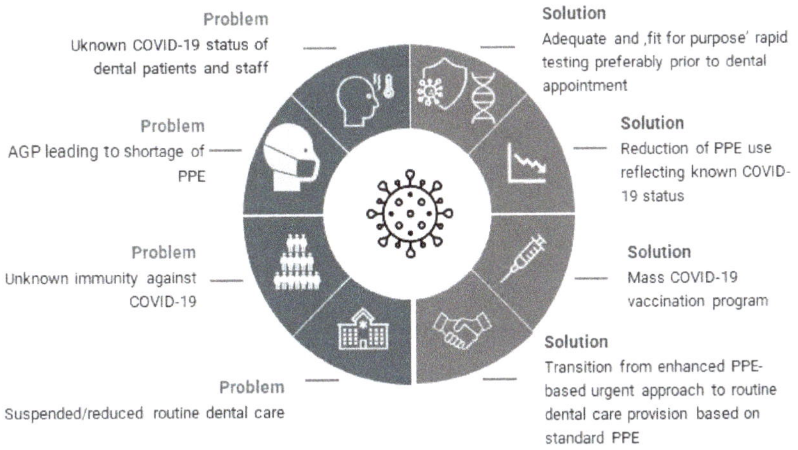

Figure 5. Resuming dental practice during the COVID-19 pandemic. Challenges and solutions.

This is the main task for governments, local authorities, health care commissioners, and professional bodies to support the full recovery of healthcare services logistically or financially [48]. Wide-scale application of these measures will provide a safe environment for treatment, securing the wellbeing of clinicians and patients. Unfortunately, the subdued response to dynamic changes in pandemics, as well as resumption of services reflects the lack of appropriate policies, deficit of expertise, funding, and infrastructure for rapid tasting [48]. We should continue to investigate further the ways to reduce the infection risk by adopting specific cross-infection protocols and by using innovative products.

It has been suggested that the resulting situation can be compared to the universal 'hierarchy of needs'. The more advanced hierarchical needs can only be considered when the basic needs have been fulfilled [49]. Similarly, in today's new reality, crucial aspects are pushed to the top of the COVID-19 dental practice and general healthcare 'hierarchy of needs'. DCWs should all be aware of this set of special measures, based on recent health authority guidelines. Four levels of tasks, from basic to advanced measures are presented in Figure 6. The introduction of each basic task should be performed permanently and effectively, which is necessary for the implementation of the next stage of tasks. Conversely, as we move away from the general policies, more emphasis should be placed on achieving more comprehensive and precise tasks, such as using rapid testing for COVID-19. Nevertheless, this stage would be inefficient without first considering the basic, universal measures.

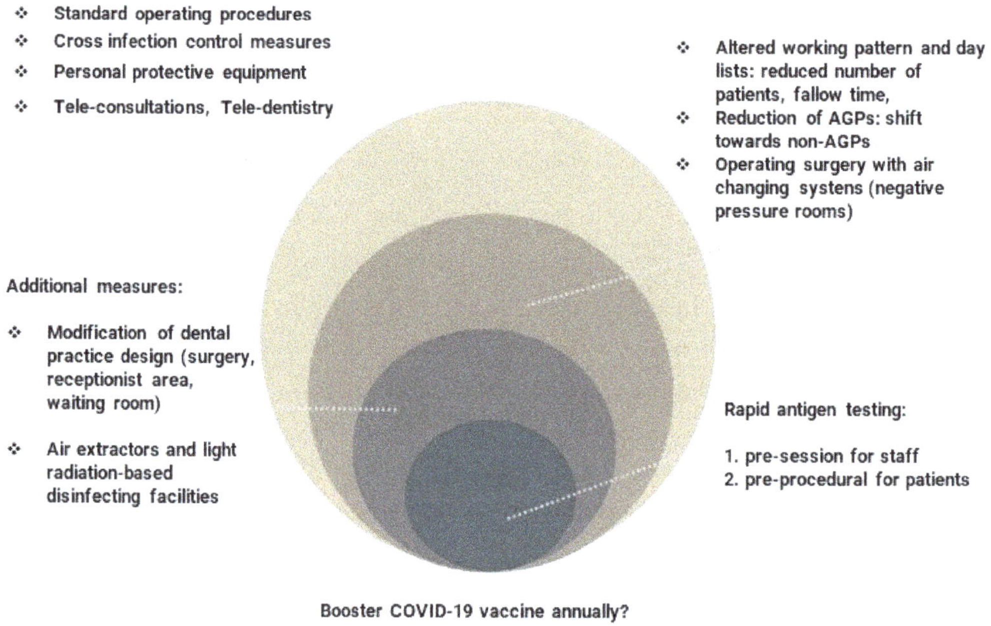

Figure 6. Prioritization of mitigation measures in dental care. The staged reinstallation of dental practice during and after the COVID-19 pandemic.

7. Long-Term Prediction: Being Prepared for Health and Dental Care Disruption

Expanded worldwide 'pan-vaccination' is considered crucial to acquire herd immunity, enabling special measures to be relaxed and safe resumption of dental activity, whilst limiting the risk of serious respiratory complications. As of 10th March 2021, there were more than 200 vaccines in pre-clinical and clinical development [50], including 21 in phase three trials, six in the early/limited use phase, and six approved for full use [51]. Equal distribution of the COVID-19 vaccine worldwide seems currently to be a major, unresolved, and time-consuming challenge [52,53]. However, this tendency related to the disproportionate vaccine delivery to different regions is escalating (Figure 7). Therefore, during the transition phase, standard and essential precautions based on SOP should be always considered to reduce the exposure of both DCWs and patients to SARS-CoV-2.

Until worldwide mass-scale vaccination is completed, preventive and diagnostic measures must be maintained in primary and secondary services based on national guidelines in order to suppress transmission of the virus. Looking ahead, oral inoculation is deemed a complementary and scalable option in preventing COVID-19 as oral vaccine formulation would ease vaccine distribution, manufacturing, and administration, which in turn shall expand immunization, especially in resource-limited populations [54]. We believe that local authorities responsible for healthcare are committed to ensuring equitable access to efficacious, affordable COVID-19 vaccines and diagnostics.

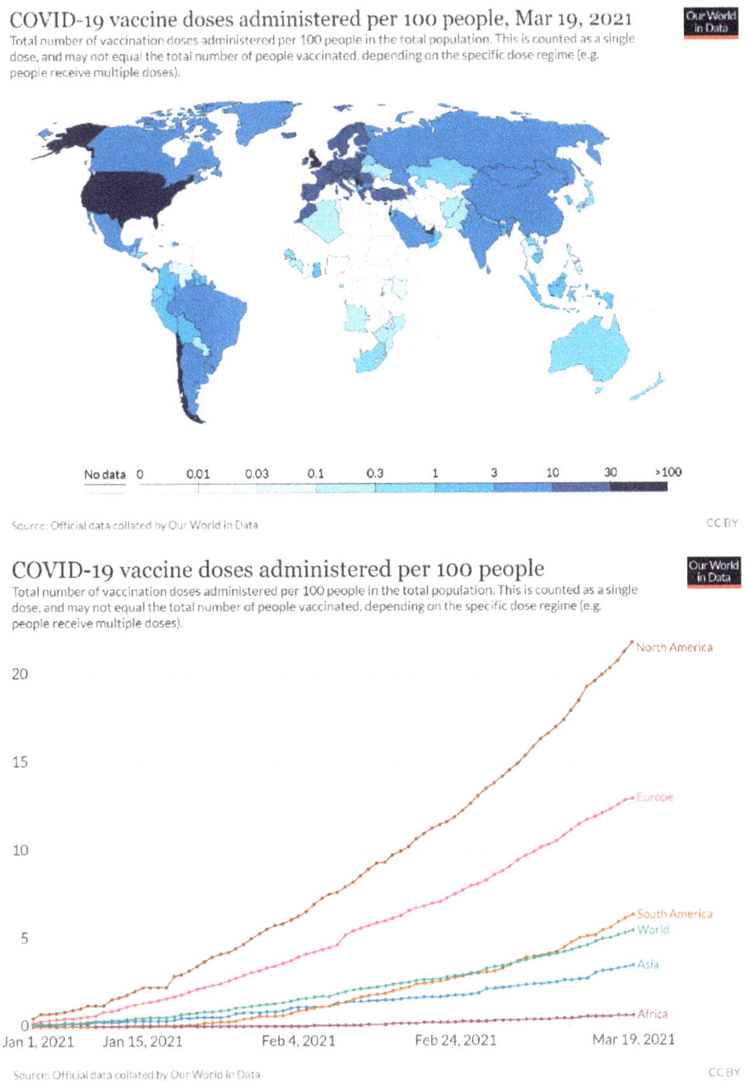

Figure 7. The rates of COVID-19 vaccine administration in different countries and continents up to 19 March 2021 (https://ourworldindata.org/covid-vaccinations).

8. The Three-Tier System of Dental Services Reinstallation in Regions Where Testing System Is Not Available

Predicting the nearest future, dental practice regarding SOP and AGP will consider primarily the regional COVID-19 cases rate, which should be monitored regularly. This is especially important as rapid testing for COVID-19 may not be available in a vast majority of regions, due to cost and infrastructure implications. Therefore, better support for developing countries is needed, including a transfer of new POCT technology and increase in testing capacity. In addition, a valid consent aspect exists, concerning personal preferences or obstacles. According to the risk assessment protocol, individuals who decline pre-procedural testing fall into the 'moderate risk category'. In these circumstances, the decision about the practice SOP involving rapid testing should rely on assessed COVID-19 risk for patients (Table 2), along with their vaccination status.

Interestingly, the COVID-19 vaccination rate as such may not be sufficient to influence decisions about reducing the use of enhanced PPE for AGPs. The new SOP designed for dental providers during post-pandemic era will have to address this concern. The proposed three-tier resumption system intends to incorporate real-time data associated with regional COVID-19 rates, the number of COVID-19 positive cases per local population, the percentage of inoculated individuals, as well as the incidence of infections with new variants.

The first, the least favorable situation involves the area with a low COVID-19 rate (R index below 1 generally), where no or only a limited number of staff and patients had been fully vaccinated, and rapid tests are not available. In this case, due to the unknown COVID-19 status of patients, preventative measures concerning AGPs should be still maintained and continued. In the area where the COVID-19 rate is low and predictable, and the staff has been vaccinated, but the dental patients have not been vaccinated yet, and rapid testing is not implemented, it is possible to reduce SOP restrictions for AGP. The decision should rely on the predicted negative COVID-19 status following the patient's risk assessment (Table 2) and dental procedures can be performed with fewer restrictions applied for AGPs. This approach would lead to a reduction in enhanced PPE usage. Finally, in an ideal scenario, both DCWs and patients are fully vaccinated in the area with low and steady COVID-19 rate. Likewise, this would minimise the risk of COVID-19 transmission in dental teams, with changes to be introduced in the protocols concerning AGP and reduction of special preventative measures (Figure 8).

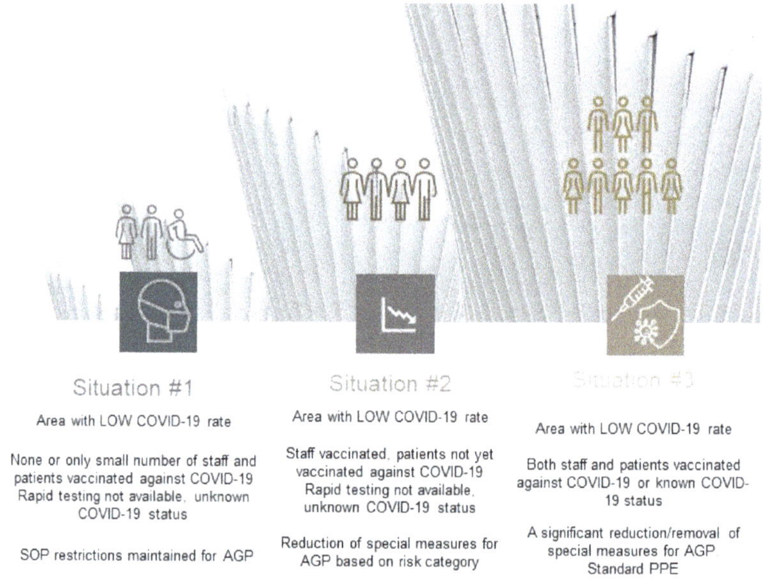

Figure 8. The proposal three-tier system in areas with low COVID-19 cases rate and testing not available. Options for change applicable for SOP depending on local COVID-19 cases rate and population immunity status. Stable, predictable COVID-19 rate locally.

In the regions with high COVID-19 rates, rapidly spreading infections, e.g., local virus resurgence, the proposed management of dental services must consider a stricter approach and risk assessment procedures (Figure 9, Table 2). The high rate of spreading COVID-19 cases spread locally may preclude permanent resumption of medical and dental services.

In areas with rapidly escalating rates of COVID-19 where only limited cohorts have been vaccinated, it would be necessary to reinforce the strict SOP and limit dental care provision to urgent and/or emergency cases only.

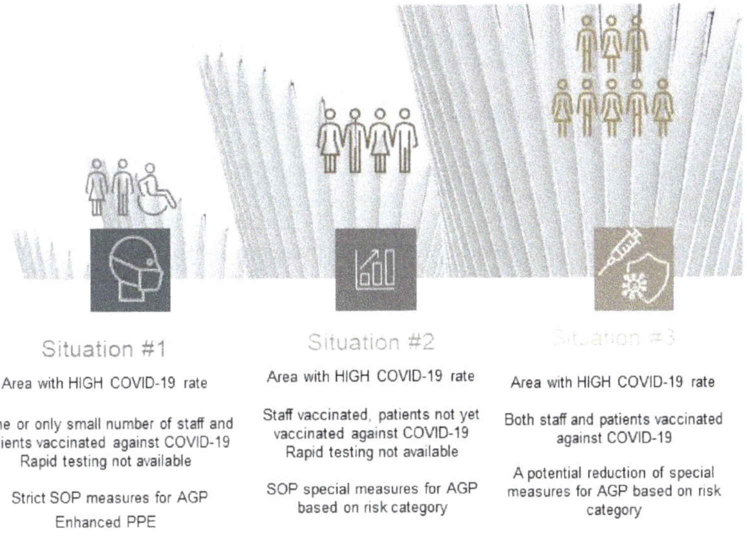

Figure 9. Proposed three-tier system in areas with high COVID-19 cases rate (new waves, local outbreaks) and rapid testing not available. Options for change applicable for SOP in future depending on local COVID-19 cases rate and population immunity status. Unstable COVID-19 rate.

Undoubtedly, whilst these options have potential limitations due to dynamic development of the pandemic, and heterogenicity between different geographical regions, they should be interpreted with caution as they may disproportionally disadvantage a considerable number of dental care providers. In the future, medical and dental care provision, resumption of healthcare services, and the need for using enhanced PPE could be graded by health policymakers using the 'traffic lights system' determined by COVID-19 rate, the proportion of the vaccinated population, and locally calculated risk of SARS-CoV-2 contraction. This approach is especially relevant during a pandemic transition time as DCWs fatigue increases while COVID-19 spread continues. It has to be highlighted, the feasibility of developing and implementing such a 'multi-pillar' protocol should be monitored, and pre-validated on a wider scale, adapting to highly specific characteristics of regional dental and medical workforces.

Our proposal for a tier-based system might vastly contribute to Public Health surveillance agendas on national levels as a response to the pandemic, monitoring the COVID-19 prevalence in local communities. This can be achieved by exchanging sets of various of COVID-19 epidemiological data from a wide range of sources. The enhanced PPE vigilance within a specific community will depend upon this information, shared with healthcare providers. Finally, this should be interpreted in the light of the dynamically changing COVID-19 pandemic and acceleration of vaccination programs. Although the proposed protocols and tiers are likely applicable by any healthcare provider, further scrutiny is required.

9. Conclusions

To the best of our knowledge, this is the first report of the easy-to-employ proposal for dental services reinstallation based on COVID-19 rates, testing accessibility, and vaccination rate. The equal distribution of the vaccine for COVID-19 around the world and in specific groups, including front-line personnel and vulnerable individuals, remains a global challenge. Before effective vaccination for various cohorts of society and different SARS-CoV-2 variants are broadly implemented, the use of adapted facilities, dentistry-specific delivery systems, altered working patterns, and operating protocols will be essential. It is necessary to pursue and deploy reliable point-of-care diagnostic countermeasures. Regardless of the expected vaccination success, the nearest future of dentistry may rely on the core operating protocols, regional COVID-19 rates, and consequently the predicted risk of infection.

Altogether, the utilization of fit-for-purpose standard operating procedures and engaging reliable rapid testing in routine practice are recommended for screening of any possible infections. Dental practice will likely emerge from the pandemic permanently changed, with new perspectives. Short and long-term re-instalment plans need to be arranged by the local authorities and government bodies.

Author Contributions: Conceptualization, N.F., D.J.; writing—original draft preparation, N.F., D.J., S.H.; writing—review and editing, N.F., D.J., S.H., A.D., M.T.; supervision, N.F., A.D.; project administration N.F.; visualization, A.D., validation, A.D. All authors have read and agreed to the published version of the manuscript.

Funding: This research received no external funding.

Institutional Review Board Statement: Not applicable.

Informed Consent Statement: Not applicable.

Data Availability Statement: Not applicable.

Conflicts of Interest: The authors declare no conflict of interest.

References

1. Rawaf, S.; Allen, L.N.; Stigler, F.L.; Kringos, D.; Quezada Yamamoto, H.; van Weel, C. Lessons on the COVID-19 pandemic, for and by primary care professionals worldwide. *Eur. J. Gen. Pract.* **2020**, *26*, 129–133. [CrossRef] [PubMed]
2. Hamedani, S.; Farshidfar, N.; Ziaei, A.; Pakravan, H. The Dilemma of COVID-19 in Dental Practice Concerning the Role of Saliva in Transmission: A Brief Review of Current Evidence. *Eur. Oral Res.* **2020**, *54*, 92–100. [CrossRef]
3. Banakar, M.; Bagheri Lankarani, K.; Jafarpour, D.; Moayedi, S.; Banakar, M.H.; Mohammadsadeghi, A. COVID-19 transmission risk and protective protocols in dentistry: A systematic review. *BMC Oral Health* **2020**, *20*, 275. [CrossRef]
4. Patini, R. How to face the post-sars-cov-2 outbreak era in private dental practice: Current evidence for avoiding cross-infections. *J. Int. Soc. Prev. Community Dent.* **2020**, *10*, 237–239. [CrossRef]
5. Bizzoca, M.E.; Campisi, G.; Lo Muzio, L. An innovative risk-scoring system of dental procedures and safety protocols in the COVID-19 era. *BMC Oral Health* **2020**, *20*, 301. [CrossRef]
6. Miller, C.S.; Carlson, C.R. A Blueprint for Recovery For The Postcoronavirus (COVID-19) World. *Oral Dis.* **2020**, *27*, 716–717. [CrossRef] [PubMed]
7. World Health Organization (WHO). *Considerations for the Provision of Essential Oral Health Services in the Context of COVID-19*; WHO: Geneva, Switzerland, 2020; p. 5.
8. Centers for Disease Control and Prevention (CDC). Interim Infection Prevention and Control Guidance for Dental Settings During the Coronavirus Disease 2019 (COVID-19) Pandemic. Available online: https://www.cdc.gov/coronavirus/2019-ncov/hcp/dental-settings.html (accessed on 1 September 2020).
9. American Dental Association (ADA). ADA Coronavirus (COVID-19) Center for Dentists. Available online: https://success.ada.org/en/practice-management/patients/infectious-diseases-2019-novel-coronavirus (accessed on 1 September 2020).
10. NHS England and NHS Improvement Coronavirus Dental Practice. Available online: https://www.englandr.nhs.uk/coronavirus/primary-care/dental-practice/ (accessed on 1 September 2020).
11. Randolph, H.E.; Barreiro, L.B. Herd Immunity: Understanding COVID-19. *Immunity* **2020**, *52*, 737–741. [CrossRef]
12. Roy, S. COVID-19 Reinfection: Myth or Truth? *SN Compr. Clin. Med.* **2020**, *2*, 710–713. [CrossRef]
13. Hoffmann, M.; Arora, P.; Groß, R.; Seidel, A.; Hörnich, B.F.; Hahn, A.S.; Krüger, N.; Graichen, L.; Hofmann-Winkler, H.; Kempf, A.; et al. SARS-CoV-2 variants B.1.351 and P.1 escape from neutralizing antibodies. *Cell* **2021**, *184*, 2384–2393. [CrossRef] [PubMed]
14. Jabbari, P.; Rezaei, N. With Risk of Reinfection, Is COVID-19 Here to Stay? *Disaster Med. Public Health Prep.* **2020**, *14*, e33. [CrossRef]
15. Williams, T.C.; Burgers, W.A. SARS-CoV-2 evolution and vaccines: Cause for concern? *Lancet Respir. Med.* **2021**, *9*, 333–335. [CrossRef]

16. Estai, M.; Kanagasingam, Y.; Xiao, D.; Vignarajan, J.; Huang, B.; Kruger, E.; Tennant, M. A proof-of-concept evaluation of a cloud-based store-and-forward telemedicine app for screening for oral diseases. *J. Telemed. Telecare* **2016**, *22*, 319–325. [CrossRef] [PubMed]
17. Martins, M.D.; Carrard, V.C.; dos Santos, C.M.; Hugo, F.N. COVID-19—Are telehealth and tele-education the answers to keep the ball rolling in Dentistry? *Oral Dis.* **2020**. [CrossRef] [PubMed]
18. Mei, X.; Lee, H.C.; Diao, K.; Huang, M.; Lin, B.; Liu, C.; Xie, Z.; Ma, Y.; Robson, P.M.; Chung, M.; et al. Artificial intelligence–enabled rapid diagnosis of patients with COVID-19. *Nat. Med.* **2020**, *26*, 1224–1228. [CrossRef] [PubMed]
19. Rahman, N.; Nathwani, S.; Kandiah, T. Teledentistry from a patient perspective during the coronavirus pandemic. *Br. Dent. J.* **2020**, 1–4. [CrossRef]
20. Giudice, A.; Barone, S.; Muraca, D.; Averta, F.; Diodati, F.; Antonelli, A.; Fortunato, L. Can teledentistry improve the monitoring of patients during the Covid-19 dissemination? A descriptive pilot study. *Int. J. Environ. Res. Public Health* **2020**, *17*, 3399. [CrossRef] [PubMed]
21. Caruso, S.; Caruso, S.; Pellegrino, M.; Skafi, R.; Nota, A.; Tecco, S. A knowledge-based algorithm for automatic monitoring of orthodontic treatment: The dental monitoring system. two cases. *Sensors* **2021**, *21*, 1856. [CrossRef]
22. Farook, T.; Jamayet, N.B.; Alam, M.K. Fatal mistake: Dentistry the next epicenter of SARS-CoV-2 spread. *Int. J. Hum. Health. Sci.* **2020**, *4*, 235. [CrossRef]
23. WHO. *Laboratory Testing for 2019 Novel Coronavirus (2019-nCoV) in Suspected Human Cases, Interim Guidance, 19 March 2020*; World Health Organization: Geneva, Switzerland, 2020.
24. Farshidfar, N.; Hamedani, S. The Potential Role of Smartphone-Based Microfluidic Systems for Rapid Detection of COVID-19 Using Saliva Specimen. *Mol. Diagnosis Ther.* **2020**, *24*, 371–373. [CrossRef]
25. Yamayoshi, S.; Sakai-Tagawa, Y.; Koga, M.; Akasaka, O.; Nakachi, I.; Koh, H.; Maeda, K.; Adachi, E.; Saito, M.; Nagai, H.; et al. Comparison of Rapid Antigen Tests for COVID-19. *Viruses* **2020**, *12*, 1420. [CrossRef] [PubMed]
26. Montesinos, I.; Gruson, D.; Kabamba, B.; Dahma, H.; Van den Wijngaert, S.; Reza, S.; Carbone, V.; Vandenberg, O.; Gulbis, B.; Wolff, F.; et al. Evaluation of two automated and three rapid lateral flow immunoassays for the detection of anti-SARS-CoV-2 antibodies. *J. Clin. Virol.* **2020**, *128*, 104413. [CrossRef]
27. Jääskeläinen, A.E.; Ahava, M.J.; Jokela, P.; Szirovicza, L.; Pohjala, S.; Vapalahti, O.; Lappalainen, M.; Hepojoki, J.; Kurkela, S. Evaluation of three rapid lateral flow antigen detection tests for the diagnosis of SARS-CoV-2 infection. *J. Clin. Virol.* **2021**, *137*, 104785. [CrossRef] [PubMed]
28. SoRelle, J.A.; Mahimainathan, L.; McCormick-Baw, C.; Cavuoti, D.; Lee, F.; Thomas, A.; Sarode, R.; Clark, A.E.; Muthukumar, A. Saliva for use with a point of care assay for the rapid diagnosis of COVID-19. *Clin. Chim. Acta* **2020**, *510*, 685–686. [CrossRef]
29. Azzi, L.; Maurino, V.; Baj, A.; Dani, M.; d'Aiuto, A.; Fasano, M.; Lualdi, M.; Sessa, F.; Alberio, T. Diagnostic Salivary Tests for SARS-CoV-2. *J. Dent. Res.* **2020**, *100*, 115–123. [CrossRef]
30. Fontana, M.; McCauley, L.; Fitzgerald, M.; Eckert, G.J.; Yanca, E.; Eber, R. Impact of COVID-19 on Life Experiences of Essential Workers Attending a Dental Testing Facility. *JDR Clin. Transl. Res.* **2021**, *6*, 24–39. [CrossRef] [PubMed]
31. NHS Lateral Flow Antigen Test FAQs for Independent Sector Providers. Available online: https://www.ox.ac.uk/news/2020-11-11-oxford-university-and-phe-confirm-high- (accessed on 25 February 2021).
32. Peeling, R.W.; Olliaro, P.L.; Boeras, D.I.; Fongwen, N. Scaling up COVID-19 rapid antigen tests: Promises and challenges. *Lancet Infect. Dis.* **2021**. [CrossRef]
33. Peto, T. COVID-19: Rapid Antigen detection for SARS-CoV-2 by lateral flow assay: A national systematic evaluation for mass-testing. *medRxiv* **2021**. [CrossRef]
34. Conway, D.I.; Culshaw, S.; Edwards, M.; Clark, C.; Watling, C.; Robertson, C.; Braid, R.; O'Keefe, E.; McGoldrick, N.; Burns, J.; et al. SARS-CoV-2 Positivity in Asymptomatic-Screened Dental Patients. *J. Dent. Res.* **2021**, 002203452110048. [CrossRef]
35. Phillips, N. The coronavirus is here to stay—Here's what that means. *Nature* **2021**, *590*, 382–384. [CrossRef]
36. Moore, S.; Hill, E.M.; Tildesley, M.J.; Dyson, L.; Keeling, M.J. Vaccination and non-pharmaceutical interventions for COVID-19: A mathematical modelling study. *Lancet Infect. Dis.* **2021**. [CrossRef]
37. Hegde, S. Which type of personal protective equipment (PPE) and which method of donning or doffing PPE carries the least risk of infection for healthcare workers? *Evid. Based Dent.* **2020**, *21*, 74–76. [CrossRef] [PubMed]
38. Bhattacharjee, S.; Joshi, R.; Chughtai, A.A.; Macintyre, C.R. Graphene Modified Multifunctional Personal Protective Clothing. *Adv. Mater. Interfaces* **2019**, *6*, 1900622. [CrossRef] [PubMed]
39. Mummolo, S.; Tieri, M.; Tecco, S.; Mattei, A.; Albani, F.; Giuca, M.R.; Marzo, G. Clinical evaluation of salivary indices and levels of Streptococcus mutans and Lactobacillus in patients treated with Occlus-o-Guide. *Eur. J. Paediatr. Dent.* **2014**, *15*, 367–370. [PubMed]
40. Benzian, H.; Niederman, R. A Dental Response to the COVID-19 Pandemic—Safer Aerosol-Free Emergent (SAFER) Dentistry. *Front. Med.* **2020**, *7*, 520. [CrossRef] [PubMed]
41. Tarraf, N.E.; Ali, D.M. Present and the future of digital orthodontics☆. *Semin. Orthod.* **2018**, *24*, 376–385. [CrossRef]
42. Kasloff, S.B.; Leung, A.; Strong, J.E.; Funk, D.; Cutts, T. Stability of SARS-CoV-2 on critical personal protective equipment. *Sci. Rep.* **2021**, *11*, 984. [CrossRef]

43. All Wales Clinical Dental Leads COVID-19 Groups Standard Operating Procedure for the Dental Management of Non-COVID-19 Patients in Wales, Version 1.01. Available online: https://bda.org/advice/Coronavirus/Documents/Wales-sops-for-agps-on-non-covid-19-patients.pdf (accessed on 25 February 2021).
44. Mupparapu, M. Aerosol reduction urgency in post-COVID-19 dental practice. *Quintessence Int. (Berl).* **2020**, *51*, 525–526.
45. Ge, Z.; Yang, L.; Xia, J.; Fu, X.; Zhang, Y. Possible aerosol transmission of COVID-19 and special precautions in dentistry. *J. Zhejiang Univ. Sci. B* **2020**, *21*, 361–368. [CrossRef]
46. Poggio, C.; Colombo, M.; Arciola, C.R.; Greggi, T.; Scribante, A.; Dagna, A. Copper-alloy surfaces and cleaning regimens against the spread of SARS-CoV-2 in dentistry and orthopedics. From fomites to anti-infective nanocoatings. *Materials* **2020**, *13*, 3244. [CrossRef] [PubMed]
47. Isha, S.N.; Ahmad, A.; Kabir, R.; Apu, E.H. Dental Clinic Architecture Prevents COVID-19-Like Infectious Diseases. *Health. Environ. Res. Des. J.* **2020**, *13*, 240–241. [CrossRef]
48. Proffitt, E. What will be the new normal for the dental industry? *Br. Dent. J.* **2020**, *228*, 678–680. [CrossRef] [PubMed]
49. Berlin-Broner, Y.; Levin, L. "Dental Hierarchy of Needs" in the COVID-19 Era—Or Why Treat When It Doesn't Hurt? *Oral Health Prev. Dent.* **2020**, *18*, 95. [CrossRef]
50. Halabi, S.; Heinrich, A.; Omer, S.B. No-Fault Compensation for Vaccine Injury — The Other Side of Equitable Access to Covid-19 Vaccines. *N. Engl. J. Med.* **2020**, *383*, e125. [CrossRef] [PubMed]
51. Corum, B.J.; Wee, S.-L.; Zimmer, C. Coronavirus Vaccine Tracker -NY Times. Available online: https://www.nytimes.com/interactive/2020/science/coronavirus-vaccine-tracker.html (accessed on 10 March 2021).
52. Wouters, O.J.; Shadlen, K.C.; Salcher-Konrad, M.; Pollard, A.J.; Larson, H.J.; Teerawattananon, Y.; Jit, M. Challenges in ensuring global access to COVID-19 vaccines: Production, affordability, allocation, and deployment. *Lancet* **2021**, *397*, 1023–1034. [CrossRef]
53. Forni, G.; Mantovani, A.; Forni, G.; Mantovani, A.; Moretta, L.; Rappuoli, R.; Rezza, G.; Bagnasco, A.; Barsacchi, G.; Bussolati, G.; et al. COVID-19 vaccines: Where we stand and challenges ahead. *Cell Death Differ.* **2021**, *28*, 626–639. [CrossRef] [PubMed]
54. Mehan, A.; Venkatesh, A.; Girish, M. COVID-19: Should oral vaccination strategies be given more consideration? *Ther. Adv. Vaccines Immunother.* **2020**, *8*, 2515135520946503. [CrossRef]

Journal of
Clinical Medicine

MDPI

Article

Prevalence of COVID-19 Vaccine Side Effects among Healthcare Workers in the Czech Republic

Abanoub Riad [1,2,*,†], Andrea Pokorná [2,3,†], Sameh Attia [4], Jitka Klugarová [1,2], Michal Koščík [1,5,‡] and Miloslav Klugar [1,2,‡]

1 Department of Public Health, Faculty of Medicine, Masaryk University, Kamenice 5, 625 00 Brno, Czech Republic; klugarova@med.muni.cz (J.K.); koscik@med.muni.cz (M.K.); klugar@med.muni.cz (M.K.)
2 Czech National Centre for Evidence-Based Healthcare and Knowledge Translation (Cochrane Czech Republic, Czech EBHC: JBI Centre of Excellence, Masaryk University GRADE Centre), Institute of Biostatistics and Analyses, Faculty of Medicine, Masaryk University, Kamenice 5, 625 00 Brno, Czech Republic; apokorna@med.muni.cz
3 Department of Nursing and Midwifery, Faculty of Medicine, Masaryk University, Kamenice 5, 625 00 Brno, Czech Republic
4 Department of Oral and Maxillofacial Surgery, Justus-Liebig-University, Klinikstrasse 33, 35392 Giessen, Germany; sameh.attia@dentist.med.uni-giessen.de
5 Czech Clinical Research Infrastructure Network, Department of Pharmacology, Faculty of Medicine, Masaryk University, Kamenice 5, 625 00 Brno, Czech Republic
* Correspondence: abanoub.riad@med.muni.cz; Tel.: +420-549-496-572
† Equal contribution as first authorship.
‡ Equal contribution as senior authorship.

Citation: Riad, A.; Pokorná, A.; Attia, S.; Klugarová, J.; Koščík, M.; Klugar, M. Prevalence of COVID-19 Vaccine Side Effects among Healthcare Workers in the Czech Republic. *J. Clin. Med.* **2021**, *10*, 1428. https://doi.org/10.3390/jcm10071428

Academic Editor: Giovanni Gabutti

Received: 9 March 2021
Accepted: 23 March 2021
Published: 1 April 2021

Abstract: Background: COVID-19 vaccine side effects have a fundamental role in public confidence in the vaccine and its uptake process. Thus far, the evidence on vaccine safety has exclusively been obtained from the manufacturer-sponsored studies; therefore, this study was designed to provide independent evidence on Pfizer–BioNTech COVID-19 vaccine side effects. Methods: A cross-sectional survey-based study was carried out between January and February 2021 to collect data on the side effects following the COVID-19 vaccine among healthcare workers in the Czech Republic. The study used a validated questionnaire with twenty-eight multiple-choice items covering the participants' demographic data, medical anamneses, COVID-19-related anamneses, general, oral, and skin-related side effects. Results: Injection site pain (89.8%), fatigue (62.2%), headache (45.6%), muscle pain (37.1%), and chills (33.9%) were the most commonly reported side effects. All the general side effects were more prevalent among the ≤43-year-old group, and their duration was mainly one day (45.1%) or three days (35.8%) following the vaccine. Antihistamines were the most common drugs associated with side effects, thus requiring further investigation. The people with two doses were generally associated with a higher frequency of side effects. Conclusions: The distribution of side effects among Czech healthcare workers was highly consistent with the manufacturer's data, especially in terms of their association with the younger age group and the second dose. The overall prevalence of some local and systemic side effects was higher than the manufacturer's report. Further independent studies on vaccine safety are strongly required to strengthen public confidence in the vaccine.

Keywords: adverse effects; BNT162 vaccine; cross-sectional studies; COVID-19; Czech Republic; drug-related side effects and adverse reactions; health personnel; mass vaccination; prevalence

1. Introduction

Vaccine hesitancy (VH) refers to the "delay in acceptance or refusal of vaccines despite availability of vaccine services"; it is an emerging public health challenge nourished by misinformation related to vaccines effectiveness and safety [1–3]. In a recent nation-wide study, aversion to vaccines' potential side effects was the most frequent cause for VH among population groups in the United Kingdom (U.K.) [4]. This finding was supported in the context of COVID-19 vaccines, because a fear of side effects was the most prominent reason to decrease the readiness of healthcare workers and students in Poland to accept the vaccination [5,6]. Consequently, a systematic review of the strategies of tackling VH revealed that raising public awareness of vaccines' effectiveness and honesty regarding their side effects is vital for improving vaccine uptake [7]. The launch of the COVID-19 vaccine rollout in December 2020 was a landmark for overcoming this pandemic crisis; therefore, it had been recommended to split the pandemic history to pre-vaccination (B.V.; before vaccine) and post-vaccination (A.V.; after vaccine) eras. COVID-19-related literature should be defined in relation to this parameter either as B.V. or A.V. [8].

In a cross-sectional study of influenza vaccine side effects, three out of thirty-seven participants who were recently influenza-vaccinated (8%) developed oral side effects, thus implying a non-statistically significant relationship between influenza vaccine and the oral cavity [9]. The short-term side effects of vaccines vary in their clinical presentation; however, they are commonly related to prophylactic vaccines' humoral immune response [10]. The oral cavity has been a locus for the adverse events of an array of vaccines, e.g., diphtheria, tetanus, acellular pertussis, and polio vaccines [9]. The COVID-19-related oral symptoms were attributed to the high expression of angiotensin-converting enzyme 2 (ACE2) receptors in the tongue's epithelial cells, buccal and gingival mucosa [11–18].

Thus far, all the available data on COVID-19 vaccine side effects has been published by manufacturer-funded studies which are in compliance with the drug authorities' guidelines and monitored by third-parties [19]. A lack of independent studies on vaccines' safety may adversely impact the vaccine uptake, which has to be accelerated in the next few months in order to escape this viscous circle of the virus and its variants [7]. Therefore, this study's primary objective was to estimate the prevalence of Pfizer–BioNTech COVID-19 vaccine side effects among the early vaccinated healthcare workers in the Czech Republic.

The secondary objectives were:

1. To identify the potential risk factors of Pfizer–BioNTech COVID-19 vaccine side effects;
2. To evaluate the correlation of general side effects, oral side effects, and skin-related side effects.

2. Materials and Methods

2.1. Study Design

This cross-sectional survey-based study was carried out from 27 January 2021 to 27 February 2021, to estimate the prevalence of COVID-19 vaccine side effects among the priority groups of the randomly selected healthcare workers in the Czech Republic. The study utilized a self-administered questionnaire of multiple-choice items which had been designed digitally using KoBoToolbox version 2.021.03 (Harvard Humanitarian Initiative. Cambridge, MA, USA, 2021).

The study protocol was registered in the trials registry of the U.S. National Library of Medicine (NLM) under the title "Oral Side Effects of COVID-19 Vaccine–OSECV" with the identifier NCT04706156; it was reported following the Strengthening the Reporting of Observational Studies in Epidemiology (STROBE) guidelines for cross-sectional studies [20,21].

After ethical clearance, invitation emails for the local coordinators of the member institutions in the Czech Clinical Research Infrastructure Network (CZECRIN; Brno, Czech Republic), the managers of all inpatient healthcare facilities within the network of the Central Adverse Events Reporting System of the Institute of Health Information and Statistics of the Czech Republic (IHIS-CR; Prague, Czech Republic), and all registered dentists through the Czech Dental Chamber (ČSK; Prague, Czech Republic) to contribute to this study by accessing the uniform resource locator (URL) of the digital questionnaire [22]. The awareness of the study was also raised by promotion on the websites and social media profiles of CZECRIN and the Faculty of Medicine [23]. The collected data are controlled by Masaryk University, and data acquisition and processing are in compliance with the General Data Protection Regulation (GDPR) [24].

2.2. Participants

Inclusion criteria for this study were Czech healthcare workers who were vaccinated with the Pfizer–BioNTech COVID-19 vaccine during the early vaccination phase of the governmental strategy (Phase 1A) [25]. The eligible participants should have received the latest dose of the vaccine, either the first or the second dose, no more than thirty days before filling in the questionnaire. Non-healthcare workers who were vaccinated during Phase 1A and the healthcare workers who were vaccinated in February 2021 by Moderna COVID-19 vaccine and Oxford/AstraZeneca COVID-19 vaccine were excluded from this report. Participation in this study was not compensated financially or by any other incentives.

2.3. Instrument

The self-administered questionnaire of this study was composed of twenty mandatory multiple-choice items and eight conditional multiple-choice items, and it was adapted from previous studies on the oral side effects of various vaccines by the authors [9,26]. A panel of four experts in oral medicine, maxillofacial surgery, and infectious diseases were formed to review the questionnaire draft and to assess its content validity. We used an iterative discussion to finalize the questionnaire. Later, the reliability of the questionnaire was evaluated by a group of eighteen recently vaccinated healthcare workers, who filled in the questionnaire twice with a minimum interval of two weeks. The result of the test re-test of the provisional instrument yielded substantial reliability, with a mean Cohen's kappa coefficient of 0.89 ± 0.13 (0.54–1) (Table 1).

Table 1. The results of test re-test reliability of the instrument of the "Oral Side Effects of COVID-19 Vaccine" study (OSECV) [1].

Participant	κ Coefficient	Participant	κ Coefficient
No. 1	0.821	No. 10	0.540
No. 2	0.842	No. 11	1.000
No. 3	0.777	No. 12	1.000
No. 4	0.940	No. 13	1.000
No. 5	1.000	No. 14	1.000
No. 6	1.000	No. 15	0.937
No. 7	0.934	No. 16	0.872
No. 8	0.758	No. 17	0.868
No. 9	1.000	No. 18	0.762

[1] Cohen's Kappa statistic (κ): 0.01–0.20 as none to slight; 0.21–0.40 as fair; 0.41–0.60 as moderate; 0.61–0.80 as substantial; and 0.81–1.00 as perfect agreement [27].

The questionnaire was divided into four main categories: (i) demographic data including gender, age, region, profession, and length of work experience; (ii) medical anamnesis including medical comorbidities and medications; (iii) COVID-19 related anamnesis including vaccination date and the number of doses, previous infection, and exposure to infected cases; and (iv) vaccine side effects including general side effects, oral side effects, and skin-related side effects (Supplementary Materials Table S1).

2.4. Ethical Considerations

The study was reviewed and approved by the Ethics Committee of the Faculty of Medicine at Masaryk University on 20 January 2021 (Ref. 2/2021). Digital informed consent had been obtained from each participant prior to participation. The participants were allowed to withdraw from the study at any moment without justifying, and no data were saved before the participant submitted their answers completely.

2.5. Statistical Analysis

All statistical tests were executed using the Statistical Package for the Social Sciences (SPSS) version 27.0 (SPSS Inc. Chicago, IL, USA, 2020). Primarily, descriptive statistics were carried out for the demographic variables (gender, age, profession, length of work experience, and region), and medical anamnesis (non-communicable diseases, and medical treatments), COVID-19-related anamnesis (number of doses, interval between doses, previous infection, patency period, and previous exposure to COVID-19 cases), and vaccine side effects (general side effects, oral side effects, and skin-related side effects) were represented by frequencies, percentages, means and standard deviations. Consequently, inferential statistics were performed to assess the association between side effects and medical anamnesis, and the association of various side effects and each other using the chi-squared test (χ^2), Student's t-test, one-way analysis of variance (ANOVA), and Pearson's correlation test (r), with a confidence level of 95% and significance value $p \leq 0.05$. Strengths of correlation are verbally described by the value of (r) 0.00–0.19 "very weak"; 0.20–0.39 "weak"; 0.40–0.59 "moderate"; 0.60–0.79 "strong"; 0.80–1.0 "very strong".

3. Results

3.1. Demographic Characteristics

A total of 922 participants filled in the questionnaire properly by 27 February 2021. Nineteen participants were administrative staff at healthcare facilities; therefore, they were vaccinated, but they did not meet the study's inclusion criteria. Similarly, twenty-eight participants received either the Moderna COVID-19 vaccine or Oxford/AstraZeneca COVID-19 vaccine; therefore, they were excluded from this report. Three participants did not submit their age properly; therefore, they were omitted from the inferential statistics based on age groups.

A total of 877 participants were included in the final analyses; 776 (88.5%) were females, 100 (11.4%) were males, and 1 (0.1%) preferred not to state their gender. Their mean age was 42.56 ± 10.5 years old, and it ranged between 19 and 78 years old with a median of 43 years old. Given the fact that the median age of this study's participants corresponds with the mean age of healthcare workers in the Czech Republic, which is between 40 and 45 years old, the sample's median age (43 years old) had been used as a cut-off to present the anamnestic characteristics and the COVID-19 vaccine side effects of the participants [28,29] (Table 2).

On comparing the number of participants to the total number of healthcare workers per region, reported by IHIS-CR, the mean density was 2.95 ± 2.22 responses per 1000 healthcare workers [30]. The highest density was in the South-Moravian region with 9.86 response per 1000 healthcare workers; the lowest was in the South Bohemian region with 1.51 response per 1000 healthcare workers (Figure 1).

3.2. Medical Anamneses

A total of 271 (31%) participants reported having at least one non-communicable disease (NCD) with a statistically significant difference between the ≤43-year-old group and the >43-year-old group: 105 (23.9%) vs. 166 (38.2%), respectively. Out of all the chronically ill participants, 100 (36.9%) reported chronic hypertension, 69 (25.6%) thyroid disease, 59 (21.8%) asthma, 23 (8.5%) diabetes mellitus type-2, 16 (5.9%) cardiac disease, 16 (5.9%) allergy, 13 (4.8%) rheumatoid arthritis, 12 (4.4%) bowel disease, 11 (4.1%) blood disease, 11 (4.1%) neurologic disease, 8 (3%) psychological distress, 6 (2.2%) renal disease, 5 (1.8%) chronic obstructive pulmonary disease (COPD), 4 (1.5%) cancer, 3 (1.1%) diabetes mellitus type-1, 2 (0.7%) hepatologic disease, and 1 (0.4%) ophthalmologic disease. Across the age groups, the total number of NCDs was significantly higher in the >43-year-old group (1.39 ± 0.66) than the ≤43-year-old group (1.22 ± 0.46) with a significance value of 0.020 (Table 3).

The chi-squared test revealed a statistically significant difference in the distribution of some NCDs between both age groups, e.g., chronic hypertension, psychological distress, blood disease, and diabetes mellitus type-2 with significance values less than 0.0001, 0.004, 0.018, and 0.028, respectively.

Table 2. Demographic characteristics of the Czech healthcare workers who received the Pfizer–BioNTech COVID-19 vaccine, January–February 2021.

Variable	Outcome	Frequency	Percentage
Gender	Female	776	88.5%
	Male	100	11.4%
	Prefer not to say	1	0.1%
Age	≤43 years old	439	50.2%
	>43 years old	435	49.8%
Profession	Registered Nurse	540	61.6%
	Physician	77	8.8%
	Practice Nurse	75	8.6%
	Lab Worker	46	5.2%
	Paramedic	26	3.0%
	Dentist	24	2.7%
	Midwife	23	2.6%
	Pharmacist	21	2.4%
	Physiotherapist	19	2.2%
	Radiological Assistant	12	1.4%
	Psychologist	8	0.9%
	Dietitian	5	0.6%
	Dental Hygienist	1	0.1%
Length of Work Experience	1–5 years	134	15.3%
	6–10 years	88	10.0%
	11–20 years	188	21.4%
	>20 years	467	53.2%
Region	South-Moravian	301	34.3%
	Prague	105	12.0%
	Moravian-Silesian	92	10.5%
	Hradec Kralove	78	8.9%
	Central Bohemian	70	8.0%
	Olomouc	51	5.8%
	Plzen	29	3.3%
	Usti nad Labem	29	3.3%
	Zlin	25	2.9%
	Vysočina	23	2.6%
	South Bohemian	22	2.5%
	Pardubice	21	2.4%
	Karlovy Vary	17	1.9%
	Liberec	14	1.6%

A total of 384 (44%) participants reported receiving at least one medical treatment at the time of filling in the questionnaire, with a statistically significant difference between the ≤43-year-old group and the >43-year-old group: 144 (32.8%) vs. 240 (55.2%), respectively. Out of all the regularly taken drugs, antihypertensive drugs were taken by 98 (25.5%), followed by thyroid hormones replacement by 90 (23.4%), antihistamine by 75 (19.6%), antidepressant by 45 (11.7%), contraceptives by 21 (5.5%), common analgesics 19 (4.9%), nonsteroidal anti-inflammatory (NSAID) by 15 (3.9%), antidiabetics by 14 (3.6%), anti-reflux by 13 (3.4%), cholesterol-lowering by 12 (3.1%), immunosuppressive by 8 (2.1%), anti-asthma by 7 (1.8%), venous insufficiency by 6 (1.6%), anticoagulants by 6 (1.6%), antiepileptics by 6 (1.6%), corticosteroids by 6 (1.6%), opioid analgesics by 3 (0.8%), antibiotics by 2 (0.5%), and other drugs by 18 (4.7%), including bronchodilators, antifungals, antidiuretic, estrogen hormone, chemotherapy, vitamin D, and interferon. Across the age groups, the total number of taken drugs was insignificantly lower in the >43-year-old group (1.20 ± 0.51) than the ≤43-year-old group (1.24 ± 0.55) (Table 4).

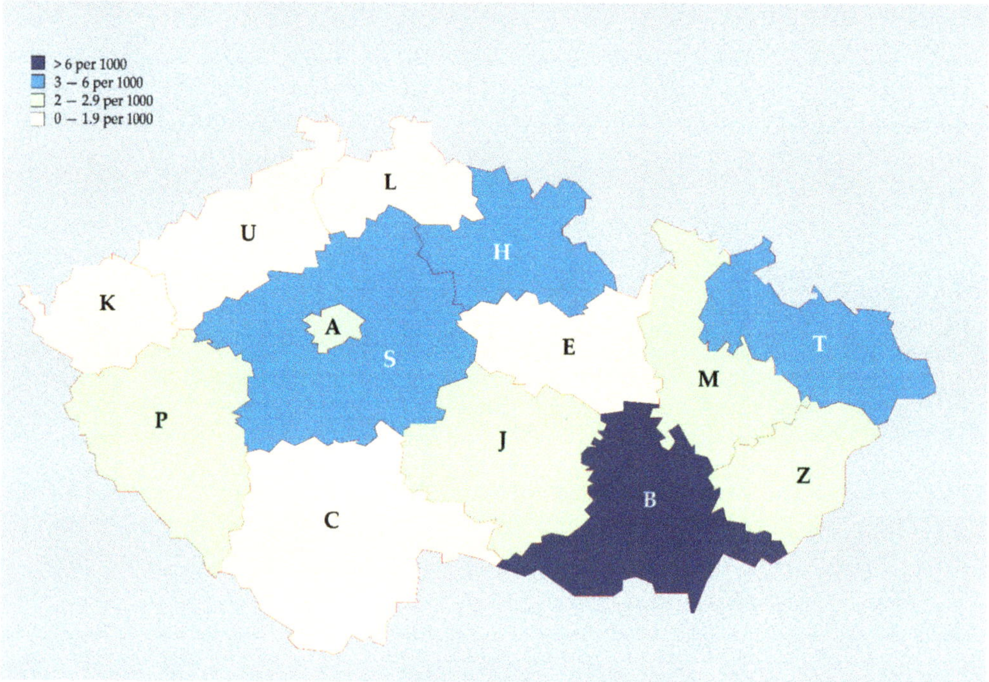

Figure 1. Regional density of the participating Czech healthcare workers; (A) Prague; (S) Central Bohemian; (C) South Bohemian; (J) Vysočina; (P) Plzen; (K) Karlovy Vary; (U) Usti nad Labem; (L) Liberec; (H) Hradec Kralove; (E) Pardubice; (M) Olomouc; (T) Moravian-Silesian; (B) South-Moravian; (Z) Zlin; January–February 2021.

Table 3. Non-communicable diseases of vaccinated healthcare workers in the Czech Republic, January–February 2021.

Disease	≤43 Years Old	>43 Years Old	Total	Significance [1]
Allergy	9 (8.6%)	7 (4.2%)	16 (5.9%)	0.138
Asthma	26 (24.8%)	33 (19.9%)	59 (21.8%)	0.343
Blood Disease	8 (7.6%)	3 (1.8%)	11 (4.1%)	**0.018**
Bowel Disease	7 (6.7%)	5 (3.0%)	12 (4.4%)	0.154
Cancer	0 (0.0%)	4 (2.4%)	4 (1.5%)	0.109
Cardiac Disease	4 (3.8%)	12 (7.2%)	16 (5.9%)	0.245
Chronic Hypertension	21 (20.0%)	79 (47.6%)	100 (36.9%)	**<0.0001**
COPD	0 (0.0%)	5 (3.0%)	5 (1.8%)	0.073
Diabetes Mellitus–I	2 (1.9%)	1 (0.6%)	3 (1.1%)	0.318
Diabetes Mellitus–II	4 (3.8%)	19 (11.4%)	23 (8.5%)	**0.028**
Hepatologic Disease	2 (1.9%)	0 (0.0%)	2 (0.7%)	0.074
Psychological Distress	7 (6.7%)	1 (0.6%)	8 (3.0%)	**0.004**
Neurologic Disease	2 (1.9%)	9 (5.4%)	11 (4.1%)	0.153
Ophthalmologic Disease	0 (0.0%)	1 (0.6%)	1 (0.4%)	0.426
Renal Disease	2 (1.9%)	4 (1.8%)	6 (2.2%)	0.783
Rheumatoid Arthritis	3 (2.9%)	10 (6%)	13 (4.8%)	0.235
Thyroid Disease	31 (29.5%)	38 (22.9%)	69 (25.5%)	0.222
Number of NCDs (1–17)	1.22 ± 0.46	1.39 ± 0.66	1.32 ± 0.59	**0.026**
Total	105 (23.9%)	166 (38.2%)	271 (31%)	**0.020**

[1] Chi-square test and Student's *t*-test were used with a significance level of <0.05. Bold format highlight the significantly different diseases across age groups.

Table 4. Regularly taken drugs by the vaccinated healthcare workers in the Czech Republic, January–February 2021.

Drug	≤43 Years Old	>43 Years Old	Total	Significance [1]
Anti-asthma	4 (2.8%)	3 (1.3%)	7 (1.8%)	0.279
Antibiotics	1 (0.7%)	1 (0.4%)	2 (0.5%)	0.714
Anticoagulant	1 (0.7%)	5 (2.1%)	6 (1.6%)	0.288
Antidepressant	19 (13.2%)	26 (10.8%)	45 (11.7%)	0.486
Antidiabetic	3 (2.1%)	11 (4.6%)	14 (3.6%)	0.206
Antiepileptic	4 (2.8%)	2 (0.8%)	6 (1.6%)	0.138
Antihistamine	37 (25.7%)	38 (15.8%)	75 (19.5%)	**0.018**
Antihypertensive	23 (16.0%)	75 (31.3%)	98 (25.5%)	**0.001**
Anti-Reflux	6 (4.2%)	7 (2.9%)	13 (3.4%)	0.512
Immunosuppressive	2 (1.4%)	6 (2.5%)	8 (2.1%)	0.460
Cholesterol-lowering	3 (2.1%)	9 (3.8%)	12 (3.1%)	0.363
Common Analgesic	7 (4.9%)	12 (5.0%)	19 (4.9%)	0.952
Contraceptive	15 (10.4%)	6 (2.5%)	21 (5.5%)	**0.001**
Corticosteroid	2 (1.4%)	4 (1.7%)	6 (1.6%)	0.832
Nonsteroidal anti-inflammatory (NSAID)	6 (4.2%)	9 (3.8%)	15 (3.9%)	0.838
Opioid Analgesic	2 (1.4%)	1 (0.4%)	3 (0.8%)	0.295
Thyroid Hormones	35 (24.3%)	55 (22.9%)	90 (23.4%)	0.756
Venous Insufficiency	4 (2.8%)	2 (0.8%)	6 (1.6%)	0.137
Other	5 (3.5%)	13 (5.4%)	18 (4.7%)	0.383
Number of Drugs (1–19)	1.24 ± 0.55	1.20 ± 0.51	1.21 ± 0.52	0.392
Total	144 (32.8%)	240 (55.2%)	384 (43.9%)	<0.0001

[1] Chi-squared test and ANOVA were used with a significance level of <0.05.

The chi-squared test revealed a statistically significant difference in the distribution of some taken drugs between both age groups, e.g., antihypertensive drugs, contraceptives, and antihistamine drugs, with significance values of 0.001, 0.001, and 0.018, respectively.

3.3. COVID-19-Related Anamnesis

By the time of filling in the questionnaire, the vast majority of the participants had received both doses of the Pfizer–BioNTech COVID-19 vaccine (93.6%), while 56 (6.4%) had received the first dose only. The interval between the first dose and the second dose ranged between 7 and 55 days, with a median of 21 days. The difference was statistically insignificant across the age groups, with a slight longer interval among the ≤43-year-old group (22.69 ± 5.14 days) compared to the >43-year-old group (22.48 ± 4.7 days).

Although 169 (19.3%) participants had been previously infected by COVID-19, the patency period between the recovery date and the first vaccine dose ranged between 7 and 270 days with a median of 65 days. Regarding the exposure to COVID-19 cases, a total of 617 (70.6%) participants reported that they had been in contact with COVID-19 cases previously: 317 (72.2%) of the ≤43-year-old group and 300 (69%) of the >43-year-old group, without statistical significance (p = 0.293) (Table 5).

Table 5. COVID-19-related anamnesis of vaccinated healthcare workers in the Czech Republic, January–February 2021.

Variable	Outcome	≤43 Years Old	>43 Years Old	Total	Significance [1]
Number of doses	One dose	26 (5.9%)	30 (6.9%)	56 (6.4%)	0.557
	Two doses	413 (94.1%)	404 (93.1%)	818 (93.6%)	
Interval	(days)	22.69 ± 5.14	22.48 ± 4.7	22.58 ± 4.92	0.551
COVID-19 infection	Yes	90 (20.5%)	79 (18.2%)	169 (19.3%)	0.381
Patency period	(days)	77.78 ± 54.69	72.44 ± 45.16	75.42 ± 50.58	0.534
Previous COVID-19 exposure	Yes	317 (72.2%)	300 (69%)	617 (70.6%)	0.293

[1] Chi-squared test and Student's t-test were used with a significance level of <0.05.

3.4. COVID-19 Vaccine Reported Side Effects

3.4.1. Prevalence of General Side Effects

A total of 814 (93.1%) participants reported having at least one side effect following the COVID-19 vaccine. The prevalence of side effects was slightly higher in the ≤43-year-old group (94.8%) than the >43-year-old group (91.5%). The most common side effect was injection site pain (89.8%), followed by fatigue (62.2%), headache (45.6%), muscle pain (37.1%), and chills (33.9%). All the reported side effects were more prevalent in the ≤43-year-old group than the >43-year-old group, with a statistically significant difference in the case of injection site pain (93.3% vs. 86.2%), headache (50.7% vs. 40.2%), fatigue (65.9% vs. 58.3%), muscle pain (40.9% vs. 33.2%), and feeling unwell (26% vs. 19.8%).

Regarding the general side effects' duration, 45.1% of them lasted for 1 day, while 35.8% lasted for 3 days, 9.4% lasted for 5 days, 5.3% lasted for one week, 3% lasted for over a week, and 1.4% for over a month. The severe side effects that required medical intervention was reported by only 1.3% of the whole study group (Table 6).

Table 6. Prevalence of the general side effects of Pfizer–BioNTech COVID-19 vaccine among healthcare workers in the Czech Republic, January–February 2021.

Variable	Outcome	≤43 Years Old	>43 Years Old	Total	Significance [1]
Side Effect	**Injection site pain**	388 (93.3%)	343 (86.2%)	731 (89.8%)	**0.001**
	Fatigue	274 (65.9%)	232 (58.3%)	506 (62.2%)	**0.026**
	Headache	211 (50.7%)	160 (40.2%)	371 (45.6%)	**0.003**
	Muscle pain	170 (40.9%)	132 (33.2%)	302 (37.1%)	**0.023**
	Chills	153 (36.8%)	123 (30.9%)	276 (33.9%)	0.077
	Joint pain	119 (28.6%)	107 (26.9%)	226 (27.8%)	0.584
	Injection site swelling	108 (26.0%)	100 (25.1%)	208 (25.6%)	0.785
	Injection site redness	106 (25.5%)	81 (20.4%)	187 (23.0%)	0.082
	Feeling unwell	108 (26.0%)	79 (19.8%)	187 (23%)	**0.038**
	Fever	101 (24.3%)	76 (19.1%)	177 (21.7%)	0.073
	Lymphadenopathy	72 (17.3%)	60 (15.1%)	132 (16.2%)	0.388
	Nausea	61 (14.7%)	45 (11.3%)	106 (13.0%)	0.155
Number of Side Effects	**(1–12)**	4.50 ± 2.596	3.87 ± 2.599	4.19 ± 2.615	**0.001**
Total		416 (94.8%)	398 (91.5%)	814 (93.1%)	0.056
Duration	1 day	196 (47.2%)	168 (42.7%)	364 (45.1%)	
	3 days	159 (38.3%)	130 (33.2%)	289 (35.8%)	
	5 days	31 (7.5%)	45 (11.5%)	76 (9.4%)	
	1 week	17 (4.1%)	26 (6.6%)	43 (5.3%)	
	>1 week	8 (1.9%)	16 (4.1%)	24 (3.0%)	
	>1 month	4 (1.0%)	7 (1.8%)	11 (1.4%)	
Severe Side Effects		5 (1.1%)	6 (1.4%)	11 (1.3%)	0.747

[1] Chi-squared test and ANOVA were used with a significance level of <0.05.

3.4.2. Prevalence of Reported Oral Side Effects

A total of 114 (13%) participants reported to have at least one oral side effect following the Pfizer–BioNTech COVID-19 vaccine. The prevalence of oral side effects was insignificantly higher in the ≤43-year-old group (13.4%) than the >43-year-old group (12.6%). The most common oral side effect was blisters (36%), followed by halitosis (25.4%), ulcers (14%), bleeding gingiva (11.4%), and white/red plaque (10.5%).

However, there were no statistically significant differences between the age groups: white/red plaque (10.9% vs. 10.2%), burning gingiva (9.1% vs. 8.5%), angular cheilitis (5.5% vs. 3.4%), tongue tingling (5.5% vs. 3.4%), taste disturbance (5.5% vs. 1.7%), vesicles (3.6% vs. 3.4%), and xerostomia (3.6% vs. 1.7%) were more prevalent in the >43-year-old group than the ≤43-year-old group. On the other hand, blisters (37.3% vs. 34.5%), halitosis (28.8% vs. 21.8%), ulcers (16.9% vs. 10.9%), bleeding gingiva (13.6% vs. 9.1%), and swollen lips (5.1% vs. 1.8%) were more prevalent in the ≤43-year-old group compared to the >43-year-old group.

Regarding oral side effects' onset, 28.6% of them emerged within the first week post-vaccination, while 26.8% emerged within 1–3 days post-vaccination, 18.8% within the third week post-vaccination, 16.1% within the second week post-vaccination, and 9.8% within the fourth week post-vaccination.

The most common location of ulcers, blisters, and vesicles was the lips (74.1%), followed by labial and buccal mucosa (14.8%), tongue (13%), palate (9.3%), and gingiva (9.3%). The difference between the age groups was statistically insignificant; however, lips were affected in 80% of the >43-year-old group versus 69% of the ≤43-year-old group. All (100%) of the >43-year-old group participants had one affected location, whereas 72.4% of the ≤43-year-old group participants had one affected location, 20.7% had two affected locations, 3.4% had three affected locations, and 3.4% had four affected locations. In the case of white/red plaque, the most common location was the tongue dorsum (75%), followed by soft palate (16.7%) and labial and buccal mucosa (8.3%) (Table 7).

Table 7. Prevalence of oral side effects of Pfizer–BioNTech COVID-19 vaccine among healthcare workers in the Czech Republic, January–February 2021.

Variable	Outcome	≤43 Years Old	>43 Years Old	Total	Significance [1]
Side Effect	Blisters	22 (37.3%)	19 (34.5%)	41 (36%)	0.760
	Halitosis	17 (28.8%)	12 (21.8%)	29 (25.4%)	0.391
	Ulcers	10 (16.9%)	6 (10.9%)	16 (14.0%)	0.354
	Bleeding gingiva	8 (13.6%)	5 (9.1%)	13 (11.4%)	0.453
	White/red plaque	6 (10.2%)	6 (10.9%)	12 (10.5%)	0.898
	Burning gingiva	5 (8.5%)	5 (9.1%)	10 (8.8%)	0.907
	Angular cheilitis	2 (3.4%)	3 (5.5%)	5 (4.4%)	0.591
	Tongue tingling	2 (3.4%)	3 (5.5%)	5 (4.4%)	0.591
	Taste disturbance	1 (1.7%)	3 (5.5%)	4 (3.5%)	0.276
	Vesicles	2 (3.4%)	2 (3.6%)	4 (3.5%)	0.943
	Swollen lips	3 (5.1%)	1 (1.8%)	4 (3.5%)	0.344
	Xerostomia	1 (1.7%)	2 (3.6%)	3 (2.6%)	0.518
Number of Side Effects	(1–12)	1.41 ± 0.098	1.22 ± 0.056	1.32 ± 0.603	0.093
Total		59 (13.4%)	55 (12.6%)	114 (13%)	0.727
Onset	1–3 days post-vaccination	10 (17.2%)	20 (37%)	30 (26.8%)	
	1st week post-vaccination	19 (32.8%)	13 (24.1%)	32 (28.6%)	
	2nd week post-vaccination	11 (19%)	7 (13.0%)	18 (16.1%)	
	3rd week post-vaccination	11 (19%)	10 (18.5%)	21 (18.8%)	
	4th week post-vaccination	7 (12.1%)	4 (7.4%)	11 (9.8%)	
Location of ulcers, vesicles, and blisters	Lips	20 (69.0%)	20 (80.0%)	40 (74.1%)	0.356
	Labial/buccal mucosa	6 (20.7%)	2 (8.0%)	8 (14.8%)	0.191
	Tongue	6 (20.7%)	1 (4.0%)	7 (13%)	0.069
	Palate	4 (13.8%)	1 (4.0%)	5 (9.3%)	0.216
	Gingiva	4 (13.8%)	1 (4.0%)	5 (9.3%)	0.216
Number of ulcers, vesicles, and blisters' locations	(1–5)	1.38 ± 0.728	1.00 ± 0.00	1.20 ± 0.562	**0.012**
	One location affected	21 (72.4%)	25 (100.0%)	46 (85.2%)	
	Two locations affected	6 (20.7%)	0 (0.0%)	6 (11.1%)	
	Three locations affected	1 (3.4%)	0 (0.0%)	1 (1.9%)	
	Four locations affected	1(3.4%)	0 (0.0%)	1 (1.9%)	
Location of white/red plaque	Tongue dorsum	5 (83.3%)	4 (66.7%)	9 (75.0%)	0.505
	Soft palate	1 (16.7%)	1 (16.7%)	2 (16.7%)	1.000
	Labial/buccal mucosa	0 (0.0%)	1 (16.7%)	1 (8.3%)	0.296

[1] Chi-squared test and ANOVA were used with a significance level of <0.05.

3.4.3. Prevalence of Skin-Related Side Effects

A total of 45 (5.2%) participants reported having at least one skin-related side effect following the COVID-19 vaccine. The prevalence of skin-related side effects was insignificantly higher in the ≤43-year-old group (6.2%) than the >43-year-old group (4.1%). The most common skin-related side effect was rash (62.2%), followed by urticaria (22.2%), and other non-specific conditions (20%). Upper limb was the most common location (60%); chest and trunk were the second most common (33.3%), and it was more common among the older age group than the younger age group (Table 8).

Table 8. Prevalence of skin-related side effects of the Pfizer–BioNTech COVID-19 vaccine among healthcare workers in the Czech Republic, January–February 2021.

Variable	Outcome	≤43 Years Old	>43 Years Old	Total	Significance [1]
Side Effect	Rash	17 (63.0%)	11 (61.1%)	28 (62.2%)	0.900
	Urticaria	7 (25.9%)	3 (16.7%)	10 (22.2%)	0.464
	Other	4 (14.8%)	5 (27.8%)	9 (20.0%)	0.287
Number of Side Effects	(1–3)	1.03 ± 0.183	1.05 ± 0.224	1.04 ± 0.198	0.774
Total		27 (6.2%)	18 (4.1%)	45 (5.2%)	0.181
Location of skin-related side effects	Upper limb	18 (66.7%)	9 (50.0%)	27 (60.0%)	0.264
	Chest/trunk	8 (29.6%)	7 (38.9%)	15 (33.3%)	0.519
	Lower limb	7 (25.9%)	3 (16.7%)	10 (22.2%)	0.464
	Face	5 (18.5%)	4 (22.2%)	9 (20.0%)	0.761
	Back	5 (18.5%)	3 (16.7%)	8 (17.8%)	0.874
Number of locations	(1–5)	1.59 ± 0.797	1.44 ± 0.856	1.53 ± 0.815	0.556

[1] Chi-squared test and ANOVA were used with a significance level of <0.05.

3.4.4. COVID-19 Vaccine Side Effects and Medical Anamneses

The correlation test between the composite variables of side effects and medical anamnesis revealed a significant direct association between the total number of general side effects and the total number of medical treatments ($r = 0.108$; $p = 0.041$). Age was significantly inversely correlated with the total number of general side effects ($r = -0.180$; $p < 0.001$).

The general side effects' duration was significantly and directly correlated with age ($r = 0.097$; $p = 0.006$), the total number of medical treatments ($r = 0.122$; $p = 0.021$), and the total number of general side effects ($r = 0.256$; $p < 0.001$). The total number of NCDs was directly correlated with age ($r = 0.182$; $p = 0.003$), the total number of medical treatments ($r = 0.232$; $p < 0.001$), and the total number of general side effects ($r = 0.072$; $p = 0.258$).

Similarly, the oral side effects were inversely, but not significantly, correlated with age ($r = -0.164$; $p = 0.086$). The total number of oral side effects was positively correlated with the total number of NCDs ($r = 0.045$; $p = 0.790$), the total number of medical treatments ($r = 0.175$; $p = 0.188$), the total number of general side effects ($r = 0.202$; $p = 0.038$), and the general side effects' duration ($r = 0.279$; $p = 0.004$).

The oral side effects' onset was inversely correlated with the ($r = -0.202$; $p = 0.033$), and directly correlated with the total number of NCDs ($r = 0.018$; $p = 0.914$), the total number of medical treatments ($r = 0.168$; $p = 0.208$), the general side effects' duration ($r = 0.025$; $p = 0.794$), and the total number of oral side effects ($r = 0.143$; $p = 0.138$) (Table 9).

Table 9. Correlation between medical anamneses and side effects of Pfizer–BioNTech COVID-19 vaccine among healthcare workers in the Czech Republic, January–February 2021.

		Age	Chronic Illnesses Number	Medical Treatments Number	General SE Number	General SE Duration	Oral SE Number	Oral SE Onset
Age	*r*	1	0.180 **	0.016	−0.180 **	0.097 **	−0.164	−0.202 *
	Sig.		0.003	0.756	0.000	0.005	0.086	0.033
	n	874	271	384	814	807	111	112
Chronic Illnesses Number	*r*	0.180 **	1	0.232 **	0.072	0.088	0.045	0.018
	Sig.	0.003		0.000	0.258	0.167	0.790	0.914
	n	271	272	249	249	246	38	37
Medical Treatments Number	*r*	0.016	0.232 **	1	0.108 *	0.122 *	0.175	0.168
	Sig.	0.756	0.000		0.041	0.021	0.188	0.208
	n	384	249	386	359	354	58	58
General SE Number	*r*	−0.180 **	0.072	0.108 *	1	0.256 **	0.202 *	−0.054
	Sig.	0.000	0.258	0.041		0.000	0.038	0.574
	n	814	249	359	817	809	106	109
General SE Duration	*r*	0.097 **	0.088	0.122 *	0.256 **	1	0.279 **	0.025
	Sig.	0.005	0.167	0.021	0.000		0.004	0.794
	n	807	246	354	809	809	106	107
Oral SE Number	*r*	−0.164	0.045	0.175	0.202 *	0.279 **	1	0.143
	Sig.	0.086	0.790	0.188	0.038	0.004		0.138
	n	111	38	58	106	106	111	109
Oral SE Onset	*r*	−0.202 *	0.018	0.168	−0.054	0.025	0.143	1
	Sig.	0.033	0.914	0.208	0.574	0.794	0.138	
	n	112	37	58	109	107	109	113

* Correlation is significant at the 0.05 level (2-tailed); ** Correlation is significant at the 0.01 level (2-tailed); SE, side effects.

3.4.5. Risk Factors of COVID-19 Vaccine Side Effects

Injection site pain was significantly more prevalent among the younger age group (p = 0.001), the healthcare workers with shorter work experience (p = 0.009), the participants with diabetes mellitus type-2 (p = 0.019), and the participants receiving antidiabetic drugs (p = 0.038) and venous insufficiency drugs (p = 0.028).

Injection site swelling was significantly more prevalent among females (p = 0.021), the participants receiving corticosteroids (p = 0.028), and the previously infected participants (p = 0.030).

Injection site redness was significantly more prevalent among the participants with allergies (p = 0.018), and the participants receiving antihistamine drugs (p = 0.013), and corticosteroids (p = 0.001). It was also significantly associated with the total number of NCDs (p = 0.010), and the total number of medical treatments (p = 0.031).

Fatigue was significantly more prevalent among the young age group (p = 0.024), the healthcare workers with shorter work experience (p = 0.026), and the participants not receiving cholesterol-lowering drugs (p = 0.010).

Headache was significantly more prevalent among females (p = 0.006), the young age group (p = 0.003), the healthcare workers with shorter work experience (p = 0.007), and the participants receiving antihistamine drugs (p = 0.007).

Nausea was significantly more prevalent among females (p = 0.015), the healthcare workers with shorter work experience (p = 0.029), and the participants receiving antihistamine drugs (p = 0.027), and antidepressants (p = 0.013).

Feeling unwell was significantly more prevalent among the younger age group (p = 0.032), the healthcare workers with shorter work experience (p = 0.003), and the participants with hepatologic disease (p = 0.006) and renal disease (p = 0.008).

Muscle pain was significantly more prevalent among the younger age group (p = 0.025), the participants receiving antidepressants (p = 0.053) and antiepileptics (p = 0.018), and the previously exposed participants to COVID-19 (p = 0.007).

Joint pain was significantly more prevalent among the participants with NCDs ($p = 0.041$) and hepatologic disease ($p = 0.041$), the participants receiving antibiotics ($p = 0.034$) and antidepressants ($p = 0.021$), and the previously exposed participants ($p = 0.027$).

Fever was significantly more prevalent among the healthcare workers with shorter work experience ($p = 0.014$), the participants with NCDs ($p = 0.033$) and asthma ($p = 0.008$), the participants receiving antihistamine drugs ($p = 0.011$) and NSAIDs ($p = 0.035$), and the previously infected participants ($p = 0.023$).

Chills were significantly more prevalent among the healthcare workers with shorter work experience ($p = 0.005$), and the participants receiving antihistamine drugs ($p = 0.014$) and NSAIDs ($p = 0.029$).

Lymphadenopathy was significantly more prevalent among the participants receiving antihistamine drugs ($p = 0.019$).

3.4.6. Number of Doses and Side Effects' Prevalence

The prevalence of injection site pain, swelling, redness, fatigue, headache, nausea, muscle pain, lymphadenopathy was higher among the participants who received two doses compared to the participants with one dose. Injection site redness was the only general side effect that was significantly more prevalent in the two-doses group (23.9%) than the one-dose group (8%), with a p-value of 0.10.

The oral side effects were insignificantly more prevalent in the one dose group, e.g., ulcers, white/red plaque, and bleeding gingiva. In contrast, vesicles, blisters, burning gingiva, swollen lips, angular cheilitis, xerostomia, taste disturbance, and tongue tingling were more common in the two-dose group. The mean total number of oral side effects was higher in the one-dose group (Table 10).

Table 10. Number of doses and the side effects of Pfizer–BioNTech COVID-19 vaccine among healthcare workers in the Czech Republic, January–February 2021.

	One Dose	Two Doses	Significance [1]
Injection site pain	44 (88%)	690 (90%)	0.657
Injection site swelling	12 (24%)	197 (25.7%)	0.791
Injection site redness	4 (8%)	183 (23.9%)	**0.010**
Fatigue	30 (60%)	477 (62.2%)	0.757
Headache	21 (42%)	353 (46%)	0.580
Nausea	6 (12%)	101 (13.2%)	0.812
Feeling unwell	16 (32%)	173 (22.6%)	0.125
Muscle pain	18 (36%)	286 (37.3%)	0.855
Chills	17 (34%)	260 (33.9%)	0.988
Joint pain	17 (34%)	210 (27.4%)	0.311
Fever	11 (22%)	168 (21.9%)	0.987
Lymphadenopathy	8 (16%)	124 (16.2%)	0.975
Number of General SE	4.08 ± 2.52	4.20 ± 2.63	0.752
Ulcers	1 (14.3%)	15 (13.9%)	0.977
Vesicles	0 (0%)	4 (3.7%)	0.604
Blisters	2 (28.6%)	39 (36.1%)	0.687
White/red plaque	1 (14.3%)	11 (10.2%)	0.731
Halitosis	4 (57.1%)	25 (23.1%)	**0.045**
Bleeding gingiva	2 (28.6%)	11 (10.2%)	0.137
Burning gingiva	0 (0%)	10 (9.3%)	0.399
Swollen lips	0 (0%)	4 (3.7%)	0.604
Angular cheilitis	0 (0%)	5 (4.6%)	0.561
Xerostomia	0 (0%)	3 (2.8%)	0.655
Taste disturbance	0 (0%)	4 (3.7%)	0.604
Tongue tingling	0 (0%)	5 (4.6%)	0.561
Number of Oral SEs	1.43 ± 1.13	1.31 ± 0.56	0.610
Rash	2 (100%)	26 (60.5%)	0.260
Urticaria	0 (0%)	10 (23.3%)	0.439
Other skin-related SEs	0 (0%)	9 (20.9%)	0.469
Number of skin-related SEs	1 ± 0	1.04 ± 0.202	0.774

[1] Chi-squared test and ANOVA were used with a significance level of <0.05.

3.4.7. Oral and General Side Effects of COVID-19 Vaccine

The emergence of oral side effects was significantly associated with some general side effects, e.g., headache ($\chi^2 = 13.18$; $p < 0.001$), nausea ($\chi^2 = 10.36$; $p = 0.001$), muscle pain ($\chi^2 = 4.56$; $p = 0.033$), fever ($\chi^2 = 4.86$; $p = 0.027$), and lymphadenopathy ($\chi^2 = 9.78$; $p = 0.002$). In addition to the association between the total number of general side effects, their duration, and the emergence of oral side effects, blisters were significantly lower among the participants receiving thyroid hormone replacements ($\chi^2 = 4.05$; $p = 0.044$). In contrast, angular cheilitis was significantly more prevalent among the participants receiving thyroid hormone replacements ($\chi^2 = 7.2$; $p = 0.007$).

4. Discussion

The first evidence to evaluate the efficacy of the Pfizer–BioNTech COVID-19 vaccine was obtained from a randomized controlled trial (RCT) which recruited 43,000 volunteers with a median age of 52 years old. The early results of this RCT showed that the vaccine's efficacy was around 95%, with several adverse reactions that occurred in the few days following the vaccine shot [19]. The vaccine's side effects could be categorized as either local or systemic reactions, and their severity varied from mild to moderate [31].

The present study reported a statistically significant difference in the prevalence of injection site pain ($p = 0.001$), fatigue ($p = 0.026$), headache ($p = 0.003$), muscle pain ($p = 0.023$), and feeling unwell ($p = 0.038$) between the ≤43-year-old group and the >43-year-old group, where the younger adults were more frequently affected. These findings are consistent with those reported by the Food and Drug Administration (FDA): injection site pain was more prevalent in the ≤55-year-old group than the >55-year-old group (80.56% vs. 68.75%); fatigue was more prevalent in the younger group (53.13% vs. 42%), headache was also more prevalent in the younger group (46.57% vs. 31.8%); and muscle pain was more prevalent in the younger group (28.94% vs. 21.03%) [19].

However, differences between the age groups in terms of fever, chills and joint pain were not statistically significant in our sample: the ≤43-year-old group was more affected by fever (9.47% vs. 5.98%), chills (36.8% vs. 30.9%) and joint pain (28.6% vs. 26.9%) than the >43-year-old group. These trends were similar to the FDA's report, where fever was more prevalent among young adults than old adults (24.3% vs. 19.1%), and the same pattern was recorded for chills (24.11% vs. 14.15%) and joint pain (16.18% vs. 13.52%). In contrast to the manufacturer's data, injection site swelling (26% vs. 25.2%) and injection site redness (25.5% vs. 20.4%) were more frequent in the younger age group of our sample. According to the FDA's report, injection site swelling was slightly less frequent among the younger adults (6.02% vs. 7.51%). Injection site redness was also slightly less frequent among the younger adults (5.37% vs. 5.92%).

The overall frequency of systemic reactions including fever, fatigue, headache, chills, vomiting, diarrhea, muscle pain and joint pain was significantly higher among the younger adults than the older adults, according to the FDA's report (82.8% vs. 70.6%). The same pattern was reported for local reactions, including injection site pain, swelling, and redness, where 88.7% of younger adults were affected compared to 79.7% of the older. This pattern was identified in our sample; the mean number of side effects (4.50 ± 2.596 vs. 3.87 ± 2.599) and the overall frequency of affected participants (94.8% vs. 91.5%) were significantly higher in the younger than the older.

The overall frequencies of injection site pain (89.8% vs. 75.35%), injection site swelling (25.6% vs. 6.44%), and injection site swelling (23% vs. 5.5%) were significantly higher among the Czech healthcare workers than the volunteers of the Pfizer–BioNTech trial [19]. In contrast, the overall frequency of headache was quite consistent between the Czech sample and the FDA's report (45.6% vs. 40.06%, respectively).

On comparing the first dose and the second dose of the vaccine, the FDA's report revealed that the frequency of local side effects was slightly higher after the second dose compared to the first dose. The same trend was more significant in the case of systemic side effects [19]. The Czech data confirmed this trend in all the reported side effects except for injection site redness, which was more frequent among the people with one dose only.

Injection site pain as a subjectively reported symptom has a number of confounders that are worth being considered for future research on vaccines' side effects, including injection technique, vaccine temperature, and injection velocity. These confounders are difficult to be standardized and will significantly impact one's experience [32]. Moreover, injection in a relaxed muscle leads to less pain compared to a tensed one; therefore, it is recommended to lower the patient's arm which will be injected. Vaccines in situ are preserved in very low temperature, including the BNT162b2 vaccine which requires −70 °C, and if injected without optimal warming up, this may increase the probability of post-vaccination pain of the injection site [33]. Additionally, muscle mass might play a role in pain perception following the injection. The healthcare workers involved in the vaccination process are highly recommended to receive appropriate training on optimal injection techniques to reduce inequalities in patients' experience of pain after vaccination [34].

The allergic population that used antihistamine drugs were the most susceptible group for experiencing side effects, because they were significantly affected by injection site redness (χ^2 = 6.27; p = 0.012), headache (χ^2 = 7.5; p = 0.006), nausea (χ^2 = 4.97; p = 0.026), fever (χ^2 = 6.62; p = 0.01), chills (χ^2 = 6.1; p = 0.014), and lymphadenopathy (χ^2 = 5.54; p = 0.019). The Centers for Disease Control and Prevention (CDC) had stated, within its interim guidelines for COVID-19 vaccine rollout, that people with a history of any immediate allergic reaction to other vaccines or injectable therapies should be vaccinated with high precaution. People with a history of severe allergic reactions such as anaphylaxis after a previous dose or to a component of the vaccine such as polyethylene glycol (PEG) are prohibited from receiving the vaccine at this stage [31]. Although people with allergies to oral medications, food, pets, insects, venom, latex, and other environmental insults and family histories are recommended to proceed with receiving the vaccine normally, it is worth noting that antihistamine consumption increases considerably in spring in Europe; therefore, special attention should be given to the prescription of these drugs during this season in the context of vaccination. This result will be further explored in our upcoming study phase.

Lymphadenopathy of the arm and neck was among the unsolicited side effects in the FDA's report with 64 cases; however, it should have been a predictable side effect due to it being common with other vaccines such as the human papillomavirus vaccine and influenza vaccine [35–37] Therefore, in this study, lymphadenopathy was among the general side effects of the COVID-19 vaccine and its overall prevalence was 16.2%, with a higher frequency among females compared to males (16.8% vs. 10.6%), young adults compared to old adults (17.3% vs. 15.1%), and people with allergies (21.4% vs. 14.5%), asthma (17.6% vs. 14.1%), bowel disease (25% vs. 14.3%), cardiac disease (25% vs. 14.2%), COPD (20% vs. 14.8%), DM type-2 (19% vs. 14.5%), and neurologic disease (30% vs. 14.2%). The majority of participants with lymphadenopathy reported that its duration was either one day (18.9%), three days (43.9%), or five days (18.2%). This finding is slightly in agreement with the FDA's report, where lymphadenopathy emerged 2–4 days post-vaccination and lasted for approximately 10 days.

The median interval between the first dose and the second dose was 21 days, which is in compliance with the recommended interval of the Czech ministry of health (MOH) [38]. The median patency period between the recovery date and the first vaccine dose was 65 days, which fulfills the recommendation of the Czech MOH for a patency period of seven days between the positive test and the vaccination [39].

The reported NCDs in our sample were generally less frequent than what is reported for the general Czech population. This difference was predictable for this special subset of the population, because medical fitness is a prerequisite for pursuing healthcare professions. Unfortunately, the data on diseases prevalence in the Czech Republic are not stratified by profession or employment sector; therefore, there is no reference prevalence for Czech healthcare workers. Diabetes Mellitus type-2 had prevalence in the Czech Republic around

7.4% (2017); however, in our sample, its prevalence was considerably lower 2.63% [40,41]. Cardiac disease and chronic hypertension had prevalence around 4.3% and 23.7%, respectively (2019), which were two-fold higher than the prevalence values of our sample, which were 1.83% and 11.44%, respectively [42,43]. In contrast, asthma had a prevalence in the Czech Republic 4.5% (2018), while in our sample it was 6.75% [44]. Thyroid disease had a prevalence in the Czech Republic in 7.5% (2015) which was similar to our sample (7.89%) [45].

4.1. Strengths and Limitations

The findings of this study should be interpreted cautiously regarding the association of side effects with the second dose of the vaccine, because we did not ask whether the side effect occurred after the first dose or the second dose. The external validity of this study is limited because the sample was not equally distributed across gender or profession. Another methodological limitation is due to the survey-based technique that may lead to self-selection bias, when perhaps only the highly motivated participants filled in the questionnaire. The self-reporting nature of the collected data compromises its objectivity when it comes to clinical evaluation and standardization. This methodological confounding had been controlled to some degree because all the study's participants were healthcare workers who have a high level of health literacy and medical expertise, so the outcomes were supposed to be accurately reported. To the best of our knowledge, this was the first independent study dealing with the BNT162b2 vaccine side effects, and the first designed study evaluating the side effects among a European population.

4.2. Study Implications

1. Further independent (non-sponsored) epidemiological studies for COVID-19 vaccine side effects should be carried out by academic institutions in the upcoming months to increase public confidence in the vaccines' safety and accelerate its uptake process.
2. The upcoming studies will benefit from comparing data of different vaccines from other manufacturers.
3. The upcoming studies of vaccine side effects should distinguish between the side effects that emerged after the first dose, the second dose, and both doses.
4. Healthcare workers and healthcare students are among the ideal population groups to participate in this type of studies due to their high level of health literacy and scientific motivation.
5. The potential association between antihistamine drugs and the vaccine side effects' frequency should be further explored.

5. Conclusions

The most common side effects of the Pfizer–BioNTech COVID-19 vaccine among Czech healthcare workers were injection site pain, fatigue, headache, muscle pain, chills, and joint pain. They were highly consistent with the data reported by the manufacturer in terms of their association with the younger age group and the second dose. The overall prevalence of some local and systemic side effects was higher than the manufacturer's report; this could be attributed to the special type of population enrolled in this study. Antihistamines were the most common drugs associated with side effect emergence, which might require special attention in the following months. The oral side effects were significantly associated with headache, nausea, muscle pain, fever, and lymphadenopathy. Further independent studies on vaccine safety are strongly required to strengthen the public confidence in the vaccine, and to provide a better understanding of the potential risk factors of vaccine side effects.

Supplementary Materials: The following are available online at https://www.mdpi.com/article/10.3390/jcm10071428/s1, Table S1: OSECV Instrument (in Czech).

Author Contributions: Conceptualization, A.R. and M.K. (Miloslav Klugar); methodology, A.R. and S.A.; validation, S.A., J.K. and M.K. (Miloslav Klugar); formal analysis, A.R. and M.K. (Miloslav Klugar); investigation, A.P. and M.K. (Michal Koščík); data curation, A.P. and M.K. (Michal Koščík); writing—original draft preparation, A.R.; writing—review and editing, A.P., S.A., J.K. and M.K. (Michal Koščík); supervision, M.K. (Miloslav Klugar); project administration, A.R.; funding acquisition, M.K. All authors have read and agreed to the published version of the manuscript.

Funding: This study was funded by Masaryk University, grant numbers MUNI/IGA/1543/2020 and MUNI/A/1608/2020. The work of A.R., A.P., J.K., and M.K. (Miloslav Klugar) was supported by the INTER-EXCELLENCE grant number LTC20031—"Towards an International Network for Evidence-based Research in Clinical Health Research in the Czech Republic". The work of M.K. (Michal Koščík) was supported by the European Regional Development Fund–Project CZECRIN_4 PACIENTY (No. CZ.02.1.01/0.0/0.0/16_013/0001826) and the project Large Research infrastructure CZECRIN (LM2018128).

Institutional Review Board Statement: The study was conducted according to the guidelines of the Declaration of Helsinki and approved by the Ethics Committee of the Faculty of Medicine, Masaryk University Ref. 2/2021 on 20 January 2021.

Informed Consent Statement: Informed consent was obtained from all participants involved in the study.

Data Availability Statement: The data that support the findings of this study are available from the corresponding author upon reasonable request.

Acknowledgments: This work is dedicated to the more than two million worldwide fatalities and their families who have fallen victim to COVID-19. The authors thank Lydie Izakovičová Hollá and Lenka Součková for their help with dissemination of questionnaires among the potential participants of the study.

Conflicts of Interest: The authors declare no conflict of interest.

References

1. Butler, R.; MacDonald, N.E.; Eskola, J.; Liang, X.; Chaudhuri, M.; Dube, E.; Gellin, B.; Goldstein, S.; Larson, H.; Manzo, M.L.; et al. Diagnosing the determinants of vaccine hesitancy in specific subgroups: The Guide to Tailoring Immunization Programmes (TIP). *Vaccine* **2015**, *33*, 4176–4179. [CrossRef]
2. Harrison, E.A.; Wu, J.W. Vaccine confidence in the time of COVID-19. *Eur. J. Epidemiol.* **2020**, *35*, 325–330. [CrossRef]
3. Dror, A.A.; Eisenbach, N.; Taiber, S.; Morozov, N.G.; Mizrachi, M.; Zigron, A.; Srouji, S.; Sela, E. Vaccine hesitancy: The next challenge in the fight against COVID-19. *Eur. J. Epidemiol.* **2020**, *35*, 775–779. [CrossRef] [PubMed]
4. Luyten, J.; Bruyneel, L.; van Hoek, A.J. Assessing vaccine hesitancy in the UK population using a generalized vaccine hesitancy survey instrument. *Vaccine* **2019**, *37*, 2494–2501. [CrossRef] [PubMed]
5. Szmyd, B.; Bartoszek, A.; Karuga, F.F.; Staniecka, K.; Błaszczyk, M.; Radek, M. Medical Students and SARS-CoV-2 Vaccination: Attitude and Behaviors. *Vaccines* **2021**, *9*, 128. [CrossRef]
6. Szmyd, B.; Karuga, F.F.; Bartoszek, A.; Staniecka, K.; Siwecka, N.; Bartoszek, A.; Błaszczyk, M.; Radek, M. Attitude and Behaviors towards SARS-CoV-2 Vaccination among Healthcare Workers: A Cross-Sectional Study from Poland. *Vaccines* **2021**, *9*, 218. [CrossRef]
7. Jarrett, C.; Wilson, R.; O'Leary, M.; Eckersberger, E.; Larson, H.J.; Eskola, J.; Liang, X.; Chaudhuri, M.; Dube, E.; Gellin, B.; et al. Strategies for addressing vaccine hesitancy—A systematic review. *Vaccine* **2015**, *33*, 4180–4190. [CrossRef]
8. Attia, S.; Howaldt, H.-P. Impact of COVID-19 on the Dental Community: Part I before Vaccine (BV). *J. Clin. Med.* **2021**, *10*, 288. [CrossRef]
9. Sawires, L. Effects of the Influenza Vaccine on the Oral Cavity. 2018. Available online: https://stars.library.ucf.edu/cgi/viewcontent.cgi?article=1306&context=honorstheses (accessed on 16 December 2020).
10. Gonçalves, A.K.; Cobucci, R.N.; Rodrigues, H.M.; De Melo, A.G.; Giraldo, P.C. Safety, tolerability and side effects of human papillomavirus vaccines: A systematic quantitative review. *Braz. J. Infect. Dis.* **2014**, *18*, 651–659. [CrossRef]
11. Riad, A.; Klugar, M.; Krsek, M. COVID-19 Related Oral Manifestations, Early Disease Features? *Oral Dis.* **2020**. [CrossRef]
12. Riad, A.; Kassem, I.; Issa, J.; Badrah, M.; Klugar, M. Angular cheilitis of COVID-19 patients: A case-series and literature review. *Oral Dis.* **2020**. [CrossRef]
13. Riad, A.; Kassem, I.; Stanek, J.; Badrah, M.; Klugarova, J.; Klugar, M. Aphthous Stomatitis in COVID-19 Patients: Case-series and Literature Review. *Dermatol. Ther.* **2021**, *34*, e14735. [CrossRef] [PubMed]
14. Riad, A.; Kassem, I.; Hockova, B.; Badrah, M.; Klugar, M. Tongue ulcers associated with SARS-CoV-2 infection: A case series. *Oral Dis.* **2020**. [CrossRef]

15. Hocková, B.; Riad, A.; Valky, J.; Šulajová, Z.; Stebel, A.; Slávik, R.; Bečková, Z.; Pokorná, A.; Klugarová, J.; Klugar, M. Oral Complications of ICU Patients with COVID-19: Case-Series and Review of Two Hundred Ten Cases. *J. Clin. Med.* **2021**, *10*, 581. [CrossRef]
16. Riad, A.; Gad, A.; Hockova, B.; Klugar, M. Oral candidiasis in non-severe COVID-19 patients: Call for antibiotic stewardship. *Oral Surg.* **2020**. [CrossRef] [PubMed]
17. Riad, A.; Kassem, I.; Badrah, M.; Klugar, M. The manifestation of oral mucositis in COVID-19 patients: A case-series. *Dermatol. Ther.* **2020**, *33*. [CrossRef] [PubMed]
18. Maspero, C.; Abate, A.; Cavagnetto, D.; El Morsi, M.; Fama, A.; Farronato, M. Available Technologies, Applications and Benefits of Teleorthodontics. A Literature Review and Possible Applications during the COVID-19 Pandemic. *J. Clin. Med.* **2020**, *9*, 1891. [CrossRef]
19. Centres for Diseases Control and Prevention (CDC). Reactions and Adverse Events of the Pfizer-BioNTech COVID-19 Vaccine. Available online: https://www.cdc.gov/vaccines/covid-19/info-by-product/pfizer/reactogenicity.html (accessed on 7 March 2021).
20. Masaryk University. Oral Side Effects of COVID-19 Vaccine (OSECV). 2021. Available online: https://clinicaltrials.gov/ct2/show/NCT04706156 (accessed on 24 February 2021).
21. Von Elm, E.; Altman, D.G.; Egger, M.; Pocock, S.J.; Gøtzsche, P.C.; Vandenbroucke, J.P. The Strengthening the Reporting of Observational Studies in Epidemiology (STROBE) Statement: Guidelines for reporting observational studies. *Ann. Int. Med.* **2007**, *147*, 573–577. [CrossRef]
22. Ústav Zdravotnických Informací a Statistiky České Republiky (ÚZIS ČR). Systém Hlášení Nežádoucích Událostí (SHNU). 2021. Available online: https://shnu.uzis.cz/ (accessed on 8 March 2021).
23. CZECRIN. Czech Clinical Research Infrastructure Network. Available online: https://czecrin.cz/en/home/ (accessed on 2 March 2021).
24. Proton Technologies AG. General Data Protection Regulation (GDPR) Compliance Guidelines. HORIZON 2020—Project REP-791727-1. Available online: https://gdpr.eu/ (accessed on 1 May 2020).
25. Ministry of Interior—Czech Republic. Who Will Be Vaccinated First? Covid Portál. Available online: https://covid.gov.cz/en/situations/register-vaccination/who-will-be-vaccinated-first (accessed on 2 March 2021).
26. Tarakji, B.; Umair, A.; Alakeel, R.; Ashok, N.; Azzeghaibi, S.; Darwish, S.; Mahmoud, R.; Elkhatat, E. Hepatitis B vaccination and associated oral manifestations: A non-systematic review of literature and case reports. *Ann. Med. Health Sci. Res.* **2014**, *4*, 829. [CrossRef]
27. McHugh, M.L. Interrater reliability: The kappa statistic. *Biochem. Med.* **2012**, *22*, 276–282. [CrossRef]
28. OECD. *Health at a Glance 2019*; OECD: Paris, France, 2019; ISBN 9789264382084.
29. Národní Pedagogický Institut České Republiky. Odborní Pracovníci v Oblasti Zdravotnictví Kromě Všeobecných Sester bez Specializace. Available online: https://www.infoabsolvent.cz/Temata/ClanekAbsolventi/8-8-17 (accessed on 8 March 2021).
30. Institute of Health Information and Statistics of the Czech Republic (UZIS). Health Yearbook of the Czech Republic 2017. 2018. Available online: https://www.uzis.cz/index-en.php?pg=record&id=8166 (accessed on 3 March 2021).
31. Oliver, S.E.; Gargano, J.W.; Marin, M.; Wallace, M.; Curran, K.G.; Chamberland, M.; McClung, N.; Campos-Outcalt, D.; Morgan, R.L.; Mbaeyi, S.; et al. The Advisory Committee on Immunization Practices' Interim Recommendation for Use of Pfizer-BioNTech COVID-19 Vaccine—United States, December 2020. *Morb. Mortal. Wkly. Rep.* **2020**, *69*, 1922–1924. [CrossRef]
32. Ozdemir, L.; Pnarc, E.; Akay, B.N.; Akyol, A. Effect of Methylprednisolone Injection Speed on the Perception of Intramuscular Injection Pain. *Pain Manag. Nurs.* **2013**, *14*, 3–10. [CrossRef]
33. Centers for Disease Control and Prevention (CDC). Interim Clinical Considerations for Use of COVID-19 Vaccines. Available online: https://www.cdc.gov/vaccines/covid-19/info-by-product/clinical-considerations.html?CDC_AA_refVal=https%3A%2F%2Fwww.cdc.gov%2Fvaccines%2Fcovid-19%2Finfo-by-product%2Fpfizer%2Fclinical-considerations.html (accessed on 7 March 2021).
34. Training and Education Resources | COVID-19 Vaccination | CDC. Available online: https://www.cdc.gov/vaccines/covid-19/training-education-resources.html (accessed on 8 March 2021).
35. Pereira, M.P.; Flores, P.; Neto, A.S. Neck and supraclavicular lymphadenopathy secondary to 9-valent human papillomavirus vaccination. *BMJ Case Rep.* **2019**, *12*, e231582. [CrossRef]
36. Shirone, N.; Shinkai, T.; Yamane, T.; Uto, F.; Yoshimura, H.; Tamai, H.; Imai, T.; Inoue, M.; Kitano, S.; Kichikawa, K.; et al. Axillary lymph node accumulation on FDG-PET/CT after influenza vaccination. *Ann. Nucl. Med.* **2012**, *26*, 248–252. [CrossRef]
37. Studdiford, J.; Lamb, K.; Horvath, K.; Altshuler, M.; Stonehouse, A. Development of Unilateral Cervical and Supraclavicular Lymphadenopathy After Human Papilloma Virus Vaccination. *Pharmacotherapy* **2008**, *28*, 1194–1197. [CrossRef]
38. Ministry of Interior—Czech Republic. Information about Available Vaccines. Covid Portál. 2021. Available online: https://covid.gov.cz/en/situations/information-about-vaccine/information-about-available-vaccines (accessed on 3 March 2021).
39. Ministry of Interior—Czech Republic. Specific Situations during Vaccination. Covid Portál. 2021. Available online: https://covid.gov.cz/en/situations/information-about-vaccine/specific-situations-during-vaccination (accessed on 3 March 2021).
40. ÚZIS-ČR. *Stručný Přehled Činnosti Oboru Diabetologie a Endokrinologie 2017*; Ústav Zdravotnických Informací a Statistiky ČR: Prague, Czech Republic, 2007.

41. Klugar, M.; Klugarová, J.; Pokorná, A.; Benešová, K.; Jarkovský, J.; Dolanová, D.; Mužík, J.; Líčeník, R.; Prázný, M.; Búřilová, P.; et al. Use of epidemiological analyses in Clinical Practice Guideline development focused on the diabetic patients treated with insulin. *Int. J. Evid. Based. Healthc.* **2019**, *17*, S48–S52. [CrossRef]
42. Klugar, M.; Hunčovský, M.; Pokorná, A.; Dolanová, D.; Benešová, K.; Jarkovský, J.; Mužík, J.; Líčeník, R.; Nečas, T.; Búřilová, P.; et al. Epidemiological analyses for preparation of Clinical Practice Guidelines related to acute coronary syndromes in the Czech Republic. *Int. J. Evid. Based. Healthc.* **2019**, *17*, S43–S47. [CrossRef]
43. ÚZIS-ČR. *Zdravotnická ročenka ČR 2018;* Ústav Zdravotnických Informací a Statistiky ČR: Prague, Czech Republic, 2018.
44. ÚZIS-ČR. *Stručný Přehled Činnosti Oboru Pneumologie a Ftizeologie za Období 2007–2019;* Ústav Zdravotnických Informací a Statistiky ČR: Prague, Czech Republic, 2007.
45. Bílek, R.; Horakova, L.; Gos, R.; Zamrazil, V. Thyroid disease in the Czech Republic: The EUthyroid project and the evaluation of the General Health Insurance Company epidemiological data for the period of 2012–2015. *Vnitř. Lék.* **2017**, *63*, 548–554.

Journal of
Clinical Medicine

MDPI

Review

Characteristics and Detection Rate of SARS-CoV-2 in Alternative Sites and Specimens Pertaining to Dental Practice: An Evidence Summary

Sajjad Shirazi [1,*], Clark M. Stanford [2] and Lyndon F. Cooper [1]

[1] Department of Oral Biology, College of Dentistry, University of Illinois at Chicago, 801 S Paulina St, Chicago, IL 60612, USA; cooperlf@uic.edu
[2] Department of Restorative Dentistry, University of Illinois at Chicago, Chicago, IL 60612, USA; cmstan60@uic.edu
* Correspondence: s.shirazi.tbzmed88@gmail.com

Abstract: Knowledge about the detection potential and detection rates of severe acute respiratory syndrome coronavirus 2 (SARS-CoV-2) in various body fluids and sites is important for dentists since they, directly or indirectly, deal with many of these fluids/sites in their daily practices. In this study, we attempt to review the latest evidence and meta-analysis studies regarding the detection rate of SARS-CoV-2 in different body specimens and sites as well as the characteristics of these sample. The presence/detection of SARS-CoV-2 viral biomolecules (nucleic acid, antigens, antibody) in different clinical specimens depends greatly on the specimen type and timing of collection. These specimens/sites include nasopharynx, oropharynx, nose, saliva, sputum, bronchoalveolar lavage, stool, urine, ocular fluid, serum, plasma and whole blood. The relative detection rate of SARS-CoV-2 viral biomolecules in each of these specimens/sites is reviewed in detail within the text. The infectious potential of these specimens depends mainly on the time of specimen collection and the presence of live replicating viral particles.

Keywords: dentistry; RT-PCR testing; antigen; antibody; saliva; aerosols; body fluids; viral load; epidemiological monitoring; COVID-19

Citation: Shirazi, S.; Stanford, C.M.; Cooper, L.F. Characteristics and Detection Rate of SARS-CoV-2 in Alternative Sites and Specimens Pertaining to Dental Practice: An Evidence Summary. *J. Clin. Med.* **2021**, *10*, 1158. https://doi.org/10.3390/jcm10061158

Academic Editor: Hans-Peter Howaldt

Received: 6 February 2021
Accepted: 8 March 2021
Published: 10 March 2021

1. Introduction

Human viral infection and transmission can occur through multiple routes, including exposure to infected blood, exchange of saliva or aerosols generated from sneezing, coughing or dental procedures, fecal–oral, ingestion of contaminated food and drinks and sexual contact. Common examples of viruses isolated from the oral cavity include coronavirus, norovirus, human immunodeficiency virus (HIV), rotavirus, hepatitis C virus, influenza viruses herpes simplex viruses 1 and 2 and Epstein–Barr virus [1].

The cause of the coronavirus disease 2019 (COVID-19) is the severe acute respiratory syndrome coronavirus 2 (SARS-CoV-2), which is an enveloped, positive-sense single-stranded ribonucleic acid (RNA) virus (+ssRNA). The genome encodes 27 proteins including a number of non-structural proteins, including an RNA-dependent RNA polymerase (RdRP), putative accessory proteins and four structural proteins, named as surface or spike glycoprotein (S), envelope protein (E), membrane protein (M) and nucleocapsid (N) proteins. The virus binds to an angiotensin-converting enzyme 2 (ACE2) receptor through S protein for host cell entry. The virus also has an RNA proofreading mechanism keeping the mutation rate relatively low.

The practice of dentistry necessitates a close contact between the dentist, patient and dental healthcare personnel for patient care and procedure support. In addition, the use of rotary and ultrasonic instruments as well as air–water syringes create aerosols containing particle droplets of water, saliva, blood, microorganisms and other debris. Therefore, the dental setting is a unique environment in the current pandemic since it potentially possesses all transmission risk factors for SARS-CoV-2 virus, as stated by the Centers for Diseases Control and Prevention (CDC). Accordingly, SARS-CoV-2 mainly spreads between people who are in close contact with each other (within 6 feet or 2 m) through respiratory droplets from an infected person. It can linger in aerosols for hours and be spread by people who are not showing symptoms. SARS-CoV-2 can sometimes be spread by airborne transmission within enclosed spaces that have inadequate ventilation within distances more than 6 feet. Contact with contaminated surfaces is another potential transmission route. The infection occurs when the virus is inhaled or deposited on mucous membranes, including that of the nose and mouth [2,3]. Currently, there is no data available to assess the risk of SARS-CoV-2 transmission during dental practice [4,5].

In a recent survey of 849 Italian dentists, a high level of concern for in-office transmission was noted. Dentists perceive needed improvement and change in screening, hygiene and testing patients for SARS-CoV-2 [6]. The Delphi mythology was used among 197 Latin American implant experts to define the importance placed on minimization of disease transmission [7]. When French dental professionals were surveyed early in the pandemic, laboratory-confirmed prevalence of COVID-19 was 1.9% among dentists. Interestingly, practice limited to endodontics (implying general use of rubber dam) was associated with reduced odds of disease [8]. The importance of protecting oral health workers was underscored. A US survey among dentists conducted in June 2020 indicated that 16.6% of participants were tested using respiratory and blood samples, and demonstrated a 0.9% infection rate [9]. A narrative review of Canadian protocols to reduce disease transmission in the dental office included eight different areas involving administrative, physical and procedural controls. The absence of testing was noted as a potential limitation of practice [10].

The presence/detection of SARS-CoV-2 viral biomolecules (nucleic acid, antigens, antibody) in different clinical specimens has been documented based on the type of fluid or material and timing of collection relative to the onset of infection [11]. An infected individual takes an average of 5–6 days (range, 1–14 days) following exposure to develop symptoms (incubation period). The virus may be detectable in the upper respiratory tract 1–3 days before the onset of symptoms, facilitating pre-symptomatic or asymptomatic transmission, but its load is highest around the time of symptom onset, after which it gradually declines [12,13]. Reports recommend that upper respiratory tract samples may have higher infectivity early in the course of the disease (0–5 days), after which the virus starts moving towards the lower parts of the respiratory system. Lower respiratory tract samples may have higher viral load later in the course of disease [14].

Current guidance from the World Health Organization (WHO) suggests that the detection of SARS-CoV-2 depends on the testing method, clinical presentation and time since symptom onset [13]. The CDC considers nasopharyngeal, oropharyngeal, nasal and saliva samples to have high viral load and infectivity [15]. In addition, positive detection of SARS-CoV-2 in other clinical samples including sputum, fecal matter, urine, ocular fluid and blood has also been highlighted [16].

In this report, we attempt to review the latest evidence regarding the detection rate of SARS-CoV-2 in different body specimens and sites. The knowledge of the detection rate and the infectivity potential of these specimens is essential. This is of particular importance for dentists because they, in their daily practices, directly or indirectly deal with these specimens/sites which might be the port of entry, or replication and transmission site for SARS-CoV-2.

2. Detection of COVID-19 in Alternative Samples/Sites

While SARS-CoV-2 can be detected in a wide range of body fluids and compartments, saliva and respiratory samples remain the main choice for diagnostics. Table 1 summarizes the characteristics of the alternative specimens/sites.

2.1. Nasopharynx/Oropharynx

The nasopharynx and oropharynx are main detection sites in early-stage infection of SARS-CoV-2 in both symptomatic and asymptomatic cases. The peak of viral load in nasopharyngeal samples occurs within the first few days after symptom onset. A special type of swabs (flocked swab, synthetic fiber swabs with plastic shafts) is used as the sample collection tool. Calcium alginate swabs or those with wooden shafts are not recommended since they may interfere with nucleic acid amplification tests (NAATs) or contain substances which inactivate the virus [17]. While dependent on the viral load, nasopharyngeal samples are generally more sensitive than oropharyngeal samples. However, the number of days passed since the onset of symptoms and disease stage influence positive testing [13,18–20]. The infectivity potential of both specimens has been demonstrated [21].

In a meta-analysis of studies comparing at least two respiratory specimen types (oropharyngeal, nasopharyngeal or sputum), the overall positive detection rate with NAATs in confirmed patients was estimated to be 43% (95% confidence interval (CI): 34–52%) for oropharyngeal swabs and 54% (95% CI: 41–67%) for nasopharyngeal swabs. The estimated percentage of positive tests were 75% (95% CI: 60–88%) between days 0–7, 35% (95% CI: 27–43%) between days 8–14 and 12% (95% CI: 2–25%) after 14 days from symptom onset for oropharyngeal swab sampling. For nasopharyngeal swabs, this figure was 80% (95% CI: 66–91%), 59% (95% CI: 53–64%) and 36% (95% CI: 18–57%) at 0–7, 8–14 and >14 days after symptom onset, respectively [20].

A recent meta-analysis of studies comparing paired oropharyngeal and nasopharyngeal samples in confirmed cases found a similar positive detection rate between oropharyngeal and nasopharyngeal swabs (84% (95% CI: 57–100%) vs. 88% (95% CI: 73–98%), respectively) using NAATs. Importantly, there is limited agreement between tests from these sites as the percent of individuals positive for both specimens was only 68% (95% CI: 36–93%) [22]. Nevertheless, combining swabs from both sites has been shown to improve sensitivity and reliability of the results [13]. In addition, a meta-analysis of studies investigating the clinical performance of antigen tests not requiring a separate reading device in confirmed COVID-19 patients revealed a pooled sensitivity of 0.747 (95% CI: 0.673–0.809) for nasopharyngeal or combined oro/nasopharyngeal samples [23].

There are some contraindications for collection of nasopharyngeal samples, including coagulopathy or anticoagulant therapy, and significant nasal septum deviation [24]. Swabs should be placed immediately into a sterile transport tube containing 2–3 mL of either viral transport medium (VTM), Amies transport medium, phosphate-buffered saline, or sterile saline, unless using a test designed to analyze a specimen directly (i.e., without placement in VTM) (Table 1).

2.2. Nasal

Nasal specimen may be obtained with swabs from two anatomical sites, nasal mid-turbinate (deep nasal) and anterior nares, or with nasal wash/aspirate [15]. There is currently no strong evidence regarding SARS-CoV-2 overall positive detection rate in nasal wash compared to other methods. However, Calame et al. [25] compared nasal wash and nasopharyngeal swab sampling and concluded that these methods have comparable clinical and analytical sensitivity.

A meta-analysis of studies comparing paired nasal (either mid-turbinate or anterior nares) and nasopharyngeal samples for NAATs in confirmed cases found that nasal swabs had substantially lower positive detection rate than the nasopharyngeal samples (82% (95% CI: 73–90%) vs. 98% (95% CI: 96–100%), respectively). The percent of individuals positive for both specimens was only 79% (95% CI: 69–88%), suggesting limited agreement. Nasal specimens collected from a single nostril seemed to perform better in comparison to swabs collected from both nares [22]. In addition, studies of only symptomatic patients had a similar positive detection rate for nasal samples as compared to studies of mixed patients. Ultimately, the use of more sensitive assays (limit of detection < 1000 copies/milliliter) for nasal samples resulted in lower positive detection in comparison to assays with limit of detection ≥ 1000 copies/mL. However, this figure was not affected by assay sensitivity in nasopharyngeal samples. This reflects lower viral burden in the mid-turbinate/anterior nares region than the nasopharynx, resulting in lower performance when using highly sensitive assays [22].

A meta-analysis of studies that compared combined oropharyngeal-nasal swabs and nasopharyngeal swabs for NAATs in confirmed cases found an identical positive detection rate (97% (95% CI: 90–100%)) between the two methods. The percent of individuals positive for both specimens was also high (90% (95% CI: 84–96%)) [22].

2.3. Saliva

The detection of SARS-CoV-2 through oral shedding and especially in saliva has been shown. The infectivity potential of saliva has also been well-demonstrated [26]. SARS-CoV-2 viral load in saliva may be a good indicator of the transmission potential of infected patients, since it is highest during the first week of infection, during which a person is most infectious.

Saliva has been shown to yield greater detection sensitivity and consistency throughout the course of infection than the nasopharyngeal samples [18,27–30]. Positive detection rate with NAATs in confirmed cases for saliva samples vary greatly in the literature but is estimated to be higher than 80% [11,31]. A recent meta-analysis of studies comparing paired saliva and nasopharyngeal samples in confirmed cases estimated a positive detection rate of 88% (95% CI: 81–93%) and 94% (95% CI: 90–98%) respectively, with no statistically significant difference. The percent of individuals positive for both the specimens was 79% (95% CI: 71–86%), indicating relatively poor agreement [22]. This study also demonstrated that positive detection rate with NAATs after 7 days from symptom onset was lower compared to ≤7 days (74% (95%CI: 62–85%) vs. 89% (95% CI: 73–99%)), which was also observed for nasopharyngeal swabs in the same patients (91% (95% CI: 82–98%) vs. 99% (95% CI: 90–100%), respectively) [22]. Another meta-analysis estimated an overall diagnostic accuracy of 92.1% (95% CI: 70–98.3%), with sensitivity of 83.9% (95% CI: 77.4–88.8%) and specificity of 96.4% (95% CI: 89.5–98.8) for saliva samples in comparison to nasopharyngeal/oropharyngeal samples in confirmed cases [32]. The sensitivity of saliva was estimated to be 3.4% lower (−3.4%, 95% CI: −9.9–3.1%) than that of nasopharyngeal swabs in another recent meta-analysis [33].

The differences in sensitivity of oral fluids' evaluations are possibly because of large differences in collection, transport, storage and processing techniques, as well as the evaluation of different testing populations and disease stage. Collection methods included spitting or drooling, coughing or clearing throat, collection with pipet or special sponges and gargling with saline solutions [22,24]. It is likely that a simple drooling technique, with no extra stimulation of saliva secretion, will provide the greatest sensitivity [24]. In addition, many studies have supported the hypothesis of coughing (likely mixed sputum and saliva specimen) or deep throat saliva being better than drool/spit. However, considerable differences have not been revealed [22].

Another difference among studies is sample collection in the morning, or avoidance of eating, drinking, or brushing teeth (30 min to 2 h before specimen collection), which lead to a slightly higher positive detection rate. The variable dilution of saliva prior to processing is another difference among the studies. However, the positivity rate is similar in studies utilizing diluted or undiluted saliva samples. Moreover, studies that directly input the saliva specimen into the amplification assay without any pre-processing showed substantially lower positive detection than those which used a nucleic acid extraction step. Additionally, a positive detection rate in saliva samples was shown to be similar between asymptomatic and symptomatic patients [22]. Ultimately, no substantial difference was detected among studies that used assays with low (<1000 copies/milliliter) or high limit of detection for saliva samples, which demonstrates high viral load in saliva samples [22].

To optimize saliva-based testing and obtain a reliable and sensitive result, a specific, standard and optimized saliva collection and transportation method should be utilized.

Also, an optimal solution should be used to collect, transport and store saliva samples. In addition, the RNA isolation and detection protocol should be optimized for saliva, using an appropriate internal control. The use of human DNA is suggested for nasopharyngeal samples but not for saliva samples [24]. The use of saliva samples is quicker, less painful and invasive and allows for higher volume testing, and collection by the patient at home or clinic without posing risks to healthcare providers. Sample includes 1–5 mL of saliva in a sterile, leak-proof screw cap container, with no preservative required (Table 1). The simplicity of saliva-based testing for large populations must be weighed against the reported differences in sensitivity when compared to nasopharyngeal samples.

2.4. Sputum

Sputum is mucus produced in the respiratory tract (the trachea and bronchi) and is collected by coughing up deeply and spitting out directly into a sterile, leak-proof, collection cup. It is indicated later in the course of the COVID-19 disease or in patients with a negative upper respiratory sample result while there is a strong clinical suspicion of COVID-19 [13]. The overall positive detection rate with NAATs in confirmed cases for sputum samples was estimated by a recent meta-analysis to be 71% (95% CI: 61–80%), which was significantly higher than that of nasopharyngeal and oropharyngeal samples in the same study. More specifically, the estimated percentage of COVID-19-positive samples was 98% (95% CI: 89–100%), 69% (95% CI: 57–80%) and 46% (95% CI: 23–70%) at 0–7 days, 8–14 days and >14 days after symptom onset, respectively [20]. In another meta-analysis, an overall accuracy of 79.7% (95% CI: 43.3–95.3%), sensitivity of 90.1% (95% CI: 83.3–96.9%) and specificity of 63.1% (95% CI: 36.8–89.3%) was estimated for deep-throat saliva/posterior oropharyngeal saliva samples in comparison to nasopharyngeal/oropharyngeal samples in confirmed cases [32].

The infectivity and transmissibility potential of sputum has been demonstrated [21]. If spontaneously produced, sputum collection is an easier process than swab sampling and can easily be done by the patient. The collection of coughed or spit samples carries the potential added risk of transmission by aerosolization [13] (Table 1).

2.5. Bronchoalveolar Lavage

Bronchoalveolar lavage is generally collected later in the course of COVID-19, from patients with severe illness or undergoing mechanical ventilation or to determine the recovery of admitted patients [13]. A meta-analysis revealed that it has a positive detection rate of 91.8% (95% CI: 79.9–103.7%) by NAATs, which was higher than that of sputum and nasopharyngeal specimen in the same review [34]. Collecting bronchoalveolar lavage is complex and with high risk of aerosolization. It includes the instillation of sterile normal saline into a sub-segment of the lung, followed by suction and collection. Endotracheal aspiration has a lower risk of aerosolization than bronchoalveolar lavage with comparable sensitivity and specificity [43] (Table 1).

Table 1. Characteristics of the alternative specimens/site for detection of severe acute respiratory syndrome coronavirus 2 (SARS-CoV-2).

Site/Fluid	Collection Method [1]	Self-Sampling	Infectivity Potential	Analyte Detected	Detection Method [2]	Analyte Load	Approximate Time to Peak	Relative Detection Rate [3]	Advantage	Disadvantage
Nasopharynx	Synthetic fiber swabs with plastic or wire shafts with	No, healthcare personnel preferred	Yes	Nucleic acid Viral antigen	NAATs IA	High	0–7 days after symptom onset	54% (95% CI: 41–67%) [20]	Gold standard specimen	Needs trained personnel. Procedure is painful and not easy. Not suitable in individuals prone to nose bleeds or has had recent facial or head injury/surgery
Oropharynx	Synthetic fiber swabs with plastic or wire shafts	Possibly, healthcare personnel preferred	Yes	Nucleic acid	NAATs	High	0–7 days after symptom onset	43% (95% CI: 34–52%) [20]	Easy to operate	Less sensitive than nasopharyngeal swab and sputum.
Nasal (mid-turbinate or anterior nares)	Flocked or spun polyester swab	Yes	Yes	Nucleic acid Viral antigen	NAATs IA	Average	0–7 days after symptom onset	82% (95% CI: 73–90%) [22]	Minimally invasive. Lower risk for healthcare infection	Less sensitive if not collected correctly. Not suitable in individuals prone to nose bleeds or has had recent facial or head injury/surgery
Sputum	Sterile container	Yes	Yes	Nucleic acid	NAATs	Average–high	3–7 days after symptom onset	71% (95% CI: 61–80%) [20]	High yield compared to upper respiratory swab	High risk of infection for operators. The high viscosity of sputum makes it difficult to extract nucleic acids.
Saliva	Sterile container	Yes	Yes	Nucleic acid	NAATs	High	3–7 days after symptom onset	>80% [11,20,31]	Not invasive. Less risk for healthcare infection. Large amount of sample	Less sensitive if not collected correctly. False negative results
Broncho-alveolar lavage fluid	Sterile container	No	Yes	Nucleic acid	NAATs	Medium	7–14 days after symptom onset	91.8% (95% CI: 79.9–103.7%) [34]	High detection rate/low limit of detection	High risk of cross-infection
Stool	Stool container	Yes	Not fully clear	Nucleic acid	NAATs	Medium	>14 days after symptom onset	51.8% (95% CI: 43.8–59.7%) [35]	Less risk for healthcare infection. Non-invasive	Might be confined to later-stage infection diagnosis
Urine	Collection tube	Yes	Not fully clear	Nucleic acid	NAATs	Low	16–21 days	5.74% (95% CI: 2.88–9.44%) [36]	Non-invasive sample collection	Limited data has been studied
Ocular fluid	Tear or conjunctival swab	Possibly, healthcare personnel preferred	Not fully clear	Nucleic acid	NAATs	Low	Unclear	0–28.57% [37–40]	Non-invasive sample collection	No conclusive data available
Blood	Collection tube with anticoagulant	No	Not fully clear	Nucleic acid Antibody	NAATs IA	Low	5–14 days for nucleic acid >10 days for antibody	10% (95% CI: 5–18%) for nucleic acid [41]	Easy to operate, low infectious concern	High false negative rate. High limit of detection.
Serum	Serum separator tubes	No	low	Antibody	IA	High	>14 days for antibody detection	61.2% (95% CI: 53.4–69.0%) for IgM, 58.8% (95% CI: 49.6–68.0%) for IgG, and 62.1% (52.7–71.4%) for IgM-IgG [42]	Rapid, simple and convenient. Sample is more stable. Low cost. Suitable for disease surveillance.	Low sensitivity in the early stage of disease. High false negative rate. Cross-reactivity of antibody and false positive.

[1] Collected specimen may be stored at room temperature for ≤4 h, at 2–8 °C if ≤72 h, and −70 °C if >72 h. Transport should be on dry ice. [2] NAATs: nucleic acid amplification tests. IA: immunoassay. [3] Detection rates are relative to other specimens/sites. See the text for detailed description.

2.6. Stool

Fecal shedding of respiratory viruses is not uncommon and stool samples may contain large viral loads of SARS-CoV-2 at early onset through the convalescent stage of illness. The World Health Organization (WHO) recommends for stool diagnostic testing to be considered from the second week after symptom onset and onwards, suggesting that this positivity is prolonged compared to that of respiratory tract specimens [13]. Detection rate of SARS-CoV-2 RNA in fecal specimens (excluding anal or rectal swabs) among patients with confirmed diagnosis has been estimated to be 43.7% (95% CI: 32.6−55.0%) in a meta-analysis [44]. This figure was 51.8% (95% CI: 43.8–59.7%) in the most recent meta-analysis which used different inclusion criteria, and also, did not exclude anal or rectal swabs. It was estimated that 64% of tested individuals had persistent positive fecal specimens test despite negative respiratory tests for a mean duration of 12.5 days after negative respiratory testing [35]. Importantly, it has been reported that SARS-CoV-2 viral shedding in stool may persist up to 6 weeks after symptom onset [36]. An overall diagnostic sensitivity of 46.0% (95% CI: 13.1–82.7%) and specificity of 91.4% (95% CI: 6.4–99.9%) has been estimated for feces/anal swab in comparison to nasopharyngeal/oropharyngeal samples in confirmed cases [32].

Fecal–oral transmission is an accepted mode of transmission for other coronaviruses such as SARS-associated coronavirus (SARS-CoV) and Middle East respiratory syndrome coronavirus (MERS-CoV) [45]. Detection of live active SARS-CoV-2 virus in stool samples has been reported in the literature, underlining the possibility of fecal–oral transmission through infected feces. However, it is unclear if the positive fecal test results are due to active virion particles or inactive viral RNA amplified by polymerase chain reaction (PCR). Therefore, the infectivity and transmissibility potential of stool has not been established [21,28,35,45]. Fecal specimens are suggested to be tested concurrently with other samples to detect false-positives and/or monitor disease progression.

Nevertheless, the viral detection rate could vary substantially due to the presence of PCR inhibitors (bile, polysaccharides, hemoglobin and bilirubin) which make the process of viral detection very difficult, susceptible to user error and requiring trained technicians and special RNA extraction kits [17,18,46,47]. Sample collection is simple and can often be performed at home by capturing a stool sample (about 10 g or peanut size) in a dry and clean container and transferring into a sterile specimen cup (Table 1).

2.7. Urine

Urinary shedding of SARS-CoV-2 has been highly correlated with disease severity in adults. A recent meta-analysis revealed that the frequency of viral shedding was 4.5% with a weighted pooled estimate of 1.18% (95% CI: 0.14–2.87%) after excluding case reports and case series with small sample size (<9 patients) [48]. The overall urinary shedding of SARS-CoV-2 in confirmed COVID-19 patients was estimated to be 8% in another meta-analysis, with a relative risk of 0.08 (95% CI: 0.05–0.16) compared to nasopharyngeal samples, 0.33 (95% CI: 0.15–0.72) compared to stool samples and 0.20 (95% CI: 0.14–0.29) compared to blood/serum samples [49]. The pooled rate of urine positivity was 5.74% (95% CI: 2.88–9.44%) in another meta-analysis based on different inclusion criteria [36]. However, it remains unclear if urine has infectivity and transmissibility potential despite containing viral genetic material [26,48] (Table 1).

2.8. Ocular Fluid

Many respiratory viruses are known to enter through eyes or utilize the eye as a replication site before causing a respiratory infection [50]. SARS-CoV-2 has been detected occasionally in tears and conjunctival swabs in confirmed patients, however, the current data is controversial. The positive detection rate varies greatly in the available studies and figures fluctuate from 0% up to 28.57% [51–54]. While there are a number of published meta-analysis studies [37–40], their search dates are not recent and may have omitted newly published studies. A recent meta-analysis reported an overall sensitivity of 17.4% (95% CI: 7.8–34.2%) and specificity of 96.1% (95% CI: 12.7–100%) for ocular fluid in comparison to nasopharyngeal/oropharyngeal samples in confirmed cases [32].

The optimal time window to detect SARS-CoV-2 on the ocular surface, and whether the viral RNA present in the ocular fluids has infectious potential, is still unclear [17,37]. A standardized sample collection method and additional sampling time points would resolve heterogeneity in positive rates and provide insightful information. It has been noted that conjunctiva, cornea or the epithelial cells of the nasolacrimal duct can take up virus and may be a port of entry or direct inoculation site of infectious droplets, leading to contraction of the infection [53]. This is of significant importance for dentists and oral health professionals due the generation of potentially infectious droplets during dental procedures. The collection method includes the use of conjunctival swabs to collect both exfoliated cells and tears, or Schirmer's test strips to collect tears (Table 1).

2.9. Serum, Plasma and Whole Blood

Serum, plasma and whole blood are primarily used in antibody (serology) tests and occasionally for nucleic acid detection for tracking COVID-19 disease progression, severity or prognosis, epidemiological studies and patient immunity [47]. According to the recent meta-analysis of diagnostic performance of serology tests for COVID-19, the pooled sensitivity of Immunoglobin G (IgG), Immunoglobin M (IgM) and combined IgM-IgG tests in confirmed COVID-19 patients was 0.76 (95% CI: 0.65–0.86), 0.69 (95% CI: 0.59–0.78) and 0.78 (95% CI: 0.70–0.85), respectively. Thus, negative serological results alone cannot exclude the diagnosis of COVID-19 [55].

It was further demonstrated that serology tests had the lowest sensitivity at 0–7 days after symptom onset, and the highest sensitivity (more than 85%) at >14 days, suggesting that serological tests might be useful for diagnosis purposes at later stages of disease. The specificity of IgG, IgM and combined IgM-IgG tests was 0.98 (95% CI: 0.96–0.99), 0.95 (95% CI: 0.91–0.98) and 0.97 (95% CI: 0.93–0.99), respectively [55]. In another meta-analysis, SARS-CoV-2 seropositivity rate was estimated to be 61.2% (95% CI: 53.4–69.0%) for IgM, 58.8% (95% CI: 49.6–68.0%) for IgG and 62.1% (52.7–71.4%) for IgM-IgG joint detection in confirmed patients. Serologic testing also yielded high values in the identification of asymptomatic infections with a seropositivity rate of 19% (95% CI: 10.0–27.0%) for combined IgM-IgG [42]. Samples for serology tests are frequently collected by a fingerstick forming the basis for a simple test that can be performed at home by the patient.

SARS-CoV-2 viral RNA has also been detected in blood, serum and plasma samples from patients. A meta-analysis estimated the positive detection rate of viral RNA in blood products up to 28 days following symptomatic onset to be 10% (95% CI: 5–18%) [41], most of which are detected with low copy numbers, at earlier time points and in more severe patients. However, it remains controversial whether the detection of viral RNA in blood samples reflects the presence of infectious virus, as this has important safety implications, especially for dental practitioners and personnel and those handling patient-related materials in clinical, laboratory and research environments [41]. For RNA detection, 5 mL of anticoagulated blood is required. Vacuum tubes containing ethylenediaminetetraacetic acid (EDTA) anticoagulant are recommended for blood collection (Table 1).

3. Discussion

Recommended infection prevention and control practices for dental treatment delivery encourage the elective procedures and non-urgent outpatient visits to be postponed in applicable circumstances, and tele-dentistry and triage protocols to be implemented prior to dental appointments. The next step is to screen and triage everyone entering the dental office for fever and symptoms consistent with COVID-19 or exposure to others with COVID-19 infection. Nevertheless, a fever might only be associated with a dental diagnosis if no other symptoms of COVID-19 are present. The patients should also be requested to contact the dental office if they develop COVID-19 signs or symptoms or are diagnosed with COVID-19 within 2 days after the dental appointment [3,56]. However, pre-symptomatic (before symptom onset), or asymptomatic patients (that account for more than 40% of confirmed cases), impose a greater challenge than symptomatic patients for dental settings in this process [57]. The high transmissibility of SARS-CoV-2 has been attributed to asymptomatic carriers and pre-symptomatic patients. These patients have similar viral load to that of symptomatic COVID-19 patients, causing comparable transmissibility [58].

There are very limited studies which reported the prevalence of COVID-19 infection among dental patients. Lamberghini et al. [59] reported an overall SARS-CoV-2 positivity rate of 2.3% in asymptomatic children attending a high-volume pediatric dental practice. Conway et al. [60] reported an overall test positivity rate of 0.6% (95% CI: 0.4–0.8%) in child and adult asymptomatic patients attending multiple dental care centers. These findings highlight that while dental practices must screen patients for signs and symptoms of COVID-19 and refer patients for appropriate medical follow-up when indicated, such screening alone will not identify all individuals who are infected. Therefore, timely, accurate (highly sensitive and specific) and rapid screening and diagnostic testing that can distinguish COVID-19 cases from healthy or other virus-infected individuals is an essential need to take required actions, optimize patient care, maintain dental patients' and treatment providers' safety and to contain and prevent disease spread. It is being recognized that dental practices would greatly benefit from the ability to evaluate the disease status of their patients by using point-of-care COVID-19 diagnostic tests.

4. Conclusions

SARS-CoV-2 can be detected in different body specimens and sites. Dentists, directly or indirectly, deal with many of these specimens/sites in their daily practices. Information regarding prevalence of SARS-CoV-2 virus among asymptomatic individuals is less well-documented but is significant in future management of the dental environment. The present literature indicates that detection of SARS-CoV-2 and the infectious potential of the tested virus is dependent on the time of specimen collection relative to symptoms/infection and the presence of actual live viral particles.

Author Contributions: Conceptualization, S.S.; methodology, S.S.; validation, S.S. and L.F.C.; formal analysis, S.S.; investigation, S.S.; writing—original draft preparation, S.S.; writing—review and editing, L.F.C. and C.M.S.; supervision, L.F.C.; funding acquisition, L.F.C. and C.M.S. All authors have read and agreed to the published version of the manuscript.

Funding: This research received no external funding.

Data Availability Statement: No new data were created or analyzed in this study. Data sharing is not applicable to this article.

Conflicts of Interest: Authors declare no conflict of interest.

References

1. Corstjens, P.L.A.M.; Abrams, W.R.; Malamud, D. Saliva and Viral Infections. *Periodontol 2000* **2016**, *70*, 93–110. [CrossRef]
2. CDC Coronavirus Disease 2019 (COVID-19)—Transmission. Available online: https://www.cdc.gov/coronavirus/2019-ncov/prevent-getting-sick/how-covid-spreads.html (accessed on 3 March 2021).
3. Guerra, F.; Mata, A.D. *COVID-19. Normas de Orientação Clínica—Medicina Dentária*; Coimbra University Press: Coimbra, Portugal, 2020; ISBN 978-989-26-1986-6. [CrossRef]
4. Ren, Y.; Feng, C.; Rasubala, L.; Malmstrom, H.; Eliav, E. Risk for Dental Healthcare Professionals during the COVID-19 Global Pandemic: An Evidence-Based Assessment. *J. Dent.* **2020**, *101*, 103434. [CrossRef] [PubMed]
5. Banakar, M.; Bagheri Lankarani, K.; Jafarpour, D.; Moayedi, S.; Banakar, M.H.; MohammadSadeghi, A. COVID-19 Transmission Risk and Protective Protocols in Dentistry: A Systematic Review. *BMC Oral Health* **2020**, *20*, 275. [CrossRef] [PubMed]
6. Amato, A.; Ciacci, C.; Martina, S.; Caggiano, M.; Amato, M. COVID-19: The Dentists' Perceived Impact on the Dental Practice. *Eur. J. Dent.* **2021**. [CrossRef]
7. Alarcón, M.A.; Sanz-Sánchez, I.; Shibli, J.A.; Santos, A.T.; Caram, S.; Lanis, A.; Jiménez, P.; Dueñas, R.; Torres, R.; Alvarado, J.; et al. Delphi Project on the Trends in Implant Dentistry in the COVID-19 Era: Perspectives from Latin America. *Clin. Oral Implant. Res.* **2021**. [CrossRef] [PubMed]

8. Jungo, S.; Moreau, N.; Mazevet, M.E.; Ejeil, A.-L.; Biosse Duplan, M.; Salmon, B.; Smail-Faugeron, V. Prevalence and Risk Indicators of First-Wave COVID-19 among Oral Health-Care Workers: A French Epidemiological Survey. *PLoS ONE* **2021**, *16*, e0246586. [CrossRef] [PubMed]
9. Estrich, C.G.; Mikkelsen, M.; Morrissey, R.; Geisinger, M.L.; Ioannidou, E.; Vujicic, M.; Araujo, M.W.B. Estimating COVID-19 Prevalence and Infection Control Practices among US Dentists. *J. Am. Dent. Assoc.* **2020**, *151*, 815–824. [CrossRef]
10. Brondani, M.; Cua, D.; Maragha, T.; Shayanfar, M.; Mathu-Muju, K.; von Bergmann, H.; Almeida, F.; Villanueva, J.; Alvarado, A.A.V.; Learey, S.; et al. A Pan-Canadian Narrative Review on the Protocols for Reopening Dental Services during the COVID-19 Pandemic. *BMC Oral Health* **2020**, *20*, 352. [CrossRef]
11. Comber, L.; Walsh, K.A.; Jordan, K.; O'Brien, K.K.; Clyne, B.; Teljeur, C.; Drummond, L.; Carty, P.G.; De Gascun, C.F.; Smith, S.M.; et al. Alternative Clinical Specimens for the Detection of SARS-CoV-2: A Rapid Review. *Rev. Med. Virol.* **2020**. [CrossRef] [PubMed]
12. Linton, N.M.; Kobayashi, T.; Yang, Y.; Hayashi, K.; Akhmetzhanov, A.R.; Jung, S.-M.; Yuan, B.; Kinoshita, R.; Nishiura, H. Incubation Period and Other Epidemiological Characteristics of 2019 Novel Coronavirus Infections with Right Truncation: A Statistical Analysis of Publicly Available Case Data. *J. Clin. Med.* **2020**, *9*, 538. [CrossRef] [PubMed]
13. World Health Organization Diagnostic Testing for SARS-CoV-2. Available online: https://www.who.int/publications-detail-redirect/diagnostic-testing-for-sars-cov-2 (accessed on 3 March 2021).
14. Dos Santos, C.C.; Zehnbauer, B.A.; Trahtemberg, U.; Marshall, J. Molecular Diagnosis of Coronavirus Disease 2019. *Crit Care Explor.* **2020**, *2*. [CrossRef]
15. CDC Interim Guidelines for Collecting, Handling, and Testing Clinical Specimens for COVID-19. Updated December 29. Available online: https://www.cdc.gov/coronavirus/2019-ncov/lab/guidelines-clinical-specimens.html (accessed on 3 March 2021).
16. Ireland Health Information and Quality Authority Evidence Summary for COVID-19 Clinical Samples | HIQA. Available online: https://www.hiqa.ie/reports-and-publications/health-technology-assessment/evidence-summary-covid-19-clinical-samples (accessed on 12 November 2020).
17. Pan, Y.; Zhang, D.; Yang, P.; Poon, L.L.M.; Wang, Q. Viral Load of SARS-CoV-2 in Clinical Samples. *Lancet Infect. Dis.* **2020**, *20*, 411–412. [CrossRef]
18. Wang, W.; Xu, Y.; Gao, R.; Lu, R.; Han, K.; Wu, G.; Tan, W. Detection of SARS-CoV-2 in Different Types of Clinical Specimens. *JAMA* **2020**, *323*, 1843–1844. [CrossRef]
19. Asselah, T.; Durantel, D.; Pasmant, E.; Lau, G.; Schinazi, R.F. COVID-19: Discovery, Diagnostics and Drug Development. *J. Hepatol.* **2020**. [CrossRef] [PubMed]
20. Mohammadi, A.; Esmaeilzadeh, E.; Li, Y.; Bosch, R.J.; Li, J.Z. SARS-CoV-2 Detection in Different Respiratory Sites: A Systematic Review and Meta-Analysis. *EBioMedicine* **2020**, *59*. [CrossRef]
21. Wölfel, R.; Corman, V.M.; Guggemos, W.; Seilmaier, M.; Zange, S.; Müller, M.A.; Niemeyer, D.; Jones, T.C.; Vollmar, P.; Rothe, C.; et al. Virological Assessment of Hospitalized Patients with COVID-2019. *Nature* **2020**, *581*, 465–469. [CrossRef]
22. Lee, R.A.; Herigon, J.C.; Benedetti, A.; Pollock, N.R.; Denkinger, C.M. Performance of Saliva, Oropharyngeal Swabs, and Nasal Swabs for SARS-CoV-2 Molecular Detection: A Systematic Review and Meta-Analysis. *medRxiv* **2020**. [CrossRef]
23. Hayer, J.; Kasapic, D.; Zemmrich, C. Real-World Clinical Performance of Commercial SARS-CoV-2 Rapid Antigen Tests in Suspected COVID-19: A Systematic Meta-Analysis of Available Data as per November 20. *medRxiv* **2020**. [CrossRef]
24. Czumbel, L.M.; Kiss, S.; Farkas, N.; Mandel, I.; Hegyi, A.; Nagy, Á.; Lohinai, Z.; Szakács, Z.; Hegyi, P.; Steward, M.C.; et al. Saliva as a Candidate for COVID-19 Diagnostic Testing: A Meta-Analysis. *Front. Med.* **2020**, *7*. [CrossRef] [PubMed]
25. Calame, A.; Mazza, L.; Renzoni, A.; Kaiser, L.; Schibler, M. Sensitivity of Nasopharyngeal, Oropharyngeal, and Nasal Wash Specimens for SARS-CoV-2 Detection in the Setting of Sampling Device Shortage. *Eur. J. Clin. Microbiol. Infect. Dis.* **2020**, 1–5. [CrossRef]
26. Jeong, H.W.; Kim, S.-M.; Kim, H.-S.; Kim, Y.-I.; Kim, J.H.; Cho, J.Y.; Kim, S.; Kang, H.; Kim, S.-G.; Park, S.-J.; et al. Viable SARS-CoV-2 in Various Specimens from COVID-19 Patients. *Clin. Microbiol. Infect.* **2020**, *26*, 1520–1524. [CrossRef]
27. Ranoa, D.R.E.; Holland, R.L.; Alnaji, F.G.; Green, K.J.; Wang, L.; Brooke, C.B.; Burke, M.D.; Fan, T.M.; Hergenrother, P.J. Saliva-Based Molecular Testing for SARS-CoV-2 That Bypasses RNA Extraction. *bioRxiv* **2020**. [CrossRef]
28. To, K.K.-W.; Tsang, O.T.-Y.; Yip, C.C.-Y.; Chan, K.-H.; Wu, T.-C.; Chan, J.M.-C.; Leung, W.-S.; Chik, T.S.-H.; Choi, C.Y.-C.; Kandamby, D.H.; et al. Consistent Detection of 2019 Novel Coronavirus in Saliva. *Clin. Infect. Dis.* **2020**, *71*, 841–843. [CrossRef]
29. Iwasaki, S.; Fujisawa, S.; Nakakubo, S.; Kamada, K.; Yamashita, Y.; Fukumoto, T.; Sato, K.; Oguri, S.; Taki, K.; Senjo, H.; et al. Comparison of SARS-CoV-2 Detection in Nasopharyngeal Swab and Saliva. *J. Infect.* **2020**, *81*, e145–e147. [CrossRef]
30. Wyllie, A.L.; Fournier, J.; Casanovas-Massana, A.; Campbell, M.; Tokuyama, M.; Vijayakumar, P.; Warren, J.L.; Geng, B.; Muenker, M.C.; Moore, A.J.; et al. Saliva or Nasopharyngeal Swab Specimens for Detection of SARS-CoV-2. *N. Engl. J. Med.* **2020**, *383*, 1283–1286. [CrossRef]
31. Lippi, G.; Henry, B.M.; Sanchis-Gomar, F.; Mattiuzzi, C. Updates on Laboratory Investigations in Coronavirus Disease 2019 (COVID-19). *Acta Bio Med.* **2020**, *91*, e2020030. [CrossRef]
32. Moreira, V.M.; Mascarenhas, P.; Machado, V.; Botelho, J.; Mendes, J.J.; Taveira, N.; Almeida, M.G. Diagnosis of SARS-Cov-2 Infection Using Specimens Other than Naso- and Oropharyngeal Swabs: A Systematic Review and Meta-Analysis. *medRxiv* **2021**. [CrossRef]

33. Bastos, M.L.; Perlman-Arrow, S.; Menzies, D.; Campbell, J.R. The Sensitivity and Costs of Testing for SARS-CoV-2 Infection With Saliva Versus Nasopharyngeal Swabs. *Ann. Intern. Med.* **2021**. [CrossRef]
34. Bwire, G.M.; Majigo, M.V.; Njiro, B.J.; Mawazo, A. Detection Profile of SARS-CoV-2 Using RT-PCR in Different Types of Clinical Specimens: A Systematic Review and Meta-Analysis. *J. Med. Virol.* **2020**. [CrossRef]
35. Van Doorn, A.S.; Meijer, B.; Frampton, C.M.A.; Barclay, M.L.; de Boer, N.K.H. Systematic Review with Meta-analysis: SARS-CoV-2 Stool Testing and the Potential for Faecal-oral Transmission. *Aliment. Pharmacol. Ther.* **2020**. [CrossRef]
36. Chan, V.W.-S.; Chiu, P.K.-F.; Yee, C.-H.; Yuan, Y.; Ng, C.-F.; Teoh, J.Y.-C. A Systematic Review on COVID-19: Urological Manifestations, Viral RNA Detection and Special Considerations in Urological Conditions. *World J. Urol.* **2020**, 1–12. [CrossRef]
37. Aggarwal, K.; Agarwal, A.; Jaiswal, N.; Dahiya, N.; Ahuja, A.; Mahajan, S.; Tong, L.; Duggal, M.; Singh, M.; Agrawal, R.; et al. Ocular Surface Manifestations of Coronavirus Disease 2019 (COVID-19): A Systematic Review and Meta-Analysis. *PLoS ONE* **2020**, *15*, e0241661. [CrossRef] [PubMed]
38. Cao, K.; Kline, B.; Han, Y.; Ying, G.; Wang, N.L. Current Evidence of 2019 Novel Coronavirus Disease (COVID-19) Ocular Transmission: A Systematic Review and Meta-Analysis. *Biomed. Res. Int.* **2020**, *2020*. [CrossRef]
39. Ling, X.C.; Kang, E.Y.-C.; Lin, J.-Y.; Chen, H.-C.; Lai, C.-C.; Ma, D.H.-K.; Wu, W.-C. Ocular Manifestation, Comorbidities, and Detection of Severe Acute Respiratory Syndrome-Coronavirus 2 from Conjunctiva in Coronavirus Disease 2019: A Systematic Review and Meta-Analysis. *Taiwan J. Ophthalmol.* **2020**, *10*, 153–166. [CrossRef]
40. Ulhaq, Z.S.; Soraya, G.V. The Prevalence of Ophthalmic Manifestations in COVID-19 and the Diagnostic Value of Ocular Tissue/Fluid. *Graefes Arch. Clin. Exp. Ophthalmol.* **2020**, *258*, 1351–1352. [CrossRef]
41. Andersson, M.; Carcamo, C.V.A.-; Auckland, K.; Baillie, J.K.; Barnes, E.; Beneke, T.; Bibi, S.; Carroll, M.; Crook, D.; Dingle, K.; et al. SARS-CoV-2 RNA Detected in Blood Samples from Patients with COVID-19 Is Not Associated with Infectious Virus. *medRxiv* **2020**. [CrossRef]
42. Guo, C.-C.; Mi, J.-Q.; Nie, H. Seropositivity Rate and Diagnostic Accuracy of Serological Tests in 2019-NCoV Cases: A Pooled Analysis of Individual Studies. *Eur. Rev. Med. Pharmacol. Sci.* **2020**, *24*, 10208–10218. [CrossRef]
43. SARS-CoV-2 Testing. Available online: https://www.covid19treatmentguidelines.nih.gov/overview/sars-cov-2-testing/ (accessed on 24 December 2020).
44. Wong, M.C.; Huang, J.; Lai, C.; Ng, R.; Chan, F.K.L.; Chan, P.K.S. Detection of SARS-CoV-2 RNA in Fecal Specimens of Patients with Confirmed COVID-19: A Meta-Analysis. *J. Infect.* **2020**, *81*, e31–e38. [CrossRef] [PubMed]
45. Kutti-Sridharan, G.; Vegunta, R.; Vegunta, R.; Mohan, B.P.; Rokkam, V.R.P. SARS-CoV2 in Different Body Fluids, Risks of Transmission, and Preventing COVID-19: A Comprehensive Evidence-Based Review. *Int. J. Prev. Med.* **2020**, *11*. [CrossRef]
46. Xie, C.; Jiang, L.; Huang, G.; Pu, H.; Gong, B.; Lin, H.; Ma, S.; Chen, X.; Long, B.; Si, G.; et al. Comparison of Different Samples for 2019 Novel Coronavirus Detection by Nucleic Acid Amplification Tests. *Int. J. Infect. Dis.* **2020**, *93*, 264–267. [CrossRef]
47. Jayamohan, H.; Lambert, C.J.; Sant, H.J.; Jafek, A.; Patel, D.; Feng, H.; Beeman, M.; Mahmood, T.; Nze, U.; Gale, B.K. SARS-CoV-2 Pandemic: A Review of Molecular Diagnostic Tools Including Sample Collection and Commercial Response with Associated Advantages and Limitations. *Anal. Bioanal. Chem.* **2020**, 1–23. [CrossRef] [PubMed]
48. Kashi, A.H.; De la Rosette, J.; Amini, E.; Abdi, H.; Fallah-Karkan, M.; Vaezjalali, M. Urinary Viral Shedding of COVID-19 and Its Clinical Associations: A Systematic Review and Meta-Analysis of Observational Studies. *Urol. J.* **2020**, *17*, 433–441. [CrossRef] [PubMed]
49. Roshandel, M.R.; Nateqi, M.; Lak, R.; Aavani, P.; Sari Motlagh, R.; Shariat, S.F.; Aghaei Badr, T.; Sfakianos, J.; Kaplan, S.A.; Tewari, A.K. Diagnostic and Methodological Evaluation of Studies on the Urinary Shedding of SARS-CoV-2, Compared to Stool and Serum: A Systematic Review and Meta-Analysis. *Cell. Mol. Biol.* **2020**, *66*, 148–156. [CrossRef]
50. Belser, J.A.; Rota, P.A.; Tumpey, T.M. Ocular Tropism of Respiratory Viruses. *Microbiol. Mol. Biol. Rev.* **2013**, *77*, 144–156. [CrossRef] [PubMed]
51. Kaya, H.; Çalışkan, A.; Okul, M.; Sarı, T.; Akbudak, İ.H. Detection of SARS-CoV-2 in the Tears and Conjunctival Secretions of Coronavirus Disease 2019 Patients. *J. Infect. Dev. Ctries* **2020**, *14*, 977–981. [CrossRef] [PubMed]
52. Mahmoud, H.; Ammar, H.; El Rashidy, A.; Ali, A.H.; Hefny, H.M.; Mounir, A. Assessment of Coronavirus in the Conjunctival Tears and Secretions in Patients with SARS-CoV-2 Infection in Sohag Province, Egypt. *Clin. Ophthalmol.* **2020**, *14*, 2701–2708. [CrossRef] [PubMed]
53. Atum, M.; Boz, A.A.E.; Çakır, B.; Karabay, O.; Köroğlu, M.; Öğütlü, A.; Alagöz, G. Evaluation of Conjunctival Swab PCR Results in Patients with SARS-CoV-2 Infection. *Ocul. Immunol. Inflamm.* **2020**, *28*, 745–748. [CrossRef]
54. Seah, I.Y.J.; Anderson, D.E.; Kang, A.E.Z.; Wang, L.; Rao, P.; Young, B.E.; Lye, D.C.; Agrawal, R. Assessing Viral Shedding and Infectivity of Tears in Coronavirus Disease 2019 (COVID-19) Patients. *Ophthalmology* **2020**, *127*, 977–979. [CrossRef]
55. Wang, H.; Ai, J.; Loeffelholz, M.J.; Tang, Y.-W.; Zhang, W. Meta-Analysis of Diagnostic Performance of Serology Tests for COVID-19: Impact of Assay Design and Post-Symptom-Onset Intervals. *Emerg. Microbes. Infect.* **2020**, *9*, 2200–2211. [CrossRef] [PubMed]
56. Centers for Disease Control and Prevention Coronavirus Disease 2019 (COVID-19)—Guidance for Dental Settings. Available online: https://www.cdc.gov/coronavirus/2019-ncov/hcp/dental-settings.html (accessed on 3 March 2021).
57. Oran, D.P.; Topol, E.J. Prevalence of Asymptomatic SARS-CoV-2 Infection: A Narrative Review. *Ann. Intern. Med.* **2020**, *173*, 362–367. [CrossRef]

58. Gandhi, M.; Yokoe, D.S.; Havlir, D.V. Asymptomatic Transmission, the Achilles' Heel of Current Strategies to Control Covid-19. *N. Engl. J. Med.* **2020**, *382*, 2158–2160. [CrossRef]
59. Lamberghini, F.; Trifan, G.; Testai, F.D. SARS-CoV-2 Infection in Asymptomatic Pediatric Dental Patients. *J. Am. Dent. Assoc.* **2021**. [CrossRef]
60. Conway, D.I.; Culshaw, S.; Edwards, M.; Clark, C.; Watling, C.; Robertson, C.; Braid, R.; O'Keefe, E.; McGoldrick, N.; Burns, J.; et al. SARS-CoV-2 Positivity in Asymptomatic-Screened Dental Patients. *medRxiv* **2021**. [CrossRef]

Journal of
Clinical Medicine

MDPI

Article

The Psychological Impact of the COVID-19 Pandemic on Dentists in Germany

Mohamed Mekhemar [1,*], Sameh Attia [2], Christof Dörfer [1] and Jonas Conrad [1]

[1] Clinic for Conservative Dentistry and Periodontology, School of Dental Medicine, Kiel University, Arnold-Heller-Str. 3, Haus B, 24105 Kiel, Germany; doerfer@konspar.uni-kiel.de (C.D.); conrad@konspar.uni-kiel.de (J.C.)

[2] Department of Cranio Maxillofacial Surgery, Justus-Liebig University Giessen, Klinik Str. 33, 35392 Giessen, Germany; sameh.attia@dentist.med.uni-giessen.de

* Correspondence: mekhemar@konspar.uni-kiel.de; Tel.: +49-431-597-2817

Abstract: Since the announcement of the coronavirus 2019 (COVID-19) outbreak as a pandemic, several studies reported increased psychological distress among healthcare workers. In this investigation, we examined the association between psychological outcomes and various factors among German dentists. Dentists from all German federal states were invited to participate in this study through a self-administered online questionnaire between July and November 2020. This questionnaire collected information on demographics, Depression Anxiety Stress Scales (DASS-21), and the Impact of Events Scale-Revised (IES-R) instrument. The associations displayed between demographic and psychological outcomes of depression, anxiety, stress, intrusion, avoidance, and hyperarousal were evaluated. Seven-hundred-and-thirty-two dentists participated in the survey and reported overall scores of (4.88 ± 4.85), (2.88 ± 3.57), (7.08 ± 5.04), (9.12 ± 8.44), (10.68 ± 8.88) and (10.35 ± 8.68) for depression, anxiety, stress, intrusion, avoidance, and hyperarousal, respectively. For females, being between 50–59 years of age, being immune deficient or chronically ill, working at a dental practice, and considering the COVID-19 pandemic a financial hazard were reported as significant associated factors ($p < 0.05$) with higher DASS-21 and IES-R scores. These findings underline the aspects which need to be taken into attention to protect the mental wellbeing of dentists in Germany during the crisis.

Keywords: COVID-19; dentistry; IES-R; DASS-21; stress; anxiety; depression; dentists; psychological impact

Citation: Mekhemar, M.; Attia, S.; Dörfer, C.; Conrad, J. The Psychological Impact of the COVID-19 Pandemic on Dentists in Germany. *J. Clin. Med.* **2021**, *10*, 1008. https://doi.org/10.3390/jcm10051008

Academic Editor: Ray Williams

Received: 11 February 2021
Accepted: 24 February 2021
Published: 2 March 2021

1. Introduction

Since the beginning of January 2020, COVID-19, a new contagious disease, has been threatening the health and welfare of humans globally. The viral pandemic was first defined in the Chinese city of Wuhan and was able to spread internationally in a few months. This rapid disease transmission with growing numbers of infected cases and associated critical health conditions or fatalities led to noticeable public anxiety and panic. Early studies examining immediate psychological impacts during the first COVID-19 wave of infection described moderate or severe psychological effects of the outbreak on the general population [1].

In addition to the psychological effects of the pandemic on the general population, healthcare workers are exposed to additional psychological difficulties due to their direct treatment of infected patients and the accompanying, increased risk of infection [2]. These include the fear of transmitting the disease to their families or loved ones [3], feeling discriminated against or rejected by society as potential carriers of the virus [4], as well as heavy workloads and time pressure, despite depleted personnel protection equipment [5].

Among all healthcare workers, the COVID-19 outbreak also negatively obstructed the activities of the dental profession [6–8]. Routine measures and dental treatments have been postponed due to the high risk of cross-infection during dental procedures [9–12].

Furthermore, oral mucosa has been described as a potential route of viral entry [13], restricting dental procedures to emergency treatments only to minimize the possible droplet infection. Dental manufacturers, companies, and some practices additionally suspended parts of their staff to counteract the financial complications during the pandemic [14]. Previous studies correspondingly described how dental professionals sense their moral responsibility to reduce their regular work to evade the cross-infection among their patients and relatives while having major concerns about the financial consequences of a lockdown or decreased patient visits [15]. Other investigations declared suspended research or educational activities [15], potential feelings of guilt among oral healthcare professionals, and scarce personal protective equipment [16] as possible causes of psychological distress among dentists during the worldwide outbreak [15].

To date, Germany has registered over one million SARS-CoV-2 infections, causing numerous fatalities related to COVID-19 health complications [17,18]. Federal states that are predominantly affected with high numbers of cumulative incidence (CI-cases per 100,000 residents) include Bavaria (CI = 1041), Baden-Württemberg, and (CI = 922) Saarland (CI = 875) [19]. In Germany, the distribution of the pandemic varies extensively across all locations of the country and is subject to dynamic change. Following the first outbreak caused by an infected traveler at the beginning of the year 2020 [20], further transborder contagions were mostly due to individuals returning from ski resorts in Italy and Austria, while local hotspots of infection have often been associated with crowded events such as carnivals or concerts [17]. Other settings related to high rates of infection within the German population were linked to working conditions, including crowded collective accommodations and workplaces [17], or working in close contact with infected individuals, as in the dental profession [21].

Germany is considered the largest member state of the European Union in terms of general population and number of oral healthcare professionals, with about 80.5 million inhabitants and nearly 70,000 dentists [22]. Under a scheme of statuary or private health insurance, general dental practitioners and dental specialists provide oral healthcare services to their patients in private practices or university clinics [23]. Although previous studies reported the financial burden affecting dental personnel in Germany during the COVID-19 pandemic [24], the psychological impact on German dentists, associated with the pandemic and its related factors, still needs to be unveiled. Therefore, this study aimed to investigate this topic using the Impact of Event Scale-Revised (IES-R) and Depression, Anxiety Stress Scale (DASS-21) surveys on a nationwide level among German dentists.

2. Materials and Methods

2.1. Study Population and Procedures

A nationwide cross-sectional survey was designed to evaluate the psychological impact of the COVID-19 pandemic and its related factors on German dentists. An online survey was created using a web-based survey tool (Unipark, QuestBack GmbH, Cologne, Germany) to diminish face to face communications and to allow easy participation for all dentists. After the approval by the University of Kiel Ethics Board (D452/18), the survey link was shared on various dental social network groups from different specialties, by different dental websites, magazines, and publishing companies, and was sent by email to registered dentists of different dental societies in Germany. The introductory text in the survey briefly clarified the research project and guaranteed anonymity and voluntary participation to the dentists. No financial incentives were promised to the contributors and no criteria of exclusion were defined (e.g., age, gender, or nationality). All participants consented at the beginning of the survey, confirming their readiness to contribute to the questionnaire. Data was collected between July 2020 and November 2020.

2.2. Survey Instruments

In the first part of the questionnaire, sociodemographic information was gathered on age, gender, federal state, marital status, number of children, workplace, comorbid medical diseases, and smoking status of the respondents. Participants were also asked whether they consider COVID-19 a personal financial threat to them or not.

In the second part of the survey, the Depression Anxiety Stress Scale (DASS-21) was provided to the participants. The Depression Anxiety Stress Scale (DASS-21) is a self-report instrument comprising 21 items that evaluate three psychological constructs: depression, anxiety, and stress [25,26]. Each subscale contains 7 statements that refer to the week before survey participation. Participants are asked to read the statements and rate them emotionally. Ratings are provided on a series of 4-point Likert-type scales from 0 (did not apply to me at all/ never) to 3 (applied to me very much/ always). Higher scores designate increased emotional and psychological distress. As previously described [27], the DASS-21 subscales were scored as follows: normal (0–4 DASS-21 points), mild (5–6 DASS-21 points), moderate (7–10 DASS-21 points), severe (11–13 DASS-21 points), and extremely severe (14+ DASS-21 points) for depression; normal (0–3 DASS-21 points), mild (4–5 DASS-21 points), moderate (6–7 DASS-21 points), severe (8–9 DASS-21 points), and extremely severe (10+ DASS-21 points) for anxiety; and normal (0–7 DASS-21 points), mild (8–9 DASS-21 points), moderate (10–12 DASS-21 points), severe (13–16 DASS-21 points), and extremely severe (17+ DASS-21 points) for stress. The German version of the DASS-21 survey was applied previously in several studies and showed good validity and reliability (78–91%) in the assessment of depression, anxiety, and stress levels [28,29].

The psychological impact of the outbreak was further assessed using the Impact of Event Scale-Revised (IES-R) tool [30,31], which is a validated 22-item self-assessment measuring the subjective psychological distress triggered by traumatic events. This assessment has 3 subscales (Intrusion, Avoidance, and Hyperarousal), which show close associations to symptoms of post-traumatic stress disorder. Respondents were requested to rate the distress level for each statement on similar Likert-type scales, also referring to the previous seven days of their survey. The IES-R subscores were categorized similar to previous investigations [31] as normal (0–23 IES-R points), mild (24–32 IES-R points), moderate (33–36 IES-R points), and severe psychological impact of events (>37 IES-R points) [30,32,33]. The German version of the IES-R survey was applied previously in several studies and presented good validity and reliability (79–90%) in the evaluation of the psychological impact of events [33–36]. Both IES-R and DASS-21 scales have been validated for use in recent investigations exploring the psychological impact of the COVID-19 outbreak on the general population and healthcare workers [1,31].

2.3. Sample Size Calculation

To determine the number of responding dentists needed for nationwide significant sample size, the following circumstances were defined for the sample size calculation:

1. The number of dentists in Germany (n = 70,000).
2. A confidence level of 95%.
3. A margin of error of 5%.

Based on these conditions it was determined that from all German federal states at least 383 dentists were needed for a statistically significant sample size.

2.4. Statistical Analysis

Data from the online questionnaire was digitally recorded by the web-based survey tool and exported afterwards for statistical analysis using SPSS software (SPSS Statistic 27, IBM, Armonk, NY, USA). Descriptive data analysis was performed on each question separately and the Shapiro–Wilk-Test was performed to test for normality of the data. Data were not normally distributed. Univariate analyses (Kruskal-Wallis and Mann-Whitney U test) were conducted to explore the associations between DASS-21/IES-R ratings and sociodemographic characteristics. In case of a significant test result post hoc, single comparisons were performed using the Dunn-Bonferroni test. Subsequently, multiple linear regression analyses were performed on DASS-21 total and subscores, as well as the IES-R subscales to identify the input of these previously identified, relevant factors. Statistical significance was set at $p < 0.05$.

3. Results

3.1. Participation and Sociodemographic Data

A total of 732 dentists participated in the survey resulting in a statistically significant sample. Participants included female (59.7%), male (40%), and third gender (0.3%) dentists from all federal states of Germany except Bremen. Almost half of the participants (53.3%) were 18–49 years old, while the other respondents were either 50–59 (31.6%) or over 60 (15.2%) years old. The majority of the contributing dentists were married or in a marriage-like relationship (82.5%) and had children (66.9%), while other participants were single (12.3%), divorced, separated, or widowed (5.2%) and had no children (33.1%). Nearly all dentists were working in private practices (95.4%), while a minority stated to work at a university clinic (2.9%) or in other institutions (1.6%). Among the respondents, around two-thirds considered the COVID-19 outbreak to be a threat to their financial security (61.3%). Moreover, the study population showed a smoking rate of 8.5% and different conditions of medical comorbidity with the highest being cardiovascular diseases (13.9%) and immunodeficiencies (4.8%) (Table 1).

Table 1. Characteristics of Participants (n = 732).

		n	%
Gender			
	Female	437	59.7
	Male	293	40
	Third Gender	2	0.3
Age			
	18–49	390	53.3
	50–59	231	31.6
	≥60	111	15.2
Marital status			
	Single	90	12.3
	Married or in a marriage-like partnership	604	82.5
	Divorced, separated, or widowed	38	5.2
Having children			
	Yes	490	66.9
	No	242	33.1
COVID-19 being a personal financial threat			
	Yes	449	61.3
	No	283	38.7
Workplace [1]			
	Dental practice	698	95.4
	University clinic	21	2.9
	other	12	1.6
Federal state			
	Hamburg	12	1.6
	Mecklenburg-Western Pomerania	17	2.3

Table 1. *Cont.*

		n	%
	Schleswig-Holstein	42	5.7
	Brandenburg	11	1.5
	Berlin	42	5.7
	Lower Saxony	32	4.4
	Baden-Württemberg	275	37.6
	Thuringia	7	1
	Hesse	37	5.1
	Saarland	7	1
	Bavaria	82	11.2
	Saxony-Anhalt	6	0.8
	Saxony	19	2.6
	North Rhine-Westphalia	117	16.0
	Rhineland-Palatinate	26	3.6
Smoker			
	Yes	62	8.5
	No	670	91.5
Medical comorbidity [2]			
	Diseases of the cardiovascular system (e.g., coronary heart disease and high blood pressure)	102	13.9
	Chronic lung diseases (e.g., COPD)	19	2.6
	Chronic liver diseases	6	0.8
	Diabetes mellitus	12	1.6
	Cancer	18	2.5
	Immunodeficiency	35	4.8

[1] Multiple choice was possible; [2] No or multiple choice was possible.

3.2. DASS-21 and IES-R Scales and Associated Factors

The findings of the analysis for psychiatric symptoms in the overall sample according to the DASS-21 and IES-R scales were presented in (Tables 2 and 3 and in association with the related factors in (Tables 4 and 5), respectively.

The total study population presented DASS-21 and IES-R scores of normal psychological behaviors with potential mild distress due to the COVID-19 pandemic (Tables 2 and 3), according to the applied scoring system.

Table 2. DASS-21 and IES-R Scores of the Study Sample.

		Mean ± SD	Interquartile Range
DASS-21 (n = 729) [1]			
	Total	14.84 ± 12.31	17
	Depression	4.88 ± 4.85	6
	Anxiety	2.88 ± 3.57	5
	Stress	7.08 ± 5.04	7
IES-R (n = 727) [1]			
	Intrusion	9.12 ± 8.44	13
	Avoidance	10.68 ± 8.88	14
	Hyperarousal	10.35 ± 8.68	13

[1] n varies because of missing data.

Table 3. Amount of dentists and total population percentage for each DASS-21 and IES-R subscale category.

	Subscale	Category	n	%
DASS-21 (n = 729) [1]				
	Depression	normal	413	56.7
		mild	105	14.4
		moderate	106	14.5
		severe	47	6.4
		extremely severe	58	8
	Anxiety	normal	506	69.4
		mild	90	12.3
		moderate	47	6.4
		severe	33	4.5
		extremely severe	53	7.3
	Stress	normal	427	58.6
		mild	86	11.8
		moderate	97	13.3
		severe	81	11.1
		extremely severe	38	5.2
IES-R (n = 727) [1]				
	Intrusion	normal	679	93.3
		mild	43	5.9
		moderate	6	0.8
		severe	0	0
	Avoidance	normal	651	89.5
		mild	68	9.4
		moderate	7	1
		severe	1	0.1
	Hyperarousal	normal	665	91.3
		mild	54	7.4
		moderate	9	1.2
		severe	0	0

[1] n varies because of missing data.

DASS-21 and IES-R scales associated factors showed significantly higher DASS-21 and IES-R total and subscale scores denoting normal or mild psychological impact on depression, anxiety, stress, intrusion, avoidance, and hyperarousal among participating females, dentists working at private practices, or having systemic diseases, as well as among the respondents considering COVID-19 to be a financial threat (Tables 4 and 5). Furthermore, the youngest and oldest groups of the participants (18–49 and ≥60 years) showed significantly lower DASS-21 and IES-R scores in comparison to the middle-aged group (50–59 years) of the survey (Tables 4 and 5).

Multiple regression analyses of DASS-21 total and sub-scores within the study model showed a significant impact of financial factors, systemic immunodeficiency diseases, and age of the participants on the psychological stress, depression, and anxiety of German dentists (Table 6). Similarly, multiple regression analyses of IES-R scores displayed significant effects of analogous factors besides gender on intrusion, avoidance, and hyperarousal of the study participants (Table 7).

Table 4. Differences between participants characteristics regarding DASS-21 total and subscale scores.

	DASS-21 Total			DASS-21 Depression			DASS-21 Anxiety			DASS-21 Stress		
	Mean ± SD	Test Statistic	*p*-Value	Mean ± SD	Test Statistic	*p*-Value	Mean ± SD	Test Statistic	*p*-Value	Mean ± SD	Test Statistic	*p*-Value
Gender												
Female	15.05 ± 11.86			4.71 ± 4.63			2.99 ± 3.50			7.35± 4.95		
Male	14.35 ± 12.84	H = 6.75	0.03	5.07 ± 5.10	H = 5.01	0.08	2.67 ± 3.65	H = 9.53	0.01	6.61 ± 5.11	H = 8.35	0.02
Third Gender	38.00 ± 7.07			15.00 ± 0			8.50 ± 0.70			14.50 ± 6.36		
Posthoc: Dunn-Bonferroni-Test												
Male-Female		23.85	0.13					36.11	0.02		36.40	0.02
Male-Third G		−330.39	0.03					−317.67	0.03		−284.25	0.06
Female-Third G		−306.54	0.04					−281.56	0.06		−247.85	0.10
Age												
18–49	14.70 ± 11.93			4.71 ± 4.73			2.86 ± 3.44			7.13 ± 4.97		
50–59	16.16 ± 12.99	H = 7.45	0.02	5.40 ± 5.12	H = 4.23	0.12	3.17 ± 3.83	H = 4.01	0.14	7.60 ± 5.16	H = 10.59	0.01
≥60	12.49 ± 11.91			4.36 ± 4.63			2.35 ± 3.41			5.78 ± 4.82		
Posthoc: Dunn-Bonferroni-Test												
≥60 - 18–49		48.04	0.11								61.40	0.02
≥60 - 50–59		66.62	0.02								78.44	0
18–49 - 50–59		−18.57	0.29								−17.05	0.99
Marital status												
Single	13.98 ± 11.65			4.68 ± 4.60			2.52 ± 3.29			6.78 ± 4.86		
Married or in a marriage-like partnership	14.91 ± 12.33	H = 0.30	0.86	4.87 ± 4.84	H = 0.10	0.95	2.93 ± 3.63	H = 1.21	0.54	7.11 ± 5.03	0.29	0.87
Divorced, separated, or widowed	15.70 ± 13.69			5.57 ± 5.59			2.89 ± 3.19			7.24 ± 5.66		
Having children												
Yes	14.52 ± 12.01	U = 60,853	0.47	4.63 ± 4.61	U = 63,074	0.12	2.84 ± 3.60	U = 60,514.50	0.54	7.04 ± 4.99	U = 59,231	0.91
No	15.47 ± 12.89			5.37 ± 5.27			2.95 ± 3.51			7.14 ± 5.14		
COVID-19 being a personal financial threat												
Yes	18.46 ± 12.68	U = 33,639	0	6.20 ± 5.08	U = 35,374.50	0	3.69 ± 3.87	U = 40,350	0	8.56 ± 5.05	U = 34,606.50	0
No	9.13 ± 9.15			2.79 ± 3.58			1.60 ± 2.56			4.74 ± 4.04		
Workplace (Multiple Choice)												
Dental practice	15.03 ± 12.24	U = 15,076	0.01	4.92 ± 4.81	U = 13,960	0.07	2.89 ± 3.54	U = 13,646	0.12	7.21 ± 5.04	U = 16,018	0
University clinic	6.29 ± 7.86	U = 3867	0	2.05 ± 2.77	U = 4652	0	1.57 ± 3.06	U = 5057	0.01	2.67 ± 2.42	U = 3289.50	0
other	16.75 ± 15.70	U = 4400.50	0.89	6.42 ± 6.64	U = 4842.50	0.45	3.75 ± 4.71	U = 4590	0.68	6.58 ± 5.35	U = 4069.50	0.74

Table 4. *Cont.*

	DASS-21 Total			DASS-21 Depression			DASS-21 Anxiety			DASS-21 Stress		
	Mean ± SD	Test Statistic	*p*-Value	Mean ± SD	Test Statistic	*p*-Value	Mean ± SD	Test Statistic	*p*-Value	Mean ± SD	Test Statistic	*p*-Value
Federal state												
Hamburg	12.17 ± 8.08			4.50 ± 3.45			2.08 ± 1.93			5.58 ± 4.19		
Mecklenburg-Western Pomerania	9.82 ± 12.81			4.18 ± 5.33			1.53 ± 3.06			4.12 ± 4.91		
Schleswig-Holstein	11.90 ± 12.32			3.83 ± 4.49			2.51 ± 3.65			5.56 ± 5.09		
Brandenburg	16.09 ± 9.19			6.09 ± 4.13			2.45 ± 2.51			7.55 ± 3.42		
Berlin	13.40 ± 12.35			4.14 ± 4.31			2.74 ± 3.92			6.52 ± 4.94		
Lower Saxony	13.12 ± 12.71			4.97 ± 5.50			1.97 ± 3.47			6.19 ± 4.94		
Baden-Württemberg	15.30 ± 12.21			4.75 ± 4.68			2.96 ± 3.56			7.58 ± 5.09		
Thuringia	14.14 ± 17.83	H = 18.38	0.19	4.29 ± 6.16	H = 13.79	0.47	3.71 ± 4.79	H = 20.93	0.10	6.14 ± 7.24	H = 23.02	0.06
Hesse	16.64 ± 12.82			5.89 ± 5.18			3.42 ± 3.64			7.33 ± 5.05		
Saarland	20.29 ± 22.77			7.43 ± 8.58			5.43 ± 7.79			7.43 ± 6.88		
Bavaria	14.21 ± 11.91			4.84 ± 5.01			2.79 ± 3.22			6.57 ± 4.97		
Saxony-Anhalt	18.00 ± 12.28			5.50 ± 4.59			3.67 ± 2.25			8.83 ± 6.15		
Saxony	12.00 ± 9.33			3.53 ± 3.79			2.11 ± 3.04			6.37 ± 3.83		
North Rhine-Westphalia	16.69 ± 12.47			5.55 ± 5.08			3.39 ± 3.64			7.75 ± 5.07		
Rhineland-Palatinate	14.19 ± 11.52			5.08 ± 4.93			2.08 ± 3.32			7.04 ± 4.37		
Smoker												
Yes	14.40 ± 12.17	U = 21,121	0.78	4.77 ± 4.56	U = 20,902.50	0.89	2.82 ± 3.80	U = 21,417	0.63	6.81 ± 4.86	U = 21,280	0.70
No	14.88 ± 12.33			4.89 ± 4.88			2.89 ± 3.55			7.10 ± 5.05		
Medical comorbidity (Multiple Choice)												
No medical comorbidities	14.24 ± 12.07			4.65 ± 4.75			2.68 ± 3.44			6.90 ± 5.03		
Diseases of the cardiovascular system (e.g., coronary heart disease and high blood pressure)	16.75 ± 13.43	U = 34,782	0.16	5.64 ± 5.27	U = 34,684.50	0.17	3.63 ± 4.08	U = 35,670.50	0.06	7.49 ± 5.18	U = 33,574.50	0.42
Chronic lung diseases (e.g., COPD)	14.11 ± 9.53	U = 6882.50	0.88	4.26 ± 3.54	U = 6628	0.90	2.95 ± 2.92	U = 7072.50	0.71	6.89 ± 4.38	U = 6811.50	0.94
Chronic liver diseases	22.50 ± 12.19	U = 2999.50	0.11	8.83 ± 4.22	U = 3303	0.03	4.33 ± 4.13	U = 2611	0.39	9.33 ± 4.76	U = 2786	0.23
Diabetes mellitus	19.17 ± 14.03	U = 5115.50	0.26	7.00 ± 5.86	U = 5180.50	0.22	3.17 ± 3.33	U = 4650.50	0.62	9.00 ± 6.27	U = 4978.50	0.35
Cancer	13.67 ± 10.45	U = 6291	0.90	4.44 ± 3.62	U = 6478.50	0.93	2.56 ± 3.52	U = 6206	0.82	6.67 ± 4.42	U = 6175.50	0.80
Immunodeficiency	19.14 ± 12.61	U = 15014	0.02	6.80 ± 5.21	U = 15,352.50	0.01	4.14 ± 4.02	U = 14791	0.03	8.20 ± 4.32	U = 14,088.50	0.11

SD = Standard deviation; H = Test statistic of Kruskal-Wallis test; U = Test statistic of Mann-Whitney U test; Significant result are highlighted.

Table 5. Differences between participants characteristics regarding IES-R subscale scores.

	IES-R Intrusion			IES-R Avoidance			IES-R Hyperarousal		
	Mean ± SD	Test Statistic	*p*-Value	Mean ± SD	Test Statistic	*p*-Value	Mean ± SD	Test Statistic	*p*-Value
Gender									
Female	9.74 ± 8.36			11.74 ± 9.12			10.87 ± 8.64		
Male	8.12 ± 8.44	H = 13.18	0.001	9.07 ± 8.26	H = 17.51	0	9.48 ± 8.65	9.59	0.01
Third Gender	20.00 ± 9.90			15.50 ± 12.02			22.50 ± 3.54		
Posthoc: Dunn-Bonferroni-Test									
Male-Female		51.60	0.001		65.27	0		39.10	0.01
Male-Third G		−271.90	0.07		−165.01	0.27		−304.00	0.04
Female-Third G		−220.30	0.14		−99.74	0.50		−264.90	0.08
Age									
18–49	8.59 ± 8.21			10.69 ± 8.78			9.88 ± 8.48		
50–59	10.38 ± 8.92	H = 6.78	0.03	11.38 ± 9.14	H = 4.52	0.10	11.78 ± 9.05	H = 9.76	0.01
≥60	8.35 ± 7.97			9.23 ± 8.60			9.04 ± 8.24		
Posthoc: Dunn-Bonferroni-Test									
≥60 - 18–49		0.62	0.98					19.53	0.39
≥60 - 50–59		44.07	0.07					65.57	0.02
18–49 - 50–59		−43.45	0.04					−46.04	0.03
Marital status									
Single	7.08 ± 7.32			10.13 ± 8.63			8.89 ± 7.50		
Married or in a marriage-like partnership	9.37 ± 8.46	H = 5.45	0.07	10.85 ± 8.95	H = 1.41	0.50	10.61 ± 8.82	H = 2.34	0.31
Divorced, separated, or widowed	10.03 ± 10.15			9.34 ± 8.38			9.76 ± 8.93		
Having children									
Yes	9.01 ± 8.38	U = 59,615	0.69	10.33 ± 8.62	U = 61,854	0.20	10.33 ± 8.58	U = 58,065	0.85
No	9.34 ± 8.57			11.41 ± 9.37			10.38 ± 8.89		
COVID-19 being a personal financial threat									
Yes	11.53 ± 8.69	U = 34,886.50	0	12.82 ± 9.00	U = 39,615	0	13.00 ± 8.83	U = 33,329	0
No	5.33 ± 6.41			7.34 ± 7.58			6.18 ± 6.55		
Workplace (Multiple Choice)									
Dental practice	9.26 ± 8.42	U = 14,933.50	0.01	10.79 ± 8.88	U = 13,820	0.09	10.54 ± 8.66	U = 15,584	0
University clinic	4.38 ± 6.31	U = 4531.50	0	7.43 ± 8.07	U = 5633	0.06	4.10 ± 5.22	U = 3917.50	0
other	6.50 ± 8.95	U = 3239	0.14	7.83 ± 8.64	U = 3388	0.21	8.58 ± 9.90	U = 3553.50	0.30

Table 5. *Cont.*

	IES-R Intrusion			IES-R Avoidance			IES-R Hyperarousal		
	Mean ± SD	Test Statistic	*p*-Value	Mean ± SD	Test Statistic	*p*-Value	Mean ± SD	Test Statistic	*p*-Value
Federal state									
Hamburg	8.00 ± 7.84	H = 14.29	0.43	10.42 ± 7.23	H = 16.88	0.26	9.58 ± 7.85	H = 17.92	0.21
Mecklenburg-Western Pomerania	5.53 ± 6.75			6.24 ± 7.09			5.88 ± 7.80		
Schleswig-Holstein	8.43 ± 8.07			9.14 ± 7.05			8.71 ± 9.35		
Brandenburg	9.36 ± 10.31			10.18 ± 11.07			9.64 ± 8.63		
Berlin	8.83 ± 9.01			11.32 ± 9.94			9.24 ± 8.78		
Lower Saxony	10.75 ± 10.28			9.53 ± 7.83			8.66 ± 8.25		
Baden-Württemberg	9.31 ± 8.35			10.90 ± 9.15			11.00 ± 8.62		
Thuringia	6.29 ± 9.46			8. 71 ± 12.33			10.00 ± 11.21		
Hesse	9.76 ± 8.43			10.30 ± 7.54			10.03 ± 7.94		
Saarland	9.43 ± 9.61			7.57 ± 7.48			11.29 ± 12.45		
Bavaria	8.26 ± 8.28			10.35 ± 9.37			9.93 ± 8.77		
Saxony-Anhalt	7.83 ± 6.56			14.00 ± 5.73			13.33 ± 6.71		
Saxony	5.89 ± 7.21			7.84 ± 8.07			9.26 ± 8.68		
North Rhine-Westphalia	10.01 ± 8.62			12.14 ± 8.94			11.72 ± 9.07		
Rhineland-Palatinate	10.58 ± 7.51			12.35± 8.98			9.12 ± 6.44		
Smoker									
Yes	9.00 ± 8.34	U = 20,444	0.95	10.41 ± 8.38	U = 20,551.50	0.88	10.49 ± 8.28	U = 19,770.50	0.72
No	9.13 ± 8.46			10.71 ± 8.93			10.34 ± 8.72		
Medical comorbidity (Multiple Choice)									
No medical comorbidities	8.85 ± 8.29			10.77 ± 8.88			10.00 ± 8.55		
Diseases of the cardiovascular system (e.g., coronary heart disease and high blood pressure)	9.34 ± 8.76	U = 31,913	0.90	9.37 ± 8.14	U = 28,785	0.15	11.18 ± 9.10	U = 33,471	0.36
Chronic lung diseases (e.g., COPD)	10.84 ± 8.24	U = 7758.50	0.26	11.37 ± 9.35	U = 7073.50	0.70	9.95 ± 6.39	U = 6952.50	0.81
Chronic liver diseases	15.00 ± 10.47	U = 2909	0.15	15.67 ± 9.42	U = 2895.50	0.15	16.83 ± 8.52	U = 3140.50	0.06
Diabetes mellitus	9.50 ± 9.60	U = 4349.50	0.94	10.25 ± 9.10	U = 4180.50	0.88	12.67 ± 10.27	U = 4853.50	0.44
Cancer	11.44 ± 9.35	U = 7469	0.22	10.83 ± 7.58	U = 6770.50	0.66	12.11 ± 9.27	U = 7188.50	0.36
Immunodeficiency	11.34 ± 9.58	U = 13,991	0.12	13.23 ± 10.49	U = 13,822.50	0.16	13.20 ± 9.84	U = 14,320	0.07

SD = Standard deviation; H = Test statistic of Kruskal-Wallis test; U = Test statistic of Mann-Whitney U test; Significant result are highlighted.

Table 6. Multiple regression analyses with relevant factors of DASS-21 total and subscores.

	B	SE	β	T	p	95% CI
DASS-21 Total						
Gender [1]	−0.04	0.88	−0	−0.04	0.97	−1.76; 1.69
Age [2]	−0.87	0.60	−0.05	−1.45	0.15	−2.04; 0.31
COVID-19 being personal financial threat [3]	−9.05	0.89	0.36	−10.20	0	−10.79; −7.31
Workplace: Dental practice [4]	−1.74	3.21	−0.03	−0.54	0.59	−8.03; 4.56
Workplace: University clinic [4]	−5.54	4.08	0.08	−1.36	0.18	−13.56; 2.48
Medical comorbidity: Immunodeficiency [4]	3.94	1.98	0.07	1.99	0.05	0.05; 7.83
DASS-21 Depression						
COVID-19 being personal financial threat [3]	−3.29	0.35	−0.33	−9.30	0	−3.98; −2.59
Workplace: University clinic [4]	−0.98	1.03	0.03	−0.96	0.34	−3.00; 1.03
Medical comorbidity: Chronic liver diseases [4]	2.76	1.87	0.05	1.48	0.14	−0.91; 6.43
Medical comorbidity: Immunodeficiency [4]	1.79	0.79	0.08	2.27	0.02	0.24; 3.33
DASS-21 Anxiety						
Gender [1]	−0.23	0.26	0.03	−0.92	0.36	−0.73; 0.27
COVID-19 being personal financial threat [3]	−2.07	0.27	−0.28	−7.81	0	−2.59; −1.55
Workplace: University clinic[4]	−0.12	0.77	−0.01	−0.15	0.88	−1.63; 1.40
Medical comorbidity: Immunodeficiency [4]	1.16	0.59	0.07	1.95	0.05	−0.01; 2.32
DASS-21 Stress						
Gender [1]	−0.44	0.35	−0.04	−1.23	0.22	−1.14; 0.26
Age [2]	−0.51	0.24	−0.07	−2.09	0.04	−0.99; −0.03
COVID-19 being personal financial threat [3]	−3.70	0.36	−0.36	−10.25	0	−4.41; −2.99
Workplace: Dental practice [4]	0.99	1.31	0.04	0.76	0.45	−1.57; 3.56
Workplace: University clinic [4]	−1.54	1.66	−0.05	−0.92	0.36	−4.80; 1.73

B = unstandardized beta coefficient; SE = standard error; β = standardized beta coefficient; p = p-value; CI: confidence interval; Significant results are highlighted; [1] 1 = female; 2 = male; 3 = third gender; [2] 1 = 18–49 years; 2 = 50–59 years; 3 = ≥ 60 years; [3] 1 = yes; 2 = no; [4] 0 = not quoted; 1 = quoted.

Table 7. Multiple regression analyses with relevant factors of IES-R scores.

IES-R Intrusion						
Gender [1]	−1.57	0.61	−0.09	2.59	0.01	−2.76; −0.38
Age [2]	0.35	0.41	0.03	0.86	0.39	−0.45; 1.16
COVID-19 being personal financial threat [3]	−6.14	0.61	−0.36	−10.05	0	−7.34; −4.94
Workplace: Dental practice [4]	0.67	2.21	0.02	0.30	0.76	−3.67; 5
Workplace: University clinic [4]	−0.35	2.81	−0.01	−0.12	0.90	−5.87; 5.17
IES-R Avoidance						
Gender [1]	−2.59	0.63	−0.15	−4.13	0	−3.82; −1.36
COVID-19 being personal financial threat [3]	−5.52	0.34	0.30	8.65	0	−6.77; −4.27
IES-R Hyperarousal						
Gender [1]	−1.21	0.62	−0.07	−1.96	0.05	−2.42; 0
Age [2]	0.04	0.42	0	0.10	0.92	−0.78; 0.86
COVID-19 being personal financial threat [3]	−6.68	0.62	−0.38	−10.74	0	−0.79; −5.46
Workplace: Dental practice [4]	1.20	2.25	0.03	0.53	0.59	−3.22; 5.61
Workplace: University clinic [4]	−1.22	2.86	−0.02	0.43	0.67	−6.84; 4.40

B = unstandardized beta coefficient; SE = standard error; β = standardized beta coefficient; p = p-value; CI: confidence interval; Significant results are highlighted; [1] 1 = female; 2 = male; 3 = third gender; [2] 1 = 18−49 years; 2 = 50−59 years; 3 = ≥ 60 years; [3] 1 = yes; 2 = no; [4] 0 = not quoted; 1 = quoted.

4. Discussion

In the early months of 2020, the first reported case of COVID-19 in Bavaria, Germany was confirmed [20]. Similar to the reactions globally, fast conversion and adaptation procedures were initiated in the healthcare system and instant steps were taken to counteract the outbreak. This severe and extraordinary crisis undoubtedly had an inevitable impact on healthcare workers nationwide. Among all healthcare divisions, the dental sector is considered highly distressed by the viral outbreak in Germany and worldwide due to various factors affecting the psychological steadiness and financial stability of dentists during the pandemic and its related lockdowns [6,26,37]. To date, this study is the first to evaluate the psychological effects of the COVID-19 pandemic on dentists in Germany nationwide.

In this survey 732 dentists participated via the online survey link and completed the online questionnaire, displaying a significant sample size and representing German dentists in the investigation. Sociodemographic data of the participants presented an analogous gender distribution compared to the dental population in Germany (60–70% female) and Europe (Table 1) with higher percentages of female dentists [23,38]. The majority of the survey participants were younger than 50 years old and working in dental practices (Table 1). This corresponds to the reported average age (48 years old) and equivalent professional characteristics among dentists in Germany [23,24,39]. Moreover, survey respondents displayed a smoking rate below 10% (Table 1) comparable to reported results of oral health professionals in Germany (5–8%), as well as in other dental communities worldwide [38,40]. Cardiovascular diseases exhibited the most prevalent systemic diseases among participating dentists, with a rate of 13.9% (Table 1), corresponding to the rates reported by previous studies on the German population (10–13%) [41].

In the current investigation, German dentists displayed overall mild psychological impact of the COVID-19 outbreak in terms of stress, anxiety, depression, intrusion, avoidance, and hyperarousal as estimated by the DASS-21 and IES-R survey systems. This presents obvious differences to healthcare professionals having higher levels of psychological distress in other countries worldwide [10,26,31,42–44] and might reflect the psychological value of Germany's reported success to contain the infection rates of COVID-19, stabilize the financial state of its population during the crisis and communicate the rationale for its policies to cope with the emergency [45–47]. Corresponding to the described high rates of infection and cumulative incidence of COVID-19 in different German federal states [17], several regions such as Saarland and other southern states displayed higher scores of psychological impacts on DASS-21 and IES-R scales (Tables 4 and 5). Furthermore, multiple associated factors seem to play an effective role in the amount of stress, anxiety, and depression, besides potential symptoms of PTSD affecting dental professionals in Germany during the crisis. Similar to previous investigations on healthcare workers and dentists, female participants in the current study exhibited significantly higher scores of anxiety, stress, and all three IES-R subscales (Tables 4 and 5) [26,48] than their male counterparts. This might be related to the fact that females generally show significantly greater risks than males to develop anxiety, stress, and depressive disorders, as well as PTSD symptoms during adulthood [49,50]. This difference was explained as being due to discrepant thought control strategies and metacognitive beliefs between genders, leading to more emotional and neurotic distress among females [50]. Although only 0.3% of the survey respondents represented the third gender (Table 1), these participants revealed very high scores of psychological distresses in comparison to both males and females (Tables 4 and 5). This result also confirms the previously described depressive symptoms, interpersonal trauma exposure, stress, anxiety, and general distress among transgender and gender non-conforming populations due to minority stress processes and multiple social factors [51]. The current investigation further showed that being single, married, or in a marriage-like relationship and having children among the participants were associated with lower total DASS-21 and IES-R scores and sub-scores compared to being divorced, separated, or widowed (Tables 4 and 5) as well as having no children. As defined by earlier studies, this observation was similar in other countries among healthcare workers [26,52] and might be due to the reported lower levels of stress and psychological disorders of couples in a relationship in comparison to divorced or widowed individuals. Moreover, intimate and family relationships facilitate dyadic coping and social support to help as a buffer against difficult situations, which can then translate into lower levels of psychological distress [53,54]. In the current survey, the age factor also demonstrated a significant role in the determination of dentists' psychological status or levels of mental tension in association with the COVID-19 outbreak. As observed in the results, respondents of the youngest age group (18–49 years) and the group over 60 years had overall lower DASS-21 and IES-R scores than the middle-aged group (50–59 years) with significant DASS-21 total, DASS-21 stress, and IES-R intrusion, as well as hyperarousal outcomes (Tables 4 and 5). As the Robert-Koch Institute, the main German federal government agency and research institute responsible for disease control and prevention, stated officially that the risk of severe COVID-19 complications and mortality increases steadily from 50 to 60 years of age [55], this aspect might increase the psychological burden upon the middle-aged group (50–59 years) due to their fear of death, illness or complications [56,57]. Moreover, older participants might have further health-associated age-dependent risk factors [55], which can increase the possibility of getting infected by COVID-19 or having dangerous health complications as medically compromised patients. Interestingly, the oldest age group (over 60 years old) of the study showed even lower DASS-21 and IES-R scores than the youngest participants (Tables 4 and 5). This finding that people aged 60 years and above displayed less psychological distress on this investigation's rating scales is very thought-provoking, as COVID-19 infections have been shown to cause significantly higher morbidity and mortality in this age group in comparison with younger individuals [58,59]. Since the media and health organizations emphasized the need for people over 60 years particularly to perform strict procedures of social distancing, as they are more likely to have underlying medical risk conditions, it may have been anticipated that older participants would be more psychologically affected during the pandemic. Nevertheless, this outcome is consistent with some previous investigations that described decreased indicator scores in stress, anxiety, and depression of younger individuals in comparison to older age groups in European and North American countries [60,61]. This observed psychological stability of the older group could be explained by the fact that many respondents of this group might be retired from the dental career, as the general age of retirement in Germany starts with 65 years [62]. Being in distance from patient treatment as a dentist during the COVID-19 crisis could eliminate multiple factors provoking the mental tension during the pandemic, as the stress and fear of getting infected during treatment or taking the infection to family members [10], the anxiety of treating patients with suspicious symptoms [6,16], or the depression and distress of losing the job and financial safety [24]. Moreover, older people incline to show less social mobility than younger individuals, which could explain their lower stress, anxiety, and depression during a pandemic lockdown [61]. People above 60 years are correspondingly expected to have experienced numerous difficult major life events in their past, such as war, past pandemics, or financial crises, therefore increasing their resilience, as observed in the current study [61]. Another theory that could be advocated to clarify this outcome is that older people usually spend less time on social media due to their frequent resistance to social networking sites [63]. High rates of news consumption about the pandemic have been linked previously with elevated levels of psychological distress [64].

The presence of medical comorbidities during the COVID-19 pandemic has often been linked to an increase in in-hospital complications and mortality rates [65,66]. Congruently, individuals with systemic diseases and medical risk-factors have reported higher rates of psychological pressure and distress [67]. According to this investigation, dentists in Germany have displayed the same significant inclination during the COVID-19 emergency among participants with chronic liver diseases or medical conditions of immune deficiency (Table 4). This outcome resembles previous findings of healthcare workers in other countries, where health professionals living among persons with immune deficiency or chronic diseases significantly reported higher stress and anxiety scores [68,69]. Indeed, both medical conditions are considered among the highest risk factors associated with severe medical complications after COVID-19 infection [70,71], which clarifies the reason for psychological distress.

Workplace-related stress, anxiety, and depression are among the most important factors affecting the mental health wellbeing of people worldwide [72]. In previous reports dentists and healthcare workers equally conveyed various stressors within their workplace including the risk of infection, constant time pressure, concern over their capability to provide dental or medical services in the future, and financial pressure [73,74]. These workplace stressors have significantly increased during the COVID-19 pandemic among dental professionals globally [26,74]. According to the current survey German dentists working in a private dental practice displayed significantly higher stress, hyperarousal, and intrusion scores on the DASS-21 and IES-R scales than their colleagues at university clinics (Tables 4 and 5). This observed outcome could be explained by different aspects. While university dentists usually have their working-time divided into three branches comprising education, research, and patient treatment, dental practices follow a policy mostly aimed to treat the maximum number of patients. This may give university dentists a feeling of safety from exposure to infection through continuous patient treatment [74]. Furthermore, previous reports described the lack of protective equipment against the COVID-19 infection in German non-university health facilities, which can confidently increase the risk of personnel infection and its related psychological distress [75]. Having to face the lockdown and lack of patients during the pandemic as employers or employees of private dental practices, this situation created a financial crisis for many German dental practices and non-university health facilities [24,75], which is considered one of the main sources of psychological distresses among healthcare workers worldwide [76,77]. This was also confirmed by the current survey as participants considering the pandemic a financial threat reported significantly higher scores on both DASS-21 and IES-R scales in all parameters (Tables 4 and 5). Notably, dentists who stated to work in other facilities (Tables 4 and 5) also showed lower psychological distress than their colleagues in dental practices. This may be due to similar factors as those stated above, as they could working at non-clinical institutions as dental companies or manufacturers.

To ascertain the independent effects of the measured significant factors of COVID-19 being a financial threat, workplace, gender, age, and medical comorbidities on the DASS-21 and IES-R scores and subscores, multiple linear regression analyses were conducted. Female gender, an age between 50–59 years, being immune deficient, and considering the COVID-19 pandemic a financial hazard were independently associated with worse psychiatric outcomes (Tables 4 and 5) marking these aspects as the most effective on German dentists and their mental health during the COVID-19 crisis.

5. Limitations

To the best of our knowledge, this investigation is the first one in Germany examining the psychological impact of COVID-19 on dentists nationwide. Nevertheless, we recognize some limitations to our study. First of all, the investigation is restricted by its cross-sectional nature and lacks the follow-up on a longitudinal level. On the other hand, misinterpretations in such investigations are known to be equally dispersed [23]. In this survey, the observed outcomes of German dentists cannot be accredited exclusively to the analyzed aspects and socio-environmental information. Additional co-variables and sociodemographic observations (including being an employer or employee, exact financial challenges, and the number of treated patients) could play an important role in changing some outcomes or interpretations of the study. The data collection phase of the study was completed within three months. Given the time-sensitivity throughout this crisis and rapid changes in regulations and infection rates, these aspects might also influence the results reported by the respondents. Furthermore, the voluntary nature of the investigation might have caused a selection bias among the German dentists. Finally, to reach the maximum number of participants and to diminish face to face conditions, we applied an online self-report questionnaire to assess psychological symptoms that do not rely on diagnostic evaluation by mental health professionals. Adding a clinical mental health evaluation by psychiatric specialists would definitely contribute to the outcome of the survey. Regardless of the above limitations, conclusions of this survey provide important information on the psychological impact of COVID-19 on dentists across Germany.

6. Conclusions

The mental wellness of dentists is vital for guaranteeing the sustainability of dental services during the struggle with the COVID-19 pandemic. Our findings among the study population display being female, in an age group between 50–59 years, being immune deficient or chronically ill, working at a dental practice, and considering the COVID-19 pandemic a financial hazard are significant factors which cause distress in German dentists during the COVID-19 crisis and reporting higher DASS-21 and IES-R scores and subscores. Analyzing these aspects can assist health authorities in Germany in implementing the needed actions to diminish the unwanted psychological effects of the pandemic and their influencing factors on the German dental community.

Author Contributions: Conceptualization, M.M., J.C., S.A. and C.D.; Data curation, J.C.; Investigation, J.C.; Methodology, M.M. and S.A.; Project administration, C.D.; Software, J.C.; Supervision, C.D.; Validation, M.M.; Writing—Original draft, M.M.; Writing—Review & editing, J.C., S.A. and C.D. All authors have read and agreed to the published version of the manuscript.

Funding: No third-party funding was obtained for this study.

Institutional Review Board Statement: The study was conducted according to the guidelines of the Declaration of Helsinki, and approved by the University of Kiel (D452/18).

Informed Consent Statement: Informed consent was obtained from all subjects involved in the study.

Data Availability Statement: The data presented in this study are available on request from the corresponding author.

Acknowledgments: The authors would like to thank every dentist who participated in this study and every institution and every person that helped in the distribution of this survey among dentists in Germany. The authors would also like to thank the state of Schleswig-Holstein and the University of Kiel for the financial support through the Open-Access Funds.

Conflicts of Interest: The authors declare no conflict of interest.

References

1. Wang, C.; Pan, R.; Wan, X.; Tan, Y.; Xu, L.; Ho, C.S.; Ho, R.C. Immediate Psychological Responses and Associated Factors during the Initial Stage of the 2019 Coronavirus Disease (COVID-19) Epidemic among the General Population in China. *Int. J. Environ. Res. Public Health* **2020**, *17*, 1729. [CrossRef]
2. Nguyen, L.H.; Drew, D.A.; Graham, M.S.; Joshi, A.D.; Guo, C.-G.; Ma, W.; Mehta, R.S.; Warner, E.T.; Sikavi, D.R.; Lo, C.-H.; et al. Risk of COVID-19 among front-line health-care workers and the general community: A prospective cohort study. *Lancet Public Health* **2020**, *5*, e475–e483. [CrossRef]
3. Cawcutt, K.A.; Starlin, R.; Rupp, M.E. Fighting fear in healthcare workers during the COVID-19 pandemic. *Infect. Control. Hosp. Epidemiol.* **2020**, *41*, 1–2. [CrossRef]
4. Abdelhafiz, A.S.; Alorabi, M. Social Stigma: The Hidden Threat of COVID-19. *Front. Public Health* **2020**, *8*, 429. [CrossRef]
5. Bielicki, J.A.; Duval, X.; Gobat, N.; Goossens, H.; Koopmans, M.; Tacconelli, E.; van der Werf, S. Monitoring approaches for health-care workers during the COVID-19 pandemic. *Lancet Infect. Dis.* **2020**, *20*, e261–e267. [CrossRef]
6. Consolo, U.; Bellini, P.; Bencivenni, D.; Iani, C.; Checchi, V. Epidemiological Aspects and Psychological Reactions to COVID-19 of Dental Practitioners in the Northern Italy Districts of Modena and Reggio Emilia. *Int. J. Environ. Res. Public Health* **2020**, *17*, 3459. [CrossRef]
7. Attia, S.; Howaldt, H.-P. Impact of COVID-19 on the Dental Community: Part I before Vaccine (BV). *J. Clin. Med.* **2021**, *10*, 288. [CrossRef] [PubMed]
8. Ammar, N.; Aly, N.; Folayan, M.; Khader, Y.; Mohebbi, S.; Attia, S.; Howaldt, H.-P.; Boettger, S.; Virtanen, J.; Madi, M.; et al. Perceived Preparedness of Dental Academic Institutions to Cope with the COVID-19 Pandemic: A Multi-Country Survey. *Int. J. Environ. Res. Public Health* **2021**, *18*, 1445. [CrossRef]

9. Meng, L.; Hua, F.; Bian, Z. Coronavirus Disease 2019 (COVID-19): Emerging and Future Challenges for Dental and Oral Medicine. *J. Dent. Res.* **2020**, *99*, 481–487. [CrossRef]
10. Ahmed, M.A.; Jouhar, R.; Ahmed, N.; Adnan, S.; Aftab, M.; Zafar, M.S.; Khurshid, Z. Fear and Practice Modifications among Dentists to Combat Novel Coronavirus Disease (COVID-19) Outbreak. *Int. J. Environ. Res. Public Health* **2020**, *17*, 2821. [CrossRef]
11. WHO. *Considerations for the Provision of Essential Oral Health Services in the Context of COVID-19*; WHO: Geneva, Switzerland, 2020.
12. Ammar, N.; Aly, N.M.; Folayan, M.O.; Mohebbi, S.Z.; Attia, S.; Howaldt, H.-P.; Boettger, S.; Khader, Y.; Maharani, D.A.; Rahardjo, A.; et al. Knowledge of dental academics about the COVID-19 pandemic: A multi-country online survey. *BMC Med. Educ.* **2020**, *20*, 1–12. [CrossRef] [PubMed]
13. Peng, X.; Xu, X.; Li, Y.; Cheng, L.; Zhou, X.; Ren, B. Transmission routes of 2019-nCoV and controls in dental practice. *Int. J. Oral Sci.* **2020**, *12*, 1–6. [CrossRef]
14. Proffitt, E. What will be the new normal for the dental industry? *Br. Dent. J.* **2020**, *228*, 678–680. [CrossRef]
15. Vergara-Buenaventura, A.; Chavez-Tuñon, M.; Castro-Ruiz, C. The Mental Health Consequences of Coronavirus Disease 2019 Pandemic in Dentistry. *Disaster Med. Public Health Prep.* **2020**, *10*, 1–4. [CrossRef]
16. Mahendran, K.; Patel, S.; Sproat, C. Psychosocial effects of the COVID-19 pandemic on staff in a dental teaching hospital. *Br. Dent. J.* **2020**, *229*, 127–132. [CrossRef]
17. Santos-Hövener, C.; Busch, M.A.; Koschollek, C.; Schlaud, M.; Hoebel, J.; Hoffmann, R.; Wilking, H.; Haller, S.; Allenj, J.; Wernitz, J.; et al. Seroepidemiological study on the spread of SARS-CoV-2 in populations in especially affected areas in Germany—Study protocol of the CORONA-MONITORING lokal study. *J. Health Monit.* **2020**. [CrossRef]
18. Robert Koch Institut. *Epidemiologisches Bulletin 49/2020*; RKI: Berlin, Germany, 2020.
19. Robert Koch Institut. *Coronavirus SARS-CoV-2*; Situation Report; RKI: Berlin, Germany, 2020.
20. Böhmer, M.M.; Buchholz, U.; Corman, V.M.; Hoch, M.; Katz, K.; Marosevic, D.V.; Böhm, S.; Woudenberg, T.; Ackermann, N.; Konrad, R.; et al. Investigation of a COVID-19 outbreak in Germany resulting from a single travel-associated primary case: A case series. *Lancet Infect. Dis.* **2020**, *20*, 920–928. [CrossRef]
21. Nienhaus, A.; Hod, R. COVID-19 among Health Workers in Germany and Malaysia. *Int. J. Environ. Res. Public Health* **2020**, *17*, 4881. [CrossRef] [PubMed]
22. Ziller, S.; Eaton, K.E.; Widström, E. The healthcare system and the provision of oral healthcare in European Union member states. Part 1: Germany. *Br. Dent. J.* **2015**, *218*, 239–244. [CrossRef] [PubMed]
23. Conrad, J.; Retelsdorf, J.; Attia, S.; Dörfer, C.; Mekhemar, M. German Dentists' Preferences for the Treatment of Apical Periodontitis: A Cross-Sectional Survey. *Int. J. Environ. Res. Public Health* **2020**, *17*, 7447. [CrossRef]
24. Schwendicke, F.; Krois, J.; Gomez, J. Impact of SARS-CoV2 (Covid-19) on dental practices: Economic analysis. *J. Dent.* **2020**, *99*, 103387. [CrossRef] [PubMed]
25. Lovibond, P.F.; Lovibond, S.H. The structure of negative emotional states: Comparison of the Depression Anxiety Stress Scales (DASS) with the Beck Depression and Anxiety Inventories. *Behav. Res. Ther.* **1995**, *33*, 335–343. [CrossRef]
26. Elbay, R.Y.; Kurtulmuş, A.; Arpacıoğlu, S.; Karadere, E. Depression, anxiety, stress levels of physicians and associated factors in Covid-19 pandemics. *Psychiatry Res.* **2020**, *290*, 113130. [CrossRef]
27. Lovibond, S.H.; Lovibond, P.F.; Psychology Foundation of Australia. *Manual for the Depression Anxiety Stress Scales*; Psychology Foundation of Australia: Sydney, Australia, 1995.
28. Nilges, P.; Essau, C.A. Die Depressions-Angst-Stress-Skalen. *Schmerz* **2015**, *29*, 649–657. [CrossRef]
29. Bibi, A.; Lin, M.; Zhang, X.C.; Margraf, J. Psychometric properties and measurement invariance of Depression, Anxiety and Stress Scales (DASS-21) across cultures. *Int. J. Psychol.* **2020**, *55*, 916–925. [CrossRef]
30. Weiss, D.S. The Impact of Event Scale: Revised. In *Cross-Cultural Assessment of Psychological Trauma and PTSD*; Wilson, J.P., Tang, C.S., Eds.; Springer: Boston, MA, USA, 2007; pp. 219–238.
31. Chew, N.W.; Lee, G.K.; Tan, B.Y.; Jing, M.; Goh, Y.; Ngiam, N.J.; Yeo, L.L.; Ahmad, A.; Khan, F.A.; Shanmugam, G.N.; et al. A multinational, multicentre study on the psychological outcomes and associated physical symptoms amongst healthcare workers during COVID-19 outbreak. *Brain Behav. Immun.* **2020**, *88*, 559–565. [CrossRef]
32. Creamer, M.; Bell, R.; Failla, S. Psychometric properties of the Impact of Event Scale—Revised. *Behav. Res. Ther.* **2003**, *41*, 1489–1496. [CrossRef] [PubMed]
33. Fröhlich-Gildhoff, K. Schutzmechanismen gegen psychische Belastungen. *DNP Der Neurol. Psychiater* **2014**, *15*, 60–64. [CrossRef]
34. Strenge, H. Selbstbeurteilung von Stressreaktionen infolge der Terroranschläge vom 11. September 2001 in New York. *Nervenarzt* **2003**, *74*, 269–273. [CrossRef] [PubMed]
35. Schnyder, U.; Moergeli, H. German version of clinician-administered PTSD scale. *J. Trauma. Stress* **2002**, *15*, 487–492. [CrossRef]
36. Angerpointner, K.; Weber, S.; Tschech, K.; Schubert, H.; Herbst, T.; Ernstberger, A.; Kerschbaum, M. Posttraumatic stress disorder after minor trauma—A prospective cohort study. *Med. Hypotheses* **2020**, *135*, 109465. [CrossRef]
37. Ghani, F. Covid-19 Outbreak—Immediate and long-term impacts on the dental profession. *Pak. J. Med Sci.* **2020**, *36*, 126. [CrossRef] [PubMed]
38. Mekhemar, M.; Conrad, J.; Attia, S.; Dörfer, C. Oral Health Attitudes among Preclinical and Clinical Dental Students in Germany. *Int. J. Environ. Res. Public Health* **2020**, *17*, 4253. [CrossRef] [PubMed]
39. Bundeszahnärztekammer—Arbeitsgemeinschaft der Deutschen Zahnärztekammern e.V. Altersverteilung. Available online: Bzaek.de (accessed on 1 March 2021).

40. Smith, D.R.; Leggat, P.A. A comparison of tobacco smoking among dentists in 15 countries. *Int. Dent. J.* **2006**, *56*, 283–288. [CrossRef] [PubMed]
41. Dornquast, C.; Kroll, L.E.; Neuhauser, H.K.; Willich, S.N.; Reinhold, T.; Busch, M.A. Regional Differences in the Prevalence of Cardiovascular Disease. *Dtsch. Aerzteblatt Online* **2016**, *113*, 704–711. [CrossRef] [PubMed]
42. Vahedian-Azimi, A.; Moayed, M.S.; Rahimibashar, F.; Shojaei, S.; Ashtari, S.; Pourhoseingholi, M.A. Comparison of the severity of psychological distress among four groups of an Iranian population regarding COVID-19 pandemic. *BMC Psychiatry* **2020**, *20*, 1–7. [CrossRef]
43. Kinariwala, N.; Samaranayake, L.P.; Perera, I.; Patel, Z. Concerns and fears of Indian dentists on professional practice during the coronavirus disease 2019 (COVID-19) pandemic. *Oral Dis.* **2020**. [CrossRef] [PubMed]
44. Martina, S.; Amato, A.; Rongo, R.; Caggiano, M.; Amato, M. The Perception of COVID-19 among Italian Dentists: An Orthodontic Point of View. *Int. J. Environ. Res. Public Health* **2020**, *17*, 4384. [CrossRef]
45. Forman, R.; Atun, R.; McKee, M.; Mossialos, E. 12 Lessons learned from the management of the coronavirus pandemic. *Health Policy* **2020**, *124*, 577–580. [CrossRef] [PubMed]
46. Kerres, M. Against All Odds: Education in Germany Coping with Covid-19. *Postdigit. Sci. Educ.* **2020**, *2*, 690–694. [CrossRef]
47. Gerke, S.; Stern, A.D.; Minssen, T. Germany's digital health reforms in the COVID-19 era: Lessons and opportunities for other countries. *NPJ Digit. Med.* **2020**, *3*, 1–6. [CrossRef]
48. De Stefani, A.; Bruno, G.; Mutinelli, S.; Gracco, A. COVID-19 Outbreak Perception in Italian Dentists. *Int. J. Environ. Res. Public Health* **2020**, *17*, 3867. [CrossRef]
49. Altemus, M.; Sarvaiya, N.; Epperson, C.N. Sex differences in anxiety and depression clinical perspectives. *Front. Neuroendocr.* **2014**, *35*, 320–330. [CrossRef]
50. Bahrami, F.; Yousefi, N. Females Are More Anxious Than Males: A Metacognitive Perspective. *Iran. J. Psychiatry Behav. Sci.* **2011**, *5*, 83–90. [PubMed]
51. Valentine, S.E.; Shipherd, J.C. A systematic review of social stress and mental health among transgender and gender non-conforming people in the United States. *Clin. Psychol. Rev.* **2018**, *66*, 24–38. [CrossRef] [PubMed]
52. Cabarkapa, S.; Nadjidai, S.E.; Murgier, J.; Ng, C.H. The psychological impact of COVID-19 and other viral epidemics on frontline healthcare workers and ways to address it: A rapid systematic review. *Brain Behav. Immun. Health* **2020**, *8*, 100144. [CrossRef]
53. Thomas, A.P.; Liu, H.; Umberson, D. Family Relationships and Well-Being. *Innov. Aging* **2017**, *1*, 025. [CrossRef] [PubMed]
54. Kowal, M.; Coll-Martín, T.; Ikizer, G.; Rasmussen, J.; Eichel, K.; Studzińska, A.; Koszałkowska, K.; Karwowski, M.; Najmussaqib, A.; Pankowski, D.; et al. Who is the Most Stressed During the COVID-19 Pandemic? Data From 26 Countries and Areas. *Appl. Psychol. Health Well Being* **2020**, *12*, 946–966. [CrossRef] [PubMed]
55. Starke, K.R.; Petereit-Haack, G.; Schubert, M.; Kämpf, D.; Schliebner, A.; Hegewald, J.; Seidler, A. The Age-Related Risk of Severe Outcomes Due to COVID-19 Infection: A Rapid Review, Meta-Analysis, and Meta-Regression. *Int. J. Environ. Res. Public Health* **2020**, *17*, 5974. [CrossRef]
56. Brown, R.S.; Lees-Haley, P.R. Fear of Future Illness, Chemical Aids, and Cancerphobia: A Review. *Psychol. Rep.* **1992**, *71*, 187–207. [CrossRef]
57. Awang, H.; Mansor, N.; Peng, T.N.; Osman, N.A.N. Understanding ageing: Fear of chronic diseases later in life. *J. Int. Med Res.* **2018**, *46*, 175–184. [CrossRef]
58. Onder, G.; Rezza, G.; Brusaferro, S. Case-Fatality Rate and Characteristics of Patients Dying in Relation to COVID-19 in Italy. *JAMA* **2020**, *323*, 1775–1776. [CrossRef]
59. The epidemiological characteristics of an outbreak of 2019 novel coronavirus diseases (COVID-19) in China. *Zhonghua Liu Xing Bing Xue Za Zhi* **2020**, *41*, 145–151. [CrossRef]
60. Ozamiz-Etxebarria, N.; Dosil-Santamaria, M.; Picaza-Gorrochategui, M.; Idoiaga-Mondragon, N. Stress, anxiety, and depression levels in the initial stage of the COVID-19 outbreak in a population sample in the northern Spain. *Cad. Saúde Pública* **2020**, *36*, e00054020. [CrossRef] [PubMed]
61. Nwachukwu, I.; Nkire, N.; Shalaby, R.; Hrabok, M.; Vuong, W.; Gusnowski, A.; Surood, S.; Urichuk, L.; Greenshaw, A.J.; Agyapong, V.I. COVID-19 Pandemic: Age-Related Differences in Measures of Stress, Anxiety and Depression in Canada. *Int. J. Environ. Res. Public Health* **2020**, *17*, 6366. [CrossRef] [PubMed]
62. Hofacker, D.; Naumann, E. The emerging trend of work beyond retirement age in Germany. *Z. Gerontol. Geriatr.* **2015**, *48*, 473–479. [CrossRef] [PubMed]
63. Xie, B.; Watkins, I.; Golbeck, J.; Huang, M. Understanding and Changing Older Adults' Perceptions and Learning of Social Media. *Educ. Gerontol.* **2012**, *38*, 282–296. [CrossRef]
64. Gao, J.; Zheng, P.; Jia, Y.; Chen, H.; Mao, Y.; Chen, S.; Wang, Y.; Fu, H.; Dai, J. Mental health problems and social media exposure during COVID-19 outbreak. *PLoS ONE* **2020**, *15*, e0231924. [CrossRef]
65. Singh, A.K.; Misra, A. Impact of COVID-19 and comorbidities on health and economics: Focus on developing countries and India. *Diabetes Metab. Syndr. Clin. Res. Rev.* **2020**, *14*, 1625–1630. [CrossRef]
66. Zhou, F.; Yu, T.; Du, R.; Fan, G.; Liu, Y.; Liu, Z.; Xiang, J.; Wang, Y.; Song, B.; Gu, X.; et al. Clinical course and risk factors for mortality of adult inpatients with COVID-19 in Wuhan, China: A retrospective cohort study. *Lancet* **2020**, *395*, 1054–1062. [CrossRef]

67. Wang, Y.; Duan, Z.; Ma, Z.; Mao, Y.; Li, X.; Wilson, A.; Qin, H.; Ou, J.; Peng, K.; Zhou, F.; et al. Epidemiology of mental health problems among patients with cancer during COVID-19 pandemic. *Transl. Psychiatry* **2020**, *10*, 1–10. [CrossRef]
68. Alenazi, T.H.; BinDhim, N.F.; Alenazi, M.H.; Tamim, H.; Almagrabi, R.S.; Aljohani, S.M.; Basyouni, M.H.; Almubark, R.A.; Althumiri, N.A.; Alqahtani, S.A. Prevalence and predictors of anxiety among healthcare workers in Saudi Arabia during the COVID-19 pandemic. *J. Infect. Public Health* **2020**, *13*, 1645–1651. [CrossRef]
69. Torun, F.; Torun, S.D. The psychological impact of the COVID-19 pandemic on medical students in Turkey. *Pak. J. Med. Sci.* **2020**, *36*, 1355–1359. [CrossRef] [PubMed]
70. Gao, Y.; Chen, Y.; Liu, M.; Shi, S.; Tian, J. Impacts of immunosuppression and immunodeficiency on COVID-19: A systematic review and meta-analysis. *J. Infect.* **2020**, *81*, e93–e95. [CrossRef] [PubMed]
71. Liu, H.; Chen, S.; Liu, M.; Nie, H.; Lu, H. Comorbid Chronic Diseases are Strongly Correlated with Disease Severity among COVID-19 Patients: A Systematic Review and Meta-Analysis. *Aging Dis.* **2020**, *11*, 668–678. [CrossRef]
72. Maulik, P.K. Workplace stress: A neglected aspect of mental health wellbeing. *Indian J. Med. Res.* **2017**, *146*, 441–444. [PubMed]
73. Pouradeli, S.; Shahravan, A.; Eskandarizdeh, A.; Rafie, F.; Hashemipour, M.A. Occupational Stress and Coping Behaviours Among Dentists in Kerman, Iran. *Sultan Qaboos Univ. Med. J. SQUMJ* **2016**, *16*, e341–e346. [CrossRef]
74. Ammar, N.; Aly, N.M.; Folayan, M.O.; Khader, Y.; Virtanen, J.I.; Al-Batayneh, O.B.; Mohebbi, S.Z.; Attia, S.; Howaldt, H.-P.; Boettger, S.; et al. Behavior change due to COVID-19 among dental academics—The theory of planned behavior: Stresses, worries, training, and pandemic severity. *PLoS ONE* **2020**, *15*, e0239961. [CrossRef]
75. Stöß, C.; Steffani, M.; Kohlhaw, K.; Rudroff, C.; Staib, L.; Hartmann, D.; Friess, H.; Müller, M.W. The COVID-19 pandemic: Impact on surgical departments of non-university hospitals. *BMC Surg.* **2020**, *20*, 1–9. [CrossRef]
76. Gasparro, R.; Scandurra, C.; Maldonato, N.M.; Dolce, P.; Bochicchio, V.; Valletta, A.; Sammartino, G.; Sammartino, P.; Mariniello, M.; Di Lauro, A.E.; et al. Perceived Job Insecurity and Depressive Symptoms Among Italian Dentists: The Moderating Role of Fear of COVID-19. *Int. J. Environ. Res. Public Health* **2020**, *17*, 5338. [CrossRef]
77. Farooq, I.; Ali, S. COVID-19 outbreak and its monetary implications for dental practices, hospitals and healthcare workers. *Postgrad. Med. J.* **2020**, *96*, 791–792. [CrossRef] [PubMed]

Journal of
Clinical Medicine

MDPI

Review

COVID-19 and Dentistry in 72 Questions: An Overview of the Literature

Stéphane Derruau [1,2,3,†], Jérôme Bouchet [4,5,†], Ali Nassif [6,7,8,†], Alexandre Baudet [9,10,†], Kazutoyo Yasukawa [9,10], Sandrine Lorimier [1,2,11], Isabelle Prêcheur [12,13,14], Agnès Bloch-Zupan [15,16,17], Bernard Pellat [4,5], Hélène Chardin [4,18,19], Sophie Jung [15,16,20,*] and on behalf of TASK FORCE COVID-19–Collège National des EnseignantS en Biologie Orale (CNESBO)—France [‡]

1 UFR Odontologie, Université de Reims Champagne-Ardenne, 51100 Reims, France; stephane.derruau@univ-reims.fr (S.D.); sandrine.lorimier@univ-reims.fr (S.L.)
2 Pôle de Médecine Bucco-dentaire, Centre Hospitalier Universitaire de Reims, 51092 Reims, France
3 BioSpecT EA-7506, UFR de Pharmacie, Université de Reims Champagne-Ardenne, 51096 Reims, France
4 UFR Odontologie-Montrouge, Université de Paris, 92120 Montrouge, France; jerome.bouchet1@u-paris.fr (J.B.); bernard.pellat@u-paris.fr (B.P.); helene.chardin@u-paris.fr (H.C.)
5 Laboratory "Orofacial Pathologies, Imaging and Biotherapies" URP 2496, University of Paris, 92120 Montrouge, France
6 UFR Odontologie-Garancière, Université de Paris, 75006 Paris, France; alinassifodf@gmail.com
7 AP-HP, Sites hospitaliers Pitié Salpêtrière et Rothschild, Service d'Orthopédie Dento-Faciale, Centre de Référence Maladies Rares Orales et Dentaires (O-Rares), 75013-75019 Paris, France
8 INSERM, UMR_S 1138, Laboratoire de Physiopathologie Orale et Moléculaire, Centre de Recherche des Cordeliers, 75006 Paris, France
9 Faculté de Chirurgie Dentaire, Université de Lorraine, 54505 Vandœuvre-lès-Nancy, France; alexandre.baudet@univ-lorraine.fr (A.B.); kazutoyo.yasukawa@univ-lorraine.fr (K.Y.)
10 Centre Hospitalier Régional Universitaire de Nancy, 54000 Nancy, France
11 Université de Reims Champagne-Ardenne, MATIM EA, UFR Sciences, 51687 Reims, France
12 Faculté de Chirurgie Dentaire, Université Côte d'Azur, 06000 Nice, France; isabelle.precheur@univ-cotedazur.fr
13 Pôle Odontologie, Centre Hospitalier Universitaire de Nice, 06000 Nice, France
14 Laboratoire Microbiologie Orale, Immunothérapie et Santé (MICORALIS EA 7354), Faculté de Chirurgie Dentaire, 06300 Nice, France
15 Faculté de Chirurgie Dentaire, Université de Strasbourg, 67000 Strasbourg, France; agnes.bloch-zupan@unistra.fr
16 Pôle de Médecine et de Chirurgie Bucco-Dentaires, Centre de Référence Maladies Rares Orales et Dentaires (O-Rares), Hôpitaux Universitaires de Strasbourg, 67000 Strasbourg, France
17 Institut de Génétique et de Biologie Moléculaire et Cellulaire (IGBMC), INSERM U 1258, CNRS UMR 7104, Université de Strasbourg, 67400 Illkirch-Graffenstaden, France
18 AP-HP, Hôpital Henri Mondor, 94010 Créteil, France
19 ESPCI, UMR CBI 8231, 75005 Paris, France
20 INSERM UMR_S 1109 «Molecular Immuno-Rheumatology», Institut Thématique Interdisciplinaire de Médecine de Précision de Strasbourg, Transplantex NG, Fédération hospitalo-universitaire OMICARE, Fédération de Médecine Translationnelle de Strasbourg, Université de Strasbourg, 67000 Strasbourg, France
* Correspondence: s.jung@unistra.fr; Tel.: +33-(0)3-68-85-38-79
† Equal contribution.
‡ on behalf of TASK FORCE COVID-19.

Citation: Derruau, S.; Bouchet, J.; Nassif, A.; Baudet, A.; Yasukawa, K.; Lorimier, S.; Prêcheur, I.; Bloch-Zupan, A.; Pellat, B.; Chardin, H.; et al. COVID-19 and Dentistry in 72 Questions: An Overview of the Literature. *J. Clin. Med.* **2021**, *10*, 779. https://doi.org/10.3390/jcm10040779

Academic Editor: Hans-Peter Howaldt

Received: 15 January 2021
Accepted: 11 February 2021
Published: 16 February 2021

Abstract: The outbreak of Coronavirus Disease 2019 (COVID-19), caused by Severe Acute Respiratory Syndrome Coronavirus 2 (SARS-CoV-2), has significantly affected the dental care sector. Dental professionals are at high risk of being infected, and therefore transmitting SARS-CoV-2, due to the nature of their profession, with close proximity to the patient's oropharyngeal and nasal regions and the use of aerosol-generating procedures. The aim of this article is to provide an update on different issues regarding SARS-CoV-2 and COVID-19 that may be relevant for dentists. Members of the French National College of Oral Biology Lecturers ("Collège National des EnseignantS en Biologie Orale"; CNESBO-COVID19 Task Force) answered seventy-two questions related to various topics, including epidemiology, virology, immunology, diagnosis and testing, SARS-CoV-2 transmission and oral cavity, COVID-19 clinical presentation, current treatment options, vaccine strategies, as well as infection prevention and control in dental practice. The questions were selected based on their relevance for dental practitioners. Authors independently extracted and gathered scientific data related to COVID-19, SARS-CoV-2 and the specific topics using scientific databases. With this review, the dental practitioners will have a general overview of the COVID-19 pandemic and its impact on their practice.

Keywords: COVID-19; dental practice; dentistry; oral health; SARS-CoV-2

1. Introduction

Severe Acute Respiratory Syndrome Coronavirus 2 (SARS-CoV-2) is the cause of the current Coronavirus Disease 2019 (COVID-19) pandemic, whose first case was reported in December 2019 in Wuhan, Hubei province, China. In January 2021, the pandemic is still ongoing and is getting worse [1]. Dental surgery is considered to be a profession at high risk for being infected, and therefore transmitting SARS-CoV-2. Our professional practice was disrupted by lockdowns, resulting in reduced activity, new dental protocols and additional costs for staff protective equipment. This has caused unexpected financial difficulties for many dental practitioners. Even with treatments or vaccines, our professional practice will probably never revert back to the previous situation, as the new constraints may become permanent.

The aim of this article is to provide an update on issues dentists may encounter with SARS-CoV-2/COVID-19 or that are not addressed in recommendations to dental professionals.

To compose this integrative review, a panel of questions susceptible to be of major interest for the dental community has been selected. The questions were selected after discussion between the members of the working group, which is mostly composed of dentists and experienced dental researchers that are members of the French National College of Oral Biology Lecturers ("Collège National des EnseignantS en Biologie Orale"; CNESBO-COVID19 Task Force). Questions were grouped in 10 different major topics that made up the different sections of the manuscript.

To answer these questions, a wide range of keywords was chosen to cover all the topics that are discussed. In total, 378 references were selected in this review. Original studies and significant reviews were included, based on their importance regarding the chosen topics, but also websites from relevant national and international health agencies (e.g., World Health Organization (WHO), Center for Disease Control and Prevention (CDC)). The time period covered by this review gathers published literature from the onset of the COVID-19 pandemic until mid-January 2021.

Q1—What is the impact of COVID-19 on dental practice?

In the Hospital of Stomatology from Wuhan, nine dental staff members and students were infected from 23 January to 4 February 2020 [2]. Chinese dental surgeons immediately responded with recommendations for the management of patients in the context of the epidemic [2,3]. Since then, recommendations have been published on professional websites in many countries, for example in the US (Centers for Disease Control and Prevention (CDC), American Dental Association), in Europe (European Centre for Disease Prevention and Control (ECDC)), in the UK (National Health Service, British Dental Association), in France (Health Ministry, French Dental Association). During the first epidemic wave, the most affected countries put in place a general lockdown, with the closure of dental offices. Only dental emergency services and teleconsultations were authorized. Then, dental offices reopened, with strict conditions for sorting and receiving patients, and detailed protocols for staff protection and to carry out dental care. These recommendations are still ongoing [4,5]. The economic impact is worrying. Besides, fear of contracting and transmitting the virus has caused work-related stress, and sometimes premature retirement of dental surgeons [6–8]

2. Worldwide COVID-19 Epidemiology

Q2—What was the starting point of the pandemic?

At the end of 2019, several cases of "pneumonia of unknown cause" were identified in Wuhan, and a new coronavirus, SARS-CoV-2, was rapidly identified [9,10]. An outbreak of zoonotic origin was suspected, as bats are the natural reservoir of many coronaviruses. Transmission to humans may be mediated by intermediate animals [11]. Attention was focused on the Wuhan wholesale market, which trades in a variety of live animals, but not bats. Genomic analysis confirmed that SARS-CoV-2 shared 96.2% identity with a bat coronavirus (BatCoV RaTG13), and 91.02% identity with a Pangolin-CoV, newly identified from Wuhan market [12]. Direct contact with pangolins, or meat consumption, were suspected to be the main source of transmission of SARS-CoV-2 [13]. However, in the initial cohort of 41 hospitalized patients, 14 patients had no direct exposure to Wuhan market [14]. In particular, the first patient identified had no reported connection with the Wuhan market, or with subsequent cases. His respiratory symptoms began on 1 December 2019, indicating that SARS-CoV-2 was circulating in Wuhan in November 2019. The 7th edition of the World Military Summer Games, which took place in Wuhan and ended October 27, is suspected to have been an early cluster. To date, the starting point of COVID-19 pandemic is still unknown [15,16].

Q3—Why did the initial outbreak turn into a pandemic?

The COVID-19 outbreak arose at the time of the Chinese New Year holidays with large movements of travelers across China. Holidays began on 21 January 2020. Chinese Authorities quarantined Wuhan on January 24 and implemented severe control measures [1,17,18]. In early 2020, Health Authorities from various countries estimated that they could stop COVID-19 by applying the same control measures as for SARS (Severe Acute Respiratory Syndrome) pandemic (2002–2003) and MERS (Middle East Respiratory Syndrome) pandemic (2012, still ongoing). However, scientific studies have progressively shown that SARS-CoV-2 was more contagious than SARS-CoV and MERS-CoV [19]. SARS-CoV-2 is easily transmitted by droplets from person to person, and via contaminated surfaces. Asymptomatic people may be contagious, and sick people are contagious before, during and after clinical symptoms onset [20]. As a result, temperature checking was not sufficient to detect virus carriers. Travelers arriving from Wuhan before January 24 were able to transmit SARS-CoV-2 throughout China and then to Thailand and other countries. In addition, on January 30, the World Health Organization (WHO) "believed that it was still possible to stop virus spread by applying strong preventive measures at the international level," but did not ban travel and trade [21]. Travel controls and preventive measures have been gradually introduced by various countries, but too late [22].

Q4—What is the extent of the pandemic today?

COVID-19 epidemiologic data vary according to sources, such as Johns Hopkins University (JHU) coronavirus resource center or WHO situation updates. Mid-January 2021, global data approached 91 million cases and 2 million deaths worldwide [23]. According to JHU [1], current global mortality rate of COVID-19 is 2.2%. As a comparison, the mortality rate of SARS was 9.6%, MERS was 34.5% and pandemic flu H1N1 (2009–2018; pdm09 virus) were 0.07% [24]. There are major differences between countries that depend on geographical and demographic factors, and on the political will to communicate the data transparently. Infection fatality rate for COVID-19 is below 1% under 50 years, with an exponential increase over 60 years, ranging from 2.5% in the age group 65–74 years, to around 28% over 80 years [25]. According to JHU reports, there was an initial epidemic peak in China on 13 February 2020, followed by three pandemic waves worldwide in April–May, August–September and November–December-January (still ongoing) [1]. A fourth wave has been described in Hong Kong. Vaccination began in some countries in December 2020, but at the beginning of January 2021, its impact is not yet noticeable. Taking into account the number of cases, the ten most affected countries are currently the US (>23 million cases, >388,000 deaths), followed by India, Brazil, Russia, United Kingdom, France, Turkey, Italy, Spain, and Germany [1].

Q5—What is the effectiveness of preventive measures implemented?

Preventive measures aim at slowing down the transmission of the virus via social distancing, face masks, hand hygiene, avoidance of crowds and poorly ventilated spaces, contact tracing, rapid testing and isolation [26]. At the beginning of the pandemic, many countries attempted to detect and quarantine at-risk travelers, identify clusters and isolate confirmed patients. This strategy was not efficient, and lockdown was imposed [26]. The aim was to "flatten the curve" of new contaminations, and to avoid the saturation of hospitals and intensive care units. Teleworking, banning cultural, sports, and family gatherings, closure of schools, universities, non-essential businesses have had a heavy psychological and economic impact. In China, lockdown and all preventive measures have been applied with highest severity. It was accepted by the population, which has made it possible to stop the virus transmission [17]. In addition, protective equipment is mostly manufactured in China [17]. Initially, in some countries, medical teams and populations could not be properly equipped [8]. In January 2021, the pandemic seems under control in China and in some other countries [1]. Elsewhere, preventive measures were implemented too late, insufficient or poorly accepted because all nations do not share the same idea of civil liberties [17]. The pandemic continues to spread rapidly [26,27].

Q6—Is there a risk to be co-infected with SARS-CoV-2 and other respiratory pathogens?

As with other acute respiratory infections, microbial superinfection is common in people infected with SARS-CoV-2 [19]. In a series of 257 subjects, 94.2% of cases had co-infection, and 9 viruses, 11 bacteria and 4 fungi were detected. The most common were bacterial superinfections due to *Streptococcus pneumoniae*, *Klebsiella pneumoniae* and *Haemophilus influenzae*. The other germs most often isolated were a fungus (*Aspergillus*) and a virus (Epstein Barr Virus; EBV). At a lower rate, other bacteria (*Escherichia coli, Staphylococcus aureus, Pseudomonas aeruginosa*), viruses (Rhinovirus, Adenovirus, Herpes virus, but rarely Influenza virus A or B) and fungi (*Mucor, Candida spp.*) were detected [28]. In a series of 2188 patients, respiratory viruses were identified, mostly Bocavirus, followed by Respiratory Syncytial and Parainfluenza viruses [29]. However, the boundaries between viral/viral co-colonization, superinfection or successive infections must be clarified. The diagnosis of bacterial or fungal superinfections is easier. Overall, co-infections aggravate respiratory signs and the risk of severe or critical COVID-19 by weakening the immune system (see Q20). There is no association between SARS-CoV-2 and specific respiratory pathogens, but influenza vaccine appears more than ever to be recommended for dental surgeons, in order to avoid two successive acute respiratory infections [28,30].

3. SARS-CoV-2 Virology

Q7—Where does the virus come from? Are there some other pathogenic coronaviruses?

Human coronaviruses, discovered in the 1960s, are part of the Coronaviridae family and the Nidovirales order [31]. These are enveloped viruses with unsegmented, single-stranded RNA of positive polarity approaching 30,000 nucleotides (Baltimore Classification Group IV [32,33]). Among the Coronaviridae, 7 strains of coronavirus are known to infect humans. Four are considered to be responsible for benign respiratory infections such as the "common colds" (HCoV-229E, -OC43, -NL63 and -HKU1) and three strains, identified more recently, can cause the development of serious, potentially fatal pneumopathies. SARS-CoV and MERS-CoV were discovered in 2002 and 2012, respectively, while SARS-CoV-2, named because of its similarity to SARS-CoV, was discovered in 2019 [34,35].

Q8—What is SARS-CoV-2 as a virus?

Coronaviruses are enveloped viruses characterized by the presence of spikes (S) made up of glycoproteins, found in trimeric form and embedded in the viral envelope. These spikes, arranged in the shape of a crown around the viral membrane, give their name to the coronaviruses. The genomic RNA (gRNA) is encapsulated in a nucleocapsid (N) of helical shape. The whole genomic RNA and the nucleocapsid (N), called ribonucleoprotein (RNP), are enveloped in the viral particle using membrane (M) and envelope (E) glycoproteins [36]. The SARS-CoV-2 genome enables the transcription of gRNA as well as of 9 major subgenomic RNAs [37]. From the complete genomic RNA, two polypeptides are translated according to their open reading frame. Their autocleavage allows the release of about 26 non-structural proteins essential for virus replication, among which are the proteins of the replicase-transcriptase complex [37]. Subgenomic RNAs allow the expression of structural proteins (N, M, E and S) common to all coronaviruses, and of certain non-structural and accessory proteins, which are all virulence factors [36,37].

Q9—How does the virus penetrate cells?

The spike (S) surface protein interacts through its receptor-binding domain (RBD) with the cell surface receptor ACE2 [38]. ACE2 is the angiotensin 2 converting enzyme, whose function is to decrease the plasma concentration of angiotensin, thereby causing vasoconstriction and regulation of blood pressure [39]. This receptor is common to several strains of coronavirus, including SARS-CoV, SARS-CoV-2 and HCoV-NL63 [38,40,41]. After SARS-CoV endocytosis, an interaction of the viral protein S with the transmembrane serine 2 protease (TMPRSS2) mediates its cleavage [42,43], thus exposing the fusogenic peptide of protein S and allowing subsequent fusion between the viral envelope and the membrane of endocytosis vesicles [38,40,44].

Q10—How does the virus replicate?

After entering the cell cytosol, viral genomic RNA, which is 3'polyadenylated, is directly translated by cellular ribosomes into non-structural polypeptides which are self-cleaved by their proteolytic activity and reassembled into a RNA-dependent replicase protein complex [45]. This allows RNA replication into genomic RNA or subgenomic RNAs. The subgenomic RNAs are then translated into structural proteins (N, M, E and S) and accessory proteins, which assemble into new virions at the level of an intermediate compartment between the endoplasmic reticulum and Golgi apparatus [46,47]. The fusion of the vesicles containing the viral particles with the cell plasma membrane allows the release by exocytosis of the virions into the extracellular medium [45].

Q11—Which cells/organs are infected by SARS-CoV-2 and how does SARS-CoV-2 spread in infected organism?

As SARS-CoV [48], SARS-CoV-2 is a multiple organ targeting virus. The abundant epithelial expression of ACE2 (angiotensin 2 converting enzyme) is thought to provide a route for virus entry into the organism, while its vascular endothelial expression may help the virus replication and spreading within the organism [49]. The importance of host proteases, mainly TMPRSS2 (transmembrane serine 2 protease), in SARS-CoV-2 entry has been evidenced [50]. Using single-cell RNA sequencing, Ziegler et al. identified the tissue-resident cells subsets expressing both ACE2 and TMPRSS2 proteins. They found that secretory goblet cells, type II pneumocytes and absorptive enterocytes were the primary targets of SARS-CoV-2, thus explaining the high replication rate of the virus in these tissues, and the associated symptoms [51]. Finally, as glial cells and neurons express ACE2, they have been suspected of being targets for SARS-CoV-2 infection [52,53], in agreement with the neurological manifestations observed in a large proportion of COVID-19 patients [54].

Q12—Does the virus evolve?

Thanks to the proofreading activity of their polymerase (nucleic acid repair activity), coronaviruses exhibit a lower mutation rate than other RNA viruses [55]. Nonetheless, several mutants of SARS-CoV-2 have been described [56]. Mutations on the S protein are closely monitored because they could involve some modification of the virus virulence, as well as the emergence of resistance against vaccines targeting this protein. Very early in the development of the epidemic, a D614G mutation (aspartic acid into glycine) was described as increasing infectivity. This mutation presented a selection advantage, as this subtype of SARS-CoV-2 is now the major variant worldwide [57]. More recently, a set of new mutations in the spike (S) protein (viral strain B.1.1.7) has been described in the UK, as probable evolutionary advantages for the virus, increasing its dissemination ability [58].

4. Immunology of COVID-19

Q13—What are the main characteristics of the innate immune response against SARS-CoV-2?

The efficacy of the innate immunity against viral infections relies on the early and robust type I interferon (IFN) responses, which promotes viral clearance and induction of adequate adaptive immunity [59,60]. SARS-CoV-2 is able to evade immune system recognition, to suppress the activation of the innate immune system, and to dampen type I IFN responses [61–65]. This is supported by the observation that very rare genetic defects causing primary immunodeficiency of type I IFN immunity and autoantibodies against type I IFNs are more commonly found in patients with life-threatening COVID-19 [66,67]. These viral immune evasion strategies allow uncontrolled SARS-CoV-2 replication without triggering the innate anti-viral response machinery of epithelial cells [63]. However, at a later stage, infected cells undergo cell death, particularly in the airways, resulting in lung injury. The important release of viral particles triggers the production of high levels of pro-inflammatory cytokines (e.g., IL-1β, IL-6, TNF-α). Failure to control SARS-CoV-2 infection at early stages in the respiratory tract may in some cases lead to a dysregulated systemic hyperinflammation called "cytokine storm", in a second phase of the disease (see Q18) [59].

Q14—What are the main characteristics of the adaptative immune response against SARS-CoV-2?

Adaptive immunity involves both humoral (mediated by antibodies) and cellular (mediated by T lymphocytes) responses. However, lymphopenia has been shown to be one of the most prominent markers of COVID-19 [59,68–71].

Humoral immunity to SARS-CoV-2 is mediated by antibodies directed against surface proteins of the virus. Antibodies are important for viral neutralization and clearance, but also play a role in the modulation of immune responses. The neutralizing antibodies mainly target the spike (S) protein (in particular the receptor-binding domain RBD), thus blocking the interaction between SARS-CoV-2 and ACE2 and inhibiting the virus entry into host cells, but also the nucleocapsid (N) protein. In most infected individuals, anti-SARS-CoV-2 IgM and IgG antibodies are detectable within 1-2 weeks (median: 11 days [72]) after symptoms onset (see Q24) [73]. IgM are typically the first produced antibodies, but some authors have found that the IgA response peaks earlier and may be more pronounced [74,75]. However, the detection of antibodies against SARS-CoV-2 does not indicate directly protective immunity and the kinetics of neutralizing antibodies is yet unclear (see Q17). A strong antibody response appeared to correlate with more severe clinical disease [76,77]. Sex differences have also been reported, with males displaying higher antibody levels shortly after infection, but a faster decrease of neutralizing antibodies at 3–6 months [78].

Regarding cellular adaptive immunity, both $CD4^+$ helper T lymphocytes and $CD8^+$ cytotoxic T lymphocytes are crucial for optimal antibody production and lysis of virus-infected cells [79]. They also secrete cytokines that drive the recruitment of other immune cells. SARS-CoV-2-specific $CD8^+$ and $CD4^+$ T-cell responses are found in most COVID-19 patients within 1–2 weeks [80,81]. Similar to other viral infections, SARS-CoV-2-specific $CD4^+$ T cells predominantly possess a Th_1 phenotype (that lead to an increased cell-mediated response) [79]. A decrease in the number of T cells has been reported in patients with more severe forms of COVID-19, suggesting that strong T-cell responses may be correlated with milder disease [59,68–70]. In addition, reduced functional diversity and elevated T-cell exhaustion (i.e., dysfunction with loss of effector functions) contribute to severe progression [80]. Some individuals exposed to SARS-CoV-2 develop specific T-cell memory responses (see Q17) but no specific antibodies, suggesting that cellular immunity might be induced in the absence of humoral immune responses [82,83].

Q15—Are there differences in the immune responses between symptomatic and asymptomatic individuals?

Approximately 45% of SARS-CoV-2 infections may be asymptomatic [84] but importantly, asymptomatic carriers have been proven to be contagious [85]. Several differences in immune responses have been observed between symptomatic and asymptomatic individuals. First, the duration of viral shedding is longer in asymptomatic individuals [86]. Second, IgG titers were reported to be significantly lower in asymptomatic individuals compared to symptomatic patients, with a faster decrease of antibody responses (40% of asymptomatic individuals become seronegative within 2–3 months versus 13% of symptomatic patients) [86]. Conversely, many individuals with asymptomatic or mild COVID-19 seem to have highly durable memory T-cell responses, even in the absence of detectable humoral responses [82]. The level of "herd immunity" (i.e., population immunity) can therefore not be extrapolated from serology studies only.

Q16—Are there differences in the immune responses between adults and children?

Children are underrepresented in the total burden of COVID-19 (about 2%; see Q37) [87]. Except rare cases of life-threatening multisystem inflammatory syndrome (MIS-C or Kawasaki-like hyperinflammatory syndrome) [88,89], children tend to develop a milder disease and a large proportion of infected children are asymptomatic (see Q37) [87,90,91], probably resulting in an under-estimation of SARS-CoV-2 infection in this population [92]. Different mechanisms have been proposed. First, the expression of ACE2 receptors in the airway epithelial cells appears to be lower in children [93,94]. Second, children may exhibit more robust innate immune responses [89,95]. They also have the ability to produce more rapidly than adults the so-called natural antibodies (IgM) that play an important role in early phases of infection as they are present prior to antigen encounter. Owing to their high reactivity, they contribute to containing the infection until specific antibodies are produced [96,97]. Third, previous infection by seasonal endemic coronaviruses, which are very frequent in children, could confer a certain degree of cross-reactive immunity to SARS-CoV-2 (see Q19) [98]. It has also been suggested that frequent vaccinations and repeated infections might result in a more "trained immunity" (i.e., form of memory exhibited by the innate immune system) [99,100]. Fourth, adaptive immune responses differ in pediatric and adult populations. In contrast with COVID-19 adult patients, which present high rates of lymphopenia [59,68], white blood cell counts are within the normal ranges in most children [90]. Both quantitative and qualitative differences have been observed in the specific antibody response. Children have a reduced breadth of anti-SARS-CoV-2 specific antibodies and a lower neutralizing activity as compared to adult COVID-19 cohorts [101]. The reduced functional antibody response could be due to a more efficient immune-mediated viral clearance [101]. Pediatric T-cell responses to SARS-CoV-2 may exceed those of adults as children present a higher number of naive T cells [102].

Q17—What do we know about long-term protective immunity to SARS-CoV-2 infection?

Long-term immunity relies on memory T and B lymphocytes, the latter being able to produce antibodies for a long time. Evaluating its duration and strength in the protection against reinfection is a key issue to predict the course of COVID-19 pandemic. Indeed, cases of SARS-CoV-2 reinfection have been reported [103–107], some resulting in worse disease outcomes than at first infection [104,105]. Insight can be gained from previous studies on other human coronaviruses [108]. Protective immunity to seasonal coronaviruses responsible for "common colds" is short-lasting with frequent reinfections [108,109]. In SARS, serum antibody titers remain elevated for the first 2 years, but then decrease significantly over time with undetectable memory B cell responses at 6 years. However, SARS-CoV specific T-cells have been shown to persist more than 10 years after infection [110–114].

Regarding SARS-CoV-2, some authors observed a decline in specific IgG and neutralizing antibodies titers after an initial peak [115]. One study revealed that 40% of asymptomatic and 13% of symptomatic infected individuals, after showing anti-SARS-CoV-2 IgG positivity, reverted back to seronegativity in the early convalescent phase [86]. In addition, antibody responses were not detectable in all patients, especially asymptomatic individuals or with mild forms of COVID-19 [86]. Other studies have however shown a relative stability of antibodies titers [116,117] for more than 6 months, with S-specific memory B cells that were more abundant at 6 months than at 1 month post symptom onset [117].

SARS-CoV-2-specific memory T cells have been detected in most convalescent individuals, including asymptomatic cases and those with undetectable antibody responses [80,82,118]. Remarkably, more than 90% of "exposed asymptomatic" individuals exhibited detectable T cell responses to SARS-CoV-2, despite 60% of them only being seropositive [82,119]. However, a recent study showed that SARS-CoV-2 specific memory T cells declined with a half-life of 3-5 months [117]. Further studies are therefore strongly needed to assess the kinetics of long-term immunity and to evaluate the efficiency of memory responses against reinfection.

Q18—What does the expression "cytokine storm" mean?

Between 5 and 10% of COVID-19 patients may develop a severe form requiring critical care management, with a high mortality rate [59,120]. Rapidly progressing clinical deterioration is generally observed in the advanced stages of COVID-19 (7-10 days after symptoms onset), with the development of acute respiratory distress syndrome (ARDS), accompanied by a state of aggressive systemic hyperinflammation in a condition termed "cytokine storm" [121]. Notably, ARDS occurs despite a decreasing viral load, suggesting that it may be due to an exuberant host immune response, rather than to viral virulence [59]. Normal anti-viral immune responses require the activation of inflammatory pathways and the production of proinflammatory cytokines (IL-1β, IL-6, TNF-α, type I IFNs) [122]. However, in some cases, a dysfunctional immune reaction can lead to an uncontrolled release of pro-inflammatory cytokines [123]. The "cytokine storm" is not a specific complication of COVID-19 and can be associated with a variety of other infectious (e.g., influenza, SARS, MERS) and non-infectious diseases [121,124]. It produces an excessive inflammatory feedforward loop, which starts at a local site (in the lungs in COVID-19) but rapidly spreads throughout the body and drives the pathology. It is responsible for vascular hyperpermeability, coagulopathy, widespread tissue damage, leading multi-organ failure with ARDS, and ultimately death [125–127]. Several factors have been involved and include rapid viral replication in the early stages of infection, resulting in high proinflammatory responses. Surprisingly, SARS-CoV-2 is also able to dampen the host immune responses, inducing a state of immunodeficiency, which contributes to a less controlled inflammatory response [126] (see Q20).

Underlying uncontrolled diseases that are characterized by an hyperinflammatory state such as diabetes, but also possibly generalized periodontitis, may increase the risk of developing severe forms of COVID-19 [128–130]. The presence of diabetes in patients with COVID-19 is associated with a significant increase in severity and mortality [129]. Various hypotheses have been proposed to explain this correlation, including a dental hypothesis [131], diabetes being a risk factor for periodontal diseases. Although there is currently insufficient evidence to link periodontal diseases with an increased risk of SARS-

CoV-2 infection, some authors have observed a higher mortality for COVID-19 patients with periodontal diseases [130,132].

The development of treatments targeting the cytokine storm (i.e., anti-cytokine therapy or immunomodulators; see Q41) will be crucial for patients with severe COVID-19. However, this strategy must be balanced with the maintenance of an adequate inflammatory response for virus clearance [127].

Q19—Can previous exposure to "common cold" coronaviruses protect against SARS-CoV-2 infection?

Four strains of coronaviruses (see Q7) have been shown to be responsible for around 15% of "common colds" in humans [108]. It has been suggested that previous infection with these seasonal endemic coronaviruses could confer a certain degree of cross-reactive immunity to SARS-CoV-2 [98]. This can be explained by a relatively high amino acid similarity between recognized SARS-CoV-2 and seasonal coronaviruses epitopes [79]. Indeed, T cells reactive to SARS-CoV-2 have been detected in 20% to 60% of healthy individuals without known exposure to the virus [80,110,133]. It has been estimated that more than 90% of adults have serum antibodies specific for the common cold coronaviruses (that could potentially cross react with SARS-CoV-2 epitopes) [108], but their titers wane rapidly within months after infection, with only a weak protection against reinfection [63,98,109]. Although we still lack direct evidence that recent exposure to seasonal coronaviruses can reduce COVID-19 severity (this could also contribute to an increase in inflammatory signals [79]), understanding the protective value of pre-existing SARS-CoV-2-reactive T cells will therefore be crucial, in particular since cross-reactive immune responses can be boosted through vaccination and contribute to an increased vaccine-induced protective immunity [63].

Q20—Are patients with immunodeficiencies/under immunosuppressants at higher risk to develop severe COVID-19?

Immunodepression may be a "double-edged sword" in SARS-CoV-2 infection [134]. On the one hand, an immunocompromised state may predispose to infections and facilitate virus spreading. Patients with a compromised immune status (e.g., HIV infection, cancer, primary immunodeficiencies, history of solid organ transplantation, immunosuppressive/modulating treatments) have been identified as being at higher risk of developing severe forms of COVID-19 both in Europe (European Centre for Disease Prevention and Control; ECDC) and the US (Centers for Disease Control and Prevention; CDC) [135,136]. The risk seems even increased as SARS-CoV-2 itself induces lymphopenia [14,71], favoring the development of secondary infections (see Q6). On the other hand, in advanced stages of COVID-19, immunosuppression may be beneficial in countering immune-mediated damage due to excessive inflammation, particularly in the context of "cytokine storm" (see Q18). Several immunosuppressive therapies are currently under investigation or at various phases of development to control or prevent the development of this complication (see Q41) [59,137]. Current knowledge on the impact of immunosuppression on SARS-CoV-2 infection is still limited with varying results between studies and depending on the cause of immunosuppression [138–148]. Patients suffering from cancer seem to represent the highest risk subgroup [140,144,145]. Regarding COVID-19 patients with primary immunodeficiencies, more than one third presented only a mild form of COVID-19 and the risk factors predisposing to severe disease were comparable to those in the general population [148]. A higher prevalence of COVID-19 has been observed in patients with systemic autoimmune diseases, particularly in those without ongoing conventional immunosuppressants [147]. However, the risk of complications appeared to be similar when compared to the general population [146]. Patients under immunosuppressive/modulating therapy without suspected or confirmed COVID-19 should continue their treatment without modification, unless otherwise indicated by the patient's expert physician, as recommended by national and international societies [149–151]. Until reliable data are available, a close clinical monitoring and social distancing should be prioritized for these patients.

Q21—What is the role played by oral/mucosal immunity in SARS-CoV-2 infection?

To date, very little is known about mucosal immune responses at the sites of SARS-CoV-2 infection. As this virus mainly penetrates mucosal epithelial cells, mucosal immunity may be an important parameter influencing the infection course. The induction of a strong local immune response may be crucial for the initial control of the virus and for paving the way to an effective adaptive immune response [152]. Mucosal immune responses are initiated at inductive sites in nasopharynx-associated lymphoid tissues and lead to the production of secretory IgA. The latter play a crucial role in the exclusion of pathogens from the upper respiratory tract mucosal surfaces. During SARS-CoV-2 infection, IgG, IgA and IgM antibodies directed against the Spike (S) protein and the receptor-binding domain (RBD) of the S protein are detectable in the saliva, but only the IgG response seems to persist beyond day 60 [153]. A better understanding of mucosal immune responses will be crucial, as they may have important implications for vaccine design, in particular for the development of mucosal immunization strategies (see Q45) [154,155].

Q22—Can the microbiota play a role in the course of SARS-CoV-2 infection?

The microbiota is crucial for maintaining mucosal homeostasis. Indeed, a persistent imbalance of microbial communities, named dysbiosis, can lead to dysregulated immune responses with hyperinflammation. A dysbiosis profile has been observed in COVID-19 patients, particularly in those presenting a severe form of the disease and/or with pre-existing comorbidities [156–159]. Future studies are needed to understand the interactions between the microbiome and SARS-CoV-2, and the influence of the microbiota on the course of the disease. The therapeutic potential of microbiota modulation should also be evaluated in this context.

5. Diagnosis and SARS-CoV-2 Detection

Q23—What are the various tests to diagnose COVID-19?

Samples are generally obtained using nasopharyngeal swabs (NPS) but also from the oral cavity, as high viral loads are found both in the respiratory tract and the saliva [160,161] (see Q31). The highest viral loads are usually detected in the airways 5 to 6 days after the onset of symptoms. The swabs are then placed in a viral transport medium and can be kept for up to 72h at 2–8 °C, but should be stored below −70 °C for longer time [162] The rRT-PCR (real-time Reverse Transcription Polymerase Chain Reaction) assay, which relies on the recognition and amplification of viral RNA, is the "gold standard" for diagnosing COVID-19 [163,164]. The interpretation of rRT-PCR results is based on the number of amplifications that are necessary to obtain a detectable fluorescent signal, named cycle threshold (Ct). The Ct is inversely proportional to the viral load of the sample but does not correlate with the severity of the disease [164]. More recently, Rapid Antigen Tests (RATs) have emerged as low-cost, fast and simple-handling tests for COVID-19 diagnosis [165]. These tests detect viral antigens using specific recombinant antibodies. RATs are less sensitive than rRT-PCR assays because they can detect the presence of high loads of viral antigens, only when the patient is most infectious. Tests that are commercially available or in development for the diagnosis of COVID-19 are listed at the following address: https://www.finddx.org/covid-19/pipeline/ (accessed on 5 December 2020) [166].

Q24—What are the roles of the serological tests? [167,168]

While the diagnosis of SARS-CoV-2 infection (acute phase) is primarily based on detection of viral RNA (see Q23), serological tests, which detect SARS-CoV-2 specific antibodies (IgM, IgG and/or IgA), are used to identify exposure to the virus. Indeed, IgM and IgG are not detectable until 1–2 weeks following the onset of symptoms [72] (see Q14). Serological assays are mainly blood tests, but they can also be performed on other body fluids, including the oral fluid (see Q25). Different types of serological assays have been developed and include quantitative assays to determine antibodies titers (enzyme-linked immunosorbent assays (ELISAs)), assays with binary results (yes/no; lateral flow assays), and assays that show Ab functionality (virus neutralization assays). In ELISA and lateral flow assays, recombinant SARS-CoV-2 antigens (spike (S) and nucleocapsid (N) proteins, receptor-binding domain (RBD) domain of the S protein) are used to detect specific antibodies. Neutralization assays are more complicated to implement as they require the use of replication-competent infectious SARS-CoV-2 (biosafety level 3 facilities). The main purpose of serological tests is to measure the antibody responses induced by SARS-CoV-2, but also by the vaccination, and to determine seroconversion. Both quantitative and functional antibody assays will be important in evaluating immune protection against reinfection, and known protective titers would be extremely beneficial, in particular for vaccine development. Serological tests also play an essential role in epidemiological studies, to evaluate the prevalence of SARS-CoV-2 infection in different populations, and to determine the level of "herd immunity".

Q25—What could be the benefits of using saliva tests?

Nasopharyngeal swab (NPS) has been recommended by the World Health Organization, especially to test early stage SARS-CoV-2 infection [169], but may be associated with pharynx irritation, pain, sneezing and cough, increasing the risk of contamination [170]. Saliva offers many advantages because its collection is easy, potentially carried out at-home by the patient, non-invasive, inexpensive, stress-free, painless, and with a minimal infection risk [171,172]. Saliva tests have also been developed and approved by the Food and Drug Administration (FDA) with an Emergency Use Authorization, as saliva contains SARS-CoV-2 (see Q30 and Q31). In fact, viral loads equivalent to those obtained from NPS are present in saliva the first week of symptoms, then decrease over time [173]. Based on the presence of viral RNA in saliva, but also of specific antibodies such as IgA (detectable 2 days after the onset of symptoms), some tests such as rRT-PCR or ELISA can be performed using saliva, but require a medical laboratory [172,174]. The promising role of saliva is highlighted by some tests that are usable in medical office as diagnostic tool, for example by colorimetric RT-LAMP (reverse transcription loop-mediated isothermal amplification) [175] or on the field (Point-Of-Need) for mass screening, in particular by lateral flow assay (Rapid Salivary Test), which detects the presence of the virus (Antigen Test), by identifying the spike (S) protein in saliva in a few minutes [176].

Q26—What are the diagnostic performances of saliva tests?

When comparing saliva with nasopharyngeal swab (NPS), the sensitivity values of salivary rRT-PCR ranged from 60% to 98% (mean sensitivity of 85%). Specificity values settled over 90% in most cases [172,177,178]. However, several studies have reported positive saliva samples from COVID-19 patients with negative NPS, suggesting that the combined use of saliva and NPS tests could increase diagnostic accuracy [172,178]. Detection of salivary IgA by ELISA tests, seems to show good diagnostic accuracy (>90% agreement with rRT-PCR) [174], as well as Point-of-Care technologies with RT-LAMP (95% agreement with rRT-PCR) [179] and Point-of-Need tools with Rapid Salivary Test (sensitivity of 93%) [176]. Further studies are needed, in particular for asymptomatic individuals, where the diagnostic accuracy of these tests is still largely under evaluation. However, these tests could be useful before aerosol-generating treatments and could reduce the risk of SARS-CoV-2 transmission in dental offices.

6. SARS-CoV-2 Transmission and Oral Cavity

Q27—Is the oral cavity a potential entry route for SARS-CoV-2?

The oral cavity can be a significant reservoir for respiratory pathogens such as *Mycobacterium tuberculosis*, Influenza virus, SARS-CoV, MERS-CoV, but also SARS-CoV-2 [180–186]. Several mechanisms could explain the ability of these oral pathogens to exacerbate lung infection including their oral inhalation into the lower respiratory tract, by swallowing contaminated oral fluid, but also by the oral localization of host receptor-proteases-mediated pathways facilitating their viral infectivity [184,187,188].

Q28—Which are the oral sites expressing receptor-proteases of SARS-CoV-2 infectivity? Other receptors?

The transmembrane protein receptor ACE2 (angiotensin 2 converting enzyme), as well as TMPRSS2 (transmembrane serine 2 protease) and furin enzymes, have been identified as critical determinants of oral SARS infectivity [189]. ACE2 is expressed on different cells of oral tissues including oral mucosa, gingiva, tongue, salivary glands, and tonsils [49,190–196] (Figure 1). Almost 96% of ACE2-positive oral cells would locate in dorsal tongue. Epithelial cells of the oral cavity showed abundant expression of ACE2 receptor, that is also expressed in T cells, B cells, and fibroblasts, although to a lesser extent [190,194]. ACE2 is reported to be predominantly localized to the basal cells of stratified squamous epithelium but was also visible in the horny layer of keratinized epithelium and finally, in tongue coating [49,190,191]. Interestingly, gingival sulcular epithelium tended to display stronger ACE2 expression than the buccal gingival epithelium [191]. The presence of ACE2 is confirmed in the taste epithelial cells of tongue fungiform papillae. The epithelial cells of salivary ducts and serous cells of human submandibular glands express abundantly ACE2 [191,195,196]. Its expression in epithelial cells of minor salivary glands is even higher than in lung cells, and could constitute a reservoir zone for SARS-CoV-2 in asymptomatic patients [193,196]. Interestingly, TMPRSS2 and furin were found to be expressed globally in the same oral tissues as ACE2 (dorsal tongue, gingiva, salivary glands, taste buds) [191,196,197]. TMPRSS2 is expressed in the squamous epithelium of the tonsils [198,199]. Oral localization of furin was not systematically associated with that of TMPRSS2 and ACE2. Furin-positive cells were neither observed on the surface of the squamous epithelium of the dorsal tongue and salivary ducts, nor on tongue coating. Conversely, furin was secreted in saliva like TMPRSS2 [191]. TMPRSS2 may play a larger role in oral infection compared to furin, and ACE2–TMPRSS2 co-expression is a privileged target for SARS-CoV-2 infection.

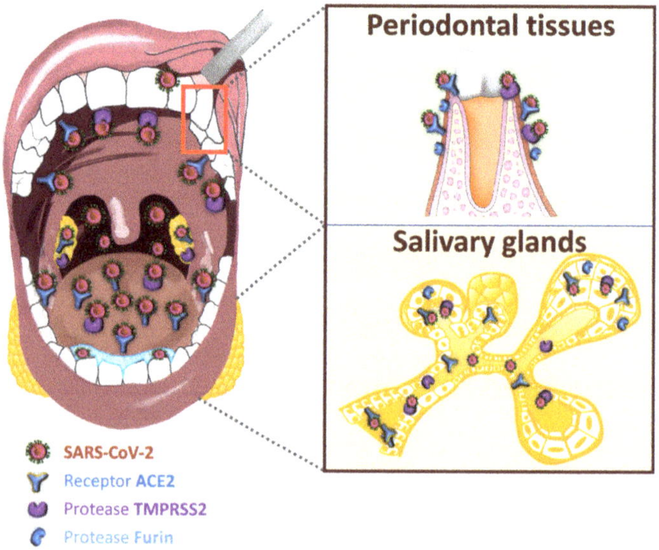

Figure 1. Potential entry routes for SARS-CoV-2.

The membrane protein neuropilin (NRP1) and extracellular MMP inducer (EMMPRIN) have been recently considered as other targets for SARS-CoV-2 infectivity. NRP1 is expressed in the differentiated epithelial cell layers of human normal tongue and in epithelial cells of human healthy salivary glands. The neuropilin-1 receptor is up-regulated in dysplastic epithelium and oral squamous cell carcinoma [200–204]. EMMPRIN expression is also up regulated in oral squamous cell carcinoma. Since ACE2 expression is depleted in oral squamous cell carcinoma, EMMPRIN receptor might be taken over for SARS-CoV-2 entry into cancer host cells [201,205]. The oral expression of all these factors indicate that oral cavity may be vulnerable to SARS-CoV-2 invasion.

Q29—Does SARS-CoV-2 penetrate the oral tissues?

While Wang et al. have reported a proliferation of SARS-CoV in exfoliated epithelial cells in saliva [184], SARS-CoV-2 is detected with a sensitivity of 89.8% on the surface of the tongue after swabbing [206]. To our knowledge, there is only one article demonstrating the direct presence of SARS-CoV-2 in COVID-19 autopsy oral tissues such as human salivary glands and mucosa. In particular, SARS-CoV-2 was detected in oral squamous keratinocytes [196].

Dysgeusia and xerostomia (early symptoms associated with SARS-CoV-2 infection) [195,207–209], but also some oral manifestations such as tongue ulcers [210], could be related to the presence of SARS-CoV-2 invasion factors (such as ACE2 and TMPRSS2) on the taste buds and dorsal tongue [196]. Interestingly, the expression of ACE2 and TMPPRSS2 in gingival sulcular epithelium (directly linked to gingivitis or periodontitis) [191], and the detection of SARS-CoV-2 in the inflammatory gingival crevicular fluid [211], raise questions on the possible role of this epithelium in SARS-CoV-2 infection. The potential passage of SARS-CoV-2 through the systemic route [212] could be considered as it has been demonstrated for periodontal bacteria such as *Porphyromonas gingivalis* [213]. It might be possible to imagine the risk of co-infection between SARS-CoV-2 and bacteria of the periodontal pocket. Co-infection of influenza virus and *Porphyromonas gingivalis* could initiate in vitro the autophagy of pulmonary epithelial cells [214].

Q30—How does saliva represent a reservoir for SARS-CoV-2?

Whole saliva is a biological fluid secreted by major and minor salivary glands and contains gingival crevicular fluid (GCF), desquamated oral epithelial cells, dental plaque, bacteria, nasal and bronchial secretions, blood and exogenous substances [215]. The detection of SARS-CoV-2 in saliva was first reported in 11 COVID-19 patients (91.7%) in Hong Kong [216]. Since then, more than 250 publications have revealed the presence of SARS-CoV-2 in saliva, in connection with the development of saliva diagnostic tests for COVID-19. At least four different pathways for SARS-CoV-2 entry are suggested into saliva: first, by major and minor salivary gland infection; second, from the lower and upper respiratory tract (sputum, oropharynx, cough); third, from the blood into the GCF and fourth, from dorsal tongue [206,217]. Since SARS-CoV has been shown to be able to infect epithelial cells in salivary gland ducts, as early as 48h after its intranasal inoculation in rhesus macaques [192], autopsy of human salivary glands from COVID-19 patients confirmed SARS-CoV-2 infection in these tissues [196]. Furthermore, SARS-CoV-2 nucleic acids were detected in pure saliva from mandibular salivary glands [195]. The salivary glands could constitute a direct source of the virions in the saliva. Saliva is principally secreted from the salivary glands but can contain secretions coming down from the nasopharynx or from the lung, especially later in infection. Saliva samples obtained by coughing up saliva from the posterior oropharynx, were collected from 23 SARS-CoV-2 infected patients. Of these, 87% were tested positive for SARS-CoV-2 [216]. Yet, it is possible that these samples included secretions from the nasopharynx or lower respiratory tract. A passive contamination of sputum could affect the kinetics of saliva [218,219]. Some SARS-CoV-2 positive ciliated cells originating from nasal cavity are found in the saliva [196]. SARS-CoV-2 infected GCF establishes the possible contribution of this fluid to the viral load of saliva [211]. Finally, the presence of SARS-CoV-2 on the dorsal tongue and in infected squamous epithelial cells in saliva [196,206] provides a potential cellular mechanism for spread and transmission of SARS-CoV-2 by saliva.

Q31—How does the profile of the viral load in oral fluid change over time?

SARS-CoV-2 viral RNA load in oral fluid globally ranged from 9.9×10^2 to 7.1×10^{10} copies/mL [161,173,176,216,220–224]. The peak was globally reached during the first week of symptom onset and declined over time with gradual symptom improvement [161,173,183,216,220–223,225,226]. A high load in the pre-symptomatic phase could also be expected [227]. During the period of virus shedding, viral RNA could be detected up to 25 days after symptom onset [161,173,184,216,219] and in one case report, up to 37 days [228], independently of the severity of the illness [184]. Few studies have reported an association between viral loads and severe symptoms [173,216,225,229]. Although in a study using posterior oropharyngeal saliva, viral loads were found higher (1 log10 higher) in patients with severe disease compared to patients with mild disease, this relationship was not statistically significant [216]. No significant difference was observed in disease severity or clinical symptoms between patients in whose saliva viral RNA was detected or undetected [225]. However, the prevalence of severe disease and cough were frequently higher in patients in whom viral RNA from saliva was detected [218]. Interestingly, several studies have reported the presence of viral RNA in the saliva of asymptomatic patients [220,225,230–232]. Salivary SARS-CoV-2 RNA was detected in more than 50% of asymptomatic patients and of patients before the symptom onset [225]. Among 98 asymptomatic health-care workers, two individuals were tested negative for matching self-collected nasopharyngeal samples, but positive in saliva [161]. Alternatively, saliva samples from symptomatic patients with negative SARS-CoV-2 NPS could also be positive [233,234]. Saliva may be more sensitive in detecting asymptomatic or pre-symptomatic infections. The timing and duration of infectivity are important to establish, especially for asymptomatic individuals, because the risk of transmission by air through salivary droplets is possible. Indeed, the relationship between SARS-CoV-2 detection, viral load and infectivity is still unclear as viral RNA may not represent infectious transmissible virus. Viral culture studies using COVID-19 patients to confirm the presence of infectious SARS-CoV-2 are limited. A positive viral culture of infectious virus was found from the saliva of three patients [221]. The infectivity of SARS-CoV-2 in saliva has been demonstrated, even 15 days after the onset of clinical symptoms, using cell culture and an animal model [235]. A recent study suggested that no viable virus could be cultured from salivary swab specimens collected from COVID-19 patients with prolonged viral RNA shedding (>20 days after diagnosis) [236]. The risk of virus transmission can therefore be expected to be low, even though late viral shedding is present in asymptomatic or mildly symptomatic patients. Further investigations with larger cohorts and standardized procedures are necessary to precise the correlation between salivary viral loads, disease severity, infectivity of salivary virus.

Q32—What are the physiological aerosolization mechanisms of oral and nasal fluids?

SARS-CoV-2 is transmitted to human either by hand carriage or by airborne route. In both cases, the virus originates from nose and/or mouth of an infected patient when breathing, speaking, sneezing, coughing or during dental treatments. By breathing, the warm (36 °C) and moist (6.2% water) gases produced in alveoli rise to the mouth and nose where they cool and condense before being expelled (0.6 to 1.4 m/s) in the form of droplets by the respiratory flow. These droplets (0.8–1 µm diameter) contain water and mucous particles from the alveolar and the upper respiratory tract, and the eventual infectious agents. They form a bio-aerosol and can contaminate nearby people but can also remain in the atmosphere (Figure 2). The questions of virus viability duration and concentration in air remain unsolved [237]. Speaking differs by the vibrations of the vocal cords, the longer exhalation time, and the typical flow and pression due to some consonants. Thus, droplets are sprayed from 0.5 to 3 m with possible contamination

(Figure 2). The same question of virus viability duration and concentration in the air remains [238]. By coughing and sneezing, air expulsion is brutal (up to 13 m/s), resulting in the transport of a large amount of alveolar, nasal/oral mucous materials and infectious agents included in very large droplets up to 100 µm [239]. In a few milliseconds, the droplets flatten and split up over a distance of 0.7 m. The heaviest particles fall down and contaminate the underlying surfaces which become fomites. In 10–20 s, the largest droplets lose water through evaporation, mostly in case of low relative humidity and high atmospheric temperature [240]. The resulting little particles with a low water content (i.e., droplet nuclei) and can stay in the atmosphere for many hours or even days (Figure 2). The aerial viral load can therefore increase over time, mostly in closed spaces without sufficient ventilation. Inhaled airborne viruses deposit directly into the human respiration tract. Finally, airborne transmission appears to be highly virulent and represents an important transmission route of the disease [241].

Q33—How is indirect viral transmission by fomites possible for COVID-19?

Direct droplet and airborne transmissions of SARS-CoV-2 occur at variable distance and extended duration [242]. The droplets and droplet nuclei containing SARS-CoV-2 fall down (<1.5 m and several meters, respectively) and contaminate the surrounding surfaces which become fomites (Figure 2). Viral transmission from contaminated surfaces or fomites has a long history, including self-inoculation of the oral, nasal and ocular mucous membranes by hands that have touched these surfaces [243]. This transmission route is important in dental settings where aerosolization of droplets containing SARS-CoV-2 is also generated by many dental instruments. The bio-aerosols produced could be found several meters from the patient's mouth and could remain in the atmosphere of the treatment room for several hours before settling on the worktops [237].

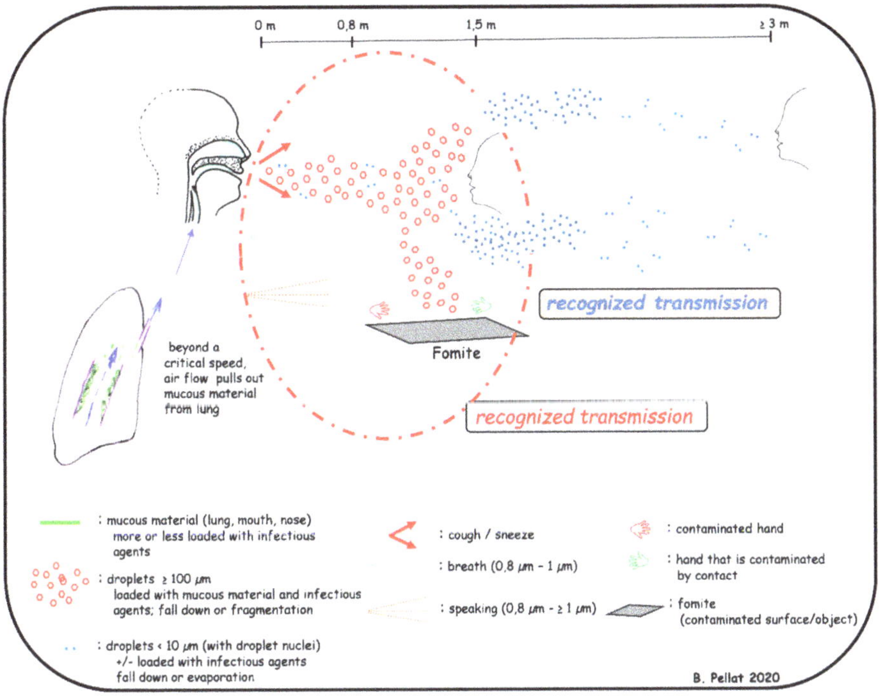

Figure 2. Aerosolization mechanisms of oral and nasal fluids.

Q34—How long can an infected surface remain contaminated?

Regarding the stability of viruses on surfaces, the persistence of SARS-CoV-2 infectivity on fomites has been analyzed by spraying a solution containing the virus onto various surfaces [244]. The stability is higher on plastic and stainless-steel surfaces, 72 h and 48 h, respectively, than on copper and cardboard, 4 h and 24 h respectively. Another study showed that internal and external protective masks may be contaminated for several days with SARS-CoV-2 [245]. These results increase the probability of transmission by contact with fomites since the virus can remain viable several days on supports (plastic, steel) that frequently found in the medical environment [245,246].

7. Clinical Presentation of COVID-19 and Risk Factors

Q35—What are the main presenting symptoms of COVID-19?

Many individual variabilities in the clinical manifestations of COVID-19 have been recorded, ranging from asymptomatic patients confirmed by rRT-PCR to severe forms of infection. The mean incubation period has been reported to be around 5.44 days [247]. The differences in clinical features are due to the age of the infected individuals, their underlying conditions, immune status, coinfection, or even the daily diet, which seems to alter ACE2 expression [248].

World Health Organization (WHO) has classified three levels of symptoms [23].

- Most common symptoms: fever, dry cough and tiredness.
- Less frequent symptoms: loss of taste or smell, nasal congestion, conjunctivitis, sore throat, headache, muscle or joint pain, skin rash, nausea/vomiting, diarrhea, chills or dizziness.
- Severe manifestations: shortness of breath, loss of appetite, confusion, persistent chest pain or pressure, high temperature (above 38 °C) that can lead to acute respiratory distress syndrome and "cytokine storm" (see Q18).

Some symptoms may persist, collectively referred as post-COVID syndrome, such as tiredness, cough, congestion, shortness of breath or even loss of taste or smell [249,250]. Additionally, COVID-19 may increase the risk of health problems by affecting certain organs such as the heart or lungs.

In the oral cavity, sudden loss of taste and smell has been suggested as an early and easy indicator of COVID-19 [251,252].

Q36—What are the main comorbidities and risk factors of COVID-19?

The links between COVID-19 severity and the presence of underlying comorbidities have been thoroughly studied [71,253,254]. Richardson et al. have concluded that hypertension, obesity (see Q38), diabetes and chronic obstructive pulmonary diseases are the most common comorbidities [255]. The risk is increased in elderly patients with weakened immune response, higher frequency of metabolic syndrome along with an increased damage of endothelial cells, as well as increased affinity and distribution of ACE2 (angiotensin 2 converting enzyme) and TMPRSS2 (transmembrane serine 2 protease) compared to children [256,257]. Stable vitamin D3 level and melatonin availability may have protective effects against COVID-19 [258,259]. Smoking and exposure to nicotine, associated with the fragility of the cardiopulmonary system, may be linked to severe COVID-19 forms. However, some studies have suggested a protective effects of smoking via the anti-inflammatory action of nicotine [260,261]. Drug–drug interactions (especially in the context of cancer and autoimmune diseases) have been also considered as a major factor affecting the circuit of COVID-19 for patients receiving these therapies [262]. The severe forms of COVID-19 in patients with underlying conditions have been explained by the availability of ACE2 in different organs (including lungs, heart, kidneys, brain and oral mucosa), the extreme immune reaction to SARS-CoV-2 (see Q18), and also the variations of microbiota (see Q22) [253,263–265]. In the oral cavity, oral submucous fibrosis seems to worsen COVID-19 by activating ACE2 [266]. Poor oral health, as an indirect cause of comorbidities, may increase the risk of severe symptoms [267].

Q37—What are the main symptoms in children and adolescents? Can they present severe forms of COVID-19?

COVID-19 is much less common in the pediatric population. In a cohort of 44,672 confirmed cases, only 2% were children and adolescents aged from 0 to 19 years [87]. Severe forms are rare within this population (0.6%) [268] with very low morbidity and mortality rates compared to the adult population (0.3% of total deaths in the US) [23]. Children tend to develop a milder disease with reduced respiratory symptoms and a very low incidence of acute respiratory distress syndrome (ARDS). Although a large proportion of infected children is asymptomatic [87,90,91], they can spread SARS-CoV-2 [269]. COVID-19 can affect children at all ages (average age: 8–9 years) with no significant sex difference [270]. Children have been typically exposed to the virus through a family member (75.6%) [271]. Fever remains the main presenting symptom together with cough, rhinorrhea and tiredness [271].

Children with other underlying conditions (e.g., congenital heart diseases, pulmonary chronic diseases, diabetes, immune-related disorders, co-infections, obesity) may however develop severe forms of COVID-19 [136,270]. In rare cases, SARS-CoV2 infection has also been associated with severe multisystem inflammatory syndrome (MIS-C or Kawasaki-like hyperinflammatory syndrome) in previously healthy children [272].

No evidence of any related oral manifestation of SARS-CoV-2 infection has been found. All reported manifestations, like fissured lips, erythema, or strawberry tongue (Kawasaki-like disease manifestations) were more related to the underlying conditions and the immune system rather than to the infection itself [273].

Maternal–fetal transmission of COVID-19 during pregnancy is about 2.67% [274], but it is unknown whether the newborns were infected during pregnancy or delivery [275]. SARS-CoV-2 infection during pregnancy seems to be associated with a higher disease severity and an increased frequency of fetal and neonatal complications [276]. However, no relationship between the exposure of newborns to SARS-CoV-2 and the severity of COVID-19 is yet well established [274].

Q38—What are the links between COVID-19, overweight and malnutrition?

The links between COVID-19, weight and nutrition are complex. On the one hand, in Europe, the first lockdown resulted in weight gain in approximately 30–40% of the population (average 2.5–3.0 kg) [277,278]. This was due to boredom or stress, resulting in an increase in calorie intake (overeating, alcohol) associated with limited outdoor exercise [279]. Besides, overweight people have an increased risk to develop a severe or lethal form of COVID-19 (see Q36) [280]. On the other hand, lockdown resulted in weight loss in approximately 10–20% of the population, in average 3 kg [278]. Loss of appetite was due to stress (fear of going out, income decrease), social isolation or a depressed state [279]. In addition, approximately 60% of people with mild to moderate forms of COVID-19 have anosmia and ageusia, which generally regress within a few weeks [281,282]. Severe or persistent forms can cause anorexia and rapid weight loss. Whether it is recent or installed, underweight is usually the sign of protein-energy malnutrition. SARS-CoV-2 infection is characterized by inflammatory syndrome leading to increased muscle catabolism and increased protein-energy needs. There is a vicious circle, because dyspnea, oxygen therapy and isolation hinder food intake [283]. In a study involving 403 patients hospitalized for COVID-19, 70% of them left the hospital with malnutrition and an average loss of 6.5 kg [284].

Q39—What are the main oral manifestations of COVID-19?

Taste impairment is considered to be one of the most common oral manifestations directly linked to SARS-CoV-2 infection, with different degrees varying from dysgeusia, hypogeusia, to ageusia [285,286]. Taste alterations can be one of the earliest signs of COVID-19 and may be the only symptom of COVID-19 in asymptomatic and mild forms of the disease [287]. Prevalence variations of taste disorders have been reported between populations [288] but no significant sex difference has been found [289]. Taste disorders seemed to affect older and hospitalized patients [290], but they can affect younger patients too [289]. First, it was proposed that taste disorders may be associated with olfactory dysfunction [289], but later with increasing case reports, it has been shown that they may happen with or without, and even before the apparition of olfactory disorders [291]. No significant association has been found between comorbidities and the development of olfactory or gustatory dysfunctions [289]. Dysgeusia was also linked to poor oral hygiene and hyposalivation [290]. Many difficulties in evaluating this dysfunction have been reported and include the lack of specific tests, the fact that some COVID-19 patients did not remember having taste disorders and that patients with severe forms were not evaluated for dysgeusia. The four taste receptors (i.e., salty, sweet, bitter, sour) can be affected [289]. Many hypotheses have been proposed to explain taste disorders in COVID-19 patients [291–293]. They may result from interactions between neurons expressing high levels of ACE2 and SARS-CoV-2, which consequently disturb the gustatory pathway by affecting gustatory cranial nerves (VII, IX, X) [292]. The tongue and taste buds' cells that highly express ACE2, interact with SARS-CoV-2, and facilitate its tissular invasion, subsequently altering taste function (see Q28). This was explained by the dysregulation of dopamine and serotonin pathway [292]. This hypothesis is based on previous findings on taste impairment with ACE inhibitors used to treat hypertension [294]. Taste disorders have also been considered as a side effect of COVID-19 treatment [292]. Finally, it has been suggested that SARS-CoV-2 binds to sialic acids of salivary mucins, which leads to their accelerated degradation and the alteration of gustative function [195]. Despite the absence of evidence, dysgeusia seems to persist in some patients, even after COVID-19 recovery [207].

Alteration of salivary glands secretion have also been reported in COVID-19 patients (about 30% of hospitalized patients) [295] but the links are not yet well established. Elderly patients and patients with other comorbidities such as hypertension or diabetes have pre-existing decreased salivary secretion, which makes it difficult to perform an objective reliable evaluation. Since ACE2 is expressed by acinar epithelial cells of major and minor salivary glands [221], some authors have hypothesized the development of acute sialadenitis during SARS-CoV-2 infection phase and chronic sialadenitis after recovery [296]. This hypothesis has been supported by series of case reports of acute parotitis and submandibular gland sialadenitis in middle-aged to elderly COVID-19 patients [297–299]. Altogether, this supports a possible direct link between SARS-CoV-2 infection and sialadenitis, but further investigations are needed in order to establish this relationship, such as eliminating all other viral co-infections of salivary glands and expand clinical observations to larger cohorts of COVID-19 patients.

Some authors have described oral manifestations close to those associated with other oral viral infections such as oral pain (burning), desquamative gingivitis, irregular ulcers and blisters, aphthous stomatitis, glossitis, mucositis, patchy tongue, recurrent herpetic stomatitis, lip semi mucosa or vesiculobullous lesions [300–303]. Increased stress and tiredness during COVID-19 course have been associated with an increased risk of developing other oral viruses like Herpes simplex virus or Varicella-zoster virus [304]. ACE2, TMPRSS2 (transmembrane serine 2 protease) and FURIN proteins are highly expressed by epithelial cells of different oral mucosae (see Q28) [190]. Despite the low number of reported cases of these manifestations, it seems that they equally affect men and women. All oral mucosa localizations were found (tongue, palate, lips, gingiva, buccal mucosa). In mild cases, oral mucosal lesions developed before or at the same time as the initial respiratory symptoms. Viral exanthem was also suggested to be a COVID-19 related clinical manifestation [305]. Due to lockdown and altered lifestyle (poor oral health or overconsumption of mouthwashes, tobacco, alcohol), some oral mucosa pathologies could find suitable conditions for their development or recurrence. Some oral manifestations such as candidiasis have been reported to be due to opportunistic infections caused by broad spectrum antibiotics prescription [306]. Similarly, halitosis was described and associated to epithelial changes of keratinized tongue desquamation [307]. Variation of oral clinical manifestations may be found even between different members of the same family infected with SARS-CoV-2 [308]. Altogether, this suggests that oral mucosal lesions should be thoroughly investigated in COVID-19 patients.

Q40—What is the impact of COVID-19 on patients with rare diseases?

As the majority of rare diseases are chronic, COVID-19 pandemic has exacerbated the difficulties encountered by this population, from potential reduced access to medical care to increased anxiety, with a significant impact on their health status and social well-being [309]. Due to the very wide number of rare diseases (over 7000) and their great variability, it is not possible to address here the impact of COVID-19 on each of these rare conditions. Expert recommendations and information regarding COVID-19 and specific rare diseases are available at the following address: http://international.orphanews.org/summary/id-200327.html (accessed on 21 January 2021).

8. Therapeutic Management of Patients with COVID-19

Q41—Which treatments have been proposed for COVID-19?

Early in the course of the infection, the disease is driven by SARS-CoV-2 replication. At advanced stages, the disease is driven by an excessive inflammatory response to the virus, leading to immune-mediated tissue damage, particularly in the context of concomitant "cytokine storm" (see Q18). It has been hypothesized that antiviral strategies would be more effective in the early course of disease, while immunosuppressive therapies may be beneficial in the later stages of COVID-19.

The National Institute of Health provides treatment guidelines available at: https://www.covid19treatmentguidelines.nih.gov/ (accessed on 6 December 2020) [310].

Several antiviral strategies have been proposed and almost all steps of viral replication have been targeted. All registered clinical trials using antiviral strategies against SARS-CoV-2 have been reviewed [311]. Chemical molecules tested in clinical trials are gathered in Table 1 and the mechanisms of action of these antivirals on viral life cycle are shown in Figure 3.

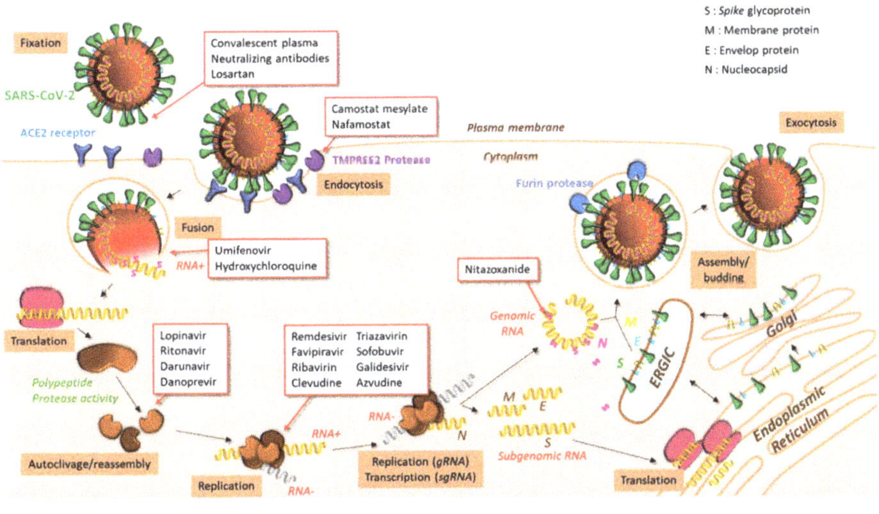

Figure 3. Mechanisms of action of the antiviral drugs on the viral life cycle.

- Serotherapies, based on the transfusion of plasma coming from convalescent patients have early been proposed [312]. This strategy assumes that convalescent plasma contains a cocktail of neutralizing antibodies against SARS-CoV-2.
- Bamlanivimab is a monoclonal antibody-based therapy, using neutralizing IgG1 targeting the receptor-binding domain (RBD) of the spike (S) protein from SARS-CoV-2. Clinical trial showed a reduction of hospitalizations for COVID-19 during the 28 days after treatment, with an improvement of symptoms [313].
- Chemical drugs (Table 1) target the different steps of the virus life cycle, from entry to virion assembly. Most of the drugs that have been tested in trials are antiviral molecules that had been developed against other viruses and reused in the fight against SARS-CoV-2.
- Type I interferons (IFN) are antiviral cytokines that have shown efficacy in the treatment of several viral diseases They trigger the regulation of more than 1000 genes involved in adaptive or innate immunity, allowing the infected cell to enter in an antiviral state, decreasing viral spreading, upregulating antigen presentation and recognition by T and B cells. While type I IFN pathways are targeted and inhibited by SARS-CoV-2 (see Q13) [314], the virus appears to be sensitive to treatment with exogenous IFN-β and IFN-α2. Hence, several clinical trials were conducted using type I IFN alone, or in association with other drugs, showing a decrease of severe symptoms or a lower mortality [315].

Table 1. Chemical drugs targeting the different steps of the virus life cycle.

Antiviral molecule	Initial Use	Target in the Viral Cycle	References
Losartan	ACE2 antagonist	ACE2 receptor: protein S binding	[316]
Camostat mesylate	TMPRSS2 protease inhibitor, recommended for the treatment of chronic pancreatitis	Protease TMPRSS2: cleavage of the S protein and release of the fusion peptide	[50]
Nafamostat	Anticoagulant, targets Factor Xa and Thrombin		[317,318]
Umifenovir	Antiviral, fusion inhibitor used against Influenzaviruses A and B	pH of endosomal compartments: fusion of viral and cellular membranes	[319,320]
Chloroquine, Hydroxychloroquine	Anti-malaria, used in the treatment of autoimmune diseases		[318,319]
Lopinavir	Antiretroviral, HIV-1 protease inhibitor	Viral protease: maturation of the viral replication/transcription complex	[321–323]
Ritonavir	Antiretroviral, HIV-1 protease inhibitor		[322,323]
Darunavir	Antiretroviral, HIV-1 protease inhibitor		[319]
Danoprevir	Antiviral, used for VHC treatment		[324,325]

Table 1. *Cont.*

Antiviral molecule	Initial Use	Target in the Viral Cycle		References
Remdesivir	Antiviral, developed against Ebolaviruses	RNA dependent RNA polymerase (RdRp)	Nucleoside analog (adenine)	[318,319]
Favipiravir	Antiviral, approved for Influenzaviruses treatment		Nucleoside analog (guanine)	[318,319,326]
Ribavirin	Antiviral, used for hepatitis C (HCV) treatment		Nucleoside analog (guanine)	[318,327]
Clevudine	Antiviral, used for hepatitis B (HBV) treatment		Nucleoside analog (pyrimidine)	[328]
Triazavirin	Antiviral, developed for Influenzaviruses treatment		Non-nucleoside inhibitor	[329]
Sofobuvir	Antiviral, used for HCV treatment		Nucleoside analog (pyrimidine)	[327,330]
Galidesivir	Antiviral, developed against HCV, used for Ebolavirus treatment		Nucleoside analog (adenine)	[330]
Azvudine	Antiviral, developed against HCV, tested against HIV-1		Nucleoside analog (cytidine),	[331]
Nitazoxanide	Antiparasitic, used to treat cryptosporidiosis and giardiasis, broad spectrum antiviral	Blocks the maturation of the viral nucleocapsid		[332,333]

Several immunosuppressive therapies are currently under investigation or at various phases of development to control or prevent the development of "cytokine storm" syndrome [59,137] (see Q18). Treatment with dexamethasone, a corticosteroid, has been shown to improve survival in patients with severe COVID-19 and receiving respiratory support [334]. Therefore, the use of dexamethasone has been strongly recommended [334,335].

COVID-19 has been associated with a prothrombotic state [336] and an increased incidence of thromboembolic disease has been reported [337]. Anticoagulant thromboprophylaxis has been recommended (in the absence of a contraindication) in acutely/critically ill hospitalized patients by different expert panels [338–340]. However, the risks and benefits of anticoagulation in COVID-19 patients must be evaluated by dedicated clinical trials.

9. Vaccine Strategies for COVID-19

At the beginning of January 2021, more than 60 candidate vaccines reached the clinical trial stage of development. Out of them, 10 reached phase III, and 5 were used for vaccination in various countries. World Health Organization maintains a landscape document referencing the candidate vaccines in development [341], available at: https://www.who.int/publications/m/item/draft-landscape-of-covid-19-candidate-vaccines (accessed on 22 November 2020).

Q42—Which are the various strategies to design vaccines to protect against SARS-CoV-2 infection? [81,342–344]

Several vaccine platforms are under development and include:

- Inactivated virus vaccines: They are produced by culturing SARS-CoV-2 in cell cultures followed by inactivation of the viral particles to prevent their replication into the host. Whole virus or subunits may be used. Three candidates are in phase III, and 5 candidates are in phases I/II.
- Viral vectored vaccines: They use viral vectors (i.e., another virus than SARS-CoV-2) engineered to express SARS-CoV-2 proteins and able to infect target cells. The latter produce viral proteins that usually induce strong humoral and cellular immunity. Non-replicating human or simian adenoviruses are used as viral vectors in several clinical trials (four in phase III). Replicating viral vectors from vesicular stomatitis virus or measles virus are also used for the development of COVID-19 vaccines (currently in phases I/II).
- Protein and peptide vaccines: Recombinant SARS-CoV-2 proteins or peptides may be used for vaccine formulations. Candidate vaccines focus on the S protein or its RBD domain subunit to obtain antibodies that neutralize virus entry in target cells. Fifteen candidates are in phases I/II, and 4 in phases II/III.
- mRNA vaccines: Viral protein-specific mRNA encapsulated into lipid nanoparticle are expected to reach the cytoplasm of target cells. Thus, cells produce and release the protein of interest, which induces both humoral and cellular immune responses. This technology is new, and mRNA vaccines pose logistical issues as they need to be stored at very low temperatures (−80 °C). Two mRNA vaccines encoding the S glycoprotein or its RBD subunit were claimed to be at least 90% protective against COVID-19 as a result of the phase III trials. Four other mRNA vaccines are under phase I/II clinical trials.
- DNA vaccines: They are based on a plasmid DNA containing the gene of the S protein or its subunits under the control of a mammalian promoter. Despite the high stability of plasmid DNA, DNA vaccines often exhibit low immunogenicity, and have to be administered via delivery devices (e.g., electroporators) to make them efficient. Yet, no DNA vaccine reached the phase III, but five are in phase I/II.

Q43—How to control vaccinal efficiency and safety? [81,343,345]

The efficiency and safety of a candidate vaccine are supported by several properties: (1) a virus-specific immunogenic preparation inducing long-term protection, (2) limited and controlled side-effects, (3) storage conditions that allow an easy distribution all around the world, (4) an easy route of administration that prevents infectious risks. Each antigenic formulation (see Q42) has interests and limitations for combining immunogenicity and tolerance. Immunogenicity is closely related to vaccine design and the presence of adjuvant. However, the adjuvant may vary depending on the route of administration (i.e., intramuscular versus mucosal). After the assessment of efficacy by in vitro and animal experiments, the efficacy and safety of a candidate vaccine for humans is determined by the 3-phase clinical trials. Phase I evaluates the safety of vaccine candidates on a limited cohort, phase II establishes formulation and dosages to optimize efficacy and to limit side-effects, and phase III demonstrates efficacy and safety in a larger cohort. In traditional vaccines development these clinical trials take 5 to 7 years, whereas they only took several months in the accelerated anti SARS-CoV-2 vaccines development. We have to keep in mind that the efficacy of a vaccine may be evaluated not only by total prevention of the disease but also by preventing the severe forms and decreasing the hospitalization rate. All vaccines that have reached phase III use the intramuscular route of delivery, which can limit their use in developing countries. However, candidate vaccines using mucosal routes are under investigation (see Q45).

Q44—What does "Vaccine-Associated Disease Enhancement" mean? [81,343,346,347]

Vaccine-associated disease enhancement (VADE) can result from Antibody-associated Disease Enhancement (ADE) and/or a Th_2 biased immune response. ADE appears when the immune response produces low titers of neutralizing IgG antibodies. Thus, the antibody response is unable to block virus entry into target cells but can even facilitate it. Antigen-Ab complexes induce the release of inflammatory cytokines by binding to Fcγ receptors on immune cells, or by activating the complement cascade. In a similar way, the bias of the helper T-cell response to Th_2 rather than to the anti-viral protective Th_1 dominant response (cell-mediated response), induces pro-inflammatory cytokines release and eosinophilic infiltration. VADE results in an increased disease severity in vaccinated animals/humans submitted to natural infection. VADE has been reported during the development of several vaccines (against Respiratory Syncytial Virus, Dengue, SARS-CoV, MERS-CoV). To control the risk of VADE, SARS-CoV-2 candidate vaccines must induce (1) high and long-lasting titers of neutralizing antibodies, (2) low titers of non-neutralizing antibodies, and (3) a strong cellular immunity. More than likely, candidate vaccines entering phase III respond to these criteria. However, the diversity of the immune responses among the population (i.e., younger versus older, male versus female, previously infected versus naïve) and its impact as regards the risk of developing VADE is still an open question. Even if phase III trials have not evidenced such side effects, the exposure of vaccinated individuals to natural infection is not easy to follow, and probably, waiting for longer periods as well as larger cohorts will be needed to evaluate the real risk.

Q45—How could oral mucosal immunity contribute to vaccine development? [155,348]

Mucosal (nasal or oral) route vaccines for COVID-19 prevention represent 5 out of the 51 vaccines in clinical trials (December 2020). The nasal/oral routes present several interests for vaccine development against viral diseases, especially those affecting the airways: (1) secretory IgAs are polymeric and efficiently neutralize virus entry in animal models of SARS, (2) nasal/oral vaccines are associated with high titers of secretory IgA and a local cytotoxic T lymphocytes activation that may prevent severe forms of respiratory diseases, (3) unlike IgG, IgA are not able to activate Fcγ receptors expressing cells or the complement cascade and thus may limit the risk of a "cytokine storm" or ADE (see Q18 and Q44), (4) mucosal vaccines are easy to administrate, do not need medical training and prevent the risks associated with needle use. However, the mucosal immune system is devoted to maintaining homeostasis through non-inflammatory processes called "immune exclusion". This immune exclusion tolerates the healthy microbiome and prevents tissue infection by pathogens. The stimulation of the mucosal immune system may induce tolerance rather than an active immunization, and the development of mucosal vaccines needs specific adjuvants.

10. Infection Prevention and Control in Dental Facilities Based on World Health Organization (WHO), European Centre for Disease Prevention and Control (ECDC) and Centers for Disease Control and Prevention (CDC) Recommendations

10.1. Identification and Management of Suspected/Confirmed COVID-19 Patients

Q46—How to identify suspected/confirmed patients with COVID-19?

Suspected COVID-19 patients are symptomatic patients showing signs of COVID-19 (see Q35) or asymptomatic patients in close contact—within the previous 14 days—with another person infected or presenting these symptoms [349]. Confirmed COVID-19 patients are symptomatic or asymptomatic patients who have been tested positive for SARS-CoV-2 with rRT-PCR or rapid antigen test [169]. The early and rapid recognition of infected patients and patients in close contact with COVID-19 infected individuals aims at limiting contacts with others to break the viral chains of transmission [349]. Screening questionnaire based on the criteria of confirmed/suspected SARS-CoV-2 infection should be carried out by telephone or by internet when a patient makes an appointment, and at the dental office entrance [350,351].

Q47—How to manage dental appointments?

Patients should access the dental office only by appointment [350]. To minimize contact with other patients, only one single patient is ideally allowed in the waiting room with waiting time as short as possible [350,352]. The planning schedule should be set with sufficient time for patients' appointments [350,351,353]. During the COVID-19 outbreak, patients should not be accompanied to the dental office unless necessary. Only essential persons such as parents of pediatric patients and guardian of patients presenting intellectual disability are allowed [350–352]. The presence of these persons is prohibited (if possible) during aerosol-generating procedures (AGPs) [352]. Patients should have their appointment be rescheduled if they show symptoms of COVID-19 within 10 days, if they have been tested positive for SARS-CoV-2 infection within 10 days, or if they have had close contact with a suspected/confirmed COVID-19 person within 14 days, prior to their scheduled appointment [353]. In case of dental emergency, their appointment must be set at the end of the day [351].

Q48—How to manage patients according to their COVID-19 status?

For patients who seem to be "negative" for COVID-19, all dental cares can be provided by applying the standard precautions and using a respirator for aerosol-generating procedures (AGPs). Patients with suspected/confirmed COVID-19 should not enter the dental facility, unless they need urgent dental care [350]. Only dental emergency should be handled minimally invasively—without AGPs if possible—in a well-ventilated room. The dental staff in the treatment room should be limited to essential personnel and the doors should always remain closed during treatment. Dental staff should apply standard, contact and droplet precautions when performing clinical exam, and add airborne precautions when performing AGPs (see Sections 10.3 and 10.4) [349,351,352]. Tele-dentistry (i.e., telephone consultations or videoconferencing) could be an alternative to face-to-face outpatient visits, providing clinical support and pharmacological treatments without direct contact with suspected/confirmed COVID-19 patients [352]. An appointment can be made after the contagiousness period (see Q47 and Q57).

10.2. Identification and Management of Suspected/Confirmed COVID-19 Dental Staff Members

Q49—How to identify a dental staff member infected with SARS-CoV-2?

Early detection of SARS-CoV-2 infection among dental staff members may be achieved through daily self-assessment for signs and symptoms of COVID-19 [351,354], and laboratory testing in case of suspected SARS-CoV-2 contamination [354].

Q50—What to do if a dental staff member is suspected/confirmed COVID-19?

Dental staff members exposed to SARS-CoV-2—due to a close contact with a COVID-19 person without appropriate personal protective equipment—should be excluded from work, self-monitor their symptoms and self-quarantine for 14 days [353,355,356]. They should be tested [353,355]. A rRT-PCR test on day 10 after exposure can be performed and if it is negative, quarantine can be discontinued earlier [356]. Dental staff member presenting symptoms that are compatible with COVID-19 should stop working, self-isolate at home [350,351,353] and get tested [350,355]. A dental staff member with a positive SARS-CoV-2 test—with or without symptoms—should self-isolate at home. The safe return to work can be achieved after at least 10 days (minimum 20 days for severe COVID-19 and for immunocompromised staff member) with an additional 24 to 72h without fever associated with improvement of respiratory symptoms [354,357].

10.3. Applying Standard Precautions for All Patients in a COVID-19 Context

Q51—What are standard precautions?

Standard precautions are designed to reduce the risk of pathogen transmission, including bloodborne and airborne pathogens. They include hand and respiratory hygiene, use of appropriate personal protective equipment based on the risk assessment [351] (see Section 10.5), care equipment and environmental cleaning, and safe waste management [358].

Q52—How to perform hand hygiene?

Hand hygiene is one of the most effective method to prevent pathogen transmission and healthcare-associated infections [358,359], including COVID-19 [353]. Dental staff members should apply WHO's "My five moments for hand hygiene" approach: before touching a patient, before a clean or aseptic procedure, after body fluid exposure risk, after touching a patient, and after touching patient surroundings (whether or not gloves are worn). In addition, hand hygiene should be performed before putting on personal protective equipment and after removing them [353,358–361]. To perform hand hygiene, nails should be kept natural (without nail polish, artificial fingernails or extenders) and short ($\leq$0.5 cm). Wearing watches, rings or other jewelry is discouraged, and long-sleeves should be avoided [360]. When hands are not visibly dirty or soiled, the preferred method is to use an alcohol-based hand rub for 20−30 s until they are dry [358–360]. Virucidal activity of hand rub agents is tested by EN 14476 (European Committee for Standardization standards) or by ASTM E1838 (American Society for Testing and Materials standards). When hands are visibly dirty or soiled with blood or other body fluids, hands must be washed with plain soap and water for 40−60 s [358–360].

Q53—How to perform respiratory hygiene?

Controlling the spread of pathogens from the source is key to avoiding any transmission. Standard respiratory hygiene precautions should be applied to every person exhibiting respiratory symptoms (coughing or sneezing) [358]. Respiratory hygiene precautions are taken during influenza and SARS-CoV epidemics. They are as follows: cover nose and mouth with a disposable/single-used tissue or bent elbow when coughing or sneezing, discard used tissues and masks, and perform hand hygiene after any contact with respiratory secretions or objects potentially contaminated with respiratory secretions [352,358,362]. During COVID-19 outbreak, patients and visitors should wear a medical or cloth mask in the dental facility to prevent the spread of respiratory secretions due to potential asymptomatic and pre-symptomatic transmission [351,353]. Patients should be provided with hand hygiene means, paper tissues and masks in common areas (i.e., reception area and waiting room) [351–353,358,363].

10.4. Implementing Additional Precautions in COVID-19 Context

Q54—What are additional precautions in COVID-19 context?

Additional precautions are supplementary infection prevention and control measures required by dental staff members to protect themselves and prevent transmission of pathogens like SARS-CoV-2 [363,364]. They include contact, droplet and airborne precautions [362]. During the COVID-19 outbreak, spatial distancing of at least 1–1.5 m should always be maintained between patients [350–353,363]. It should be also maintained between dental staff members when they need to be unmasked (when eating and drinking) [351]. It can be only broken by dental staff members during a patient's dental treatment. In addition, use of physical barriers such as glass or plastic panels as protection against respiratory droplets can reduce dental staff members' exposure to SARS-CoV-2, especially in the reception area [350–352,363]. It does not exempt patients and dental staff members from respecting spatial distancing and the use of masks [350].

Q55—How to implement contact and droplet precautions in COVID-19 context?

SARS-CoV-2 is mainly transmitted through respiratory droplets (>5 µm in diameter) and contact routes (see Q32 and Q33). Droplet transmission occurs when a person is in close contact (within 1 m) of infected people. Their mucosae (mouth, nose, eyes) are therefore exposed to infectious respiratory droplets. Transmission can also occur through direct contact with infected people and indirect contact with surfaces (fomites) in the immediate environment or with medical devices previously used on an infected person [352]. Therefore, contact and droplet precautions should be implemented by dental staff caring for each suspected/confirmed COVID-19 patient [349]. They comprise the use of appropriate personal protective equipment (PPE): medical mask, eye protection, non-sterile long-sleeved gown, and medical gloves (see Section 10.5) [352,365]. PPE must fulfil quality standards (European Committee for Standardization [CEN] or American Society for Testing and Materials [ASTM] standards for instance) [354]. A new set of PPE is needed when providing care to a different patient. Dental staff members should refrain from touching their eyes, nose or mouth with potentially contaminated gloved or bare hands [352].

Q56—How to implement airborne precautions in COVID-19 context?

Airborne transmission refers to the presence of droplet nuclei (<5 μm in diameter) which can remain in the air for longer periods of time and can be transmitted to others for distances greater than 1m (see Q32). Airborne transmission of SARS-CoV-2 is possible in settings where aerosol-generating procedures (AGPs) are performed [352]. During the COVID-19 outbreak, airborne precautions should be applied by dental staff for each AGP [350] (e.g., use of high-speed dental turbine and handpiece, air/water syringe, ultrasonic scaler, air polishing, and air abrasion) [351]. They rely on the use of appropriate personal protective equipment: respirator, eye protection, non-sterile long-sleeved gown, and medical gloves. If gowns are not fluid resistant, dental staff members should use an additional water-resistant apron. In addition, the dental treatment room should be ventilated [352].

Q57—When discharging patients from additional precautions?

To relieve patients from isolation, negative rRT-PCR tests are not required [366]. Indeed, the detection of viral RNA does not necessarily mean that a person is contagious. The duration of rRT-PCR positivity generally appears to be 1-2 weeks for asymptomatic patients, and up to 3 weeks or more for symptomatic patients [349].

Criteria for releasing COVID-19 patients from isolation are:

- For symptomatic patients: at least 10 days after symptoms onset (14 to 20 days for severe COVID-19, and 20 days for immunocompromised patients) with an additional 24 to 72 h without fever associated with improvement of respiratory symptoms.
- For asymptomatic cases: 10 days after positive SARS-CoV-2 test [366–368].

10.5. Using Personal Protective Equipment

Q58—Why using personal protective equipment in COVID-19 context?

Appropriate use of personal protective equipment aims to reduce, but not eliminate, the risks of transmission of respiratory pathogens to dental staff [362].

Q59—How to use gloves in dental facility?

According to standard precautions, medical gloves are indicated in all clinical situations at risk of contact with blood, body fluids, secretions, excretions and items visibly soiled by body fluids, and in cases of contact with mucosae and non-intact skin of patients [359,360,369]. In addition, they are indicated for handling/cleaning instruments, handling waste and cleaning environmental surfaces in the dental facility [359,360]. Their use does not replace the need for proper hand hygiene [359,364]. It is recommended to change them between each patient, and to perform hand hygiene immediately after their removal [358]. Washing or decontaminating gloved hands is strictly prohibited [360,369]. The double gloving is not recommended for COVID-19 patients [363]. Gloves should be removed as soon as they are damaged (or non-integrity suspected). They should also be removed as soon as dental treatment has been completed, and when there is an indication for hand hygiene [356,360].

Q60—Which mask for which situation in dental facility?

Masks are indicated for the protection of healthy people. Wearing a mask allows to protect oneself in case of contact with a COVID-19 patient, and prevents onward transmission of the virus when used by a COVID-19 patient [365].

For the general population, the cloth mask is recommended as an alternative to the medical mask during COVID-19 outbreak in public places where there is community transmission and where other prevention measures, such as physical distancing, are not possible [349,365]. Patients and visitors should wear their own cloth mask upon arrival and throughout their stay in the dental facility. Patients may remove them in the dental treatment room, but they must put it back on at the end of dental treatment [351]. For dental staff, the use of cloth masks as an alternative to medical masks is not considered appropriate [363,365] because cloth masks are not personal protective equipment [351]. In addition, cloth masks are not fluid-resistant and thus may retain moisture, become contaminated, and act as a potential source of infection [363].

Medical masks—also known as surgical masks—are indicated for dental staff member and at-risk individuals [365]. Continued use of a medical mask by dental staff members is recommended during all routine activities throughout the entire shift [349,351,353]. Dental staff members caring for COVID-19 patients without aerosol-generating procedures (AGPs) may wear a medical mask. Medical masks should be type IIR (EN 14683 [European Committee for Standardization standards] or tested by ASTM F2100 [American Society for Testing and Materials standards]) [365].

Particulate respirators—also known as filtering facepiece respirator—offer greater filtration capacity. Whereas medical masks filter 3 µm droplets, respirators filter out 0.075 µm solid particles [365]. Thus, medical masks do not offer adequate respiratory protection against aerosols (droplet nuclei), especially due to leaks around the edge of the mask when the user inhales [362]. Use of a respirator is required in dental treatment room where AGPs are performed, especially for COVID-19 patients [351,353,365,370]. In addition, according to ECDC and CDC, respirators are indicated when managing a suspected/confirmed COVID-19 patient (with or without AGPs) [351,353,370]. Respirators should be FFP2 or FFP3 (EN 149; European standards), N95 (NIOSH-42CFR84.181; US standards), or KN95 (GB 2626-2006; Chinese standard) [365]. Moreover, respirators with exhalation valves should not be used during surgical procedures as they allow unfiltered exhaled breath to escape [351,352].

To date, WHO, ECDC and CDC recommendations did not change regarding mask use despite the emergence of new SARS-CoV-2 variants, which have led to increased transmissibility [371–373]. However, some countries no longer accept cloth mask for the general population in certain places (e.g., hospitals, public transportation) and extend the use of respirators.

Q61—How to use a mask/respirator?

Correct use of mask/respirator consists in performing hand hygiene before putting on the mask, then placing the mask/respirator on carefully, ensuring it covers the mouth and nose, adjusting it to the nose bridge, and tying it securely to minimize any gaps between the face and the mask/respirator, and finally avoiding touching the mask/respirator while wearing it [365]. Regarding respirator, an initial fit testing is needed before use [352,370]. If the dental staff member has a beard, this may prevent proper fit of the respirator [352]. Mask/respirator should be removed if it is wet, soiled or damaged, if it is exposed to splashes, if it is touched or displaced from face for any reason [363,365]. The use of the same medical mask/respirator by a dental staff member between a confirmed/suspected COVID-19 patient and a patient who does not have COVID-19 is not recommended due to the risk of transmission [363]. Mask/respirator should be removed without touching their front, then a hand hygiene should be performed [365].

Q62—Can dental staff members extend the period of use of their masks/respirators?

Medical mask and respirator are single-used personal protective equipment (PPE). They should ideally be changed after each patient [351,362]. However, during COVID-19 outbreak, which created severe shortages of PPE, medical masks and respirator could be used by dental staff without removing them for up to 6h and 4h, respectively [363,364]. However, wearing medical mask during a prolonged period increases the risk of contamination of the mask/respirator with SARS-CoV-2 and other pathogens. There is a risk that dental staff members will contaminate their hand by touching the front of the mask/respirator. If it is touched/adjusted, hand hygiene must be performed immediately [363]. The risk of contamination can be reduced by wearing a face shield over the mask [356]. Finally, wearing the same medical mask/respirator is only allowed to treat several patients who have the same COVID-19 status [356,364]. Methods of reprocessing medical mask/respirator—by disinfection or sterilization—are neither well established nor standardized. No evidence is available to date on the reprocessing of medical mask/respirator [363].

Q63—How to use eye protection?

Eye protection—such as goggles and face shield—are indicated to reduce the risk of droplets transmission and splashes to the ocular mucosa [365,370]. Face shield covers and protects the entire face from splashes, including the side of the face and the chin [363]. Conventional eye glasses should not be used as eye protection [362]. During COVID-19 outbreak, dental staff should wear eye protection associated with their medical mask/respirator during all patient care [351]. Immediately after removal, goggles and face shield should be decontaminated, and hand hygiene should be performed [363].

Q64—How to use gowns?

According to the additional precautions, a long-sleeved water-resistant non-sterile gown is indicated to protect skin and prevent soiling of work clothes during treatment and activities that may generate splashes of blood or body fluids, and during aerosol-generating procedures (AGPs) [356,358,370]. When used, gowns should always be changed after each patient contact [356]. Immediately after removal, single-use gowns should be discarded and hand hygiene is required [358]. Cloth gowns can be decontaminated for reprocessing by machine washing them at high temperature (60–90 °C) and laundry detergent [363]. If gowns are not water-resistant, dental staff should use an additional disposable water-resistant apron over the gown [352,370]. Water-resistant plastic aprons should not be used alone when performing AGPs on COVID-19 patient [363].

Q65—In which order should personal protective equipment be put on and removed during dental treatments?

Before dental cares, CDC and ECDC suggest the following sequence to put on personal protective equipment (PPE): (1) perform hand hygiene, (2) put on a clean gown or apron, (3) put on a medical mask/respirator, (4) put on eye protection, and (5) put on clean gloves [351,370]. After completion of dental cares, CDC suggests the following sequence to remove PPE: (1) remove gloves, (2) remove gown or apron, (3) perform hand hygiene, (4) remove eye protection, (5) remove and discard surgical mask/respirator, and (6) perform hand hygiene [351].

10.6. Environmental Cleaning and Disinfection, and Waste Management

Q66—How to perform environmental cleaning and disinfection in COVID-19 context?

Procedures for cleaning and disinfecting the dental environment aim to reduce any role fomites may play in the transmission of SARS-CoV-2. The SARS-CoV-2 virus remained viable for up to a few days on surfaces, but it is an enveloped virus with a fragile outer lipid envelope that makes it sensitive to disinfectants [374]. Materials, objects, and devices should be stored in a way that facilitates environmental cleaning and disinfection [350]. In the waiting room, toys, magazines, books or other non-essential items that patients may touch should be removed [350,351]. All surfaces in dental facility should be regularly cleaned and disinfected, especially high-touch surfaces, and whenever they are visibly soiled or contaminated with body fluids [352,363]. In common areas, high-touch surfaces require regular cleaning at least twice a day. In dental treatment rooms, high-touch surfaces should be disinfected after each patient visit [350,374] and terminal cleaning is required for low-touch surfaces, high-touch surfaces and floors at least once a day [374].

After ventilation, surfaces should be thoroughly cleaned using a detergent-disinfectant product effective against viruses following the manufacturer's instructions [350,351,375]. Virucidal activity of disinfectants is tested by EN 14476 (European Committee for Standardization standards) or by ASTM E1053 (American Society for Testing and Materials standards). Cleaning should progress systematically to avoid missing areas, from the least soiled (cleanest) to the most soiled (dirtiest), and from higher to lower levels [374]. Cleaners should wear adequate personal protective equipment: water-resistant apron (or a long-sleeves water-resistant gown after a suspected/infected COVID-19 patient), gloves, medical mask (or respirator in a room were aerosol-generating procedures have been performed) and eye protection [374,375].

No-touch disinfection technology, such as UV irradiation or vaporized hydrogen peroxide, can complement but not replace the first manual cleaning of environmental surfaces that are required to remove organic material [374]. The effectiveness of alternative disinfection methods (e.g., ultrasonic waves, UV irradiation, and blue LED light) against SARS-CoV-2 are not known [351].

Q67—Should sterilization protocols be adapted for SARS-CoV-2?

Dental staff should perform routine cleaning, disinfection, and sterilization protocols of medical devices [351].

Q68—How to laundry work clothes?

To decontaminate work clothes, machine wash at high temperature (60–90 °C) for at least 30 min and the use of laundry detergent is recommended [361]. If a hot-water cycle cannot be used, bleach or other laundry products for decontamination of textiles should be added to the wash cycle [375].

Q69—How to manage waste?

Healthcare waste generated during the care of suspected/confirmed COVID-19 patients are considered as infectious clinical waste and should be collected safely in clearly marked lined containers and sharp safe boxes [352,356,361,375]. Waste are disposed at least once a day [374]. Waste generated in the waiting room can be classified as non-hazardous and should be disposed of in sturdy black bags before being collected by municipal waste management services [361].

10.7. Limiting Indoor Air Contamination during the COVID-19 Outbreak

Q70—How to minimize indoor air contamination during dental cares?

For suspected/confirmed COVID-19 patients, aerosol-generating procedures (AGPs) should be avoided as much as possible. When the AGP is required for dental treatment and cannot be postponed, the risk can be minimized by performing a preprocedural mouth rinse, applying rubber dam isolation, using evacuation aspirators/suction and practicing four-handed dentistry [350,351]. If an AGP was performed, the dental treatment room needs to be naturally or mechanically ventilated before admitting a new patient [350].

Q71—How to ventilate the dental treatment room?

Adequate ventilation with fresh and clean outdoor air can play an important role to prevent the spread of airborne infections by reducing the concentration of infectious respiratory aerosols in indoor air. There are three methods for ventilating: natural (window), mechanical, and mixed-mode ventilation [352,362,376]. In dental treatment rooms, a minimum of 6 (ideally 12) air changes per hour is recommended by CDC and ECDC [350,351]. WHO recommends an average natural ventilation rate $\geq$ 60 L/s/patient or $\geq$ 12 air changes per hour for mechanical ventilation in an outpatient room with airborne precautions [376].

Q72—Are air cleaners helpful to decontaminate the indoor air?

Air cleaners using a high-efficiency particulate air (HEPA) filter may be effective in reducing the concentrations of infectious aerosols for dental offices without adequate natural or mechanical ventilation [352,375,377]. However, the evidence for the effectiveness of HEPA filters in preventing coronavirus transmission is currently limited [352,356]. If used, the CDC recommends placing the HEPA unit near the dental chair—but not between a dental staff member and the patient's mouth—and it should not draw air into or through the breathing zone of the dental staff [351].

Air cleaners using ultraviolet germicidal irradiation, air ionizers using negative ion and ozone generators have been proposed in addition to ventilation [351,354,376]. However, the evidence on their effectiveness is currently limited and they are potentially hazardous to human health [377].

11. Conclusions

In the course of twelve months, this new virus will have devasted the world order and challenged our medical practices. Starting from virtually nothing, knowledge about SARS-CoV-2 is enriching daily, often overthrowing the approaches of the day before.

The answers to these 72 questions were submitted to give the reader a current state of science in this field. With this review, we have given a broad overview about SARS-CoV-2, in particular its behavior and transmission abilities, and COVID-19 on a global scale. This manuscript briefly explains how the patients respond to the infection, the symptoms with a focus on oral manifestations, the risk factors and comorbidities, but also the strategies that have been developed to counter the viral spread. As dental professionals are particularly exposed to COVID-19, due to their practice in a potentially contaminated environment, one of the objectives of this review was to inform them of the risks of being infected and therefore transmitting the virus. Thus, we focused on the role played by the oral route in the infection and transmission of SARS-CoV-2, leading to recommendations related to infection prevention and control in dental facilities based on guideline from national and international health agencies.

Finally, the only attitude to be held is to consider each patient as a potential carrier of the SARS-CoV-2 or of another infectious agent. From these data, the reader should be able to master the further knowledge and fully play his role as health actor with his patients. With the difficulties to provide dental healthcare in these specific conditions and the requirement to mobilize all the sanitary resources, it is essential to rethink the role of dentists and to give them a greater space in an integrated medical model.

Author Contributions: S.D. wrote, reviewed the manuscript, and conducted the final editing. J.B. wrote, reviewed the manuscript, and prepared the figures and table. A.N. wrote and reviewed the manuscript. A.B. wrote and reviewed the manuscript. K.Y. wrote and reviewed the manuscript. S.L. wrote, reviewed the manuscript, and prepared the figures. I.P. wrote and reviewed the manuscript. A.B.-Z. wrote, reviewed the manuscript, and managed the whole process. B.P. wrote, reviewed the manuscript, and prepared the figures. H.C. wrote, reviewed the manuscript, and managed the whole process. S.J. wrote, reviewed the manuscript, managed the whole process, and conducted the final editing. All authors have read and agreed to the published version of the manuscript.

Funding: This work has been supported by "Collège National des EnseignantS en Biologie Orale (CNESBO)" (publication fees).

Acknowledgments: The authors thank the "Collège National des EnseignantS en Biologie Orale (CNESBO)" and the "Académie Nationale de Chirurgie Dentaire (ANCD)" for their support. They also thank Yannick Dieudonné (Hôpitaux Universitaires de Strasbourg, France) for proofreading of the manuscript and Ganesh D. Sockalingum (Université de Reims Champagne-Ardenne, UFR Pharmacie, EA7506-Biospectroscopie Translationnelle (BioSpecT)) and Martine Spina (Lycée Masséna, Nice, France) for careful English language editing.

Conflicts of Interest: The authors declare no conflict of interest within the scope of the submitted work.

References

1. COVID-19 Map. Available online: https://coronavirus.jhu.edu/map.html (accessed on 15 January 2021).
2. Meng, L.; Hua, F.; Bian, Z. Coronavirus Disease 2019 (COVID-19): Emerging and Future Challenges for Dental and Oral Medicine. *J. Dent. Res.* **2020**, *99*, 481–487. [CrossRef]
3. Peng, X.; Xu, X.; Li, Y.; Cheng, L.; Zhou, X.; Ren, B. Transmission Routes of 2019-NCoV and Controls in Dental Practice. *Int. J. Oral Sci.* **2020**, *12*, 9. [CrossRef] [PubMed]
4. Bizzoca, M.E.; Campisi, G.; Muzio, L.L. Covid-19 Pandemic: What Changes for Dentists and Oral Medicine Experts? A Narrative Review and Novel Approaches to Infection Containment. *Int. J. Environ. Res. Public Health* **2020**, *17*, 3793. [CrossRef] [PubMed]
5. Barabari, P.; Moharamzadeh, K. Novel Coronavirus (COVID-19) and Dentistry-A Comprehensive Review of Literature. *Dent. J.* **2020**, *8*, 53. [CrossRef] [PubMed]
6. Mijiritsky, E.; Hamama-Raz, Y.; Liu, F.; Datarkar, A.N.; Mangani, L.; Caplan, J.; Shacham, A.; Kolerman, R.; Mijiritsky, O.; Ben-Ezra, M.; et al. Subjective Overload and Psychological Distress among Dentists during COVID-19. *Int. J. Environ. Res. Public Health* **2020**, *17*, 5074. [CrossRef]
7. Chamorro-Petronacci, C.; Martin Carreras-Presas, C.; Sanz-Marchena, A.; Rodríguez-Fernández, M.A.; Suárez-Quintanilla, J.M.; Rivas-Mundiña, B.; Suárez-Quintanilla, J.; Pérez-Sayáns, M. Assessment of the Economic and Health-Care Impact of COVID-19 (SARS-CoV-2) on Public and Private Dental Surgeries in Spain: A Pilot Study. *Int. J. Environ. Res. Public Health* **2020**, *17*, 5139. [CrossRef]
8. Schwendicke, F.; Krois, J.; Gomez, J. Impact of SARS-CoV2 (Covid-19) on Dental Practices: Economic Analysis. *J. Dent.* **2020**, *99*, 103387. [CrossRef] [PubMed]
9. Peiris, J.S.M.; Lai, S.T.; Poon, L.L.M.; Guan, Y.; Yam, L.Y.C.; Lim, W.; Nicholls, J.; Yee, W.K.S.; Yan, W.W.; Cheung, M.T.; et al. Coronavirus as a Possible Cause of Severe Acute Respiratory Syndrome. *Lancet* **2003**, *361*, 1319–1325. [CrossRef]
10. Zhu, N.; Zhang, D.; Wang, W.; Li, X.; Yang, B.; Song, J.; Zhao, X.; Huang, B.; Shi, W.; Lu, R.; et al. A Novel Coronavirus from Patients with Pneumonia in China, 2019. *N. Engl. J. Med.* **2020**, *382*, 727–733. [CrossRef] [PubMed]
11. Dawson, P.; Malik, M.R.; Parvez, F.; Morse, S.S. What Have We Learned About Middle East Respiratory Syndrome Coronavirus Emergence in Humans? A Systematic Literature Review. *Vector Borne Zoonotic Dis.* **2019**, *19*, 174–192. [CrossRef]
12. Zhang, T.; Wu, Q.; Zhang, Z. Probable Pangolin Origin of SARS-CoV-2 Associated with the COVID-19 Outbreak. *Curr. Biol.* **2020**, *30*, 1346–1351.e2. [CrossRef]
13. Guo, Y.-R.; Cao, Q.-D.; Hong, Z.-S.; Tan, Y.-Y.; Chen, S.-D.; Jin, H.-J.; Tan, K.-S.; Wang, D.-Y.; Yan, Y. The Origin, Transmission and Clinical Therapies on Coronavirus Disease 2019 (COVID-19) Outbreak—An Update on the Status. *Mil. Med. Res.* **2020**, *7*, 11. [CrossRef]
14. Huang, C.; Wang, Y.; Li, X.; Ren, L.; Zhao, J.; Hu, Y.; Zhang, L.; Fan, G.; Xu, J.; Gu, X.; et al. Clinical Features of Patients Infected with 2019 Novel Coronavirus in Wuhan, China. *Lancet* **2020**, *395*, 497–506. [CrossRef]
15. Park, M.; Thwaites, R.S.; Openshaw, P.J.M. COVID-19: Lessons from SARS and MERS. *Eur. J. Immunol.* **2020**, *50*, 308–311. [CrossRef]
16. Yan, Y.; Shin, W.I.; Pang, Y.X.; Meng, Y.; Lai, J.; You, C.; Zhao, H.; Lester, E.; Wu, T.; Pang, C.H. The First 75 Days of Novel Coronavirus (SARS-CoV-2) Outbreak: Recent Advances, Prevention, and Treatment. *Int. J. Environ. Res. Public Health* **2020**, *17*, 2323. [CrossRef]
17. Burki, T. China's Successful Control of COVID-19. *Lancet Infect. Dis.* **2020**, *20*, 1240–1241. [CrossRef]
18. Abebe, E.C.; Dejenie, T.A.; Shiferaw, M.Y.; Malik, T. The Newly Emerged COVID-19 Disease: A Systemic Review. *Virol. J.* **2020**, *17*, 96. [CrossRef]
19. Petersen, E.; Koopmans, M.; Go, U.; Hamer, D.H.; Petrosillo, N.; Castelli, F.; Storgaard, M.; Al Khalili, S.; Simonsen, L. Comparing SARS-CoV-2 with SARS-CoV and Influenza Pandemics. *Lancet Infect. Dis.* **2020**, *20*, e238–e244. [CrossRef]
20. Singhal, T. A Review of Coronavirus Disease-2019 (COVID-19). *Indian J. Pediatr.* **2020**, *87*, 281–286. [CrossRef]
21. World Health Organization (WHO). Statement on the Second Meeting of the International Health Regulations (2005) Emergency Committee Regarding the Outbreak of Novel Coronavirus (2019-NCoV). Available online: https://www.who.int/news/item/30-01-2020-statement-on-the-second-meeting-of-the-international-health-regulations-(2005)-emergency-committee-regarding-the-outbreak-of-novel-coronavirus-(2019-ncov) (accessed on 4 November 2020).
22. Olsen, S.J.; Chen, M.-Y.; Liu, Y.-L.; Witschi, M.; Ardoin, A.; Calba, C.; Mathieu, P.; Masserey, V.; Maraglino, F.; Marro, S.; et al. Early Introduction of Severe Acute Respiratory Syndrome Coronavirus 2 into Europe. *Emerg. Infect. Dis.* **2020**, *26*, 1567–1570. [CrossRef]
23. World Health Organization (WHO). WHO Coronavirus Disease (COVID-19) Dashboard. Available online: https://covid19.who.int (accessed on 15 January 2021).

24. Park, M.; Cook, A.R.; Lim, J.T.; Sun, Y.; Dickens, B.L. A Systematic Review of COVID-19 Epidemiology Based on Current Evidence. *J. Clin. Med.* **2020**, *9*, 967. [CrossRef]
25. Levin, A.T.; Hanage, W.P.; Owusu-Boaitey, N.; Cochran, K.B.; Walsh, S.P.; Meyerowitz-Katz, G. Assessing the Age Specificity of Infection Fatality Rates for COVID-19: Systematic Review, Meta-Analysis, and Public Policy Implications. *Eur. J. Epidemiol.* **2020**, *35*, 1123–1138. [CrossRef] [PubMed]
26. Alwan, N.A.; Burgess, R.A.; Ashworth, S.; Beale, R.; Bhadelia, N.; Bogaert, D.; Dowd, J.; Eckerle, I.; Goldman, L.R.; Greenhalgh, T.; et al. Scientific Consensus on the COVID-19 Pandemic: We Need to Act Now. *Lancet* **2020**, *396*, e71–e72. [CrossRef]
27. Bambra, C.; Riordan, R.; Ford, J.; Matthews, F. The COVID-19 Pandemic and Health Inequalities. *J. Epidemiol. Community Health* **2020**, *74*, 964–968. [CrossRef]
28. Zhu, X.; Ge, Y.; Wu, T.; Zhao, K.; Chen, Y.; Wu, B.; Zhu, F.; Zhu, B.; Cui, L. Co-Infection with Respiratory Pathogens among COVID-2019 Cases. *Virus Res.* **2020**, *285*, 198005. [CrossRef]
29. Si, Y.; Zhao, Z.; Chen, R.; Zhong, H.; Liu, T.; Wang, M.; Song, X.; Li, W.; Ying, B. Epidemiological Surveillance of Common Respiratory Viruses in Patients with Suspected COVID-19 in Southwest China. *BMC Infect. Dis.* **2020**, *20*, 688. [CrossRef]
30. Wu, X.; Cai, Y.; Huang, X.; Yu, X.; Zhao, L.; Wang, F.; Li, Q.; Gu, S.; Xu, T.; Li, Y.; et al. Co-Infection with SARS-CoV-2 and Influenza A Virus in Patient with Pneumonia, China. *Emerg. Infect. Dis.* **2020**, *26*, 1324–1326. [CrossRef]
31. McIntosh, K.; Becker, W.B.; Chanock, R.M. Growth in Suckling-Mouse Brain of "IBV-like" Viruses from Patients with Upper Respiratory Tract Disease. *Proc. Natl. Acad. Sci. USA* **1967**, *58*, 2268–2273. [CrossRef] [PubMed]
32. Baltimore, D. Expression of Animal Virus Genomes. *Bacteriol. Rev.* **1971**, *35*, 235–241. [CrossRef]
33. Woo, P.C.Y.; Huang, Y.; Lau, S.K.P.; Yuen, K.-Y. Coronavirus Genomics and Bioinformatics Analysis. *Viruses* **2010**, *2*, 1804–1820. [CrossRef]
34. Wu, F.; Zhao, S.; Yu, B.; Chen, Y.-M.; Wang, W.; Song, Z.-G.; Hu, Y.; Tao, Z.-W.; Tian, J.-H.; Pei, Y.-Y.; et al. A New Coronavirus Associated with Human Respiratory Disease in China. *Nature* **2020**, *579*, 265–269. [CrossRef]
35. Wang, C.; Horby, P.W.; Hayden, F.G.; Gao, G.F. A Novel Coronavirus Outbreak of Global Health Concern. *Lancet* **2020**, *395*, 470–473. [CrossRef]
36. Chen, Y.; Liu, Q.; Guo, D. Emerging Coronaviruses: Genome Structure, Replication, and Pathogenesis. *J. Med. Virol.* **2020**, *92*, 418–423. [CrossRef]
37. Kim, D.; Lee, J.-Y.; Yang, J.-S.; Kim, J.W.; Kim, V.N.; Chang, H. The Architecture of SARS-CoV-2 Transcriptome. *Cell* **2020**, *181*, 914–921.e10. [CrossRef]
38. Ou, X.; Liu, Y.; Lei, X.; Li, P.; Mi, D.; Ren, L.; Guo, L.; Guo, R.; Chen, T.; Hu, J.; et al. Characterization of Spike Glycoprotein of SARS-CoV-2 on Virus Entry and Its Immune Cross-Reactivity with SARS-CoV. *Nat. Commun.* **2020**, *11*, 1620. [CrossRef]
39. Donoghue, M.; Hsieh, F.; Baronas, E.; Godbout, K.; Gosselin, M.; Stagliano, N.; Donovan, M.; Woolf, B.; Robison, K.; Jeyaseelan, R.; et al. A Novel Angiotensin-Converting Enzyme-Related Carboxypeptidase (ACE2) Converts Angiotensin I to Angiotensin 1-9. *Circ. Res.* **2000**, *87*, E1–E9. [CrossRef]
40. Hofmann, H.; Pyrc, K.; van der Hoek, L.; Geier, M.; Berkhout, B.; Pöhlmann, S. Human Coronavirus NL63 Employs the Severe Acute Respiratory Syndrome Coronavirus Receptor for Cellular Entry. *Proc. Natl. Acad. Sci. USA* **2005**, *102*, 7988–7993. [CrossRef]
41. Li, W.; Moore, M.J.; Vasilieva, N.; Sui, J.; Wong, S.K.; Berne, M.A.; Somasundaran, M.; Sullivan, J.L.; Luzuriaga, K.; Greenough, T.C.; et al. Angiotensin-Converting Enzyme 2 Is a Functional Receptor for the SARS Coronavirus. *Nature* **2003**, *426*, 450–454. [CrossRef]
42. Huang, I.-C.; Bosch, B.J.; Li, F.; Li, W.; Lee, K.H.; Ghiran, S.; Vasilieva, N.; Dermody, T.S.; Harrison, S.C.; Dormitzer, P.R.; et al. SARS Coronavirus, but Not Human Coronavirus NL63, Utilizes Cathepsin L to Infect ACE2-Expressing Cells. *J. Biol. Chem.* **2006**, *281*, 3198–3203. [CrossRef] [PubMed]
43. Simmons, G.; Gosalia, D.N.; Rennekamp, A.J.; Reeves, J.D.; Diamond, S.L.; Bates, P. Inhibitors of Cathepsin L Prevent Severe Acute Respiratory Syndrome Coronavirus Entry. *Proc. Natl. Acad. Sci. USA* **2005**, *102*, 11876–11881. [CrossRef]
44. Glowacka, I.; Bertram, S.; Müller, M.A.; Allen, P.; Soilleux, E.; Pfefferle, S.; Steffen, I.; Tsegaye, T.S.; He, Y.; Gnirss, K.; et al. Evidence That TMPRSS2 Activates the Severe Acute Respiratory Syndrome Coronavirus Spike Protein for Membrane Fusion and Reduces Viral Control by the Humoral Immune Response. *J. Virol.* **2011**, *85*, 4122–4134. [CrossRef]
45. Fehr, A.R.; Perlman, S. Coronaviruses: An Overview of Their Replication and Pathogenesis. *Methods Mol. Biol.* **2015**, *1282*, 1–23. [CrossRef]
46. Klumperman, J.; Locker, J.K.; Meijer, A.; Horzinek, M.C.; Geuze, H.J.; Rottier, P.J. Coronavirus M Proteins Accumulate in the Golgi Complex beyond the Site of Virion Budding. *J. Virol.* **1994**, *68*, 6523–6534. [CrossRef]
47. De Haan, C.A.M.; Rottier, P.J.M. Molecular Interactions in the Assembly of Coronaviruses. *Adv. Virus Res.* **2005**, *64*, 165–230. [CrossRef]
48. Gu, J.; Gong, E.; Zhang, B.; Zheng, J.; Gao, Z.; Zhong, Y.; Zou, W.; Zhan, J.; Wang, S.; Xie, Z.; et al. Multiple Organ Infection and the Pathogenesis of SARS. *J. Exp. Med.* **2005**, *202*, 415–424. [CrossRef]
49. Hamming, I.; Timens, W.; Bulthuis, M.L.C.; Lely, A.T.; Navis, G.J.; van Goor, H. Tissue Distribution of ACE2 Protein, the Functional Receptor for SARS Coronavirus. A First Step in Understanding SARS Pathogenesis. *J. Pathol.* **2004**, *203*, 631–637. [CrossRef] [PubMed]

50. Hoffmann, M.; Kleine-Weber, H.; Schroeder, S.; Krüger, N.; Herrler, T.; Erichsen, S.; Schiergens, T.S.; Herrler, G.; Wu, N.-H.; Nitsche, A.; et al. SARS-CoV-2 Cell Entry Depends on ACE2 and TMPRSS2 and Is Blocked by a Clinically Proven Protease Inhibitor. *Cell* **2020**, *181*, 271–280.e8. [CrossRef]
51. Ziegler, C.G.K.; Allon, S.J.; Nyquist, S.K.; Mbano, I.M.; Miao, V.N.; Tzouanas, C.N.; Cao, Y.; Yousif, A.S.; Bals, J.; Hauser, B.M.; et al. SARS-CoV-2 Receptor ACE2 Is an Interferon-Stimulated Gene in Human Airway Epithelial Cells and Is Detected in Specific Cell Subsets across Tissues. *Cell* **2020**, *181*, 1016–1035.e19. [CrossRef] [PubMed]
52. Parsamanesh, N.; Pezeshgi, A.; Hemmati, M.; Jameshorani, M.; Saboory, E. Neurological Manifestations of Coronavirus Infections: Role of Angiotensin-Converting Enzyme 2 in COVID-19. *Int. J. Neurosci.* **2020**, 1–11. [CrossRef]
53. Baig, A.M.; Khaleeq, A.; Ali, U.; Syeda, H. Evidence of the COVID-19 Virus Targeting the CNS: Tissue Distribution, Host-Virus Interaction, and Proposed Neurotropic Mechanisms. *ACS Chem. Neurosci.* **2020**, *11*, 995–998. [CrossRef] [PubMed]
54. Mao, L.; Jin, H.; Wang, M.; Hu, Y.; Chen, S.; He, Q.; Chang, J.; Hong, C.; Zhou, Y.; Wang, D.; et al. Neurologic Manifestations of Hospitalized Patients with Coronavirus Disease 2019 in Wuhan, China. *JAMA Neurol.* **2020**, *77*, 683–690. [CrossRef] [PubMed]
55. Peck, K.M.; Lauring, A.S. Complexities of Viral Mutation Rates. *J. Virol.* **2018**, *92*. [CrossRef] [PubMed]
56. Phan, T. Genetic Diversity and Evolution of SARS-CoV-2. *Infect. Genet. Evol.* **2020**, *81*, 104260. [CrossRef]
57. Leung, K.; Pei, Y.; Leung, G.M.; Lam, T.T.Y.; Wu, J.T. Empirical Transmission Advantage of the D614G Mutant Strain of SARS-CoV-2. *MedRxiv* **2020**. [CrossRef]
58. Rambaut, A.; Loman, N.; Pybus, O.; Barclay, W.; Barrett, J.; Carabelli, A.; Connor, T.; Peacock, T.; Robertson, D.; Volz, E.; et al. Preliminary Genomic Characterisation of an Emergent SARS-CoV-2 Lineage in the UK Defined by a Novel Set of Spike Mutations. Available online: https://virological.org/t/preliminary-genomic-characterisation-of-an-emergent-sars-cov-2-lineage-in-the-uk-defined-by-a-novel-set-of-spike-mutations/563 (accessed on 22 December 2020).
59. Jamilloux, Y.; Henry, T.; Belot, A.; Viel, S.; Fauter, M.; El Jammal, T.; Walzer, T.; François, B.; Sève, P. Should We Stimulate or Suppress Immune Responses in COVID-19? Cytokine and Anti-Cytokine Interventions. *Autoimmun. Rev.* **2020**, *19*, 102567. [CrossRef]
60. Crouse, J.; Kalinke, U.; Oxenius, A. Regulation of Antiviral T Cell Responses by Type I Interferons. *Nat. Rev. Immunol.* **2015**, *15*, 231–242. [CrossRef]
61. Blanco-Melo, D.; Nilsson-Payant, B.E.; Liu, W.-C.; Uhl, S.; Hoagland, D.; Møller, R.; Jordan, T.X.; Oishi, K.; Panis, M.; Sachs, D.; et al. Imbalanced Host Response to SARS-CoV-2 Drives Development of COVID-19. *Cell* **2020**, *181*, 1036–1045.e9. [CrossRef]
62. Felsenstein, S.; Herbert, J.A.; McNamara, P.S.; Hedrich, C.M. COVID-19: Immunology and Treatment Options. *Clin. Immunol.* **2020**, *215*, 108448. [CrossRef]
63. Jeyanathan, M.; Afkhami, S.; Smaill, F.; Miller, M.S.; Lichty, B.D.; Xing, Z. Immunological Considerations for COVID-19 Vaccine Strategies. *Nat. Rev. Immunol.* **2020**, 1–18. [CrossRef] [PubMed]
64. Trouillet-Assant, S.; Viel, S.; Gaymard, A.; Pons, S.; Richard, J.-C.; Perret, M.; Villard, M.; Brengel-Pesce, K.; Lina, B.; Mezidi, M.; et al. Type I IFN Immunoprofiling in COVID-19 Patients. *J. Allergy Clin. Immunol.* **2020**, *146*, 206–208.e2. [CrossRef]
65. Channappanavar, R.; Fehr, A.R.; Vijay, R.; Mack, M.; Zhao, J.; Meyerholz, D.K.; Perlman, S. Dysregulated Type I Interferon and Inflammatory Monocyte-Macrophage Responses Cause Lethal Pneumonia in SARS-CoV-Infected Mice. *Cell Host Microbe* **2016**, *19*, 181–193. [CrossRef]
66. Zhang, Q.; Bastard, P.; Liu, Z.; Le Pen, J.; Moncada-Velez, M.; Chen, J.; Ogishi, M.; Sabli, I.K.D.; Hodeib, S.; Korol, C.; et al. Inborn Errors of Type I IFN Immunity in Patients with Life-Threatening COVID-19. *Science* **2020**, *370*. [CrossRef]
67. Bastard, P.; Rosen, L.B.; Zhang, Q.; Michailidis, E.; Hoffmann, H.-H.; Zhang, Y.; Dorgham, K.; Philippot, Q.; Rosain, J.; Béziat, V.; et al. Autoantibodies against Type I IFNs in Patients with Life-Threatening COVID-19. *Science* **2020**, *370*, eabd4585. [CrossRef]
68. Qin, C.; Zhou, L.; Hu, Z.; Zhang, S.; Yang, S.; Tao, Y.; Xie, C.; Ma, K.; Shang, K.; Wang, W.; et al. Dysregulation of Immune Response in Patients with Coronavirus 2019 (COVID-19) in Wuhan, China. *Clin. Infect. Dis.* **2020**, *71*, 762–768. [CrossRef] [PubMed]
69. Jiang, M.; Guo, Y.; Luo, Q.; Huang, Z.; Zhao, R.; Liu, S.; Le, A.; Li, J.; Wan, L. T-Cell Subset Counts in Peripheral Blood Can Be Used as Discriminatory Biomarkers for Diagnosis and Severity Prediction of Coronavirus Disease 2019. *J. Infect. Dis.* **2020**, *222*, 198–202. [CrossRef]
70. Chen, G.; Wu, D.; Guo, W.; Cao, Y.; Huang, D.; Wang, H.; Wang, T.; Zhang, X.; Chen, H.; Yu, H.; et al. Clinical and Immunological Features of Severe and Moderate Coronavirus Disease 2019. *J. Clin. Investig.* **2020**, *130*, 2620–2629. [CrossRef]
71. Wang, D.; Hu, B.; Hu, C.; Zhu, F.; Liu, X.; Zhang, J.; Wang, B.; Xiang, H.; Cheng, Z.; Xiong, Y.; et al. Clinical Characteristics of 138 Hospitalized Patients With 2019 Novel Coronavirus–Infected Pneumonia in Wuhan, China. *JAMA* **2020**, *323*, 1061. [CrossRef]
72. Huang, A.T.; Garcia-Carreras, B.; Hitchings, M.D.T.; Yang, B.; Katzelnick, L.C.; Rattigan, S.M.; Borgert, B.A.; Moreno, C.A.; Solomon, B.D.; Trimmer-Smith, L.; et al. A Systematic Review of Antibody Mediated Immunity to Coronaviruses: Kinetics, Correlates of Protection, and Association with Severity. *Nat. Commun.* **2020**, *11*, 4704. [CrossRef]
73. Zhao, J.; Yuan, Q.; Wang, H.; Liu, W.; Liao, X.; Su, Y.; Wang, X.; Yuan, J.; Li, T.; Li, J.; et al. Antibody Responses to SARS-CoV-2 in Patients of Novel Coronavirus Disease 2019. *Clin. Infect. Dis.* **2020**, *71*, 2027–2034. [CrossRef]
74. Padoan, A.; Sciacovelli, L.; Basso, D.; Negrini, D.; Zuin, S.; Cosma, C.; Faggian, D.; Matricardi, P.; Plebani, M. IgA-Ab Response to Spike Glycoprotein of SARS-CoV-2 in Patients with COVID-19: A Longitudinal Study. *Clin. Chim. Acta* **2020**, *507*, 164–166. [CrossRef]

75. Yu, H.; Sun, B.; Fang, Z.; Zhao, J.; Liu, X.; Li, Y.; Sun, X.; Liang, H.; Zhong, B.; Huang, Z.; et al. Distinct Features of SARS-CoV-2-Specific IgA Response in COVID-19 Patients. *Eur. Respir. J.* **2020**, *56*. [CrossRef]
76. Chen, X.; Pan, Z.; Yue, S.; Yu, F.; Zhang, J.; Yang, Y.; Li, R.; Liu, B.; Yang, X.; Gao, L.; et al. Disease Severity Dictates SARS-CoV-2-Specific Neutralizing Antibody Responses in COVID-19. *Signal Transduct. Target. Ther.* **2020**, *5*, 1–6. [CrossRef] [PubMed]
77. Lynch, K.L.; Whitman, J.D.; Lacanienta, N.P.; Beckerdite, E.W.; Kastner, S.A.; Shy, B.R.; Goldgof, G.M.; Levine, A.G.; Bapat, S.P.; Stramer, S.L.; et al. Magnitude and Kinetics of Anti-SARS-CoV-2 Antibody Responses and Their Relationship to Disease Severity. *Clin. Infect. Dis.* **2020**. [CrossRef]
78. Grzelak, L.; Velay, A.; Madec, Y.; Gallais, F.; Staropoli, I.; Schmidt-Mutter, C.; Wendling, M.-J.; Meyer, N.; Planchais, C.; Rey, D.; et al. Sex Differences in the Decline of Neutralizing Antibodies to SARS-CoV-2. *MedRxiv* **2020**. [CrossRef]
79. Karlsson, A.C.; Humbert, M.; Buggert, M. The Known Unknowns of T Cell Immunity to COVID-19. *Sci. Immunol.* **2020**, *5*. [CrossRef]
80. Grifoni, A.; Weiskopf, D.; Ramirez, S.I.; Mateus, J.; Dan, J.M.; Moderbacher, C.R.; Rawlings, S.A.; Sutherland, A.; Premkumar, L.; Jadi, R.S.; et al. Targets of T Cell Responses to SARS-CoV-2 Coronavirus in Humans with COVID-19 Disease and Unexposed Individuals. *Cell* **2020**, *181*, 1489–1501. [CrossRef]
81. Poland, G.A.; Ovsyannikova, I.G.; Kennedy, R.B. SARS-CoV-2 Immunity: Review and Applications to Phase 3 Vaccine Candidates. *Lancet* **2020**, *396*, 1595–1606. [CrossRef]
82. Sekine, T.; Perez-Potti, A.; Rivera-Ballesteros, O.; Strålin, K.; Gorin, J.-B.; Olsson, A.; Llewellyn-Lacey, S.; Kamal, H.; Bogdanovic, G.; Muschiol, S.; et al. Robust T Cell Immunity in Convalescent Individuals with Asymptomatic or Mild COVID-19. *Cell* **2020**, *183*, 158–168. [CrossRef]
83. Gallais, F.; Velay, A.; Wendling, M.-J.; Nazon, C.; Partisani, M.; Sibilia, J.; Candon, S.; Fafi-Kremer, S. Intrafamilial Exposure to SARS-CoV-2 Induces Cellular Immune Response without Seroconversion. *Emerg. Infect. Dis.* **2021**, *27*, 113–121. [CrossRef]
84. Oran, D.P.; Topol, E.J. Prevalence of Asymptomatic SARS-CoV-2 Infection: A Narrative Review. *Ann. Intern. Med.* **2020**, *173*, 362–367. [CrossRef]
85. Gao, M.; Yang, L.; Chen, X.; Deng, Y.; Yang, S.; Xu, H.; Chen, Z.; Gao, X. A Study on Infectivity of Asymptomatic SARS-CoV-2 Carriers. *Respir. Med.* **2020**, *169*. [CrossRef]
86. Long, Q.-X.; Tang, X.-J.; Shi, Q.-L.; Li, Q.; Deng, H.-J.; Yuan, J.; Hu, J.-L.; Xu, W.; Zhang, Y.; Lv, F.-J.; et al. Clinical and Immunological Assessment of Asymptomatic SARS-CoV-2 Infections. *Nat. Med.* **2020**, *26*, 1200–1204. [CrossRef]
87. Wu, Z.; McGoogan, J.M. Characteristics of and Important Lessons from the Coronavirus Disease 2019 (COVID-19) Outbreak in China: Summary of a Report of 72314 Cases from the Chinese Center for Disease Control and Prevention. *JAMA* **2020**, *323*, 1239–1242. [CrossRef] [PubMed]
88. Akca, U.K.; Kesici, S.; Ozsurekci, Y.; Aykan, H.H.; Batu, E.D.; Atalay, E.; Demir, S.; Sag, E.; Vuralli, D.; Bayrakci, B.; et al. Kawasaki-like Disease in Children with COVID-19. *Rheumatol. Int.* **2020**, *40*, 2105–2115. [CrossRef]
89. Consiglio, C.R.; Cotugno, N.; Sardh, F.; Pou, C.; Amodio, D.; Rodriguez, L.; Tan, Z.; Zicari, S.; Ruggiero, A.; Pascucci, G.R.; et al. The Immunology of Multisystem Inflammatory Syndrome in Children with COVID-19. *Cell* **2020**. [CrossRef] [PubMed]
90. Liguoro, I.; Pilotto, C.; Bonanni, M.; Ferrari, M.E.; Pusiol, A.; Nocerino, A.; Vidal, E.; Cogo, P. SARS-COV-2 Infection in Children and Newborns. A Systematic Review. *Eur. J. Pediatr.* **2020**, *179*, 1029–1046. [CrossRef]
91. Lu, X.; Zhang, L.; Du, H.; Zhang, J.; Li, Y.Y.; Qu, J.; Zhang, W.; Wang, Y.; Bao, S.; Li, Y.; et al. SARS-CoV-2 Infection in Children. *N. Engl. J. Med.* **2020**, *382*, 1663–1665. [CrossRef]
92. Lu, X.; Xiang, Y.; Du, H.; Wing-Kin Wong, G. SARS-CoV-2 Infection in Children—Understanding the Immune Responses and Controlling the Pandemic. *Pediatr. Allergy Immunol.* **2020**, *31*, 449–453. [CrossRef] [PubMed]
93. Bunyavanich, S.; Do, A.; Vicencio, A. Nasal Gene Expression of Angiotensin-Converting Enzyme 2 in Children and Adults. *JAMA* **2020**, *323*, 2427–2429. [CrossRef]
94. Saheb Sharif-Askari, N.; Saheb Sharif-Askari, F.; Alabed, M.; Temsah, M.-H.; Al Heialy, S.; Hamid, Q.; Halwani, R. Airways Expression of SARS-CoV-2 Receptor, ACE2, and TMPRSS2 Is Lower in Children Than Adults and Increases with Smoking and COPD. *Mol. Ther. Methods Clin. Dev.* **2020**, *18*, 1–6. [CrossRef]
95. Pierce, C.A.; Preston-Hurlburt, P.; Dai, Y.; Aschner, C.B.; Cheshenko, N.; Galen, B.; Garforth, S.J.; Herrera, N.G.; Jangra, R.K.; Morano, N.C.; et al. Immune Responses to SARS-CoV-2 Infection in Hospitalized Pediatric and Adult Patients. *Sci. Transl. Med.* **2020**, *12*. [CrossRef]
96. Holodick, N.E.; Rodríguez-Zhurbenko, N.; Hernández, A.M. Defining Natural Antibodies. *Front. Immunol.* **2017**, *8*, 872. [CrossRef]
97. Carsetti, R.; Quintarelli, C.; Quinti, I.; Piano Mortari, E.; Zumla, A.; Ippolito, G.; Locatelli, F. The Immune System of Children: The Key to Understanding SARS-CoV-2 Susceptibility? *Lancet Child Adolesc. Health* **2020**, *4*, 414–416. [CrossRef]
98. Doshi, P. Covid-19: Do Many People Have Pre-Existing Immunity? *BMJ* **2020**, *370*. [CrossRef] [PubMed]
99. Lyu, J.; Miao, T.; Dong, J.; Cao, R.; Li, Y.; Chen, Q. Reflection on Lower Rates of COVID-19 in Children: Does Childhood Immunizations Offer Unexpected Protection? *Med. Hypotheses* **2020**, *143*, 109842. [CrossRef] [PubMed]
100. Felsenstein, S.; Hedrich, C.M. SARS-CoV-2 Infections in Children and Young People. *Clin. Immunol.* **2020**, *220*, 108588. [CrossRef]
101. Weisberg, S.P.; Connors, T.J.; Zhu, Y.; Baldwin, M.R.; Lin, W.-H.; Wontakal, S.; Szabo, P.A.; Wells, S.B.; Dogra, P.; Gray, J.; et al. Distinct Antibody Responses to SARS-CoV-2 in Children and Adults across the COVID-19 Clinical Spectrum. *Nat. Immunol.* **2020**. [CrossRef]

102. Kumar, B.V.; Connors, T.J.; Farber, D.L. Human T Cell Development, Localization, and Function throughout Life. *Immunity* **2018**, *48*, 202–213. [CrossRef]
103. AlFehaidi, A.; Ahmad, S.A.; Hamed, E. SARS-CoV-2 Re-Infection: A Case Report from Qatar. *J. Infect.* **2020**. [CrossRef] [PubMed]
104. Tillett, R.L.; Sevinsky, J.R.; Hartley, P.D.; Kerwin, H.; Crawford, N.; Gorzalski, A.; Laverdure, C.; Verma, S.C.; Rossetto, C.C.; Jackson, D.; et al. Genomic Evidence for Reinfection with SARS-CoV-2: A Case Study. *Lancet Infect. Dis.* **2021**, *21*, 52–58. [CrossRef]
105. Prado-Vivar, B.; Becerra-Wong, M.; Guadalupe, J.J.; Marquez, S.; Gutierrez, B.; Rojas-Silva, P.; Grunauer, M.; Trueba, G.; Barragan, V.; Cardenas, P. *COVID-19 Re-Infection by a Phylogenetically Distinct SARS-CoV-2 Variant, First Confirmed Event in South America*; Social Science Research Network: Rochester, NY, USA, 2020. [CrossRef]
106. To, K.K.-W.; Hung, I.F.-N.; Ip, J.D.; Chu, A.W.-H.; Chan, W.-M.; Tam, A.R.; Fong, C.H.-Y.; Yuan, S.; Tsoi, H.-W.; Ng, A.C.-K.; et al. Coronavirus Disease 2019 (COVID-19) Re-Infection by a Phylogenetically Distinct Severe Acute Respiratory Syndrome Coronavirus 2 Strain Confirmed by Whole Genome Sequencing. *Clin. Infect. Dis.* **2020**. [CrossRef]
107. Van Elslande, J.; Vermeersch, P.; Vandervoort, K.; Wawina-Bokalanga, T.; Vanmechelen, B.; Wollants, E.; Laenen, L.; André, E.; Van Ranst, M.; Lagrou, K.; et al. Symptomatic SARS-CoV-2 Reinfection by a Phylogenetically Distinct Strain. *Clin. Infect. Dis.* **2020**. [CrossRef]
108. Sariol, A.; Perlman, S. Lessons for COVID-19 Immunity from Other Coronavirus Infections. *Immunity* **2020**, *53*, 248–263. [CrossRef] [PubMed]
109. Edridge, A.W.D.; Kaczorowska, J.; Hoste, A.C.R.; Bakker, M.; Klein, M.; Loens, K.; Jebbink, M.F.; Matser, A.; Kinsella, C.M.; Rueda, P.; et al. Seasonal Coronavirus Protective Immunity Is Short-Lasting. *Nat. Med.* **2020**, 1–3. [CrossRef] [PubMed]
110. Le Bert, N.; Tan, A.T.; Kunasegaran, K.; Tham, C.Y.L.; Hafezi, M.; Chia, A.; Chng, M.H.Y.; Lin, M.; Tan, N.; Linster, M.; et al. SARS-CoV-2-Specific T Cell Immunity in Cases of COVID-19 and SARS, and Uninfected Controls. *Nature* **2020**, *584*, 457–462. [CrossRef] [PubMed]
111. Ng, O.-W.; Chia, A.; Tan, A.T.; Jadi, R.S.; Leong, H.N.; Bertoletti, A.; Tan, Y.-J. Memory T Cell Responses Targeting the SARS Coronavirus Persist up to 11 Years Post-Infection. *Vaccine* **2016**, *34*, 2008–2014. [CrossRef] [PubMed]
112. Tang, F.; Quan, Y.; Xin, Z.-T.; Wrammert, J.; Ma, M.-J.; Lv, H.; Wang, T.-B.; Yang, H.; Richardus, J.H.; Liu, W.; et al. Lack of Peripheral Memory B Cell Responses in Recovered Patients with Severe Acute Respiratory Syndrome: A Six-Year Follow-Up Study. *J. Immunol.* **2011**, *186*, 7264–7268. [CrossRef]
113. Cao, W.-C.; Liu, W.; Zhang, P.-H.; Zhang, F.; Richardus, J.H. Disappearance of Antibodies to SARS-Associated Coronavirus after Recovery. *N. Engl. J. Med.* **2007**, *357*, 1162–1163. [CrossRef]
114. Wu, L.-P.; Wang, N.-C.; Chang, Y.-H.; Tian, X.-Y.; Na, D.-Y.; Zhang, L.-Y.; Zheng, L.; Lan, T.; Wang, L.-F.; Liang, G.-D. Duration of Antibody Responses after Severe Acute Respiratory Syndrome. *Emerg. Infect. Dis.* **2007**, *13*, 1562–1564. [CrossRef]
115. Seow, J.; Graham, C.; Merrick, B.; Acors, S.; Pickering, S.; Steel, K.J.A.; Hemmings, O.; O'Byrne, A.; Kouphou, N.; Galao, R.P.; et al. Longitudinal Observation and Decline of Neutralizing Antibody Responses in the Three Months Following SARS-CoV-2 Infection in Humans. *Nat. Microbiol.* **2020**. [CrossRef]
116. Wajnberg, A.; Amanat, F.; Firpo, A.; Altman, D.R.; Bailey, M.J.; Mansour, M.; McMahon, M.; Meade, P.; Mendu, D.R.; Muellers, K.; et al. Robust Neutralizing Antibodies to SARS-CoV-2 Infection Persist for Months. *Science* **2020**. [CrossRef]
117. Dan, J.M.; Mateus, J.; Kato, Y.; Hastie, K.M.; Yu, E.D.; Faliti, C.E.; Grifoni, A.; Ramirez, S.I.; Haupt, S.; Frazier, A.; et al. Immunological Memory to SARS-CoV-2 Assessed for up to 8 Months after Infection. *Science* **2021**. [CrossRef]
118. Ni, L.; Ye, F.; Cheng, M.-L.; Feng, Y.; Deng, Y.-Q.; Zhao, H.; Wei, P.; Ge, J.; Gou, M.; Li, X.; et al. Detection of SARS-CoV-2-Specific Humoral and Cellular Immunity in COVID-19 Convalescent Individuals. *Immunity* **2020**, *52*, 971–977. [CrossRef]
119. Cañete, P.F.; Vinuesa, C.G. COVID-19 Makes B Cells Forget, but T Cells Remember. *Cell* **2020**, *183*, 13–15. [CrossRef]
120. Fu, L.; Wang, B.; Yuan, T.; Chen, X.; Ao, Y.; Fitzpatrick, T.; Li, P.; Zhou, Y.; Lin, Y.; Duan, Q.; et al. Clinical Characteristics of Coronavirus Disease 2019 (COVID-19) in China: A Systematic Review and Meta-Analysis. *J. Infect.* **2020**, *80*, 656–665. [CrossRef] [PubMed]
121. Fajgenbaum, D.C.; June, C.H. Cytokine Storm. *N. Engl. J. Med.* **2020**, *383*, 2255–2273. [CrossRef] [PubMed]
122. Aoshi, T.; Koyama, S.; Kobiyama, K.; Akira, S.; Ishii, K.J. Innate and Adaptive Immune Responses to Viral Infection and Vaccination. *Curr. Opin. Virol.* **2011**, *1*, 226–232. [CrossRef]
123. Ragab, D.; Salah Eldin, H.; Taeimah, M.; Khattab, R.; Salem, R. The COVID-19 Cytokine Storm; What We Know So Far. *Front. Immunol.* **2020**, *11*, 1446. [CrossRef] [PubMed]
124. Tisoncik, J.R.; Korth, M.J.; Simmons, C.P.; Farrar, J.; Martin, T.R.; Katze, M.G. Into the Eye of the Cytokine Storm. *Microbiol. Mol. Biol. Rev.* **2012**, *76*, 16–32. [CrossRef]
125. Hu, B.; Huang, S.; Yin, L. The Cytokine Storm and COVID-19. *J. Med. Virol.* **2020**. [CrossRef]
126. De la Rica, R.; Borges, M.; Gonzalez-Freire, M. COVID-19: In the Eye of the Cytokine Storm. *Front. Immunol.* **2020**, *11*. [CrossRef]
127. Jose, R.J.; Manuel, A. COVID-19 Cytokine Storm: The Interplay between Inflammation and Coagulation. *Lancet Respir. Med.* **2020**, *8*, e46–e47. [CrossRef]
128. Singh, A.K.; Gupta, R.; Ghosh, A.; Misra, A. Diabetes in COVID-19: Prevalence, Pathophysiology, Prognosis and Practical Considerations. *Diabetes Metab. Syndr.* **2020**, *14*, 303–310. [CrossRef]
129. Kumar, A.; Arora, A.; Sharma, P.; Anikhindi, S.A.; Bansal, N.; Singla, V.; Khare, S.; Srivastava, A. Is Diabetes Mellitus Associated with Mortality and Severity of COVID-19? A Meta-Analysis. *Diabetes Metab. Syndr.* **2020**, *14*, 535–545. [CrossRef]

130. Larvin, H.; Wilmott, S.; Wu, J.; Kang, J. The Impact of Periodontal Disease on Hospital Admission and Mortality During COVID-19 Pandemic. *Front. Med.* **2020**, *7*, 604980. [CrossRef]
131. Pfützner, A.; Lazzara, M.; Jantz, J. Why Do People with Diabetes Have a High Risk for Severe COVID-19 Disease?—A Dental Hypothesis and Possible Prevention Strategy. *J. Diabetes Sci. Technol.* **2020**, *14*, 769–771. [CrossRef]
132. Pitones-Rubio, V.; Chávez-Cortez, E.G.; Hurtado-Camarena, A.; González-Rascón, A.; Serafín-Higuera, N. Is Periodontal Disease a Risk Factor for Severe COVID-19 Illness? *Med. Hypotheses* **2020**, *144*, 109969. [CrossRef]
133. Braun, J.; Loyal, L.; Frentsch, M.; Wendisch, D.; Georg, P.; Kurth, F.; Hippenstiel, S.; Dingeldey, M.; Kruse, B.; Fauchere, F.; et al. SARS-CoV-2-Reactive T Cells in Healthy Donors and Patients with COVID-19. *Nature* **2020**. [CrossRef]
134. Ritchie, A.I.; Singanayagam, A. Immunosuppression for Hyperinflammation in COVID-19: A Double-Edged Sword? *Lancet* **2020**, *395*, 1111. [CrossRef]
135. Rapid Risk Assessment: Coronavirus Disease 2019 (COVID-19) Pandemic: Increased Transmission in the EU/EEA and the UK—Eighth Update. Available online: https://www.ecdc.europa.eu/en/publications-data/rapid-risk-assessment-coronavirus-disease-2019-covid-19-pandemic-eighth-update (accessed on 9 November 2020).
136. CDC Coronavirus Disease 2019 (COVID-19). Available online: https://www.cdc.gov/coronavirus/2019-ncov/need-extra-precautions/people-with-medical-conditions.html (accessed on 9 November 2020).
137. De Stefano, L.; Bobbio-Pallavicini, F.; Manzo, A.; Montecucco, C.; Bugatti, S. A "Window of Therapeutic Opportunity" for Anti-Cytokine Therapy in Patients with Coronavirus Disease 2019. *Front. Immunol.* **2020**, *11*, 572635. [CrossRef]
138. Xu, Z.; Zhang, C.; Wang, F.-S. COVID-19 in People with HIV. *Lancet HIV* **2020**, *7*, e524–e526. [CrossRef]
139. Sigel, K.; Swartz, T.; Golden, E.; Paranjpe, I.; Somani, S.; Richter, F.; De Freitas, J.K.; Miotto, R.; Zhao, S.; Polak, P.; et al. Coronavirus 2019 and People Living With Human Immunodeficiency Virus:: Outcomes for Hospitalized Patients in New York City. *Clin. Infect. Dis.* **2020**, *71*, 2933–2938. [CrossRef]
140. Razanamahery, J.; Soumagne, T.; Humbert, S.; Brunel, A.S.; Lepiller, Q.; Daguindau, E.; Mansi, L.; Chirouze, C.; Bouiller, K. Does Type of Immunosupression Influence the Course of Covid-19 Infection? *J. Infect.* **2020**, *81*, e132–e135. [CrossRef]
141. Gao, Y.; Chen, Y.; Liu, M.; Shi, S.; Tian, J. Impacts of Immunosuppression and Immunodeficiency on COVID-19: A Systematic Review and Meta-Analysis. *J. Infect.* **2020**, *81*, e93–e95. [CrossRef] [PubMed]
142. Minotti, C.; Tirelli, F.; Barbieri, E.; Giaquinto, C.; Donà, D. How Is Immunosuppressive Status Affecting Children and Adults in SARS-CoV-2 Infection? A Systematic Review. *J. Infect.* **2020**, *81*, e61–e66. [CrossRef]
143. Nacif, L.S.; Zanini, L.Y.; Waisberg, D.R.; Pinheiro, R.S.; Galvão, F.; Andraus, W.; D'Albuquerque, L.C. COVID-19 in Solid Organ Transplantation Patients: A Systematic Review. *Clinics* **2020**, *75*, e1983. [CrossRef] [PubMed]
144. Liang, W.; Guan, W.; Chen, R.; Wang, W.; Li, J.; Xu, K.; Li, C.; Ai, Q.; Lu, W.; Liang, H.; et al. Cancer Patients in SARS-CoV-2 Infection: A Nationwide Analysis in China. *Lancet Oncol.* **2020**, *21*, 335–337. [CrossRef]
145. Wang, H.; Zhang, L. Risk of COVID-19 for Patients with Cancer. *Lancet Oncol.* **2020**, *21*, e181. [CrossRef]
146. Emmi, G.; Bettiol, A.; Mattioli, I.; Silvestri, E.; Di Scala, G.; Urban, M.L.; Vaglio, A.; Prisco, D. SARS-CoV-2 Infection among Patients with Systemic Autoimmune Diseases. *Autoimmun. Rev.* **2020**, *19*, 102575. [CrossRef]
147. Ferri, C.; Giuggioli, D.; Raimondo, V.; L'Andolina, M.; Tavoni, A.; Cecchetti, R.; Guiducci, S.; Ursini, F.; Caminiti, M.; Varcasia, G.; et al. COVID-19 and Rheumatic Autoimmune Systemic Diseases: Report of a Large Italian Patients Series. *Clin. Rheumatol.* **2020**, *39*, 3195–3204. [CrossRef] [PubMed]
148. Meyts, I.; Bucciol, G.; Quinti, I.; Neven, B.; Fischer, A.; Seoane, E.; Lopez-Granados, E.; Gianelli, C.; Robles-Marhuenda, A.; Jeandel, P.-Y.; et al. Coronavirus Disease 2019 in Patients with Inborn Errors of Immunity: An International Study. *J. Allergy Clin. Immunol.* **2020**. [CrossRef]
149. European Alliance of Associations for Rheumatology (EULAR). EULAR Guidance for Patients COVID-19 Outbreak. Available online: https://www.eular.org/eular_guidance_for_patients_covid19_outbreak.cfm (accessed on 9 November 2020).
150. Wahezi, D.M.; Lo, M.S.; Rubinstein, T.B.; Ringold, S.; Ardoin, S.P.; Downes, K.J.; Jones, K.B.; Laxer, R.M.; Pellet Madan, R.; Mudano, A.S.; et al. American College of Rheumatology Guidance for the Management of Pediatric Rheumatic Disease During the COVID-19 Pandemic: Version 1. *Arthritis Rheumatol.* **2020**, *72*, 1809–1819. [CrossRef] [PubMed]
151. ESID—European Society for Immunodeficiencies. Available online: https://esid.org/News-Events/Joint-statement-on-the-current-epidemics-of-new-Coronavirus (accessed on 9 November 2020).
152. Rodríguez-Argente, F.; Alba-Domínguez, M.; Ortiz-Muñoz, E.; Ortega-González, Á. Oromucosal Immunomodulation as Clinical Spectrum Mitigating Factor in SARS-CoV-2 Infection. *Scand. J. Immunol.* **2020**, e12972. [CrossRef]
153. Isho, B.; Abe, K.T.; Zuo, M.; Jamal, A.J.; Rathod, B.; Wang, J.H.; Li, Z.; Chao, G.; Rojas, O.L.; Bang, Y.M.; et al. Persistence of Serum and Saliva Antibody Responses to SARS-CoV-2 Spike Antigens in COVID-19 Patients. *Sci. Immunol.* **2020**, *5*. [CrossRef]
154. Mudgal, R.; Nehul, S.; Tomar, S. Prospects for Mucosal Vaccine: Shutting the Door on SARS-CoV-2. *Hum. Vaccines Immunother.* **2020**, 1–11. [CrossRef]
155. Moreno-Fierros, L.; García-Silva, I.; Rosales-Mendoza, S. Development of SARS-CoV-2 Vaccines: Should We Focus on Mucosal Immunity? *Expert Opin. Biol. Ther.* **2020**, *20*, 831–836. [CrossRef] [PubMed]
156. Aktas, B.; Aslim, B. Gut-Lung Axis and Dysbiosis in COVID-19. *Turk. J. Biol.* **2020**, *44*, 265–272. [CrossRef]
157. Khatiwada, S.; Subedi, A. Lung Microbiome and Coronavirus Disease 2019 (COVID-19): Possible Link and Implications. *Hum. Microbiome J.* **2020**, *17*, 100073. [CrossRef] [PubMed]

158. Gu, S.; Chen, Y.; Wu, Z.; Chen, Y.; Gao, H.; Lv, L.; Guo, F.; Zhang, X.; Luo, R.; Huang, C.; et al. Alterations of the Gut Microbiota in Patients with COVID-19 or H1N1 Influenza. *Clin. Infect. Dis.* **2020**. [CrossRef]
159. Ferreira, C.; Viana, S.D.; Reis, F. Gut Microbiota Dysbiosis–Immune Hyperresponse–Inflammation Triad in Coronavirus Disease 2019 (COVID-19): Impact of Pharmacological and Nutraceutical Approaches. *Microorganisms* **2020**, *8*, 1514. [CrossRef] [PubMed]
160. Wang, W.; Xu, Y.; Gao, R.; Lu, R.; Han, K.; Wu, G.; Tan, W. Detection of SARS-CoV-2 in Different Types of Clinical Specimens. *JAMA* **2020**, *323*, 1843–1844. [CrossRef] [PubMed]
161. Wyllie, A.L.; Fournier, J.; Casanovas-Massana, A.; Campbell, M.; Tokuyama, M.; Vijayakumar, P.; Warren, J.L.; Geng, B.; Muenker, M.C.; Moore, A.J.; et al. Saliva or Nasopharyngeal Swab Specimens for Detection of SARS-CoV-2. *N. Engl. J. Med.* **2020**, *383*, 1283–1286. [CrossRef] [PubMed]
162. Ghoshal, U.; Vasanth, S.; Tejan, N. A Guide to Laboratory Diagnosis of Corona Virus Disease-19 for the Gastroenterologists. *Indian J. Gastroenterol.* **2020**, *39*, 236–242. [CrossRef]
163. Sheridan, C. Coronavirus and the Race to Distribute Reliable Diagnostics. *Nat. Biotechnol.* **2020**, *38*, 382–384. [CrossRef] [PubMed]
164. Corman, V.M.; Landt, O.; Kaiser, M.; Molenkamp, R.; Meijer, A.; Chu, D.K.; Bleicker, T.; Brünink, S.; Schneider, J.; Schmidt, M.L.; et al. Detection of 2019 Novel Coronavirus (2019-NCoV) by Real-Time RT-PCR. *Euro Surveill.* **2020**, *25*, 2000045. [CrossRef]
165. European Centre For Diseases Prevention and Control. Options for the Use of Rapid Antigen Tests for COVID-19 in the EU/EEA and the UK. Available online: https://www.ecdc.europa.eu/Sites/Default/Files/Documents/Options-Use-of-Rapid-Antigen-Tests-for-COVID-19.Pdf (accessed on 5 December 2020).
166. SARS-CoV-2 Diagnostic Pipeline. Available online: https://www.finddx.org/Covid-19/Pipeline/.FIND (accessed on 5 December 2020).
167. Peeling, R.W.; Wedderburn, C.J.; Garcia, P.J.; Boeras, D.; Fongwen, N.; Nkengasong, J.; Sall, A.; Tanuri, A.; Heymann, D.L. Serology Testing in the COVID-19 Pandemic Response. *Lancet Infect. Dis.* **2020**, *20*, e245–e249. [CrossRef]
168. Krammer, F.; Simon, V. Serology Assays to Manage COVID-19. *Science* **2020**, *368*, 1060–1061. [CrossRef]
169. World Health Organization Diagnostic Testing for SARS-CoV-2: Interim Guidance, 11 September 2020. Available online: https://apps.who.int/iris/bitstream/handle/10665/334254/WHO-2019-nCoV-laboratory-2020.6-eng.pdf?sequence=1&isAllowed=y (accessed on 8 November 2020).
170. Ng, K.; Poon, B.H.; Kiat Puar, T.H.; Shan Quah, J.L.; Loh, W.J.; Wong, Y.J.; Tan, T.Y.; Raghuram, J. COVID-19 and the Risk to Health Care Workers: A Case Report. *Ann. Intern. Med.* **2020**. [CrossRef]
171. Streckfus, C.F. *Advances in Salivary Diagnostics*; Springer: Berlin/Heidelberg, Germany, 2015; ISBN 978-3-662-45398-8.
172. Azzi, L.; Maurino, V.; Baj, A.; Dani, M.; d'Aiuto, A.; Fasano, M.; Lualdi, M.; Sessa, F.; Alberio, T. Diagnostic Salivary Tests for SARS-CoV-2. *J. Dent. Res.* **2020**. [CrossRef]
173. Zhu, J.; Guo, J.; Xu, Y.; Chen, X. Viral Dynamics of SARS-CoV-2 in Saliva from Infected Patients. *J. Infect.* **2020**, *81*, e48–e50. [CrossRef] [PubMed]
174. Varadhachary, A.; Chatterjee, D.; Garza, J.; Garr, R.P.; Foley, C.; Letkeman, A.F.; Dean, J.; Haug, D.; Breeze, J.; Traylor, R.; et al. Salivary Anti-SARS-CoV-2 IgA as an Accessible Biomarker of Mucosal Immunity against COVID-19. *MedRxiv* **2020**. [CrossRef]
175. L'Helgouach, N.; Champigneux, P.; Santos-Schneider, F.; Molina, L.; Espeut, J.; Alali, M.; Baptiste, J.; Cardeur, L.; Dubuc, B.; Foulongne, V.; et al. EasyCOV: LAMP Based Rapid Detection of SARS-CoV-2 in Saliva. *MedRxiv* **2020**. [CrossRef]
176. Azzi, L.; Baj, A.; Alberio, T.; Lualdi, M.; Veronesi, G.; Carcano, G.; Ageno, W.; Gambarini, C.; Maffioli, L.; Saverio, S.D.; et al. Rapid Salivary Test Suitable for a Mass Screening Program to Detect SARS-CoV-2: A Diagnostic Accuracy Study. *J. Infect.* **2020**, *81*, e75–e78. [CrossRef] [PubMed]
177. Riccò, M.; Ranzieri, S.; Peruzzi, S.; Valente, M.; Marchesi, F.; Balzarini, F.; Bragazzi, N.L.; Signorelli, C. RT-QPCR Assays Based on Saliva Rather than on Nasopharyngeal Swabs Are Possible but Should Be Interpreted with Caution: Results from a Systematic Review and Meta-Analysis. *Acta Bio Medica Atenei Parm.* **2020**, *91*, e2020025. [CrossRef]
178. Czumbel, L.M.; Kiss, S.; Farkas, N.; Mandel, I.; Hegyi, A.; Nagy, Á.; Lohinai, Z.; Szakács, Z.; Hegyi, P.; Steward, M.C.; et al. Saliva as a Candidate for COVID-19 Diagnostic Testing: A Meta-Analysis. *Front. Med.* **2020**, *7*. [CrossRef]
179. Lamb, L.E.; Bartolone, S.N.; Ward, E.; Chancellor, M.B. Rapid Detection of Novel Coronavirus/Severe Acute Respiratory Syndrome Coronavirus 2 (SARS-CoV-2) by Reverse Transcription-Loop-Mediated Isothermal Amplification. *PLoS ONE* **2020**, *15*, e0234682. [CrossRef]
180. Hanada, S.; Pirzadeh, M.; Carver, K.Y.; Deng, J.C. Respiratory Viral Infection-Induced Microbiome Alterations and Secondary Bacterial Pneumonia. *Front. Immunol.* **2018**, *9*, 2640. [CrossRef] [PubMed]
181. Yu, I.T.S.; Li, Y.; Wong, T.W.; Tam, W.; Chan, A.T.; Lee, J.H.W.; Leung, D.Y.C.; Ho, T. Evidence of Airborne Transmission of the Severe Acute Respiratory Syndrome Virus. *N. Engl. J. Med.* **2004**, *350*, 1731–1739. [CrossRef]
182. Xu, R.; Cui, B.; Duan, X.; Zhang, P.; Zhou, X.; Yuan, Q. Saliva: Potential Diagnostic Value and Transmission of 2019-NCoV. *Int. J. Oral Sci.* **2020**, *12*, 11. [CrossRef]
183. Zhang, W.; Du, R.-H.; Li, B.; Zheng, X.-S.; Yang, X.-L.; Hu, B.; Wang, Y.-Y.; Xiao, G.-F.; Yan, B.; Shi, Z.-L.; et al. Molecular and Serological Investigation of 2019-NCoV Infected Patients: Implication of Multiple Shedding Routes. *Emerg. Microbes Infect.* **2020**, *9*, 386–389. [CrossRef]

184. Wang, W.-K.; Chen, S.-Y.; Liu, I.-J.; Chen, Y.-C.; Chen, H.-L.; Yang, C.-F.; Chen, P.-J.; Yeh, S.-H.; Kao, C.-L.; Huang, L.-M.; et al. Detection of SARS-Associated Coronavirus in Throat Wash and Saliva in Early Diagnosis. *Emerg. Infect. Dis.* **2004**, *10*, 1213–1219. [CrossRef]
185. Laheij, A.M.G.A.; Kistler, J.O.; Belibasakis, G.N.; Välimaa, H.; de Soet, J.J.; European Oral Microbiology Workshop (EOMW) 2011. Healthcare-Associated Viral and Bacterial Infections in Dentistry. *J. Oral Microbiol.* **2012**, *4*. [CrossRef]
186. Adhikari, U.; Chabrelie, A.; Weir, M.; Boehnke, K.; McKenzie, E.; Ikner, L.; Wang, M.; Wang, Q.; Young, K.; Haas, C.N.; et al. A Case Study Evaluating the Risk of Infection from Middle Eastern Respiratory Syndrome Coronavirus (MERS-CoV) in a Hospital Setting Through Bioaerosols. *Risk Anal.* **2019**, *39*, 2608–2624. [CrossRef]
187. Herrera, D.; Serrano, J.; Roldán, S.; Sanz, M. Is the Oral Cavity Relevant in SARS-CoV-2 Pandemic? *Clin. Oral Investig.* **2020**, *24*, 2925–2930. [CrossRef]
188. Segal, L.N.; Clemente, J.C.; Tsay, J.-C.J.; Koralov, S.B.; Keller, B.C.; Wu, B.G.; Li, Y.; Shen, N.; Ghedin, E.; Morris, A.; et al. Enrichment of the Lung Microbiome with Oral Taxa Is Associated with Lung Inflammation of a Th17 Phenotype. *Nat. Microbiol.* **2016**, *1*, 16031. [CrossRef]
189. Hasan, A.; Paray, B.A.; Hussain, A.; Qadir, F.A.; Attar, F.; Aziz, F.M.; Sharifi, M.; Derakhshankhah, H.; Rasti, B.; Mehrabi, M.; et al. A Review on the Cleavage Priming of the Spike Protein on Coronavirus by Angiotensin-Converting Enzyme-2 and Furin. *J. Biomol. Struct. Dyn.* **2020**, 1–9. [CrossRef]
190. Xu, H.; Zhong, L.; Deng, J.; Peng, J.; Dan, H.; Zeng, X.; Li, T.; Chen, Q. High Expression of ACE2 Receptor of 2019-NCoV on the Epithelial Cells of Oral Mucosa. *Int. J. Oral Sci.* **2020**, *12*, 8. [CrossRef] [PubMed]
191. Sakaguchi, W.; Kubota, N.; Shimizu, T.; Saruta, J.; Fuchida, S.; Kawata, A.; Yamamoto, Y.; Sugimoto, M.; Yakeishi, M.; Tsukinoki, K. Existence of SARS-CoV-2 Entry Molecules in the Oral Cavity. *Int. J. Mol. Sci.* **2020**, *21*, 6000. [CrossRef] [PubMed]
192. Liu, L.; Wei, Q.; Alvarez, X.; Wang, H.; Du, Y.; Zhu, H.; Jiang, H.; Zhou, J.; Lam, P.; Zhang, L.; et al. Epithelial Cells Lining Salivary Gland Ducts Are Early Target Cells of Severe Acute Respiratory Syndrome Coronavirus Infection in the Upper Respiratory Tracts of Rhesus Macaques. *J. Virol.* **2011**, *85*, 4025–4030. [CrossRef] [PubMed]
193. Xu, J.; Li, Y.; Gan, F.; Du, Y.; Yao, Y. Salivary Glands: Potential Reservoirs for COVID-19 Asymptomatic Infection. *J. Dent. Res.* **2020**, *99*, 989. [CrossRef] [PubMed]
194. Descamps, G.; Verset, L.; Trelcat, A.; Hopkins, C.; Lechien, J.R.; Journe, F.; Saussez, S. ACE2 Protein Landscape in the Head and Neck Region: The Conundrum of SARS-CoV-2 Infection. *Biology* **2020**, *9*, 235. [CrossRef]
195. Chen, L.; Zhao, J.; Peng, J.; Li, X.; Deng, X.; Geng, Z.; Shen, Z.; Guo, F.; Zhang, Q.; Jin, Y.; et al. Detection of SARS-CoV-2 in Saliva and Characterization of Oral Symptoms in COVID-19 Patients. *Cell Prolif.* **2020**. [CrossRef] [PubMed]
196. Huang, N.; Perez, P.; Kato, T.; Mikami, Y.; Okuda, K.; Gilmore, R.C.; Conde, C.D.; Gasmi, B.; Stein, S.; Beach, M.; et al. Integrated Single-Cell Atlases Reveal an Oral SARS-CoV-2 Infection and Transmission Axis. *MedRxiv* **2020**. [CrossRef]
197. López de Cicco, R.; Watson, J.C.; Bassi, D.E.; Litwin, S.; Klein-Szanto, A.J. Simultaneous Expression of Furin and Vascular Endothelial Growth Factor in Human Oral Tongue Squamous Cell Carcinoma Progression. *Clin. Cancer Res.* **2004**, *10*, 4480–4488. [CrossRef]
198. Böttcher, E.; Matrosovich, T.; Beyerle, M.; Klenk, H.-D.; Garten, W.; Matrosovich, M. Proteolytic Activation of Influenza Viruses by Serine Proteases TMPRSS2 and HAT from Human Airway Epithelium. *J. Virol.* **2006**, *80*, 9896–9898. [CrossRef] [PubMed]
199. Bertram, S.; Heurich, A.; Lavender, H.; Gierer, S.; Danisch, S.; Perin, P.; Lucas, J.M.; Nelson, P.S.; Pöhlmann, S.; Soilleux, E.J. Influenza and SARS-Coronavirus Activating Proteases TMPRSS2 and HAT Are Expressed at Multiple Sites in Human Respiratory and Gastrointestinal Tracts. *PLoS ONE* **2012**, *7*, e35876. [CrossRef]
200. Kielian, M. Enhancing Host Cell Infection by SARS-CoV-2. *Science* **2020**, *370*, 765–766. [CrossRef]
201. Varadarajan, S.; Balaji, T.M.; Sarode, S.C.; Sarode, G.S.; Sharma, N.K.; Gondivkar, S.; Gadbail, A.; Patil, S. EMMPRIN/BASIGIN as a Biological Modulator of Oral Cancer and COVID-19 Interaction: Novel Propositions. *Med. Hypotheses* **2020**, *143*, 110089. [CrossRef] [PubMed]
202. Shahrabi-Farahani, S.; Gallottini, M.; Martins, F.; Li, E.; Mudge, D.R.; Nakayama, H.; Hida, K.; Panigrahy, D.; D'Amore, P.A.; Bielenberg, D.R. Neuropilin 1 Receptor Is Up-Regulated in Dysplastic Epithelium and Oral Squamous Cell Carcinoma. *Am. J. Pathol.* **2016**, *186*, 1055–1064. [CrossRef] [PubMed]
203. Daly, J.L.; Simonetti, B.; Klein, K.; Chen, K.-E.; Williamson, M.K.; Antón-Plágaro, C.; Shoemark, D.K.; Simón-Gracia, L.; Bauer, M.; Hollandi, R.; et al. Neuropilin-1 Is a Host Factor for SARS-CoV-2 Infection. *Science* **2020**, *370*, 861–865. [CrossRef]
204. Cantuti-Castelvetri, L.; Ojha, R.; Pedro, L.D.; Djannatian, M.; Franz, J.; Kuivanen, S.; van der Meer, F.; Kallio, K.; Kaya, T.; Anastasina, M.; et al. Neuropilin-1 Facilitates SARS-CoV-2 Cell Entry and Infectivity. *Science* **2020**, *370*, 856–860. [CrossRef] [PubMed]
205. Wang, K.; Chen, W.; Zhou, Y.-S.; Lian, J.-Q.; Zhang, Z.; Du, P.; Gong, L.; Zhang, Y.; Cui, H.-Y.; Geng, J.-J.; et al. SARS-CoV-2 Invades Host Cells via a Novel Route: CD147-Spike Protein. *BioRxiv* **2020**. [CrossRef]
206. Tu, Y.-P.; Jennings, R.; Hart, B.; Cangelosi, G.A.; Wood, R.C.; Wehber, K.; Verma, P.; Vojta, D.; Berke, E.M. Swabs Collected by Patients or Health Care Workers for SARS-CoV-2 Testing. *N. Engl. J. Med.* **2020**, *383*, 494–496. [CrossRef]
207. Pellegrino, R.; Cooper, K.W.; Di Pizio, A.; Joseph, P.V.; Bhutani, S.; Parma, V. Corona Viruses and the Chemical Senses: Past, Present, and Future. *Chem. Senses* **2020**. [CrossRef] [PubMed]
208. Freni, F.; Meduri, A.; Gazia, F.; Nicastro, V.; Galletti, C.; Aragona, P.; Galletti, C.; Galletti, B.; Galletti, F. Symptomatology in Head and Neck District in Coronavirus Disease (COVID-19): A Possible Neuroinvasive Action of SARS-CoV-2. *Am. J. Otolaryngol.* **2020**, *41*, 102612. [CrossRef] [PubMed]

209. Capocasale, G.; Nocini, R.; Faccioni, P.; Donadello, D.; Bertossi, D.; Albanese, M.; Zotti, F. How to Deal with Coronavirus Disease 2019: A Comprehensive Narrative Review about Oral Involvement of the Disease. *Clin. Exp. Dent. Res.* **2020**. [CrossRef]
210. Brandão, T.B.; Gueiros, L.A.; Melo, T.S.; Prado-Ribeiro, A.C.; Nesrallah, A.C.F.A.; Prado, G.V.B.; Santos-Silva, A.R.; Migliorati, C.A. Oral Lesions in Patients with SARS-CoV-2 Infection: Could the Oral Cavity Be a Target Organ? *Oral Surg. Oral Med. Oral Pathol. Oral Radiol.* **2020**. [CrossRef] [PubMed]
211. Gupta, S.; Mohindra, R.; Chauhan, P.K.; Singla, V.; Goyal, K.; Sahni, V.; Gaur, R.; Verma, D.K.; Ghosh, A.; Soni, R.K.; et al. SARS-CoV-2 Detection in Gingival Crevicular Fluid. *J. Dent. Res.* **2020**, 22034520970536. [CrossRef]
212. Badran, Z.; Gaudin, A.; Struillou, X.; Amador, G.; Soueidan, A. Periodontal Pockets: A Potential Reservoir for SARS-CoV-2? *Med. Hypotheses* **2020**, *143*, 109907. [CrossRef]
213. Fiorillo, L.; Cervino, G.; Laino, L.; D'Amico, C.; Mauceri, R.; Tozum, T.F.; Gaeta, M.; Cicciù, M. Porphyromonas Gingivalis, Periodontal and Systemic Implications: A Systematic Review. *Dent. J.* **2019**, *7*, 114. [CrossRef]
214. Li, X.; Li, C.; Liu, J.-C.; Pan, Y.-P.; Li, Y.-G. In Vitro Effect of Porphyromonas Gingivalis Combined with Influenza A Virus on Respiratory Epithelial Cells. *Arch. Oral Biol.* **2018**, *95*, 125–133. [CrossRef]
215. Kaczor-Urbanowicz, K.E.; Martin Carreras-Presas, C.; Aro, K.; Tu, M.; Garcia-Godoy, F.; Wong, D.T. Saliva Diagnostics—Current Views and Directions. *Exp. Biol. Med. (Maywood)* **2017**, *242*, 459–472. [CrossRef] [PubMed]
216. To, K.K.-W.; Tsang, O.T.-Y.; Leung, W.-S.; Tam, A.R.; Wu, T.-C.; Lung, D.C.; Yip, C.C.-Y.; Cai, J.-P.; Chan, J.M.-C.; Chik, T.S.-H.; et al. Temporal Profiles of Viral Load in Posterior Oropharyngeal Saliva Samples and Serum Antibody Responses during Infection by SARS-CoV-2: An Observational Cohort Study. *Lancet Infect. Dis.* **2020**, *20*, 565–574. [CrossRef]
217. Sabino-Silva, R.; Jardim, A.C.G.; Siqueira, W.L. Coronavirus COVID-19 Impacts to Dentistry and Potential Salivary Diagnosis. *Clin. Oral Investig.* **2020**, *24*, 1619–1621. [CrossRef]
218. Wölfel, R.; Corman, V.M.; Guggemos, W.; Seilmaier, M.; Zange, S.; Müller, M.A.; Niemeyer, D.; Jones, T.C.; Vollmar, P.; Rothe, C.; et al. Virological Assessment of Hospitalized Patients with COVID-2019. *Nature* **2020**, *581*, 465–469. [CrossRef] [PubMed]
219. Kim, S.E.; Lee, J.Y.; Lee, A.; Kim, S.; Park, K.H.; Jung, S.I.; Kang, S.J.; Oh, T.H.; Kim, U.J.; Lee, S.Y.; et al. Viral Load Kinetics of SARS-CoV-2 Infection in Saliva in Korean Patients: A Prospective Multi-Center Comparative Study. *J. Korean Med. Sci.* **2020**, *35*, e287. [CrossRef] [PubMed]
220. Han, M.S.; Seong, M.-W.; Kim, N.; Shin, S.; Cho, S.I.; Park, H.; Kim, T.S.; Park, S.S.; Choi, E.H. Viral RNA Load in Mildly Symptomatic and Asymptomatic Children with COVID-19, Seoul, South Korea. *Emerg. Infect. Dis.* **2020**, *26*, 2497–2499. [CrossRef]
221. To, K.K.-W.; Tsang, O.T.-Y.; Yip, C.C.-Y.; Chan, K.-H.; Wu, T.-C.; Chan, J.M.-C.; Leung, W.-S.; Chik, T.S.-H.; Choi, C.Y.-C.; Kandamby, D.H.; et al. Consistent Detection of 2019 Novel Coronavirus in Saliva. *Clin. Infect. Dis.* **2020**, *71*, 841–843. [CrossRef]
222. Iwasaki, S.; Fujisawa, S.; Nakakubo, S.; Kamada, K.; Yamashita, Y.; Fukumoto, T.; Sato, K.; Oguri, S.; Taki, K.; Senjo, H.; et al. Comparison of SARS-CoV-2 Detection in Nasopharyngeal Swab and Saliva. *J. Infect.* **2020**, *81*, e145–e147. [CrossRef]
223. Yoon, J.G.; Yoon, J.; Song, J.Y.; Yoon, S.Y.; Lim, C.S.; Seong, H.; Noh, J.Y.; Cheong, H.J.; Kim, W.J. Clinical Significance of a High SARS-CoV-2 Viral Load in the Saliva. *J. Korean Med. Sci.* **2020**, *35*, e195. [CrossRef]
224. Cheng, V.C.C.; Wong, S.-C.; Chen, J.H.K.; Yip, C.C.Y.; Chuang, V.W.M.; Tsang, O.T.Y.; Sridhar, S.; Chan, J.F.W.; Ho, P.-L.; Yuen, K.-Y. Escalating Infection Control Response to the Rapidly Evolving Epidemiology of the Coronavirus Disease 2019 (COVID-19) Due to SARS-CoV-2 in Hong Kong. *Infect. Control Hosp. Epidemiol.* **2020**, *41*, 493–498. [CrossRef] [PubMed]
225. Nagura-Ikeda, M.; Imai, K.; Tabata, S.; Miyoshi, K.; Murahara, N.; Mizuno, T.; Horiuchi, M.; Kato, K.; Imoto, Y.; Iwata, M.; et al. Clinical Evaluation of Self-Collected Saliva by Quantitative Reverse Transcription-PCR (RT-QPCR), Direct RT-QPCR, Reverse Transcription-Loop-Mediated Isothermal Amplification, and a Rapid Antigen Test to Diagnose COVID-19. *J. Clin. Microbiol.* **2020**, *58*. [CrossRef] [PubMed]
226. Williams, E.; Isles, N.; Chong, B.; Bond, K.; Yoga, Y.; Druce, J.; Catton, M.; Ballard, S.A.; Howden, B.P.; Williamson, D.A. Detection of SARS-CoV-2 in Saliva: Implications for Specimen Transport and Storage. *J. Med. Microbiol.* **2020**. [CrossRef]
227. Walsh, K.A.; Jordan, K.; Clyne, B.; Rohde, D.; Drummond, L.; Byrne, P.; Ahern, S.; Carty, P.G.; O'Brien, K.K.; O'Murchu, E.; et al. SARS-CoV-2 Detection, Viral Load and Infectivity over the Course of an Infection. *J. Infect.* **2020**, *81*, 357–371. [CrossRef]
228. Tajima, Y.; Suda, Y.; Yano, K. A Case Report of SARS-CoV-2 Confirmed in Saliva Specimens up to 37 Days after Onset: Proposal of Saliva Specimens for COVID-19 Diagnosis and Virus Monitoring. *J. Infect. Chemother.* **2020**, *26*, 1086–1089. [CrossRef] [PubMed]
229. Azzi, L.; Carcano, G.; Gianfagna, F.; Grossi, P.; Gasperina, D.D.; Genoni, A.; Fasano, M.; Sessa, F.; Tettamanti, L.; Carinci, F.; et al. Saliva Is a Reliable Tool to Detect SARS-CoV-2. *J. Infect.* **2020**, *81*, e45–e50. [CrossRef]
230. Kojima, N.; Turner, F.; Slepnev, V.; Bacelar, A.; Deming, L.; Kodeboyina, S.; Klausner, J.D. Self-Collected Oral Fluid and Nasal Swab Specimens Demonstrate Comparable Sensitivity to Clinician-Collected Nasopharyngeal Swab Specimens for the Detection of SARS-CoV-2. *Clin. Infect. Dis.* **2020**. [CrossRef]
231. Bosworth, A.; Whalley, C.; Poxon, C.; Wanigasooriya, K.; Pickles, O.; Aldera, E.L.; Papakonstantinou, D.; Morley, G.L.; Walker, E.M.; Zielinska, A.E.; et al. Rapid Implementation and Validation of a Cold-Chain Free SARS-CoV-2 Diagnostic Testing Workflow to Support Surge Capacity. *J. Clin. Virol.* **2020**, *128*, 104469. [CrossRef]
232. Yokota, I.; Shane, P.Y.; Okada, K.; Unoki, Y.; Yang, Y.; Inao, T.; Sakamaki, K.; Iwasaki, S.; Hayasaka, K.; Sugita, J.; et al. Mass Screening of Asymptomatic Persons for SARS-CoV-2 Using Saliva. *Clin. Infect. Dis.* **2020**. [CrossRef]
233. Landry, M.L.; Criscuolo, J.; Peaper, D.R. Challenges in Use of Saliva for Detection of SARS CoV-2 RNA in Symptomatic Outpatients. *J. Clin. Virol.* **2020**, *130*, 104567. [CrossRef]

234. Azzi, L.; Carcano, G.; Dalla Gasperina, D.; Sessa, F.; Maurino, V.; Baj, A. Two Cases of COVID-19 with Positive Salivary and Negative Pharyngeal or Respiratory Swabs at Hospital Discharge: A Rising Concern. *Oral Dis.* **2020**. [CrossRef]
235. Jeong, H.W.; Kim, S.-M.; Kim, H.-S.; Kim, Y.-I.; Kim, J.H.; Cho, J.Y.; Kim, S.; Kang, H.; Kim, S.-G.; Park, S.-J.; et al. Viable SARS-CoV-2 in Various Specimens from COVID-19 Patients. *Clin. Microbiol. Infect.* **2020**, *26*, 1520–1524. [CrossRef]
236. Sohn, Y.; Jeong, S.J.; Chung, W.S.; Hyun, J.H.; Baek, Y.J.; Cho, Y.; Kim, J.H.; Ahn, J.Y.; Choi, J.Y.; Yeom, J.-S. Assessing Viral Shedding and Infectivity of Asymptomatic or Mildly Symptomatic Patients with COVID-19 in a Later Phase. *J. Clin. Med.* **2020**, *9*, 2924. [CrossRef] [PubMed]
237. Papineni, R.S.; Rosenthal, F.S. The Size Distribution of Droplets in the Exhaled Breath of Healthy Human Subjects. *J. Aerosol Med.* **1997**, *10*, 105–116. [CrossRef] [PubMed]
238. Abkarian, M.; Mendez, S.; Xue, N.; Yang, F.; Stone, H.A. Speech Can Produce Jet-like Transport Relevant to Asymptomatic Spreading of Virus. *Proc. Natl. Acad. Sci. USA* **2020**, *117*, 25237–25245. [CrossRef] [PubMed]
239. Fahy, J.V.; Dickey, B.F. Airway Mucus Function and Dysfunction. *N. Engl. J. Med.* **2010**, *363*, 2233–2247. [CrossRef] [PubMed]
240. Xie, X.; Li, Y.; Chwang, A.T.Y.; Ho, P.L.; Seto, W.H. How Far Droplets Can Move in Indoor Environments—Revisiting the Wells Evaporation-Falling Curve. *Indoor Air* **2007**, *17*, 211–225. [CrossRef]
241. Zhang, R.; Li, Y.; Zhang, A.L.; Wang, Y.; Molina, M.J. Identifying Airborne Transmission as the Dominant Route for the Spread of COVID-19. *Proc. Natl. Acad. Sci. USA* **2020**, *117*, 14857–14863. [CrossRef]
242. Seminara, G.; Carli, B.; Forni, G.; Fuzzi, S.; Mazzino, A.; Rinaldo, A. Biological Fluid Dynamics of Airborne COVID-19 Infection. *Rend. Lincei Sci. Fis. Nat.* **2020**, 1–33. [CrossRef]
243. Kampf, G.; Todt, D.; Pfaender, S.; Steinmann, E. Persistence of Coronaviruses on Inanimate Surfaces and Their Inactivation with Biocidal Agents. *J. Hosp. Infect.* **2020**, *104*, 246–251. [CrossRef]
244. Van Doremalen, N.; Bushmaker, T.; Morris, D.H.; Holbrook, M.G.; Gamble, A.; Williamson, B.N.; Tamin, A.; Harcourt, J.L.; Thornburg, N.J.; Gerber, S.I.; et al. Aerosol and Surface Stability of SARS-CoV-2 as Compared with SARS-CoV-1. *N. Engl. J. Med.* **2020**, *382*, 1564–1567. [CrossRef]
245. Chin, A.W.H.; Chu, J.T.S.; Perera, M.R.A.; Hui, K.P.Y.; Yen, H.-L.; Chan, M.C.W.; Peiris, M.; Poon, L.L.M. Stability of SARS-CoV-2 in Different Environmental Conditions. *Lancet Microbe* **2020**, *1*, e10. [CrossRef]
246. Santarpia, J.L.; Rivera, D.N.; Herrera, V.L.; Morwitzer, M.J.; Creager, H.M.; Santarpia, G.W.; Crown, K.K.; Brett-Major, D.M.; Schnaubelt, E.R.; Broadhurst, M.J.; et al. Aerosol and Surface Contamination of SARS-CoV-2 Observed in Quarantine and Isolation Care. *Sci. Rep.* **2020**, *10*, 12732. [CrossRef]
247. Wang, Y.; Cao, Z.; Zeng, D.; Zhang, Q.; Luo, T. The Collective Wisdom in the COVID-19 Research: Comparison and Synthesis of Epidemiological Parameter Estimates in Preprints and Peer-Reviewed Articles. *Int. J. Infect. Dis.* **2020**, *104*, 1–6. [CrossRef]
248. Li, Y.; Zhou, W.; Yang, L.; You, R. Physiological and Pathological Regulation of ACE2, the SARS-CoV-2 Receptor. *Pharmacol. Res.* **2020**, *157*, 104833. [CrossRef] [PubMed]
249. World Health Organization (WHO). Coronavirus Disease (COVID-19). Available online: https://www.who.int/news-room/q-a-detail/coronavirus-disease-covid-19 (accessed on 28 December 2020).
250. Carvalho-Schneider, C.; Laurent, E.; Lemaignen, A.; Beaufils, E.; Bourbao-Tournois, C.; Laribi, S.; Flament, T.; Ferreira-Maldent, N.; Bruyère, F.; Stefic, K.; et al. Follow-up of Adults with Noncritical COVID-19 Two Months after Symptom Onset. *Clin. Microbiol. Infect.* **2020**. [CrossRef]
251. Pierron, D.; Pereda-Loth, V.; Mantel, M.; Moranges, M.; Bignon, E.; Alva, O.; Kabous, J.; Heiske, M.; Pacalon, J.; David, R.; et al. Smell and Taste Changes Are Early Indicators of the COVID-19 Pandemic and Political Decision Effectiveness. *Nat. Commun.* **2020**, *11*, 5152. [CrossRef]
252. Biadsee, A.; Biadsee, A.; Kassem, F.; Dagan, O.; Masarwa, S.; Ormianer, Z. Olfactory and Oral Manifestations of COVID-19: Sex-Related Symptoms—A Potential Pathway to Early Diagnosis. *Otolaryngol. Head Neck Surg.* **2020**. [CrossRef] [PubMed]
253. Alyammahi, S.K.; Abdin, S.M.; Alhamad, D.W.; Elgendy, S.M.; Altell, A.T.; Omar, H.A. The Dynamic Association between COVID-19 and Chronic Disorders: An Updated Insight into Prevalence Mechanism and Therapeutic Modalities. *Infect. Genet. Evol.* **2020**. [CrossRef]
254. Xu, X.-W.; Wu, X.-X.; Jiang, X.-G.; Xu, K.-J.; Ying, L.-J.; Ma, C.-L.; Li, S.-B.; Wang, H.-Y.; Zhang, S.; Gao, H.-N.; et al. Clinical Findings in a Group of Patients Infected with the 2019 Novel Coronavirus (SARS-Cov-2) Outside of Wuhan, China: Retrospective Case Series. *BMJ* **2020**, *368*, m606. [CrossRef]
255. Richardson, S.; Hirsch, J.S.; Narasimhan, M.; Crawford, J.M.; McGinn, T.; Davidson, K.W.; The Northwell COVID-19 Research Consortium. Presenting Characteristics, Comorbidities, and Outcomes Among 5700 Patients Hospitalized With COVID-19 in the New York City Area. *JAMA* **2020**, *323*, 2052–2059. [CrossRef] [PubMed]
256. Yifan, C.; Jun, P. Understanding the Clinical Features of Coronavirus Disease 2019 from the Perspective of Aging: A Systematic Review and Meta-Analysis. *Front. Endocrinol.* **2020**, *11*, 557333. [CrossRef] [PubMed]
257. Yanai, H. Metabolic Syndrome and COVID-19. *Cardiol. Res.* **2020**, *11*, 360–365. [CrossRef]
258. Cardinali, D.P.; Brown, G.M.; Pandi-Perumal, S.R. Can Melatonin Be a Potential "Silver Bullet" in Treating COVID-19 Patients? *Diseases* **2020**, *8*, 44. [CrossRef] [PubMed]
259. Zimmermann, P.; Curtis, N. Why Is COVID-19 Less Severe in Children? A Review of the Proposed Mechanisms Underlying the Age-Related Difference in Severity of SARS-CoV-2 Infections. *Arch. Dis. Child.* **2020**. [CrossRef] [PubMed]

260. Lombardi, C.; Roca, E.; Ventura, L.; Cottini, M. Smoking and COVID-19, the Paradox to Discover: An Italian Retrospective, Observational Study in Hospitalized and Non-Hospitalized Patients. *Med. Hypotheses* **2020**. [CrossRef]
261. Gupta, A.K.; Nethan, S.T.; Mehrotra, R. Tobacco Use as a Well-Recognized Cause of Severe COVID-19 Manifestations. *Respir. Med.* **2020**, *176*, 106233. [CrossRef]
262. Baburaj, G.; Thomas, L.; Rao, M. Potential Drug Interactions of Repurposed COVID-19 Drugs with Lung Cancer Pharmacotherapies. *Arch. Med. Res.* **2020**. [CrossRef]
263. Chee, Y.J.; Ng, S.J.H.; Yeoh, E. Diabetic Ketoacidosis Precipitated by Covid-19 in a Patient with Newly Diagnosed Diabetes Mellitus. *Diabetes Res. Clin. Pract.* **2020**, *164*, 108166. [CrossRef]
264. Guo, T.; Fan, Y.; Chen, M.; Wu, X.; Zhang, L.; He, T.; Wang, H.; Wan, J.; Wang, X.; Lu, Z. Cardiovascular Implications of Fatal Outcomes of Patients with Coronavirus Disease 2019 (COVID-19). *JAMA Cardiol.* **2020**, *5*, 811–818. [CrossRef]
265. Xu, Z.; Shi, L.; Wang, Y.; Zhang, J.; Huang, L.; Zhang, C.; Liu, S.; Zhao, P.; Liu, H.; Zhu, L.; et al. Pathological Findings of COVID-19 Associated with Acute Respiratory Distress Syndrome. *Lancet Respir. Med.* **2020**, *8*, 420–422. [CrossRef]
266. Sarode, S.C.; Sarode, G.S.; Gondivkar, S.; Gadbail, A.; Gopalakrishnan, D.; Patil, S. Oral Submucous Fibrosis and COVID-19: Perspective on Comorbidity. *Oral Oncol.* **2020**, *107*, 104811. [CrossRef]
267. Botros, N.; Iyer, P.; Ojcius, D.M. Is There an Association between Oral Health and Severity of COVID-19 Complications? *Biomed. J.* **2020**, *43*, 325–327. [CrossRef]
268. Victor, G. COVID-19 Admissions Calculators: General Population and Paediatric Cohort. *Early Hum. Dev.* **2020**, *145*, 105043. [CrossRef]
269. Rohani, P.; Ahmadi Badi, S.; Moshiri, A.; Siadat, S.D. Coronavirus Disease 2019 (COVID-19) and Pediatric Gastroenterology. *Gastroenterol. Hepatol. Bed Bench* **2020**, *13*, 351–354. [PubMed]
270. Eastin, C.; Eastin, T. Epidemiological Characteristics of 2143 Pediatric Patients with 2019 Coronavirus Disease in China. *J. Emerg. Med.* **2020**, *58*, 712–713. [CrossRef]
271. Hoang, A.; Chorath, K.; Moreira, A.; Evans, M.; Burmeister-Morton, F.; Burmeister, F.; Naqvi, R.; Petershack, M.; Moreira, A. COVID-19 in 7780 Pediatric Patients: A Systematic Review. *EClinicalMedicine* **2020**, *24*, 100433. [CrossRef] [PubMed]
272. Schvartz, A.; Belot, A.; Kone-Paut, I. Pediatric Inflammatory Multisystem Syndrome and Rheumatic Diseases During SARS-CoV-2 Pandemic. *Front. Pediatr.* **2020**, *8*, 605807. [CrossRef] [PubMed]
273. Verdoni, L.; Mazza, A.; Gervasoni, A.; Martelli, L.; Ruggeri, M.; Ciuffreda, M.; Bonanomi, E.; D'Antiga, L. An Outbreak of Severe Kawasaki-like Disease at the Italian Epicentre of the SARS-CoV-2 Epidemic: An Observational Cohort Study. *Lancet* **2020**, *395*, 1771–1778. [CrossRef]
274. Amaral, W.N.D.; Moraes, C.L.; Rodrigues, A.P.D.S.; Noll, M.; Arruda, J.T.; Mendonça, C.R. Maternal Coronavirus Infections and Neonates Born to Mothers with SARS-CoV-2: A Systematic Review. *Healthcare* **2020**, *8*, 511. [CrossRef]
275. Qiao, J. What Are the Risks of COVID-19 Infection in Pregnant Women? *Lancet* **2020**, *395*, 760–762. [CrossRef]
276. Allotey, J.; Stallings, E.; Bonet, M.; Yap, M.; Chatterjee, S.; Kew, T.; Debenham, L.; Llavall, A.C.; Dixit, A.; Zhou, D.; et al. Clinical Manifestations, Risk Factors, and Maternal and Perinatal Outcomes of Coronavirus Disease 2019 in Pregnancy: Living Systematic Review and Meta-Analysis. *BMJ* **2020**, *370*, m3320. [CrossRef]
277. Di Renzo, L.; Gualtieri, P.; Pivari, F.; Soldati, L.; Attinà, A.; Cinelli, G.; Leggeri, C.; Caparello, G.; Barrea, L.; Scerbo, F.; et al. Eating Habits and Lifestyle Changes during COVID-19 Lockdown: An Italian Survey. *J. Transl. Med.* **2020**, *18*, 229. [CrossRef]
278. Sidor, A.; Rzymski, P. Dietary Choices and Habits during COVID-19 Lockdown: Experience from Poland. *Nutrients* **2020**, *12*, 1657. [CrossRef] [PubMed]
279. Owen, A.; Tran, T.; Hammarberg, K.; Kirkman, M.; Fisher, J. Poor Appetite and Overeating Reported by Adults in Australia during the Coronavirus-19 Disease Pandemic: A Population-Based Study. *Public Health Nutr.* **2021**, *24*, 275–281. [CrossRef]
280. Petrakis, D.; Margină, D.; Tsarouhas, K.; Tekos, F.; Stan, M.; Nikitovic, D.; Kouretas, D.; Spandidos, D.A.; Tsatsakis, A. Obesity—A Risk Factor for Increased COVID-19 Prevalence, Severity and Lethality (Review). *Mol. Med. Rep.* **2020**, *22*, 9–19. [CrossRef]
281. Yan, C.H.; Faraji, F.; Prajapati, D.P.; Boone, C.E.; DeConde, A.S. Association of Chemosensory Dysfunction and COVID-19 in Patients Presenting with Influenza-like Symptoms. *Int. Forum Allergy Rhinol.* **2020**, *10*, 806–813. [CrossRef]
282. Makaronidis, J.; Mok, J.; Balogun, N.; Magee, C.G.; Omar, R.Z.; Carnemolla, A.; Batterham, R.L. Seroprevalence of SARS-CoV-2 Antibodies in People with an Acute Loss in Their Sense of Smell and/or Taste in a Community-Based Population in London, UK: An Observational Cohort Study. *PLoS Med.* **2020**, *17*, e1003358. [CrossRef] [PubMed]
283. Thibault, R.; Coëffier, M.; Joly, F.; Bohé, J.; Schneider, S.M.; Déchelotte, P. How the Covid-19 Epidemic Is Challenging Our Practice in Clinical Nutrition—Feedback from the Field. *Eur. J. Clin. Nutr.* **2020**, 1–10. [CrossRef] [PubMed]
284. Semaine Nationale de La Dénutrition 2020. Available online: https://www.subscribepage.com/semainedenutrition2020 (accessed on 5 December 2020).
285. Amorim Dos Santos, J.; Normando, A.G.C.; Carvalho da Silva, R.L.; Acevedo, A.C.; De Luca Canto, G.; Sugaya, N.; Santos-Silva, A.R.; Guerra, E.N.S. Oral Manifestations in Patients with COVID-19: A Living Systematic Review. *J. Dent. Res.* **2021**, *100*, 141–154. [CrossRef] [PubMed]
286. Jang, Y.; Son, H.-J.; Lee, S.; Lee, E.J.; Kim, T.H.; Park, S.Y. Olfactory and Taste Disorder: The First and Only Sign in a Patient with SARS-CoV-2 Pneumonia. *Infect. Control Hosp. Epidemiol.* **2020**, *41*, 1103. [CrossRef]
287. Spinato, G.; Fabbris, C.; Polesel, J.; Cazzador, D.; Borsetto, D.; Hopkins, C.; Boscolo-Rizzo, P. Alterations in Smell or Taste in Mildly Symptomatic Outpatients With SARS-CoV-2 Infection. *JAMA* **2020**, *323*, 2089–2090. [CrossRef] [PubMed]

288. Cao, Y.; Li, L.; Feng, Z.; Wan, S.; Huang, P.; Sun, X.; Wen, F.; Huang, X.; Ning, G.; Wang, W. Comparative Genetic Analysis of the Novel Coronavirus (2019-NCoV/SARS-CoV-2) Receptor ACE2 in Different Populations. *Cell Discov.* **2020**, *6*. [CrossRef]
289. Lechien, J.R.; Chiesa-Estomba, C.M.; De Siati, D.R.; Horoi, M.; Le Bon, S.D.; Rodriguez, A.; Dequanter, D.; Blecic, S.; El Afia, F.; Distinguin, L.; et al. Olfactory and Gustatory Dysfunctions as a Clinical Presentation of Mild-to-Moderate Forms of the Coronavirus Disease (COVID-19): A Multicenter European Study. *Eur. Arch. Otorhinolaryngol.* **2020**, *277*, 2251–2261. [CrossRef]
290. Solemdal, K.; Sandvik, L.; Willumsen, T.; Mowe, M.; Hummel, T. The Impact of Oral Health on Taste Ability in Acutely Hospitalized Elderly. *PLoS ONE* **2012**, *7*, e36557. [CrossRef] [PubMed]
291. Vaira, L.A.; Salzano, G.; Fois, A.G.; Piombino, P.; De Riu, G. Potential Pathogenesis of Ageusia and Anosmia in COVID-19 Patients. *Int. Forum Allergy Rhinol.* **2020**, *10*, 1103–1104. [CrossRef] [PubMed]
292. Finsterer, J.; Stollberger, C. Causes of Hypogeusia/Hyposmia in SARS-CoV2 Infected Patients. *J. Med. Virol.* **2020**. [CrossRef]
293. Lozada-Nur, F.; Chainani-Wu, N.; Fortuna, G.; Sroussi, H. Dysgeusia in COVID-19: Possible Mechanisms and Implications. *Oral Surg. Oral Med. Oral Pathol. Oral Radiol.* **2020**, *130*, 344–346. [CrossRef]
294. Unnikrishnan, D.; Murakonda, P.; Dharmarajan, T.S. If It Is Not Cough, It Must Be Dysgeusia: Differing Adverse Effects of Angiotensin-Converting Enzyme Inhibitors in the Same Individual. *J. Am. Med. Dir. Assoc.* **2004**, *5*, 107–110. [CrossRef]
295. Sinjari, B.; D'Ardes, D.; Santilli, M.; Rexhepi, I.; D'Addazio, G.; Di Carlo, P.; Chiacchiaretta, P.; Caputi, S.; Cipollone, F. SARS-CoV-2 and Oral Manifestation: An Observational, Human Study. *J. Clin. Med.* **2020**, *9*, 3218. [CrossRef]
296. Wang, C.; Wu, H.; Ding, X.; Ji, H.; Jiao, P.; Song, H.; Li, S.; Du, H. Does Infection of 2019 Novel Coronavirus Cause Acute and/or Chronic Sialadenitis? *Med. Hypotheses* **2020**, *140*, 109789. [CrossRef] [PubMed]
297. Capaccio, P.; Pignataro, L.; Corbellino, M.; Popescu-Dutruit, S.; Torretta, S. Acute Parotitis: A Possible Precocious Clinical Manifestation of SARS-CoV-2 Infection? *Otolaryngol. Head Neck Surg.* **2020**, *163*, 182–183. [CrossRef] [PubMed]
298. Fisher, J.; Monette, D.L.; Patel, K.R.; Kelley, B.P.; Kennedy, M. COVID-19 Associated Parotitis: A Case Report. *Am. J. Emerg. Med.* **2020**. [CrossRef]
299. Chern, A.; Famuyide, A.O.; Moonis, G.; Lalwani, A.K. Sialadenitis: A Possible Early Manifestation of COVID-19. *Laryngoscope* **2020**. [CrossRef] [PubMed]
300. Kitakawa, D.; Oliveira, F.E.; Neves de Castro, P.; Carvalho, L.F.C.S. Short Report—Herpes Simplex Lesion in the Lip Semimucosa in a COVID-19 Patient. *Eur. Rev. Med. Pharmacol. Sci.* **2020**, *24*, 9151–9153. [CrossRef] [PubMed]
301. Martín Carreras-Presas, C.; Amaro Sánchez, J.; López-Sánchez, A.F.; Jané-Salas, E.; Somacarrera Pérez, M.L. Oral Vesiculobullous Lesions Associated with SARS-CoV-2 Infection. *Oral Dis.* **2020**. [CrossRef] [PubMed]
302. Hedou, M.; Carsuzaa, F.; Chary, E.; Hainaut, E.; Cazenave-Roblot, F.; Masson Regnault, M. Comment on "Cutaneous Manifestations in COVID-19: A First Perspective" by Recalcati, S. *J. Eur. Acad. Dermatol. Venereol.* **2020**, *34*, e299–e300. [CrossRef] [PubMed]
303. Nuno-Gonzalez, A.; Martin-Carrillo, P.; Magaletsky, K.; Martin Rios, M.D.; Herranz Mañas, C.; Artigas Almazan, J.; García Casasola, G.; Perez Castro, E.; Gallego Arenas, A.; Mayor Ibarguren, A.; et al. Prevalence of Mucocutaneous Manifestations in 666 Patients with COVID-19 in a Field Hospital in Spain: Oral and Palmoplantar Findings. *Br. J. Dermatol.* **2020**. [CrossRef]
304. Forbes, H.; Warne, B.; Doelken, L.; Brenner, N.; Waterboer, T.; Luben, R.; Wareham, N.J.; Warren-Gash, C.; Gkrania-Klotsas, E. Risk Factors for Herpes Simplex Virus Type-1 Infection and Reactivation: Cross-Sectional Studies among EPIC-Norfolk Participants. *PLoS ONE* **2019**, *14*, e0215553. [CrossRef]
305. Su, C.-J.; Lee, C.-H. Viral Exanthem in COVID-19, a Clinical Enigma with Biological Significance. *J. Eur. Acad. Dermatol. Venereol.* **2020**, *34*, e251–e252. [CrossRef]
306. Riad, A.; Gad, A.; Hockova, B.; Klugar, M. Oral Candidiasis in Non-Severe COVID-19 Patients: Call for Antibiotic Stewardship. *Oral Surg.* **2020**. [CrossRef] [PubMed]
307. Riad, A.; Kassem, I.; Hockova, B.; Badrah, M.; Klugar, M. Halitosis in COVID-19 Patients. *Spec. Care Dentist.* **2020**. [CrossRef] [PubMed]
308. Ho, B.E.; Ho, A.P.; Ho, M.A.; Ho, E.C. Case Report of Familial COVID-19 Cluster Associated with High Prevalence of Anosmia, Ageusia, and Gastrointestinal Symptoms. *IDCases* **2020**, *22*, e00975. [CrossRef] [PubMed]
309. Chung, C.C.; Wong, W.H.; Fung, J.L.; Hong Kong, R.D.; Chung, B.H. Impact of COVID-19 Pandemic on Patients with Rare Disease in Hong Kong. *Eur. J. Med. Genet.* **2020**, *63*, 104062. [CrossRef] [PubMed]
310. National Institute of Health (NIH). Information on COVID-19 Treatment, Prevention and Research. Available online: https://www.covid19treatmentguidelines.nih.gov/ (accessed on 6 December 2020).
311. Babaei, F.; Mirzababaei, M.; Nassiri-Asl, M.; Hosseinzadeh, H. Review of Registered Clinical Trials for the Treatment of COVID-19. *Drug Dev. Res.* **2020**. [CrossRef]
312. Zumla, A.; Hui, D.S.; Azhar, E.I.; Memish, Z.A.; Maeurer, M. Reducing Mortality from 2019-NCoV: Host-Directed Therapies Should Be an Option. *Lancet* **2020**, *395*, e35–e36. [CrossRef]
313. Chen, P.; Nirula, A.; Heller, B.; Gottlieb, R.L.; Boscia, J.; Morris, J.; Huhn, G.; Cardona, J.; Mocherla, B.; Stosor, V.; et al. SARS-CoV-2 Neutralizing Antibody LY-CoV555 in Outpatients with Covid-19. *N. Engl. J. Med.* **2020**. [CrossRef]
314. Lei, X.; Dong, X.; Ma, R.; Wang, W.; Xiao, X.; Tian, Z.; Wang, C.; Wang, Y.; Li, L.; Ren, L.; et al. Activation and Evasion of Type I Interferon Responses by SARS-CoV-2. *Nat. Commun.* **2020**, *11*, 3810. [CrossRef] [PubMed]
315. Schreiber, G. The Role of Type I Interferons in the Pathogenesis and Treatment of COVID-19. *Front. Immunol.* **2020**, *11*, 595739. [CrossRef]
316. Gurwitz, D. Angiotensin Receptor Blockers as Tentative SARS-CoV-2 Therapeutics. *Drug Dev. Res.* **2020**, *81*, 537–540. [CrossRef]

317. Hoffmann, M.; Schroeder, S.; Kleine-Weber, H.; Müller, M.A.; Drosten, C.; Pöhlmann, S. Nafamostat Mesylate Blocks Activation of SARS-CoV-2: New Treatment Option for COVID-19. *Antimicrob. Agents Chemother.* **2020**, *64*. [CrossRef]
318. Wang, M.; Cao, R.; Zhang, L.; Yang, X.; Liu, J.; Xu, M.; Shi, Z.; Hu, Z.; Zhong, W.; Xiao, G. Remdesivir and Chloroquine Effectively Inhibit the Recently Emerged Novel Coronavirus (2019-NCoV) in Vitro. *Cell Res.* **2020**, *30*, 269–271. [CrossRef] [PubMed]
319. Ahsan, W.; Javed, S.; Bratty, M.A.; Alhazmi, H.A.; Najmi, A. Treatment of SARS-CoV-2: How Far Have We Reached? *Drug Discov. Ther.* **2020**, *14*, 67–72. [CrossRef] [PubMed]
320. Vankadari, N. Arbidol: A Potential Antiviral Drug for the Treatment of SARS-CoV-2 by Blocking Trimerization of the Spike Glycoprotein. *Int. J. Antimicrob. Agents* **2020**, *56*, 105998. [CrossRef]
321. De Wilde, A.H.; Jochmans, D.; Posthuma, C.C.; Zevenhoven-Dobbe, J.C.; van Nieuwkoop, S.; Bestebroer, T.M.; van den Hoogen, B.G.; Neyts, J.; Snijder, E.J. Screening of an FDA-Approved Compound Library Identifies Four Small-Molecule Inhibitors of Middle East Respiratory Syndrome Coronavirus Replication in Cell Culture. *Antimicrob. Agents Chemother.* **2014**, *58*, 4875–4884. [CrossRef] [PubMed]
322. Chu, C.M.; Cheng, V.C.C.; Hung, I.F.N.; Wong, M.M.L.; Chan, K.H.; Chan, K.S.; Kao, R.Y.T.; Poon, L.L.M.; Wong, C.L.P.; Guan, Y.; et al. Role of Lopinavir/Ritonavir in the Treatment of SARS: Initial Virological and Clinical Findings. *Thorax* **2004**, *59*, 252–256. [CrossRef] [PubMed]
323. Cao, B.; Wang, Y.; Wen, D.; Liu, W.; Wang, J.; Fan, G.; Ruan, L.; Song, B.; Cai, Y.; Wei, M.; et al. A Trial of Lopinavir-Ritonavir in Adults Hospitalized with Severe Covid-19. *N. Engl. J. Med.* **2020**, *382*, 1787–1799. [CrossRef] [PubMed]
324. Chen, H.; Zhang, Z.; Wang, L.; Huang, Z.; Gong, F.; Li, X.; Chen, Y.; Wu, J.J. First Clinical Study Using HCV Protease Inhibitor Danoprevir to Treat COVID-19 Patients. *Medicine* **2020**, *99*, e23357. [CrossRef] [PubMed]
325. Seiwert, S.D.; Andrews, S.W.; Jiang, Y.; Serebryany, V.; Tan, H.; Kossen, K.; Rajagopalan, P.T.R.; Misialek, S.; Stevens, S.K.; Stoycheva, A.; et al. Preclinical Characteristics of the Hepatitis C Virus NS3/4A Protease Inhibitor ITMN-191 (R7227). *Antimicrob. Agents Chemother.* **2008**, *52*, 4432–4441. [CrossRef]
326. Delang, L.; Abdelnabi, R.; Neyts, J. Favipiravir as a Potential Countermeasure against Neglected and Emerging RNA Viruses. *Antivir. Res.* **2018**, *153*, 85–94. [CrossRef]
327. Elfiky, A.A. Anti-HCV, Nucleotide Inhibitors, Repurposing against COVID-19. *Life Sci.* **2020**, *248*, 117477. [CrossRef]
328. Asselah, T.; Lada, O.; Moucari, R.; Marcellin, P. Clevudine: A Promising Therapy for the Treatment of Chronic Hepatitis, B. *Expert Opin. Investig. Drugs* **2008**, *17*, 1963–1974. [CrossRef]
329. Rusinov, V.L.; Sapozhnikova, I.M.; Ulomskii, E.N.; Medvedeva, N.R.; Egorov, V.V.; Kiselev, O.I.; Deeva, E.G.; Vasin, A.V.; Chupakhin, O.N. Nucleophilic Substitution of Nitro Group in Nitrotriazolotriazines as a Model of Potential Interaction with Cysteine-Containing Proteins. *Chem. Heterocycl. Compd.* **2015**, *51*, 275–280. [CrossRef]
330. Elfiky, A.A. Ribavirin, Remdesivir, Sofosbuvir, Galidesivir, and Tenofovir against SARS-CoV-2 RNA Dependent RNA Polymerase (RdRp): A Molecular Docking Study. *Life Sci.* **2020**, *253*, 117592. [CrossRef]
331. Harrison, C. Coronavirus Puts Drug Repurposing on the Fast Track. *Nat. Biotechnol.* **2020**, *38*, 379–381. [CrossRef] [PubMed]
332. Rossignol, J.-F. Nitazoxanide: A First-in-Class Broad-Spectrum Antiviral Agent. *Antivir. Res.* **2014**, *110*, 94–103. [CrossRef]
333. Rossignol, J.-F. Nitazoxanide, a New Drug Candidate for the Treatment of Middle East Respiratory Syndrome Coronavirus. *J. Infect. Public Health* **2016**, *9*, 227–230. [CrossRef]
334. Group, T.R.C. Dexamethasone in Hospitalized Patients with Covid-19—Preliminary Report. *N. Engl. J. Med.* **2020**. [CrossRef]
335. Tomazini, B.M.; Maia, I.S.; Cavalcanti, A.B.; Berwanger, O.; Rosa, R.G.; Veiga, V.C.; Avezum, A.; Lopes, R.D.; Bueno, F.R.; Silva, M.V.A.O.; et al. Effect of Dexamethasone on Days Alive and Ventilator-Free in Patients with Moderate or Severe Acute Respiratory Distress Syndrome and COVID-19: The CoDEX Randomized Clinical Trial. *JAMA* **2020**, *324*, 1307–1316. [CrossRef] [PubMed]
336. Han, H.; Yang, L.; Liu, R.; Liu, F.; Wu, K.-L.; Li, J.; Liu, X.-H.; Zhu, C.-L. Prominent Changes in Blood Coagulation of Patients with SARS-CoV-2 Infection. *Clin. Chem. Lab. Med.* **2020**, *58*, 1116–1120. [CrossRef]
337. Helms, J.; Tacquard, C.; Severac, F.; Leonard-Lorant, I.; Ohana, M.; Delabranche, X.; Merdji, H.; Clere-Jehl, R.; Schenck, M.; Fagot Gandet, F.; et al. High Risk of Thrombosis in Patients with Severe SARS-CoV-2 Infection: A Multicenter Prospective Cohort Study. *Intensive Care Med.* **2020**, 1–10. [CrossRef]
338. Moores, L.K.; Tritschler, T.; Brosnahan, S.; Carrier, M.; Collen, J.F.; Doerschug, K.; Holley, A.B.; Jimenez, D.; Le Gal, G.; Rali, P.; et al. Prevention, Diagnosis, and Treatment of VTE in Patients with Coronavirus Disease 2019: CHEST Guideline and Expert Panel Report. *Chest* **2020**, *158*, 1143–1163. [CrossRef]
339. Thachil, J.; Tang, N.; Gando, S.; Falanga, A.; Cattaneo, M.; Levi, M.; Clark, C.; Iba, T. ISTH Interim Guidance on Recognition and Management of Coagulopathy in COVID-19. *J. Thromb. Haemost.* **2020**, *18*, 1023–1026. [CrossRef]
340. Marietta, M.; Ageno, W.; Artoni, A.; De Candia, E.; Gresele, P.; Marchetti, M.; Marcucci, R.; Tripodi, A. COVID-19 and Haemostasis: A Position Paper from Italian Society on Thrombosis and Haemostasis (SISET). *Blood Transfus.* **2020**, *18*, 167–169. [CrossRef]
341. World Health Organization Draft Landscape of COVID-19 Candidate Vaccines. Available online: https://www.who.int/publications/m/item/draft-landscape-of-covid-19-candidate-vaccines (accessed on 22 November 2020).
342. Krammer, F. SARS-CoV-2 Vaccines in Development. *Nature* **2020**, *586*, 516–527. [CrossRef]
343. Flanagan, K.L.; Best, E.; Crawford, N.W.; Giles, M.; Koirala, A.; Macartney, K.; Russell, F.; Teh, B.W.; Wen, S.C. Progress and Pitfalls in the Quest for Effective SARS-CoV-2 (COVID-19) Vaccines. *Front. Immunol.* **2020**, *11*. [CrossRef]
344. Jain, S.; Batra, H.; Yadav, P.; Chand, S. COVID-19 Vaccines Currently under Preclinical and Clinical Studies, and Associated Antiviral Immune Response. *Vaccines* **2020**, *8*, 649. [CrossRef]

345. Amanat, F.; Krammer, F. SARS-CoV-2 Vaccines: Status Report. *Immunity* **2020**, *52*, 583–589. [CrossRef]
346. Su, S.; Du, L.; Jiang, S. Learning from the Past: Development of Safe and Effective COVID-19 Vaccines. *Nat. Rev. Microbiol.* **2020**, 1–9. [CrossRef]
347. Bournazos, S.; Gupta, A.; Ravetch, J.V. The Role of IgG Fc Receptors in Antibody-Dependent Enhancement. *Nat. Rev. Immunol.* **2020**, *20*, 633–643. [CrossRef]
348. Travis, C.R. As Plain as the Nose on Your Face: The Case for a Nasal (Mucosal) Route of Vaccine Administration for Covid-19 Disease Prevention. *Front. Immunol.* **2020**, *11*, 591897. [CrossRef]
349. World Health Organization. *Transmission of SARS-CoV-2: Implications for Infection Prevention Precautions: Scientific Brief., 9 July 2020*; WHO: Geneva, Switzerland, 2020.
350. European Centre for Disease Prevention and Control. *COVID-19 Infection Prevention and Control. Measures for Primary Care, Including General Practitioner Practices, Dental Clinics and Pharmacy Settings: First Update—19 October 2020*; ECDC: Stockholm, Sweden, 2020.
351. Centers for Disease Control and Prevention. Interim Infection Prevention and Control Guidance for Dental Settings during the Coronavirus Disease 2019 (COVID-19) Pandemic—28 August 2020. Available online: https://www.cdc.gov/coronavirus/2019-ncov/hcp/dental-settings.html (accessed on 23 November 2020).
352. World Health Organization. *Infection Prevention and Control during Health Care When Coronavirus Disease (COVID-19) Is Suspected or Confirmed: Interim Guidance, 29 June 2020*; WHO: Geneva, Switzerland, 2020.
353. Centers for Disease Control and Prevention. Infection Control Guidance—4 November 2020. Available online: https://www.cdc.gov/coronavirus/2019-ncov/hcp/infection-control-recommendations.html (accessed on 8 November 2020).
354. World Health Organization. *Prevention, Identification and Management of Health Worker Infection in the Context of COVID-19: Interim Guidance, 30 October 2020*; WHO: Geneva, Switzerland, 2020.
355. Centers for Disease Control and Prevention Testing Healthcare Personnel—17 July 2020. Available online: https://www.cdc.gov/coronavirus/2019-ncov/hcp/testing-healthcare-personnel.html (accessed on 23 November 2020).
356. European Centre for Disease Prevention and Control. *Infection Prevention and Control and Preparedness for COVID-19 in Healthcare Settings—Fifth Update—6 October 2020*; ECDC: Stockholm, Sweden, 2020.
357. Centers for Disease Control and Prevention Return-to-Work Criteria—10 August 2020. Available online: https://www.cdc.gov/coronavirus/2019-ncov/hcp/return-to-work.html (accessed on 23 November 2020).
358. World Health Organization. *Standard Precautions in Health Care*; WHO: Geneva, Switzerland, 2007.
359. World Health Organization. *Hand Hygiene: Why, How & When?* WHO: Geneva, Switzerland, 2009.
360. World Health Organization. *WHO Guidelines on Hand Hygiene in Health Care*; WHO: Geneva, Switzerland, 2009.
361. World Health Organization. *Water, Sanitation, Hygiene, and Waste Management for SARS-CoV-2, the Virus That Causes COVID-19: Interim Guidance, 29 July 2020*; WHO: Geneva, Switzerland, 2020.
362. World Health Organization. *Infection Prevention and Control of Epidemic—And Pandemic—Prone Acute Respiratory Infections in Health Care: WHO Guidelines*; WHO: Geneva, Switzerland, 2014.
363. World Health Organization. *Rational Use of Personal Protective Equipment for Coronavirus Disease (COVID-19) and Considerations during Severe Shortages: Interim Guidance, 6 April 2020*; WHO: Geneva, Switzerland, 2020.
364. World Health Organization. *Rational Use of Personal Protective Equipment (PPE) for Coronavirus Disease (COVID-19): Interim Guidance, 19 March 2020*; WHO: Geneva, Switzerland, 2020.
365. World Health Organization. *Advice on the Use of Masks in the Context of COVID-19: Interim Guidance, 5 June 2020*; WHO: Geneva, Switzerland, 2020.
366. World Health Organization. *Criteria for Releasing COVID-19 Patients from Isolation: Scientific Brief., 17 June 2020*; WHO: Geneva, Switzerland, 2020.
367. European Centre for Disease Prevention and Control. *Guidance for Discharge and Ending of Isolation of People with COVID-19—16 October 2020*; ECDC: Stockholm, Sweden, 2020.
368. Centers for Disease Control and Prevention. Ending Home Isolation: Interim Guidance, 20 July 2020. Available online: https://www.cdc.gov/coronavirus/2019-ncov/hcp/disposition-in-home-patients.html (accessed on 23 November 2020).
369. European Centre for Disease Prevention and Control. *Use of Gloves in Healthcare and Non-Healthcare Settings in the Context of the COVID 19 Pandemic—2 July 2020*; ECDC: Stockholm, Sweden, 2020.
370. European Centre for Disease Prevention and Control. *Guidance for Wearing and Removing Personal Protective Equipment in Healthcare Settings for the Care of Patients with Suspected or Confirmed COVID-19—February 2020*; ECDC: Stockholm, Sweden, 2020.
371. European Centre for Disease Prevention and Control. *Risk Related to Spread of New SARS-CoV-2 Variants of Concern in the EU/EEA—First Update—21 January 2021*; ECDC: Stockholm, Sweden, 2021.
372. Centers for Disease Control and Prevention. COVID-19 and Your Health—Your Guide to Masks—January 2021. Available online: https://www.cdc.gov/coronavirus/2019-ncov/prevent-getting-sick/about-face-coverings.html (accessed on 21 January 2021).
373. World Health Organization. *Mask Use in the Context of COVID-19: Interim Guidance*; WHO: Geneva, Switzerland, 2020.
374. World Health Organization. *Cleaning and Disinfection of Environmental Surfaces in the Context of COVID-19: Interim Guidance, 15 May 2020*; WHO: Geneva, Switzerland, 2020.
375. European Centre for Disease Prevention and Control. *Disinfection of Environments in Healthcare and Non-Healthcare Settings Potentially Contaminated with SARS-CoV-2—March 2020*; ECDC: Stockholm, Sweden, 2020.

376. World Health Organization. *Natural Ventilation for Infection Control in Health Care Settings*; WHO: Geneva, Switzerland, 2009.
377. European Centre for Disease Prevention and Control. *Heating, Ventilation and Air-Conditioning Systems in the Context of COVID-19: First Update—10 November 2020*; ECDC: Stockholm, Sweden, 2020.

Journal of
Clinical Medicine

MDPI

Review

Oral Complications of ICU Patients with COVID-19: Case-Series and Review of Two Hundred Ten Cases

Barbora Hocková [1,2,†], Abanoub Riad [3,4,*,†], Jozef Valky [5], Zuzana Šulajová [5], Adam Stebel [1], Rastislav Slávik [1], Zuzana Bečková [6,7], Andrea Pokorná [3,8], Jitka Klugarová [3,4] and Miloslav Klugar [3,4]

1 Department of Maxillofacial Surgery, F. D. Roosevelt University Hospital, 975 17 Banska Bystrica, Slovakia; bhockova@nspbb.sk (B.H.); astebel@nspbb.sk (A.S.); rslavik@nspbb.sk (R.S.)
2 Department of Prosthetic Dentistry, Faculty of Medicine and Dentistry, Palacky University, 775 15 Olomouc, Czech Republic
3 Czech National Centre for Evidence-Based Healthcare and Knowledge Translation (Cochrane Czech Republic, Czech EBHC: JBI Centre of Excellence, Masaryk University GRADE Centre), Institute of Biostatistics and Analyses, Faculty of Medicine, Masaryk University, 625 00 Brno, Czech Republic; apokorna@med.muni.cz (A.P.); klugarova@med.muni.cz (J.K.); klugar@med.muni.cz (M.K.)
4 Department of Public Health, Faculty of Medicine, Masaryk University, 625 00 Brno, Czech Republic
5 Department of Anaesthesiology, F. D. Roosevelt University Hospital, 975 17 Banska Bystrica, Slovakia; jvalky@nspbb.sk (J.V.); zsulajova@nspbb.sk (Z.Š.)
6 Department of Clinical Microbiology, F. D. Roosevelt University Hospital, 975 17 Banska Bystrica, Slovakia; zbeckova@nspbb.sk
7 St. Elizabeth University of Health and Social Work, 812 50 Bratislava, Slovakia
8 Department of Nursing and Midwifery, Faculty of Medicine, Masaryk University, 625 00 Brno, Czech Republic
* Correspondence: abanoub.riad@med.muni.cz; Tel.: +420-721-046-024
† These authors contributed equally to this work.

Citation: Hocková, B.; Riad, A.; Valky, J.; Šulajová, Z.; Stebel, A.; Slávik, R.; Bečková, Z.; Pokorná, A.; Klugarová, J.; Klugar, M. Oral Complications of ICU Patients with COVID-19: Case-Series and Review of Two Hundred Ten Cases. *J. Clin. Med.* **2021**, *10*, 581. https://doi.org/10.3390/jcm10040581

Academic Editor: Sameh Attia
Received: 14 January 2021
Accepted: 1 February 2021
Published: 4 February 2021

Abstract: Background: The critically ill patients suffering from coronavirus disease (COVID-19) and admitted to the intensive care units (ICUs) are susceptible to a wide array of complications that can be life-threatening or impose them to long-term complications. The COVID-19 oral mucocutaneous complications require multidisciplinary management and research for their pathophysiological course and epidemiological significance; therefore, the objective of this study was to evaluate the prevalence and characteristics of the critically ill COVID-19 patients with oral complications. Methods: We described the clinical and microbiological characteristics of the critically ill COVID-19 patients in our ICU department (Banska Bystrica, Slovakia). In addition, we reviewed the current body of evidence in Ovid MEDLINE®, Embase, Cochrane Library, and Google Scholar for the oral mucocutaneous complications of ICU patients with COVID-19. Results: Three out of nine critically ill patients (33.3%) in our ICU department presented with oral complications including haemorrhagic ulcers and necrotic ulcers affecting the lips and tongue. The microbiological assessment revealed the presence of opportunistic pathogens, confirming the possibility of co-infection. On reviewing the current literature, two hundred ten critically ill patients were reported to have oral complications due to their stay in the ICU setting. Perioral pressure ulcers were the most common complication, followed by oral candidiasis, herpetic and haemorrhagic ulcers, and acute onset macroglossia. The prolonged prone positioning and mechanical ventilation devices were the primary risk factors for those oral complications, in addition to the immunosuppressive drugs. Conclusions: The multidisciplinary approach is strongly advocated for monitoring and management of COVID-19 patients, thus implying that dermatology and oral healthcare specialists and nurses should be integrated within the ICU teams.

Keywords: candidiasis; COVID-19; critical care; macroglossia; oral manifestations; pressure ulcer; prone position

1. Introduction

The patients with coronavirus disease (COVID-19) have been diagnosed with an array of oral and dermatologic symptoms in addition to their typical respiratory manifestations [1–7]. These oral symptoms were equally distributed across the gender and had higher prevalence among older patients and the patients with higher severity of the COVID-19 infection [1,2]. However, there is still a question about the pathophysiologic origin of these symptoms, whether they are due to direct viral infection, co-infections, drug reactions, iatrogenic complications, or stress [2]. Current research shows that coronavirus damage to respiratory and other organs could be related to the distribution of angiotensin-converting enzyme 2 (ACE-2) receptors in the human body [8]. The high expression of ACE-2 in the epithelial cells of the tongue and the salivary glands may explain the development of dysgeusia and the mucocutaneous oral lesions in patients with COVID-19 [9].

The epidemiologic evidence reveals that up to one-quarter of the hospitalised COVID-19 patients need intensive care unit (ICU) admission, making them more vulnerable to secondary pneumonia, cardiac injury, sepsis, kidney injury, and neurologic disorders [10]. The ICU-related cutaneous and mucosal complications, including contact dermatitis, cutaneous candidiasis, pressure ulcers, and hospital-acquired infections (HAIs) have been well documented, and they require a multidisciplinary approach for timely diagnosis and treatment [11].

The association of oral health and critical care can be depicted as a bidirectional relationship because frequent toothbrushing and the use of chlorhexidine were found by a recent Cochrane review to be effective in preventing ventilator-associated pneumonia in critically ill patients [12]. Moreover, in a national retrospective analysis of ICU patients in the Czech Republic, facial pressure ulcers including perioral ulcers were significantly associated with the length of stay in the ICU [13].

The severity and frequency of dermatologic disorders increase dramatically in the patients with prolonged ICU stay; therefore, a tight collaboration among intensivists, anesthesiologists, dermatologists, nurses, and oral healthcare professionals cannot be emphasised enough especially for critically ill COVID-19 patients [14].

In compliance with this guideline, we performed an oral examination for all the patients at our ICU department with COVID-19 in order to evaluate the hypothesis of critical care impact on oral mucocutaneous conditions emergence.

The primary objectives of this study were to evaluate the prevalence of oral complications in ICU patients with COVID-19 and to describe these oral mucocutaneous conditions clinically and microbiologically if present. The secondary objective was to review the current body of evidence regarding the oral mucocutaneous complications of ICU patients with COVID-19.

2. Materials and Methods

On 8 December 2020, there were nine critically ill COVID-19 patients at the ICU department of F.D. Roosevelt Teaching Hospital (Banska Bystrica, Slovakia). All the patients underwent a complete oral examination by the same investigator who also took nasopharyngeal and lingual swabs for microbiological assessment and reverse transcription-polymerase chain reaction (RT-PCR) testing.

The samples were collected under sterile conditions in the morning on an empty stomach using a cotton swab with a solid transport medium for microbiological assessment. On standard culture media prepared by MASTERCLAVE 10® (Biomérieux, Marcy-l'Étoile, France), the upper respiratory tract's biological materials were cultivated using Columbia agar base dehydrated with sheep blood (Columbia 64674 Bio-Rad, Marnes-la-Coquette, France), chocolate agar base dehydrated with horse blood (Columbia 64678 Bio-Rad, Marnes-la-Coquette, France), and Sabouraud dextrose agar base dehydrated (Sabouraud 64494 Bio-Rad, Marnes-la-Coquette, France) in a biological thermostat for 18–24 h at a temperature of 35–37 °C. In the case of pathogenic microorganisms, sensitivity to antibiotics was determined qualitatively by the disk diffusion method and quantitatively by estimating minimum inhibitory concentration (MIC) using the modified microdilution method.

For RT-PCR testing, a viral transport medium (VTM) compatible with the isolation kit, inactivating the accompanying microbial flora and stabilising the nucleic acid, was used. The samples were collected in the morning on an empty stomach, and the patients coughed before swabbing. The collection set included two pieces of Dacron collection tampons. Firstly, the investigator wiped the palatal arches with a tampon in a circular motion without touching the tonsils. Secondly, the investigator wiped the mucosa of the nasal dome back through both nostrils. The samples were transported within one hour to the microbiology laboratory of the hospital to be tested using an RT-PCR system with a thermal cycler and QuantStudio™ 5 (Thermo Fisher Scientific Inc., Waltham, MA, USA). VERSANT® Sample Preparation 1.0 Reagents Kit (Siemens AG. Munich, Germany) was used to isolate the viral RNA, which was transcribed into complementary DNA (cDNA) and amplified by standard polymerase chain reaction methods. For viral detection, the FTD SARS-CoV-2 Assay (Siemens AG. Munich, Germany) kit which identifies N and ORF1ab genes was used.

The oral cavity was systematically examined—beginning with palatoglossal arch, followed by mucosa of palatum durum et molle, upper and lower gingiva, dorsum of the tongue, buccal mucosa, and floor of the mouth. In intubated patients, the examination was more challenging to perform. The patients' medical and oral anamneses had been reported according to the CARE guidelines and in full accordance with the Declaration of Helsinki for medical research involving human subjects [15,16].

In the second part of this study, we searched the literature from inception until 30 December 2020 for ICU-related oral conditions in COVID-19 patients. An electronic search strategy composed of a combination of keywords ((COVID-19 OR SARS-CoV-2 OR coronavirus) AND (candidiasis OR ulcer OR macroglossia OR xerostomia)) was developed and carried out in Ovid MEDLINE®, Embase, Cochrane Library, and Google Scholar. The inclusion criteria were admission to ICU and COVID-19 confirmation by RT-PCR testing. The outcomes of interest included all oral mucocutaneous conditions regardless of their severity and duration. No restrictions for language or study type were applied.

3. Results

In our examined series of cases, various oral conditions were found in three (33.3%) of them. The most common condition was haemorrhagic ulceration. On microbiological assessment, *Pseudomonas aeruginosa* was cultivated in two (22.2%) patients, and *Klebsiella pneumoniae* and *Enterococcus faecalis* were cultivated in one (11.1%) patient. The RT-PCR testing yielded positive results in both nasopharyngeal swabs and lingual swabs of 66.6% of the patients with oral conditions who are further described in detail (Table 1).

Table 1. Critically ill COVID-19 patients at F.D. Roosevelt Teaching Hospital (SK)—8 December 2020.

	Patient No. 1	**Patient No. 2**	**Patient No. 3**
Age, gender	68-year-old, Male	61-year-old, Male	64-year-old, Male
Medical anamnesis	Arterial hypertension, chronic hepatopathy, hypercholesterolemia, and gastroesophageal reflux disease.	Obesity, arterial hypertension, and a history of myocardial infarction and septic shock. **Chronic medications**: Egiramlon (Ramipril), Ebrantil (Urapidil), Tenaxum (Rilmenidine), and Metoprolol.	**Chronic medications**: Coaxil (Tianeptine), Trittico (Trazodone), and Cefixime.

Table 1. *Cont.*

	Patient No. 1	Patient No. 2	Patient No. 3
COVID-19-related treatment before ICU admission	Ceftriaxone, Klacid (Clarithromycin), Remdesivir, Paracetamol, Solumedrol (Methylprednisolone), Vitamin C, Vitamin B1, and Fraxiparine (Nadroparin calcium). **Nasogastric tube**: Isoprinosine (Inosine pranobex), Atorvastatin, Lagosa, Vigantol (Cholecalciferol), Zinc, and Quamatel (Famotidine).	Ceftriaxone, Remdesivir, Dexamethasone, Polyoxidonium, Vitamin C, Vitamin B1, and Fraxiparine (Nadroparin calcium). **Nasogastric tube**: Isoprinosine (Inosine pranobex), Atorvastatin, Lagosa, Vigantol (Cholecalciferol), Zinc, and Quamatel (Famotidine).	Cefixime, Remdesivir, Solumedrol (Methylprednisolone).
Date of ICU admission	8 November 2020	12 November 2020	14 November 2020
Dermatologic complications (extraoral)	No	Yes	Yes
Oral examination	Haemorrhagic ulcers in the middle third of the dorsal surface of the tongue.	Haemorrhagic ulcers along the lips and focal necrosis affecting the anterior third of the dorsal surface of the tongue accompanied by white patches.	Painful haemorrhagic ulcers along the upper and lower lips. Viral exanthem on the skin in the form of painless macules.
Reverse transcription-polymerase chain reaction (RT-PCR) [1]	LRTS: positive Nasopharyngeal: positive Lingual: positive	LRTS: positive Nasopharyngeal: negative Lingual: negative	LRTS: positive Nasopharyngeal: positive Lingual: positive
Microbiological assessment	*Pseudomonas aeruginosa*	Gram-positive cocci, *Enterococcus faecalis*, and *Pseudomonas aeruginosa*	*Klebsiella pneumoniae*
Post-ICU outcomes	Deceased on 11 December 2020 due to septic shock and multiple organ dysfunction syndrome.	Released from ICU on 21 December 2020 in good condition and without intubation.	Released from ICU on 17 December 2020 after two consecutive negative RT-PCR results on December 14th and 16th, 2020.

[1] LRTS: lower respiratory tract sputum.

3.1. Case-Series of ICU Patients in Banska Bystrica

3.1.1. Case Report No. 1

A 68-year-old male patient with arterial hypertension, chronic hepatopathy, hypercholesterolemia, and gastroesophageal reflux disease tested positive during the mass antigen-based testing in Slovakia on 31 October 2020 [17]. Three days later, he progressed with headache, fever, dry cough, and dyspnoea. He was transferred on 8 November 2020 from his district hospital in west Slovakia to our ICU department due to an occupancy issue. At our ICU department, the patient was continuously under analgosedation by Tramadol and *Tiapridal* (Tiapride; Sanofi-Aventis, Bratislava, Slovakia), and he began to receive *Entizol* (Metronidazole; Polpharma, Warsaw, Poland) because of clostridium difficile from 12 November 2020. Two days later, he began to receive Cefepime and Colistin due to *Pseudomonas aeruginosa* which were replaced by Vancomycin and Meropenem on 16 November 2020. To control hypercoagulation, the patient received *Fraxiparine* (Nadroparin calcium; GlaxoSmithKline Slovakia, Bratislava, Slovakia) which was replaced by Heparin, and to control clostridia infection, the patient was prescribed Noradrenalin, Dobutamine, and *Embesin* (Vasopressin; Orpha-Devel Handels und Vertriebs GmbH, Purkersdorf, Austria). By 29 November 2020, the clinical condition worsened, and the inflammatory parameters increased; therefore, Piperacillin/tazobactam, Linezolid, and Voriconazole were administered.

On 8 December 2020, the patient was intubated, under sedation and without tracheostomy. Our oral examination found out oral lesions at the dorsal surface of the tongue, specifically in the middle third, in the form of haemorrhagic ulcerations. Oral mucosa of the mouth in other places was free of lesions. The microbiological assessment for the swab of tongue dorsum showed *Pseudomonas aeruginosa*, and the RT-PCR testing for severe acute respiratory syndrome coronavirus 2 (SARS-CoV-2) was positive for both nasopharyngeal and lingual swabs. During the evening check-up, oedema of the masseter region was observed bilaterally with pain on palpation which was examined by the head of the maxillofacial surgery department who confirmed an acute form of bilateral parotitis. Non-invasive treatment was carried out using a sterile swab from the exudate for cultivation then administering antibiotic therapy.

The patient deceased on 11 December 2020 due to septic shock and multiple organ dysfunction syndrome induced by enterocolitis. According to the Committee on Publication Ethics' (COPE) Code of Conduct, the permission of the patient's next of kin was granted [18].

3.1.2. Case Report No. 2

A 61-year-old male polymorbid obese patient with arterial hypertension and a history of myocardial infarction and septic shock was admitted to the ICU department with bilateral COVID-19-related pneumonia on 12 November 2020. After two weeks, tracheostomy was done by an otolaryngologist. On 2 December 2020, a dermatologist was consulted due to exanthema on the skin of shoulders and back which was diagnosed as viral exanthema commonly observed in COVID-19 patients [19]. A topical treatment protocol was composed of *bisulepin* (Dithiaden; Zentiva, Prague, Czech Republic), *loratadine* (Flonidan; TEVA Pharmaceuticals Slovakia, Bratislava, Slovakia), and *betamethasone* (Beloderm; Fagron, Olomouc, Czech Republic).

During the oral examination, the patient was not under sedation. The microbiological assessment confirmed the presence of *Enterococcus faecalis* and *Pseudomonas aeruginosa*. However, his RT-PCR testing for lower respiratory tract sputum yielded a positive result on December 7th and 14th, the results of nasopharyngeal and lingual swabs negative. The intraoral examination revealed multiple lesions located on the tongue dorsum and labial mucosa. The lesions were mainly haemorrhagic ulcerations along the lips and focal necrosis affecting the anterior third of tongue dorsum accompanied by white patches. On December 18th, tracheostomy cannula was removed, and three days later, the patient tested negative and was transferred to the non-COVID-19 department.

3.1.3. Case Report No. 3

A 64-year-old male patient who had had contact with his COVID-19 positive daughter was examined at the emergency department of our hospital with moderate symptoms of COVID-19; therefore, he was treated at home due to persistent fever, dyspnoea, and dry cough. The general practitioner prescribed him an antibiotic treatment of cefixime one week before performing an antigen test for SARS-CoV-2, which yielded a positive result. On 14 November 2020, the patient was admitted to our ICU department, where a computed tomography (CT) scan revealed severe bronchopneumonia requiring oxygen supplement. During his ICU stay, the patient was intubated and treated with Methylprednisolone and Remdesivir.

On 8 December 2020, the patient was not under sedation; therefore, he was able to communicate nonverbally. The extraoral examination showed viral exanthem in the form of painless macules on the skin, while the intraoral examination yielded focal painful lesions located mainly along the upper and lower lip with a maximum diameter of 7 mm and erythema around them thus resembling haemorrhagic ulcerations. The oral lesions developed simultaneously with ICU admission. On 14th and 16th December 2020, the patient tested negative; therefore, he was transferred to the non-COVID-19 department.

3.2. Literature Review

On reviewing the emerging evidence on ICU-related complications in COVID-19 patients, fourteen studies (one cohort study [20], two case-control studies [21,22], one cross-sectional study [23], two case-series [24,25], and eight case-reports [26–33]) with two hundred ten patients met the inclusion criteria. The majority of the cases were from the Americas (USA n = 103, 49.5%; Brazil n = 4, 1.9%), followed by Europe (Spain n = 57, 27.1%; UK n = 16, 7.6%; France n = 2, 1%; and Italy n = 2, 1%), and Middle East (Iran n = 26, 12.4%). The demographic characteristics of 85 cases were described in the primary studies, sixty-two of them (72.9%) were males, and twenty-three (27.1%) were females. The reported cases' average age was 60.2 years old (min: 27, max: 81 years old). All the patients had been defined as critically ill according to the Australian guidelines for the clinical care of people with COVID-19 [34]. On their hospital admission, the patients were initially treated with antibiotics, corticosteroids, and hydroxychloroquine sulphate just before transferring to the ICU department. During their ICU stay, one hundred eighty patients (85.7%) underwent prone positioning in addition to mechanical ventilation (Table 2).

The reported oral complications were mainly perioral pressure ulcers (n = 179, 85.2%), intraoral candidiasis (n = 27, 12.9%), other intraoral ulcers (n = 3, 1.4%), and macroglossia (n = 1, 0.5%). While the onset ranged between four and twenty-four days after ICU admission, the duration ranged between one and two weeks. The medical treatments included dressings, position adjustment, antifungals, antivirals, and surgical interventions including full-thickness excisions. Regarding the suggested aetiology, most of the complications were caused by the prone positioning which is an essential procedure for some cases in critical care. Prolonged pronation cycles, pronation monitored by less experienced staff, and use of respiratory support equipment were risk factors to increase the incidence of pressure ulcers among ICU patients who underwent pronation. The use of broad-spectrum antibiotics and immunosuppressive drugs was associated with co-infections such as fungal, bacterial, or viral infections in the hospital setting (Figure 1).

3.2.1. Perioral Pressure Ulcers (ICD-11: EH90)

The perioral (facial) pressure ulcers have been the most prevalent ICU-related oral complication in COVID-19 patients reported by ten studies in one hundred seventy-nine patients; 73.75% of them were males, and the vast majority were of old age [20–23,25,29–33]. Prolonged pronation and endotracheal intubation were the most evident risk factors for perioral pressure ulcers. Given the long-term psychological impact of scarring caused by perioral ulcers, and their interference with mechanical ventilation equipment in the critical care setting, an array of interventions and prophylactic precautions has been proposed to prevent this potential epidemic [35–37].

3.2.2. Oral Candidiasis (ICD-11: 1F23.0)

Oral (oropharyngeal) candidiasis has been reported by two studies with twenty-seven patients who have been treated initially by broad-spectrum antibiotics and immunosuppressants, which are believed to cause immune dysregulation [24,26]. Therefore, the reported patients were more susceptible to get secondary infections and HAIs, and they were managed by either systemic fluconazole or topical nystatin according to the infection severity and lesion surface. In addition to our included cases, there were thirty-six COVID-19 patients with milder clinical courses who experienced oral candidiasis and were not admitted to the ICU [24,38–43]. The most common risk factor among mild, moderate, and critically ill COVID-19 patients with fungal co-infection, e.g., oral candidiasis, was the prolonged use of antibiotics.

Table 2. Summary of the oral complications of ICU patients with COVID-19.

Study, Location	*N*	Gender	Age	MED-COVID-19	Complication	Onset	Duration	MED-Oral	Aetiology
Amorim dos Santos et al. [26] 2020; Brasilia (Brazil)	1	Male	67	Initially: hydroxychloroquine sulphate, ceftriaxone sodium, and azithromycin. Later: meropenem, sulfamethoxazole, trimethoprim, immunosuppressants, and anticoagulants.	Oral Candidiasis	After 24 days of ICU admission.	2 weeks.	Systemic fluconazole and oral nystatin.	Opportunistic fungal infection due to COVID-19 treatments (antibiotics) which lead to immune dysregulation.
Andrews et al. [27] 2020; (Michigan, USA)	1	Female	40	Initially: hydroxychloroquine sulphate, methylprednisolone, and tocilizumab. Later: 16 h. prone/8 h. supine (11 days).	Acute Macroglossia	After 11 days of prone position.	11 days.	Lingual compression.	Prolonged course of prone positioning for treatment of COVID-19.
Brandao et al. [28] 2020; (Sao Paolo, Brazil)	3	1 Female 2 Male	81, 71, and 72	Azithromycin, piperacillin/tazobactam, and ceftriaxone.	Herpetic Ulcers and Haemorrhagic Ulcers	After 5, 4, and 5 days of respiratory symptoms.	11, >15, and 7 days.	Acyclovir and PBMT.	The ICU admission leads to immune dysfunction.
Ibarra et al. [22] 2020; (Madrid, Spain)	57	16 Female 41 Male	μ = 61 years old (56–69)	16 h. prone/8 h. supine (μ = 6 days).	Perioral Pressure Ulcers	N/A	N/A	All the cases were managed with dressings.	Prone position pressure ulcers are dependent on the clinical manoeuvre.
Martel et al. [21] 2020; (Massachusetts, USA)	18	N/A	N/A	N/A	Perioral Pressure Ulcers	N/A	N/A	All the cases were managed with dressings.	Prolonged placement in a prone position and use of respiratory support equipment.
Perrillat et al. [29] 2020; (Marseille, France)	2	2 Male	27, 50	6 prone sessions (12 h. each) 9 prone sessions (12 h. each)	Perioral Pressure Ulcers	N/A	N/A	Debridement of necrotic tissue and paraffin gauze dressing.	Prone positioning monitored by less experienced staff.
Ramondetta et al. [30] 2020; (Turin, Italy)	1	Male	48	Initially: hydroxychloroquine and antiviral treatment. Later: prone positioning cycles (5 days).	Perioral Pressure Ulcers	After 15 days of ICU admission.	N/A	Advanced dressings.	The pressure exercised during the prone positioning phases.
Rekhtman et al. [20] 2020 (New York, USA)	13	N/A	N/A	Mechanical ventilation.	Perioral Pressure Ulcers	N/A	N/A	N/A	Increased pressure from endotracheal tubes or medical equipment used to hold tubes in place.
Salehi et al. [24] 2020; (Tehran, Iran)	26	N/A	N/A	Antiviral, antibacterial, and corticosteroids.	Oropharyngeal Candidiasis	N/A	N/A	Fluconazole, nystatin and caspofungin.	Immune dysregulation due to ICU admission and broad-spectrum antibiotic.

Table 2. *Cont.*

Study, Location	N	Gender	Age	MED-COVID-19	Complication	Onset	Duration	MED-Oral	Aetiology
Shearer et al. [23] 2020; (Washington DC, USA)	68	N/A	N/A	Mechanical ventilation. µ of prone positioning = 5.14 days (1–26).	Perioral Pressure Ulcers	N/A	N/A	Antimicrobial dressings.	Longer duration of prone position appears to confer greater risk for developing these pressure injuries.
Singh et al. [31] 2020; (California, USA)	2	1 Female 1 Male	44, 71	Directly admitted to the ICU, a course of azithromycin and prednisone at home. Mechanical ventilation.	Perioral Pressure Ulcers	4 days after prone positioning; 5 days after prone positioning.	N/A	Pressure-relieving turns and position system, bordered foam dressings, fluidised positioners.	Prone positioning.
Siotos et al. [32] 2020; (Illinois, USA)	1	Female	82	Mechanical ventilation.	Perioral Pressure Ulcers	10 days after prone positioning.	N/A	Surgical removal by full-thickness excision.	Prone positioning.
Sleiwah et al. [25] 2020; (London, UK)	16	2 Female 14 Male	µ = 58.6 years old (40–77)	Mechanical ventilation, and vasopressors. µ of prone positioning = 5.2 days (2–7).	Perioral Pressure Ulcers	N/A	N/A	N/A	Prone positioning.
Zingarelli et al. [33] 2020; (Alessandria, Italy)	1	Female	50	Initially: acetaminophen and antibiotics. Later: ICU admission, mechanical ventilation.	Perioral Pressure Ulcers	After 15 days of ICU admission.	1 week	Advanced dressings.	Prone positioning.
Total	210	23 Female 62 Male	µ = 60.2 years old (27–81)	Antibiotics, hydroxychloroquine, corticosteroids, mechanical ventilation, and prone positioning.	Perioral pressure ulcers, candidiasis, stomatitis, and macroglossia.	Range 4–24 days after ICU admission.	Range 1–2 weeks.	Dressings, position change, antifungals, and antivirals.	Prone positioning, mechanical ventilation, antibiotic therapy, HAIs.

N: number of patients; MED-COVID-19: medical treatment for COVID-19 and its complications; MED-Oral: medical treatment for the oral complications; N/A: not reported by the authors; PBMT: photobiomodulation therapy.

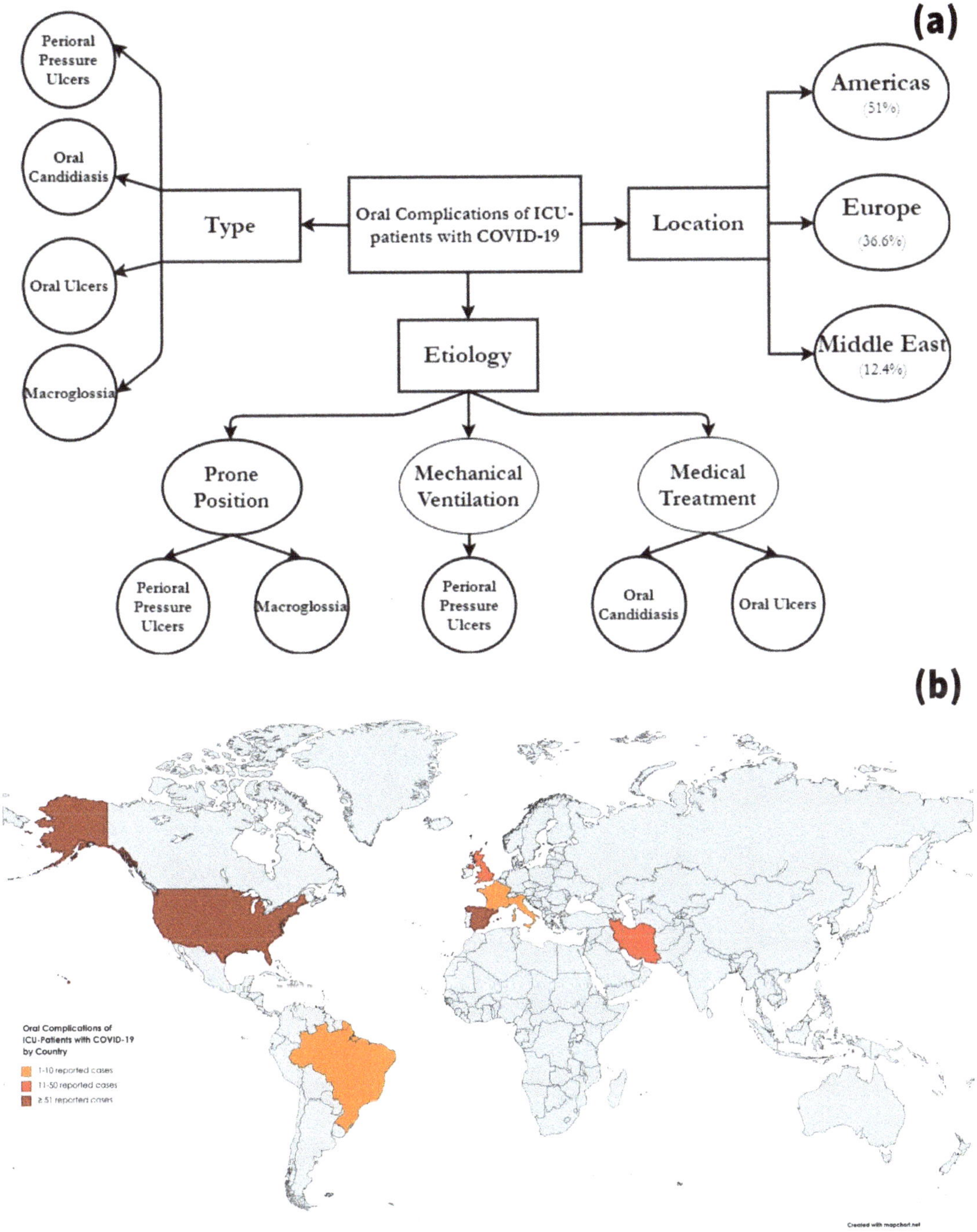

Figure 1. Summary of the oral complications which were reported in the ICU patients with COVID-19; (**a**) by type, aetiology, and region; (**b**) frequency of reported cases by country.

3.2.3. Oral Ulcers (ICD-11: DA01)

Herpetic ulcers and haemorrhagic necrotic ulcers were reported by Brandao et al. 2020 in three patients above 70 years old [28]. The ulcers emerged four-to-five days after the respiratory symptoms, and they were treated by antivirals and photobiomodulation therapy. The lesions were suggested to be triggered by the ICU admission and the pre-admission antibiotics, which may have caused immune dysregulation, thus promoting HAIs.

3.2.4. Macroglossia (ICD-11: DA03.5)

Acute macroglossia has been reported by Andrews et al. 2020 in a 40-year-old male patient who experienced prolonged pronation cycles for eleven days [27]. Endotracheal tubes and throat packing as well had been associated with lingual oedema as a result of disruption of venous drainage [44]. There has been a number of ICU cases with acute macroglossia before the COVID-19 pandemic; therefore, the emergence of this rare but devastating complication was anticipated, and its non-invasive management is deemed required [27].

4. Discussion

The emerging evidence on COVID-19 related oral manifestations had triggered a broad debate regarding the pathophysiological course and the epidemiological significance of these mucocutaneous symptoms, given that the case definition of COVID-19 needs to be as sensitive as possible [1–7,43]. The current case definitions of COVID-19 are exclusively dependent on the typical pulmonary symptoms common with other respiratory diseases. Meanwhile, from the laboratory perspective, leukopenia with lymphopenia, thrombocytopenia, high values of C-reactive proteins, and low levels of procalcitonin are well-established diagnostic aids for case triage [45]. In the review of Iranmanesh et al. 2020, direct viral enanthem, inflammatory response secondary to the viral infection, opportunistic infections, lack of oral hygiene, and stress were suggested aetiologies for the oral symptoms in COVID-19 patients which were equally distributed across the gender and associated with older age and more severe clinical courses of the disease [1]. As highlighted by Riad et al. 2020, the lack of reference time point consistency among the COVID-19 case-reports and case-series has undermined the efforts for accurate estimation of the onset of the COVID-19 related oral symptoms and their epidemiological significance [2]. Therefore, following the reporting guidelines was and is still strongly advocated for COVID-19 clinical literature.

The COVID-19 critically ill population imposed an unprecedented challenge for the health systems worldwide due to the supply/demand ratio which has been further complicated by lack of evidence on the clinical prognosis of COVID-19 cases and their post-admission complications including the life-threatening ones [46]. However, the common terminating complications are related to acute respiratory distress syndrome (ARDS) like multi-organ failure, kidney injury, sepsis, atrial arrhythmias, and myocardial infarction, the dermatological complications like candidiasis, and perioral ulcers can become life-threatening if left untreated [10]. Therefore, the multidisciplinary approach of managing COVID-19 patients in ICU units, the use of teledermatology and teledentistry, the allied staff's awareness of those mucocutaneous complications are highly recommended while navigating through this pandemic [47–49].

The primary objective of this study was to share our clinical experience with critically ill COVID-19 patients in a central European country with 120,203 detected cases (63,818 females and 56,385 males), 1046 deceased cases, and 30,753 active cases on the day of our clinical examination—8 December 2020 [50]. The oral complications of our ICU patients were similar to those described by Brandao et al. 2020 from Brazil, as both groups of patients experienced haemorrhagic ulcers related to the lips and labial mucosa [28]. All the patients were above 60 years old, and they were mainly males with a pre-ICU antibiotic therapeutic course which had been extended during their ICU stay; therefore, immune dysregulation was suggested as a pathophysiological pathway. This suggestion was supported by the microbiological results of our patients which revealed the increase of opportunistic species, e.g., *Pseudomonas aeruginosa*, *Klebsiella pneumoniae*, and *Enterococcus faecalis*.

One of the limitations of this case-series is that the microbiological assessment of the lingual swabs was carried out for the patients with oral complications only, and it was not possible to take clinical photographs because of infection control guidelines and the fact that there was only one clinical investigator permitted to examine all the patients.

Provided that prone positioning-related complications were the most prevalent ICU-related oral complications, Moore et al. 2020 systematically reviewed the current body of evidence and recommended to use pressure redistribution support surface/positioning devices, use protective coverings during pronation, and carry out simple and frequent changes in the posture of the patient and the device positioning. The clinicians are strongly advised to assess the common risk areas for pressure ulcers frequently and to keep the skin clean and moisturized [35]. This practice recommendation requires a close collaboration between intensivists, anaesthesiologists, nurses, dermatologists, and dentists to monitor and manage the pressure ulcers at an early stage. Overloaded healthcare systems for the long-term by COVID-19 might be one of the reasons for the high prevalence of perioral pressure ulcers as in many countries less experienced healthcare staff might be present in the ICU as retrieved by our literature review [22,29].

The immune dysregulation was suggested as a pathophysiological pathway for the emergence of oral ulcers in COVID-19 patients, especially in the severely affected ones. This hypothesis was supported by several cases where recurrent aphthous stomatitis and traumatic ulcerations were ruled out based on rigorous clinical and laboratory investigation, while herpes simplex virus was detected in the vast majority of the old and immunocompromised patients [28,51]. Reflecting on other immune dysregulation-related oral complications like the opportunistic infections especially those that emerge in the hospital setting, the review of Rawson et al. 2020 recommended to develop antimicrobial stewardship protocols for managing COVID-19 patients in order to support the optimal treatment outcomes and prevent the potential bacterial/fungal co-infection in critically ill COVID-19 patients [52].

Although it is currently confirmed by several high-quality clinical practice guidelines that hydroxychloroquine should not be used as the treatment for COVID-19 [34,53,54]. This research waste was identified in treatment protocols of cases from Brazil, Italy, and the USA. Higher awareness and evidence-based medicine principles about COVID-19 treatment should be advocated in all countries. A very useful tool that can inform practice by best available evidence might be the recently published living COVID-19 recommendation map [55,56].

5. Conclusions

Perioral pressure ulcers, oral candidiasis, herpetic and haemorrhagic oral ulcers, and acute macroglossia were the commonly reported complications in critically ill COVID-19 patients. These oral mucocutaneous complications were caused by the prolonged prone positioning and mechanical ventilation devices in the ICU setting, in addition to the immunosuppressive treatments prescribed for this special cohort of patients. Therefore, a multidisciplinary approach is strongly advocated for monitoring and management of COVID-19 thus implying that dermatology and oral healthcare specialists and nurses should be integrated within the ICU teams.

Author Contributions: Conceptualisation, A.R. and B.H.; methodology, A.R. and M.K.; formal analysis, A.R. and Z.Š.; investigation, B.H., Z.Š., and Z.B.; writing—original draft preparation, A.R. and B.H.; writing—review and editing, J.V., A.S., Z.B., A.P., J.K., and M.K.; supervision, R.S. and M.K.; funding acquisition, J.V. and A.P. All authors have read and agreed to the published version of the manuscript.

Funding: The work of A.R. was supported by Masaryk University grants MUNI/A/1608/2020 and MU-NI/IGA/1543/2020. A.R., A.P., J.K., and M.K. were supported by the INTER-EXCELLENCE grant number LTC20031—"Towards an International Network for Evidence-based Research in Clinical Health Research in the Czech Republic".

Institutional Review Board Statement: The study was conducted according to the guidelines of the Declaration of Helsinki, and it was exempted from ethical approval due to its observational nature and the use of publicly accessible data.

Informed Consent Statement: Informed consent was obtained from all subjects involved in the study.

Data Availability Statement: The data that support the findings of this study are available from the corresponding author upon reasonable request.

Conflicts of Interest: The authors declare no conflict of interest.

References

1. Iranmanesh, B.; Khalili, M.; Amiri, R.; Zartab, H.; Aflatoonian, M. Oral manifestations of COVID -19 disease: A review article. *Dermatol. Ther.* **2020**, 14578. [CrossRef]
2. Riad, A.; Klugar, M.; Krsek, M. COVID-19-Related Oral Manifestations: Early Disease Features? *Oral Dis.* **2020**, 13516. [CrossRef] [PubMed]
3. Riad, A.; Kassem, I.; Badrah, M.; Klugar, A.M. The manifestation of oral mucositis in COVID-19 patients: A case-series. *Dermatol. Ther.* **2020**, *33*, e14479. [CrossRef]
4. Riad, A.; Kassem, I.; Issa, J.; Badrah, M.; Klugar, M. Angular cheilitis of COVID-19 patients: A case-series and literature review. *Oral Dis.* **2020**, 13675. [CrossRef]
5. Riad, A.; Kassem, I.; Stanek, J.; Badrah, M.; Klugarova, J.; Klugar, M. Aphthous Stomatitis in COVID -19 Patients: Case-series and Literature Review. *Dermatol. Ther.* **2021**, e14735. [CrossRef]
6. Riad, A.; Kassem, I.; Badrah, M.; Klugar, M. Acute parotitis as a presentation of COVID-19? *Oral Dis.* **2020**, 13571. [CrossRef]
7. Riad, A.; Kassem, I.; Hockova, B.; Badrah, M.; Klugar, M. Tongue Ulcers Associated with SARS-COV-2 Infection: A case-series. *Oral Dis.* **2020**, 13635. [CrossRef]
8. Xu, H.; Zhong, L.; Deng, J.; Peng, J.; Dan, H.; Zeng, X.; Li, T.; Chen, Q. High expression of ACE2 receptor of 2019-nCoV on the epithelial cells of oral mucosa. *Int. J. Oral Sci.* **2020**, *12*, 1–5. [CrossRef]
9. Dziedzic, A.; Wojtyczka, R.D. The impact of coronavirus infectious disease 19 (COVID-19) on oral health. *Oral Dis.* **2020**, 13359. [CrossRef]
10. UpToDate Coronavirus Disease 2019 (COVID-19): Critical Care and Airway Management Issues. Available online: https://www.uptodate.com/contents/coronavirus-disease-2019-covid-19-critical-care-and-airway-management-issues (accessed on 7 January 2021).
11. Wollina, U.; Nowak, A. Dermatology in the Intensive Care Unit. *Our Dermatol. Online* **2012**, *3*, 298–303. [CrossRef]
12. Zhao, T.; Wu, X.; Zhang, Q.; Li, C.; Worthington, H.V.; Hua, F. Oral hygiene care for critically ill patients to prevent ventilator-associated pneumonia. *Cochrane Database Syst. Rev.* **2020**, *12*, CD008367. [CrossRef]
13. Pokorná, A.; Benešová, K.; Jarkovský, J.; Mužík, J.; Beeckman, D. Pressure Injuries in Inpatient Care Facilities in the Czech Republic. *J. Wound, Ostomy Cont. Nurs.* **2017**, *44*, 331–335. [CrossRef]
14. Badia, M.; Trujillano, J.; Gascó, E.; Casanova, J.M.; Alvarez, M.; León, M. Skin lesions in the ICU. *Intensiv. Care Med.* **1999**, *25*, 1271–1276. [CrossRef]
15. Gagnier, J.J.; Kienle, G.; Altman, D.G.; Moher, D.; Sox, H.; Riley, D.; Allaire, A.; The CARE Group. The CARE guidelines: Consensus-based clinical case reporting guideline development. *BMJ Case Rep.* **2013**, *53*, 1541–1547. [CrossRef]
16. World Medical Association. World medical association declaration of Helsinki: Ethical principles for medical research involving human subjects. *JAMA* **2013**, *310*, 2191–2194. [CrossRef]
17. Holt, E. COVID-19 testing in Slovakia. *Lancet Infect. Dis.* **2021**, *21*, 32. [CrossRef]
18. Committee on Publication Ethics (COPE). Core Practices. Available online: https://publicationethics.org/core-practices (accessed on 7 January 2021).
19. Seirafianpour, F.; Sodagar, S.; Pour Mohammad, A.; Panahi, P.; Mozafarpoor, S.; Almasi, S.; Goodarzi, A. Cutaneous manifestations and considerations in COVID-19 pandemic: A systematic review. *Dermatol. Ther.* **2020**, *33*, e13986. [CrossRef]
20. Rekhtman, S.; Tannenbaum, R.; Strunk, A.; Birabaharan, M.; Wright, S.; Grbic, N.; Joseph, A.; Lin, S.K.; Zhang, A.C.; Lee, E.C.; et al. Eruptions and Related Clinical Course Among 296 Hospitalized Adults with Confirmed COVID-19. *J. Am. Acad. Dermatol.* **2020**. [CrossRef]
21. Martel, T.; Orgill, D.P. Medical Device–Related Pressure Injuries during the COVID-19 Pandemic. *J. Wound Ostomy Cont. Nurs.* **2020**, *47*, 430–434. [CrossRef]
22. Ibarra, G.; Rivera, A.; Fernandez-Ibarburu, B.; Lorca-García, C.; Garcia-Ruano, A. Prone position pressure sores in the COVID-19 pandemic: The Madrid experience. *J. Plast. Reconstr. Aesthetic Surg.* **2020**. [CrossRef]
23. Shearer, S.C.; Parsa, K.M.; Bs, A.N.; Bs, T.P.; Walsh, A.R.; Fernandez, S.; Gao, W.Z.; Pierce, M.L. Facial Pressure Injuries from Prone Positioning in the COVID-19 Era. *Laryngoscope* **2021**, 29374. [CrossRef]

24. Salehi, M.; Ahmadikia, K.; Mahmoudi, S.; Kalantari, S.; Siahkali, S.J.; Izadi, A.; Kord, M.; Manshadi, S.A.D.; Seifi, A.; Ghiasvand, F.; et al. Oropharyngeal candidiasis in hospitalised COVID-19 patients from Iran: Species identification and antifungal susceptibility pattern. *Mycoses* **2020**, *63*, 771–778. [CrossRef]
25. Sleiwah, A.; Nair, G.; Mughal, M.; Lancaster, K.; Ahmad, I. Perioral pressure ulcers in patients with COVID-19 requiring invasive mechanical ventilation. *Eur. J. Plast. Surg.* **2020**, *43*, 727–732. [CrossRef]
26. Dos Santos, J.A.; Normando, A.G.C.; Da Silva, R.L.C.; De Paula, R.M.; Cembranel, A.C.; Santos-Silva, A.R.; Guerra, E.N.S. Oral mucosal lesions in a COVID-19 patient: New signs or secondary manifestations? *Int. J. Infect. Dis.* **2020**, *97*, 326–328. [CrossRef]
27. Andrews, E.; Lezotte, J.; Ackerman, A.M. Lingual compression for acute macroglossia in a COVID-19 positive patient. *BMJ Case Rep.* **2020**, *13*, e237108. [CrossRef] [PubMed]
28. Brandão, T.B.; Gueiros, L.A.; Melo, T.S.; Prado-Ribeiro, A.C.; Nesrallah, A.C.F.A.; Prado, G.V.B.; Santos-Silva, A.R.; Migliorati, C.A. Oral lesions in patients with SARS-CoV-2 infection: Could the oral cavity be a target organ? *Oral Surgery Oral Med. Oral Pathol. Oral Radiol.* **2020**. [CrossRef] [PubMed]
29. Perrillat, A.; Foletti, J.-M.; Lacagne, A.-S.; Guyot, L.; Graillon, N. Facial pressure ulcers in COVID-19 patients undergoing prone positioning: How to prevent an underestimated epidemic? *J. Stomatol. Oral Maxillofac. Surg.* **2020**, *121*, 442–444. [CrossRef]
30. Ramondetta, A.; Ribero, S.; Costi, S.; Dapavo, P. Pression-induced facial ulcers by prone position for COVID -19 mechanical ventilation. *Dermatol. Ther.* **2020**, *33*, e13748. [CrossRef]
31. Singh, C.; Tay, J.; Shoqirat, N. Skin and Mucosal Damage in Patients Diagnosed With COVID-19. *J. Wound Ostomy Cont. Nurs.* **2020**, *47*, 435–438. [CrossRef] [PubMed]
32. Siotos, C.; Bonett, A.M.; Hansdorfer, M.A.; Siotou, K.; Kambeyanda, R.H.; Dorafshar, A. Medical Device Related Pressure Ulcer of the Lip in a Patient with COVID-19: Case Report and Review of the Literature. *J. Stomatol. Oral Maxillofac. Surg.* **2020**. [CrossRef]
33. Zingarelli, E.M.; Ghiglione, M.; Pesce, M.; Orejuela, I.; Scarrone, S.; Panizza, R. Facial Pressure Ulcers in a COVID-19 50-year-old Female Intubated Patient. *Indian J. Plast. Surg.* **2020**, *53*, 144–146. [CrossRef]
34. Australian Government National Health and Medical Research Council (NHMRC). Australian Guidelines for the Clinical Care of People with COVID-19. Australian Clinical Practice Guidelines. Available online: https://www.clinicalguidelines.gov.au/register/australian-guidelines-clinical-care-people-covid-19 (accessed on 17 September 2020).
35. Moore, Z.; Patton, D.; Avsar, P.; McEvoy, N.L.; Curley, G.; Budri, A.; Nugent, L.; Walsh, S.; O'Connor, T. Prevention of pressure ulcers among individuals cared for in the prone position: Lessons for the COVID-19 emergency. *J. Wound Care* **2020**, *29*, 312–320. [CrossRef]
36. Pokorná, A.; Saibertová, S.; Velichová, R.; Vasmanská, S. Sorrorigenní rány, jejich identifikace a pruběh péce. In *Proceedings of the Ceska a Slovenska Neurologie a Neurochirurgie*; Purkyne, J.E., Ed.; Czech Medical Association: Prague, Czechia, 2016; Volume 78, pp. S31–S36.
37. Kambová, V.; Pokorná, A.; Saibertová, S. The knowledge and practises of nurses in the prevention of medical devices related injuries in intensive care—Questionnaire survey. *Česká Slov. Neurol. Neurochir.* **2019**, *82*, S19–S22. [CrossRef]
38. Baraboutis, I.G.; Gargalianos, P.; Aggelonidou, E.; Adraktas, A. Initial Real-Life Experience from a Designated COVID-19 Centre in Athens, Greece: A Proposed Therapeutic Algorithm. *SN Compr. Clin. Med.* **2020**, *2*, 689–693. [CrossRef]
39. Cantini, F.; Niccoli, L.; Matarrese, D.; Nicastri, E.; Stobbione, P.; Goletti, D. Baricitinib therapy in COVID-19: A pilot study on safety and clinical impact. *J. Infect.* **2020**, *81*, 318–356. [CrossRef] [PubMed]
40. Corchuelo, J.; Ulloa, F.C. Oral manifestations in a patient with a history of asymptomatic COVID-19: Case report. *Int. J. Infect. Dis.* **2020**, *100*, 154–157. [CrossRef] [PubMed]
41. Rodríguez, M.D.; Romera, A.J.; Villarroel, M. Oral manifestations associated with COVID-19. *Oral Dis.* **2020**, 13555. [CrossRef] [PubMed]
42. Dima, M.; Enatescu, I.; Craina, M.; Petre, I.; Iacob, E.R.; Iacob, D. First neonates with severe acute respiratory syndrome coronavirus 2 infection in Romania. *Medicine* **2020**, *99*, e21284. [CrossRef] [PubMed]
43. Riad, A.; Gad, A.; Hockova, B.; Klugar, M. Oral candidiasis in non-severe COVID-19 patients: Call for antibiotic stewardship. *Oral Surg.* **2020**, 12561. [CrossRef] [PubMed]
44. DePasse, J.M.; Palumbo, M.A.; Haque, M.; Eberson, C.P.; Daniels, A.H. Complications associated with prone positioning in elective spinal surgery. *World J. Orthop.* **2015**, *6*, 351–359. [CrossRef]
45. Zeidler, A.; Karpiński, T.M. SARS-CoV, MERS-CoV, SARS-CoV-2 Comparison of Three Emerging Coronaviruses. *Jundishapur J. Microbiol.* **2020**, *13*, 1–8. [CrossRef]
46. Ma, X.; Vervoort, D. Critical care capacity during the COVID-19 pandemic: Global availability of intensive care beds. *J. Crit. Care* **2020**, *58*, 96–97. [CrossRef] [PubMed]
47. Wollina, U. Challenges of COVID-19 pandemic for dermatology. *Dermatol. Ther.* **2020**, *33*, e13430. [CrossRef] [PubMed]
48. Attia, S.; Howaldt, H.-P. Impact of COVID-19 on the Dental Community: Part I before Vaccine (BV). *J. Clin. Med.* **2021**, *10*, 288. [CrossRef] [PubMed]
49. Maspero, C.; Maspero, C.; Cavagnetto, D.; El Morsi, M.; Fama, A.; Farronato, M. Available Technologies, Applications and Benefits of Teleorthodontics. A Literature Review and Possible Applications during the COVID-19 Pandemic. *J. Clin. Med.* **2020**, *9*, 1891. [CrossRef]

50. Ministry of Investments Regional Development and Informatization of the Slovak Republic (MIRRI) Coronavirus (COVID-19) in the Slovak Republic in numbers. Koronavírus a Slovensko. Available online: https://korona.gov.sk/en/coronavirus-covid-19-in-the-slovak-republic-in-numbers/ (accessed on 10 January 2021).
51. Bezerra, T.M.M.; Feitosa, S.G.; Carneiro, D.T.O.; Costa, F.-W.-G.; Pires, F.R.; Pereira, K.M.A. Oral lesions in COVID-19 infection: Is long-term follow-up important in the affected patients? *Oral Dis.* **2020**, 13705. [CrossRef]
52. Rawson, T.M.; Moore, L.S.P.; Zhu, N.; Ranganathan, N.; Skolimowska, K.; Gilchrist, M.; Satta, G.; Cooke, G.; Holmes, A. Bacterial and Fungal Coinfection in Individuals With Coronavirus: A Rapid Review To Support COVID-19 Antimicrobial Prescribing. *Clin. Infect. Dis.* **2020**, *71*. [CrossRef]
53. Bhimraj, A.; Morgan, R.L.; Shumaker, A.H.; Lavergne, V.; Baden, L.; Cheng, V.C.-C.; Edwards, K.M.; Gandhi, R.; Muller, W.J.; O'Horo, J.C.; et al. Infectious Diseases Society of America Guidelines on the Treatment and Management of Patients With Coronavirus Disease 2019 (COVID-19). *Clin. Infect. Dis.* **2020**. [CrossRef]
54. World Health Organization (WHO). Clinical Management of COVID-19—Interim Guidance. COVID-19: Clinical Care. Available online: https://www.who.int/publications/i/item/clinical-management-of-covid-19 (accessed on 13 January 2021).
55. CIHR COVID19 Recommendations. Evidenceprime. Available online: https://covid19.qa.evidenceprime.com/ (accessed on 13 January 2021).
56. Stevens, A.; Lotfi, T.; Akl, E.A.; Falavigna, M.; Kredo, T.; Mathew, J.L.; Avey, M.T.; Brignardello-Petersen, R.; Chu, D.K.; Dewidar, O.; et al. The eCOVID-19 living recommendations map and gateway to contextualisation. Introduction and background. *Cochrane Database Syst. Rev.* **2020**. [CrossRef]

Journal of
Clinical Medicine

MDPI

Review

SARS-CoV-2 Infection and Oral Health: Therapeutic Opportunities and Challenges

Christopher J. Coke [1], Brandon Davison [1], Niariah Fields [1], Jared Fletcher [1], Joseph Rollings [1], Leilani Roberson [1], Kishore B. Challagundla [2,3], Chethan Sampath [1], James Cade [1], Cherae Farmer-Dixon [1] and Pandu R. Gangula [1,*]

1 Department of Oral Diagnostic Sciences & Research, School of Dentistry, Meharry Medical College, Nashville, TN 37208, USA; ccoke20@email.mmc.edu (C.J.C.); bdavison19@email.mmc.edu (B.D.); nfields19@email.mmc.edu (N.F.); jfletcher19@email.mmc.edu (J.F.); jrollings15@email.mmc.edu (J.R.); lroberson20@email.mmc.edu (L.R.); csampath@mmc.edu (C.S.); jcade@mmc.edu (J.C.); cdixon@mmc.edu (C.F.-D.)
2 Department of Biochemistry & Molecular Biology, The Fred and Pamela Buffet Cancer Center, University of Nebraska Medical Center, Omaha, NE 68198, USA; kishore.challagundla@unmc.edu
3 The Children's Health Research Institute, University of Nebraska Medical Center, Omaha, NE 68198, USA
* Correspondence: pgangula@mmc.edu

Abstract: The novel corona virus, Severe Acute Respiratory Syndrome Coronavirus-2 (SARS-CoV-2), and the disease it causes, COVID-19 (Coronavirus Disease-2019) have had multi-faceted effects on a number of lives on a global scale both directly and indirectly. A growing body of evidence suggest that COVID-19 patients experience several oral health problems such as dry mouth, mucosal blistering, mouth rash, lip necrosis, and loss of taste and smell. Periodontal disease (PD), a severe inflammatory gum disease, may worsen the symptoms associated with COVID-19. Routine dental and periodontal treatment may help decrease the symptoms of COVID-19. PD is more prevalent among patients experiencing metabolic diseases such as obesity, diabetes mellitus and cardiovascular risk. Studies have shown that these patients are highly susceptible for SARS-CoV-2 infection. Pro-inflammatory cytokines and oxidative stress known to contribute to the development of PD and other metabolic diseases are highly elevated among COVID-19 patients. Periodontal health may help to determine the severity of COVID-19 infection. Accumulating evidence shows that African-Americans (AAs) and vulnerable populations are disproportionately susceptible to PD, metabolic diseases and COVID-19 compared to other ethnicities in the United States. Dentistry and dental healthcare professionals are particularly susceptible to this virus due to the transferability via the oral cavity and the use of aerosol creating instruments that are ubiquitous in this field. In this review, we attempt to provide a comprehensive and updated source of information about SARS-CoV-2/COVID-19 and the various effects it has had on the dental profession and patients visits to dental clinics. Finally, this review is a valuable resource for the management of oral hygiene and reduction of the severity of infection.

Keywords: COVID-19; periodontitis; Angiotensin Converting Enzyme 2 (ACE-2); saliva; inflammation; oxidative stress; dental practice

Citation: Coke, C.J.; Davison, B.; Fields, N.; Fletcher, J.; Rollings, J.; Roberson, L.; Challagundla, K.B.; Sampath, C.; Cade, J.; Farmer-Dixon, C.; et al. SARS-CoV-2 Infection and Oral Health: Therapeutic Opportunities and Challenges. *J. Clin. Med.* **2021**, *10*, 156. https://doi.org/10.3390/jcm10010156

Received: 11 November 2020
Accepted: 30 December 2020
Published: 5 January 2021

1. Introduction

Corona viruses are a diversified class of viruses with zoonotic origin, highly transmitted in humans, causing mild to severe respiratory infections. In 2002 and 2012, respectively, two highly pathogenic coronaviruses emerging in humans were (a) severe acute respiratory syndrome coronavirus (SARS-CoV) and (b) Middle East respiratory syndrome coronavirus (MERS-CoV), causing deadly respiratory illness. At the end of 2019, a novel coronavirus designated as SARS-CoV-2 emerged as a pneumonia of the lower respiratory tract in a patient in Wuhan, China on December 29, 2019 [1,2]. The World Health Organization (WHO) classified COVID-19, the disease associated with the virus SARS-CoV-2, as a global pandemic. Several patients with pneumonia were then reported to have contracted the novel virus, linked to a Hunan South Province China Seafood Market in Wuhan, Hubei Province, China [3]. This virus has currently spread to approximately 215 countries with over forty nine million cases and over 1.24 million deaths worldwide [4].

SARS-CoV-2 differs from SARS-CoV due to its higher level of transmissibility and pandemic risk. SARS-CoV-2 has a greater significant reproductive number (R), the statistic used to determine how infectious the agent is, at 2.9. SARS-CoV had an R of (1.77) [2,5,6]. It is this specific trait of SARS-CoV-2 that makes it more of a global concern than SARS-CoV. SARS-CoV-2, like SARS-CoV, is transmitted via aerosols and can pass from human to human [7]. The incubation period for the virus is from 1–14 days and the infected patient can remain contagious even through its latency period. Once symptoms are observed, a positive diagnosis is achieved by performing real-time PCR (RT-PCR) to positively detect SARS-CoV-2 RNA in various bodily fluids, including sputum, throat swabs, and secretions of the lower respiratory tract and from fecal and blood samples [2,5]. Alternative detection methods using serological/antibody testing are also employed but there are conflicting conclusions about these methods' effectiveness. Due to the recent discovery of this virus, its full effects on the body are not yet totally understood. However, scientists and dentists believe the oral cavity may play a crucial role in the early diagnosis and treatment of this disease [8,9].

The pneumonia-like symptoms of COVID-19 include fever, cough, myalgia or fatigue, and complicated dyspnea. However, there are reported symptoms including headache, diarrhea, hemoptysis, runny nose, and phlegm-producing cough [2]. Symptoms in the most severe cases rapidly progress to acute respiratory distress syndrome, respiratory failure, multiple organ failure and death [5]. These patients often experience oral and gastrointestinal complications, loss of taste and smell [2]. Patients having underlying health complications such as diabetes, cancer, cardiovascular diseases (CVD) and hypertension are more susceptible to developing COVID-19 [2,5]. In this Review, we summarize the current understanding of the nature of SARS-CoV-2/COVID-19 and its link to oral health. Based on recently published findings, this comprehensive Review covers the epidemiology/origin, cellular pathways involved, and drug–drug interactions of SARS-CoV-2 with respect to oral health and dentist perspectives.

2. Epidemiological/Viral Origin Data

SARS-CoV-2 was first discovered and isolated in Wuhan, China. The virus was isolated from a patient who suffered from pneumonia-like symptoms including fever, cough, and myalgia/fatigue. Three other cases were soon found and the outbreak was linked to a local "wet market". To confirm the infection source of SARS-Cov-2, Centers for Disease Control and Prevention (CDC) researchers collected 585 samples from the Huanan Seafood Market in Wuhan, Hubei Province, China between January 1–12, 2020. Though the original transmission is thought to be animal-to-human in nature, it is now clear that the virus has adapted a human-to-human transmission pattern. With a now recognized effective reproductive number(R) of 2.9, researchers declared SARS-CoV-2 as one of the more transmissible viruses. Other studies suggested that the basic reproduction range (R_0) is between 2.6–4.71 with an average incubation time within the range of 2–11 days [2,5,6].

Important epidemiological factors include age, sex, race, age at death, susceptible populations, and mortality rate. To date COVID-19 affects populations regardless of age, with most cases between 35 and 55 years [2,10,11]. Susceptible to death from a COVID-19 related infection are patients 75 years and older. As of Nov 4, 2020 in the mortality rate for all 75+ years, COVID-19 patients are at 57% (Figure 1A) [12]. With age a susceptibility factor, healthcare workers and researchers have also noted that people with co-morbidities, poor immune function, long-term use of immunosuppressants, and surgery history before admission are also more susceptible to worse outcomes from a COVID-19 infection [2,13–17]. There are higher rates of infection in males (~59–68%) compared to females suggesting that female sex hormones may have a beneficial role in protecting against COVID-19 [2,6,14].

The mortality rate for COVID-19 is one factor that is under dispute. Between 29 December 2019–28 January 2020, the mortality rate was estimated at between 2.3–11% [2,14,18,19]. As of 1 May 2020 the Infection Fatality Rate (IFR) was 1.4%, meaning 1.4% of people infected with SARS-CoV-2 have a fatal outcome, while 98.6% recover [2,19,20]. The total number of deaths from COVID-19 in United States alone is around 231,988 as of 4 November 2020 (Figure 1A) [12]. A comprehensive review by Alcendor provided in-depth information on the factors associated with morbidity and mortality among minority populations [21]. African Americans (AAs) and Hispanics/Latinos were disproportionately impacted by COVID-19 infection when compared with non-Hispanic Whites (Figure 1B) [21–23]. U.S. counties such as Hancock and Randolph County, Georgia, with majority AA population are experiencing a three-fold higher infection rate and six-fold higher death rate than White counties. The death rate in AAs ranges from 40–70% due to COVID-19. Comorbidities like hypertension and diabetes, which are tied to COVID-19 complications, disproportionately affect the AA community [21].

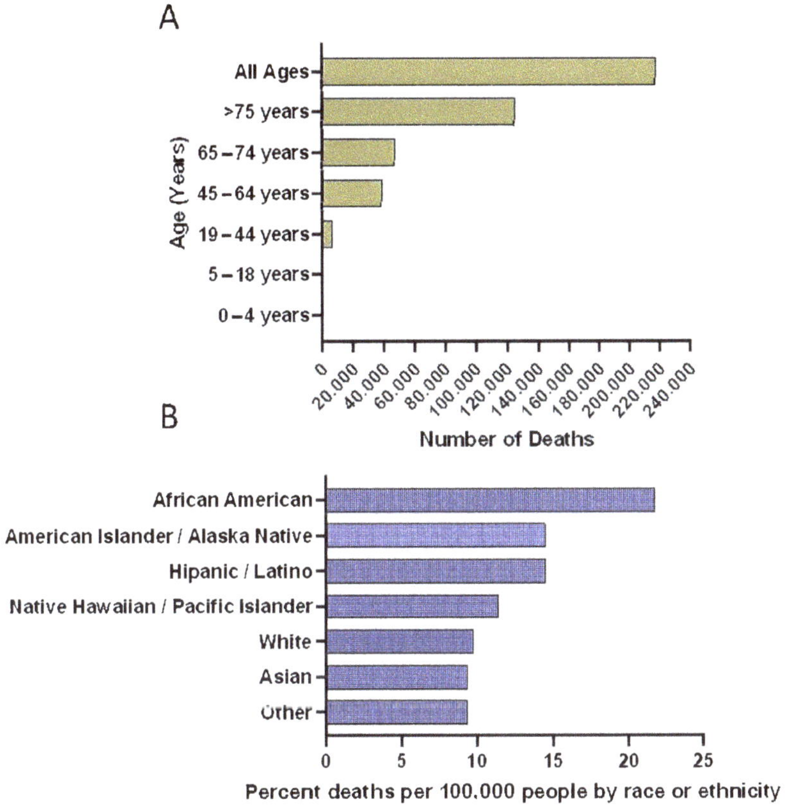

Figure 1. Cumulative confirmed cases of COVID-19 in United States as of November 4, 2020. The number of confirmed COVID-19 deaths by age (**A**) [12], and the number of confirmed COVID-19 deaths by race and ethnicity (**B**) [22] are presented.

However, the alarming rates at which COVID-19 is causing mortality in AAs extends beyond these comorbidities and can be attributed to decades of spatial segregation and inequitable access to testing and treatment [21]. Periodontal disease (PD) and metabolic syndrome such as obesity, diabetes and hypertension are known to be higher among this population. Therefore, it is not surprising that the morbidity and mortality rate from COVID-19 is greater in the AA population. These populations are located in poor accommodation, and have less access to health care and education with high unemployment rates. Low socioeconomic status is a risk factor for poorer health outcomes and is forcing some individuals residing in these communities out of their homes and into the workforce. Therefore, there is an unmet need to increase the access to and effectiveness of diagnostic testing interventions and provide various educational strategies by understanding the social, ethical, and behavioral implications of testing among underserved and vulnerable populations. In addition, biomarker evaluation may also help early diagnosis and identify the risk factors associated with COVID-19 [21].

3. Mechanism of Infection in Oral and Overall Body Health

Poor oral health may adversely influence other parts of the body. Recent studies showed that oral manifestations are commonly noticed in about 45% of COVID-19 patients [24–26]. Salivary glands, tonsils, and tongue are highly sensitive for SARS-CoV-2 infection [27–29]. The development of infection causes loss of taste, smell, and blisters on the tongue in COVID-19 patients [30,31]. It has been reported that the pathogenic microbiome found in different parts of the body such as the oral cavity, lungs and gut enhances inflammation and oxidative burden (Figures 2 and 3). Studies show PD that occurs due to gram negative bacteria can aggravate COVID-19 symptoms [32–34]. Co-infection with the SARS-CoV-2 virus and the pathobionts of the oral cavity plays a critical role in increasing the inflammatory response and cytokine storm. Poor oral health shows a direct connection to COVID-19 infection and to a higher risk of severe illness in patients with COVID-19 [35]. In addition, the SARS-CoV-2 virus stimulates lesions on the skin, hand, foot and mouth disease which resemble those of other viral infections [35]. Further investigations need to done to determine if the virus in COVID-19 patients causes oral manifestations [36,37].

SARS-CoV 2 is classified as a β coronavirus that infects its host by five sequential steps: attachment, penetration, biosynthesis, maturation, and release, like many viruses. There are four structural proteins identified in the nucleocapsids of coronaviruses; Spike (S), membrane (M), envelope (E), and nucleocapsid (N). The Spike is a glycoprotein that protrudes from the viral surface, contributing to diversity between coronaviruses, and setting tropism. The Spike is composed of subunits S_1 and S_2. S_1 binds the host cell while S_2 acts to fuse the host cell membrane with the viral membrane [38].

It was proposed that upon binding of the Spike protein, protease cleavage occurs at the S_1/S_2 that triggers priming and activation [38]. Upon cleavage, the subunits remain non-covalently bound, and S_1 assists in the stabilization of the S_2 subunit. In contrast, cleavage at this site allows for fusion via conformation changes that were found to be irreversible [38]. The receptor binding domain in the study done by Shang et al. was found to switch between a standing-up position and a lying-down position, more binding occurring when this domain was lying down [39]. Yuki et al. proposed that many different proteases were found to have the capability of cleaving and activating the Spike, but the furin cleavage site, specifically at the S_1/S_2, is believed to make coronaviruses pathogenic [39]. Another protein, pro-protein convertase (PPC) found at the Spike protein site, was found not to enhance the entry of SARS-CoV2 into the cell; however, when PCC was mutated at the site, cleavage was found not to occur, thus decreasing SARS-CoV2's ability to enter the cell. Though researchers have elucidated most of the SARS-CoV2 mechanism of infection, work continues to use what is known to develop strategies to combat the infection and disease effectively [38,39].

According to Yuki et al., Angiotensin Converting Enzyme 2 (ACE-2) was identified as one of the key targets for SARS-CoV 2, in which its expression is high among lung epithelial cells [39]. Shang et al. were amongst a group that discovered that HeLa cells (human cervical cells), Calu-3 cells (human lung epithelial cells), and MRC-5 cells (human lung fibroblast cells) were all cells that could effectively be infected by SARS-CoV-2 due to its increased affinity for hACE2, which all of these cells either exogenously or endogenously express [38]. Studies have shown that the ACE-2 receptor is a binding site for SARS-CoV2 and helps facilitate the virus's entry into cells [40]. ACE-2 counters the activation of the

Renin-Angiotensin-Aldosterone System [41]. Discussions revolve around ACE-inhibitors potentially modifying ACE-2 receptors and the effect on the virulence of COVID-19 [41,42]. Since the SARS-Coronavirus 2 disease (COVID-19) is primarily a respiratory infection, it is worth noting that ACE2 receptors are expressed on the lung alveolar epithelial cells. Lung alveolar epithelial cells were implicated as target cells for SARS-CoV 2 [41–43]. While ACE inhibitor use was widely examined due to its effects on ACE2 receptors, another class of antihypertensive drugs was also investigated for similar effects.

The coronavirus infection triggers endoplasmic reticulum (ER) stress responses in infected cells, associated with increased levels of reactive oxygen species (ROS) and unfolded protein response (UPR). ER stress has an important role in cardiovascular and metabolic disease, obesity and in diabetes. NRF2 (NF-E2-related factor 2) is a redox-sensitive, basic leucine zipper transcriptional factor that upregulates antioxidant gene expression by binding to the promoter region of the antioxidant response element (ARE) [44]. NRF2 controls the expression array of the detoxifying and antioxidant defense gene in multiple tissue damage during infection [44]. In addition to regulating antioxidant genes and suppressing oxidative burden, NRF2 also regulates inflammation in the pathogenesis of various disease complications including periodontitis [45]. That SARS-CoV-2 inhibits NRF2 indicates that the virus deprives the host cells of an essential cytoprotective pathway, and it will be crucial to determine how and when during the process of the viral infection this takes place, and the underlying mechanism [44]. Binding of viral protein to ACE-2 leads to virus entry. ACE-2 gene expression in oral tissues [46,47], lungs [48,49], kidney [50], stomach [51], and colon [52] has been shown to repress NRF2 [53]. The role of NRF2 in viral infections was investigated in the context of both DNA and RNA viruses [54]. In general, viruses can benefit from either activating or inhibiting NRF2 in host cells [53]. The receptor-binding domain (RBD) located in the S protein of SARS-CoV-2 interacts with the angiotensin-converting enzyme 2 (ACE-2) of host cells to allow viral entry [55]. NRF2 is the most potent antioxidant in humans and can block the AT1R axis. NRF2 plays a key role in protecting tissue destruction by excess reactive oxygen species (ROS) and suppressing inflammation occurring in periodontitis [56]. NRF2 deficiency is known to upregulate ACE-2, whereas its activator oltipraz reduces ACE2 levels, suggesting that NRF2 activation might reduce the availability of ACE-2 for SARS-CoV-2 entry into the cell [57]. The upregulation of NRF2 signaling inhibits the overproduction of IL-6, pro-inflammatory cytokines and chemokines as well as limiting the activation of NFkB [58]. Glycogen synthase kinase 3 beta (GSK-3β) has been reported to be elevated in adipose tissue of insulin-resistant obese rodent models and in skeletal muscle of diabetic patients [59]. GSK-3β participates in the cellular response to oxidative stress, a hallmark of several nervous system disorders through its interaction with NRF2 [59].

Angiotensin-converting enzyme 2, which is the receptor for SARS-CoV-2, is a regulator of vascular function by modulating nitric oxide (NO) release and oxidative stress [60,61]. NO reportedly interferes with the interaction between coronavirus viral S-protein and its cognate host receptor, ACE-2 [62]. Nitric oxide-mediated S-nitro-sylation of viral cysteine proteases and host serine protease, TMPRSS2, which are both critical in viral cellular entry, appear to be nitric oxide sensitive [60,63,64]. COVID-19 patients often experience periodontal disease [65,66], and vascular [67,68] and gastrointestinal (GI) [69,70] complications, perhaps because ACE2 receptors are widely expressed among these tissues [71,72]. A hyposalivation symptom is exhibited highly in COVID-19 patients [73,74]. Hyposalivation is severe in older ages and can be linked to higher COVID-19 infection and mortality rate [74]. ACE-2 has been reported to be present in epithelial cells of the salivary gland and clinical manifestation observed in COVID-19 patients has been linked to xerostomia [75]. The expression of ACE-2 in the minor salivary glands was higher than the lungs (lung medium post-translational modifications (PTM, transcripts per kilobase of exon model per Million mapped reads) = 1.010, minor salivary gland medium PTM = 2.013), which suggests that salivary glands could be a potential target for COVID-19 [76]. SARS-CoV RNA can also be detected in saliva before lung lesions appear [77]. The positive rate of COVID-19 in patients' saliva can reach 91.7%, and saliva samples can also cultivate the live virus [78]. This suggests that COVID-19 transmitted by asymptomatic infection may originate from infected saliva. Most importantly, SARS-CoV-2 infection may cause only GI symptoms such as nausea, vomiting and diarrhea in some of these patients [79]. Microbial symbiosis is very common with viral infection and SARS-CoV-2 RNA has been detected in feces of COVID-19 patients [80]. NRF2 and NO synthesis can be modulated by bacterial dysbiosis [81–83]. Our laboratory showed that Nrf2 and NO signaling play a role in maintaining vascular and gastrointestinal function in diabetic and oral infection animal models in vivo and in vitro [84–86]. The above data collectively suggest that infection with SARS-Cov-2 disrupts healthy microbiome and elevates inflammation and oxidative stress. This in turn modulate Nrf2 and NO signaling and may cause abnormalities in multiple organ function including respiratory, cardiovascular and gastrointestinal function in COVID-19 patients (Figure 3).

Al-Lami et al. discussed a higher rates of SARS-CoV-2 infection in adult males (~59–68%) compared to females [87]. This observation is due to the elevated levels of endogenous sex steroid hormones such as estrogen and progesterone known to play a critical role in viral defense in premenopausal women. In contrast, testosterone may be a culprit for the viral infection in males. Higher morbidity and mortality rate due to COVID-19 observed in postmenopausal women is probably due to the decrease in endogenous sex steroid hormones [87]. Sex hormones regulate multiple organ (cardiovascular, renal, GI, etc.) functions through antioxidant and anti-inflammatory properties in various disease conditions in human and rodent models [88]. The above data suggest that elevated endogenous sex hormones are more protective against SARS-CoV-2 infection in female than in male patients. In addition, the available data strongly suggest that a common mechanism of action on cytokine storm, lung injury and endothelial damage observed in most of the co-morbidities were also noticed with COVID-19 infection. Therefore, investigating the changes in these mechanisms may help to better assess the potential severity of COVID-19 infection in both sexes.

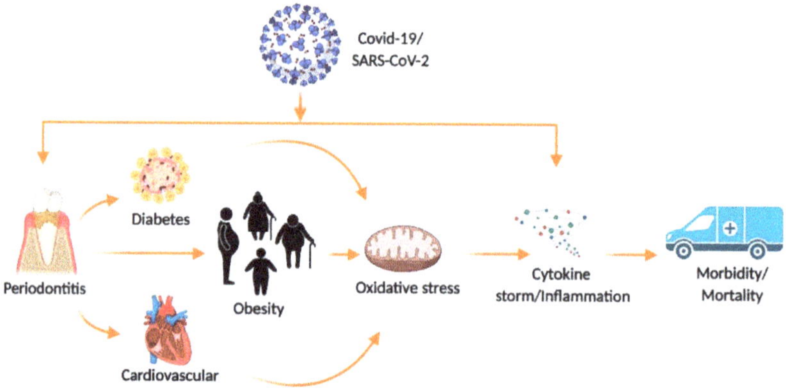

Figure 2. An overview of COVID-19 infection. COVID-19 infection is more pronounced in populations with comorbidities such as periodontitis, obesity, diabetes and cardiovascular disease. COVID-19 infection induces oxidative stress, triggers unregulated cytokine production (cytokine storm) and inflammation [89–91]. These events enhance the risk of morbidity and mortality rate in most vulnerable populations [21,23].

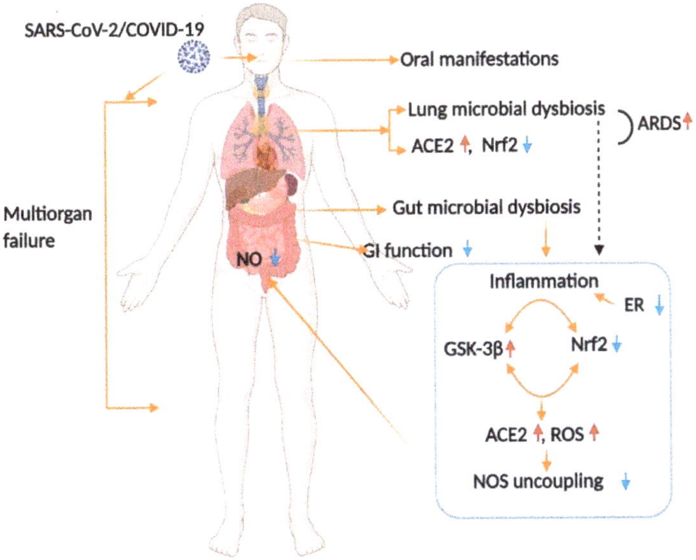

Figure 3. Schematic representation of the proposed mechanism involved in COVID-19-infection inducing multiple organ failure. Binding of viral protein to Angiotensin Converting Enzyme 2 (ACE-2) leads to virus entry. ACE-2 gene expression in oral tissues [46,47], lungs [48,49], vascular [71], kidney [50], stomach [51], and colon [52] has been shown to repress nuclear factor erythroid 2–related factor 2 (NRF2) [53]. A possible mechanism of ACE-2 and reactive oxygen species (ROS) activation by COVID-19 and the repressing of NRF2 executes oral manifestations, acute respiratory distress syndrome (ARDS) in lungs, inflammation and oxidative stress in multiple organs. Suppression of estrogen receptors (ER) by COVID-19 infection elevates inflammation in multiple organs. Suppression of NRF2 by COVID-19 infection reduces tetrahydrobiopterin (BH_4, a cofactor for nitric oxide synthase) availability, nitric oxide synthases (NOS) uncoupling, thus altering overall gastrointestinal (GI) function.

4. Pre-Exiting Condition Effect on COVID-19 Outcome

There is an abundance of information available regarding the effects of pre-existing medical conditions on patients' COVID-19 infection outcomes. Of the pre-existing conditions that researchers suspect may have an impact on the outcome of patients infected with COVID-19, hypertension has been frequently mentioned. The primary association between patients with pre-existing hypertension and COVID-19 is related to the use of Angiotensin Converting Enzyme (ACE) inhibitors, a common anti-hypertensive medication [21,40,41,60,92].

In a Japanese study, it was determined that Olmesartan, an Angiotensin Receptor Blocker that is prescribed as an antihypertensive medication, resulted in a higher urinary ACE-2 receptor than individuals not taking the medication [41,93]. Individuals with pre-existing hypertension that are currently taking one of these medications and are subsequently infected with SARS-CoV2 may be more susceptible to severe complications.

Obesity is one of the significant independent risk factor for COVID-19 infection [94]. Obesity itself promotes chronic inflammation, vitamin D deficiency, impairs immune response and causes atelectasis [95]. Hypoxemia with impaired ventilation has been associated with abdominal obesity, which increases the severity of COVID-19 infection. SARS-CoV-2 interacts with the renin–angiotensin–aldosterone system and impairs blood potassium levels, with increased susceptibility to tachyarrhythmias, possessing a potential risk of respiratory distress syndrome [95]. Therefore, COVID-19 infected obese individuals are at an additional risk of an elevated inflammatory influx and electrolyte imbalance that proves to be a potentially deadly outcome [95].

Current evidence demonstrates that patients with diabetes are more likely to experience severe symptoms and complications than patients without diabetes due to COVID-19 infection. Hyperglycemia facilitates the virus entry into the cells since ACE2 and virus both need glucose for their function [96]. Patients with poorly controlled hyperglycemia have higher pro-apoptotic factors as well as apoptosis dependent cell death in kidneys, liver, lungs, and brain [96]. Diabetic patients are prone to more severe degrees of COVID-19 infection due to their altered Renin-angiotensin-aldosterone system (RAAS) functions which facilitate viral invasion [96].

Besides, PD may also be a pre-existing condition that worsens COVID-19 outcomes [35,37]. Inflammation present in periodontal infections is often caused by an immune response known as a cytokine storm [89,90]. This immune response facilitates the release of cytokines locally into the gingival causing inflammation in periodontitis; however, increased cytokine levels are also observed systemically [97]. The cytokine storm was frequently identified as a cause of adverse outcomes in COVID-19 infections including Acute Respiratory Disease and Multiple Organ Failure [97,98]. Since patients with existing PD prior to SARS-CoV2 infection are likely to have elevated cytokine levels, they may be susceptible to more severe, and fatal, outcomes. To support this, lung tissues from COVID-19 patients express the pro-inflammatory cytokines that play an essential role in the development of PD [98]. Prevalence of severe periodontitis in diabetics and non-diabetics has been found to be 59.6% and 39%, respectively [99]. Another pre-existing condition pertaining to oral health is halitosis, which occurs due to an infection either in lungs, ears, nose, throat or gastrointestinal disease. COVID-19 infection is highly prevalent in subjects with halitosis [100]. The finding of Riad et al. suggest that SARS-CoV-2 affects the upper side of the tongue epithelial cells. The proposed alteration is due to the high expression of ACE 2 receptors in the dorsal part of the tongue and around the oral mucosa [101]. Evidence suggests that the mouth is a powerful source of SARS-CoV-2 infection and transmission. The presence of underlying co-morbidities synergistically affect the clinical outcomes of COVID-19 infection.

5. COVID-19 from a Dental Perspective

As a profession, dentistry deals with the human oral cavity, the main route for the spread of this disease (sneezing and coughing) [102]. This puts dentists and dental offices particularly at risk of being hubs for the spread of infection, from patients to doctors, and patients to other patients. As we learn more about this infection, it is important for dentists and dental practices to update and become as familiar as possible with all aspects of this disease (Table 1). COVID-19 infection spreads mainly through droplets that remain suspended as an aerosol [36,103,104]. Dental procedures create an increased risk for infection to patients, doctors, and staff by producing aerosols and the presence of saliva. Dental practices should have procedures in place for the prevention of transmission of biological agents. "However, the procedures adopted routinely to date have not been specifically designed for the prevention of pathogens transmissible by aerosol. Therefore, there are currently no specific guidelines for the protection of dentists against SARS-CoV-2." [26]. In addition, there are no specific procedures that are in place to prevent transmission by aerosol, so extra precautions must be taken to help prevent the spread of COVID-19 [36,103]. Fortunately, the latest statistics show that only 0.9% of dentists surveyed ($N = 2195$) had contracted COVID-19 infection. This implies that the recommended current PPE and social distancing precautions may be sufficient in dental practices to control transmission of SARS-CoV-2 [105].

Table 1. Effective COVID-19 Practices for a Dental Office.

Procedures	Details	Ref
PPE, Decontamination and Sterilization Procedures	• All equipment surfaces should be protected with barrier film, cleaned with hydroalcoholic disinfectants at concentrations above 60%, and then changed after every patient. • It is suggested that patients use a mouth rinse of 1% hydrogen peroxide or 1% iodopovidone for 30 secs to help lower virus concentration in the mouth.	[36,103,106]
Fresh Air or Medical Grade Air Purifiers	• Allow fresh air between patients either by open windows or medical-grade air purifiers.	[107]
Telephone Triage	• Performing a telephone triage with patients to determine if they have symptoms or have come into contact with COVID-19 will allow dental providers the ability to screen patients. • If a patient has responses that indicate, they might have come in contact inform the patent and defer treatment unless it is an emergency case.	[108]
Social Distancing	• Dental offices should adhere to social distancing in the waiting room. Minimize the amount of people who have entry into operatory rooms to individual patients or a single adult for minors. • All personal items should be left in the waiting room.	[105]
Temperatures of all patients, dentists, and staff are required	• If the patient's/staff/dentists' temperatures are less than 100 °F and no COVID-19 symptoms, patients may be treated, and the dental staff and dentist may perform treatment.	[109]

In dental practice, prevention of transmission of biological agents take place by use of PPE, decontamination and sterilization procedures. The SARS-CoV-2 virus is sensitive to ultraviolet rays and heat. If exposed to temperatures of at least 56 °Celsius (132.8 °Fahrenheit) for at least 30 min it becomes inactive. Performing a telephone triage with patients to determine if they have symptoms or have come into contact with COVID-19 will allow dental providers the ability to screen patients [108]. If a patient has responses that indicate, they might have come in contact, the patient should be informed and treatment deferred unless it is an emergency case. Dental offices should adhere to social distancing in the waiting room. The number of people who have entry into operatory rooms should be minimized to individual patients, or a single adult to accompany minors. All personal items should be left in the waiting room. Allow fresh air between patients either by open windows or medical-grade air purifiers [107]. All staff should use PPE (gloves, gowns, face shields, surgical masks, FFP1,2,3 grade masks) and dispose into medical waste bins to prevent transmission by aerosol [36,103]. Temperatures of all patients, dentists, and staff are required, additionally to proper use of PPE, and disinfection. If the patient's/staff/dentists' temperatures are less than 100 °F and there are no COVID-19 symptoms, patients may be treated, and the dental staff and dentist may perform treatment [109]. All equipment surfaces should be protected with barrier film, cleaned with hydroalcoholic disinfectants at concentrations above 60%, and then changed after every patient. It is suggested that patients use a mouth rinse of 1% hydrogen peroxide or 1% iodopovidone for 30 s to help lower virus concentration in the mouth [106]. Providers should perform extra-oral exams over intra-oral exams when possible to prevent stimulation of coughing. Besides, dental treatment may reduce the virus burden for several hours among infected patients. Oral hygiene and mouthwashes are being looked at for their effect on reducing the viral load of COVID-19. Chlorhexidine, a common oral rinse, demonstrates substantive uses intra-orally. However, it appears not to be effective in reducing viral load. Combining chlorhexidine with ethanol at appropriate concentrations may be a useful strategy to reduce the viral load as this utilizes the effectiveness of chlorhexidine within the mouth [35,37].

6. Psychological Effects on Dental Patients and HealthCare Providers

Within the dental community, the psychological impacts of COVID-19 are vast. They affect not only dentists and patients, but also dentists' family, and staff. As stated earlier, the nature of the profession places dentists at an increased risk of becoming exposed to COVID-19 and spreading it to their patients, families, and peers. Fears that dentists have been reported to experience include carrying the virus to family, getting infected while treating coughing patients, and getting infected by coworkers. These fears can lead patients to undergo treatment delays, which is why it is important to develop psychological coping mechanisms and strategies to keep the practice running [110].

Countrywide shutdowns due to COVID-19 caused many to undergo a mandated quarantine. The effects of quarantine can have severe impacts on an individual. It increases the possibility of psychological and mental problems because people lack interpersonal communication, are distant from those they care about, and psychological treatment resources are severely limited [111,112]. With that in mind, it becomes essential to look for warning signs and symptoms that show someone may be suffering from mental trauma. Some may experience anxiety, depression, nervousness, anger, rumination, hopelessness, decreased concentration, insomnia, and fear [113,114]. These are some of the emotions that dentists need to be looking for, not only in their patients but also in themselves and their staff.

Psychological distress, which often presents as fear amongst dentists, was a common experience during this pandemic. A study reported that many dentists may experience fear, anxiety, concern, sadness, and anger, but only a small percentage (8.7%) feel these intensely [10]. Another psychological effect the dental community may experience is high overload and low self-efficacy, which were associated with psychological distress amongst dentists and dental hygienists [114]. Dentists also reported fear for their professional future, such as inability to pay expenses leading them to go out of business [10,115]. The financial impact that dentists may experience has both short and long-term impacts. Some providers will go out of business, which will lead to a shortage of providers [115]. Some of this psychological distress must be ameliorated by professional improvement, such as better PPE, body temperature checks, and waiting room access. Jordanian dentists reported that they lack the minimum PPE and precaution to control infection, with 71% viewing the virus as moderately dangerous and seeing the importance of social distancing [116].

The psychological fear that both patients and dentists experience can ultimately influence the patients' health outcomes. Improvements ibn oral health reduces their risk of developing the non-oral systemic disease [117]. This is why it is crucial that patients must receive care while under pandemic conditions. The American Dental Association (ADA) has created guidelines for dentists to utilize in dental emergencies. These recommendations take into account the psychological conditions of a patient. Phone triage is being used to assess the patients' psychological and neurological functioning, resulting in patient triaging based on anxiety risk assessment. Though this cannot solely dictate if a patient has a dental emergency, it can influence the overall score [118].

Available data demonstrate that higher infection rates and the majority of deaths due to COVID-19 occur in assisted living homes and underserved communities due to lack of awareness, education and various psychosocial burdens [119–121]. As the pandemic continues, new ways to deal with dental concerns, especially in assisted living homes and underserved communities, are being implemented. As mentioned previously, telemedicine became an essential tool during COVID-19, assessing and triaging patients while also limiting contact [5,119,122]. In addition, since smokers were determined to be a high-risk group for COVID-19 complications, students and medical practitioners need to develop skills in providing smoking cessation. It is expected to see a trend towards more people wanting to quit smoking [123].

Korea is an example of implementing psychological well-being in the treatment of COVID-19. Korea has deployed mental health professionals to assist during quarantine because feelings of distress and anxiety can be exacerbated when experiencing symptoms or receiving treatment for COVID-19 [113]. Some strategies to help cope during this time are self-care and psychological flexibility. Establishing guidelines for dentists and a survey checking their mental status is an important next step for the dental community [111]. With these changing dynamics, there is a need to establish safe and secure methods for services to provide psychological counseling. In summary, high anxiety levels and significant psychosocial implications were noted among dental staff and health care workers during this pandemic. Our findings add to a growing body of data on the psychosocial impact of virus outbreaks on healthcare workers and highlight the importance of wellbeing initiatives for healthcare workers to be placed at the forefront of future pandemic crisis planning.

7. Potential Drugs for Fighting SARS-CoV-2 Infection and Their Interaction with Oral Health Medications

It is clinically important for oral health professionals to be aware of possible drug interactions that may occur between drugs commonly prescribed in dentistry, in order to prevent adverse reactions that may even endanger the life of a patient with COVID-19.

The ongoing pandemic caused by the SARS-CoV-2 virus has proven to be challenging in the pharmaceutical pursuit of a successful drug for treatment. New discoveries unveiling the details of the virus's biochemical and molecular nature have helped to determine potential drugs for treatment of the COVID-19 infection. However, the need for successful clinical trials to substantiate these drugs remains. Therefore, no official FDA approved drug for the treatment of COVID-19 currently exists. There are currently several drugs being researched for treatment which will be discussed.

Perhaps the most promising drug investigated for the treatment of COVID-19 is the antiviral drug known as remdesivir [124]. Remdesivir's overall mechanism disrupts viral replication by acting as an adenosine analog. It enters the body as a prodrug but, in its active form, can incorporate into the viral RNA via RNA-dependent RNA polymerases. This blocks the enzyme's activity, which stops RNA synthesis in the virus [125]. The drug was noted to block the virus in vitro. It also improved the condition of an infected patient via intravenous administration [126]. Other drugs similar to remdesivir include favipiravir and ribavirin. Both of these drugs are guanine analogs that are currently approved for the treatment of other infections. There is still not enough evidence to support their use in the treatment of COVID-19 [127].

Lopinavir is a protease inhibitor that targets the major coronavirus protease, 3CLpro. 3CLpro is responsible for processing the polypeptide translation product from the genomic RNA into the protein components. By blocking 3CLpro the virus is unable to complete normal protein translation and cannot replicate [128]. With ritonavir as a booster, lopinavir and/or ritonavir have been shown to possess anti coronavirus activity in vitro. The efficacy of the drug has been tested in vitro and studies have shown that SARS-CoV-2 could be inhibited by lopinavir and that the drug has an acceptable EC50 [129]. However, most clinical trial studies assess the drug in combination, or in the late stages of the disease progression. Therefore, it is difficult to assess whether lopinavir/ritonavir can treat COVID-19 as a monotherapy or combined with additional drugs [129].

Chloroquine and hydroxychloroquine are classified as aminoquinolines and are typically used to treat malaria and autoimmune diseases such as systemic lupus erythematosus. In the treatment of SARS-CoV-2 infections, they can block the glycosylation of cell receptors of the virus. They also increases the endosomal pH required for viral fusion and have the potential to be used as broad-spectrum antiviral drugs. The use of these two drugs is included in COVID-19 treatment guidelines internationally; however, additional evidential support is needed. Clinical trials are currently being conducted to assess how safe and effective the drug is against COVID-19. One study with more than 100 patients found that chloroquine was more successful at inhibiting the exacerbation of pneumonia than the control treatment [129]. An additional study found hydroxychloroquine was even more potent than chloroquine with an EC_{50} of 0.72 μM,n possibly rendering it more effective at inhibiting the virus in vitro [130].

In addition, some of the medicines such as ketoconazole and erythromycin, used for dental treatment may interfere with remdesivir, lopinavir and hydroxychloroquine [131–133]. This in turn may worsen COVID-19 symptoms. Therefore, dental professionals should be aware of the underlying comorbidities, discuss possible drug interactions and provide an appropriate treatment regimen for COVID-19 patients visiting dental clinics.

DMF, the only drug approved by the US Food and Drug Administration (FDA) and the European Medicines Agency (EMA) that targets the NRF2/KEAP1 axis [134], and two types of NRF2 activator were tested in advanced clinical trials, and thus can be immediately expedited to examine their therapeutic efficacy in patients with COVID-19. NRF2 activators such as sulforaphane and bardoxolone methyl are already in advanced clinical trials for other indications, providing a clear route for their testing in randomized clinical trials in patients with COVID-19.

Inhaled Nitric Oxide (iNO) is also being developed as a potential treatment for the pulmonary symptoms of COVID-19 [135]. NO is a potent vasodilator but when it is administered to a patient intravenously, it is quickly inactivated by hemoglobin. When NO is aerosolized, it can directly access lung tissue and exert its vasodilator effects on the lung's vasculature [135]. iNO has six beneficial effects in COVID-19 patients including, anti-thrombin effects, anti-inflammatory effects, ventilation/perfusion effects, bronchodilatory effects and microbicidal effects. This gas allows patients to have a better chance of recovery from COVID-19 while on ventilators and other ventilation aids [135].

Corticosteroids such as hydrocortisone and dexamethasone are also being tried out as they have shown some benefits in pneumonia and ARDS patients [136]. Corticosteroids were found to be less promising when treated for SARS and MERS [136]. In Covid-19 patients who received corticosteroids for 3–12 days mortality rate was higher than those who were not treated with corticosteroids in a meta-analysis study of about 21,350 patients [137]. Hence, there is a need to explore for an optimal duration for the use of corticosteroids in the treatment of SARS-CoV-2.

Sex steroid hormones, especially estrogen, mount a stronger immune response in females when compared to males. As estrogen levels fall during menopause, women become more vulnerable to numerous health issues, including loss of bone mineral density which can lead to osteoporosis. Around the same time, changes in oral health are also common as teeth and gums become more susceptible to disease, which can lead to inflammation, pain, bleeding, and eventually lost or missing teeth. Estrogen therapy was shown to be effective in reducing tooth and gum diseases in postmenopausal women [138–140]. This protective role is lost in older adults or postmenopausal women due to decreased levels of endogenous sex hormones among COVID-19 patients [87,88]. Several clinical trials are underway using sex hormones (estrogen and progesterone) as a potential drug candidate to combat COVID-19. Jarvis et al. have discussed the combination of estrogen and progesterone to improve the immune abnormalities due to cytokine storm in COVID-19 patients [141]. Our study demonstrated that in vivo supplementation of estrogen attenuated rapid gastric emptying and restored gastric relaxation, serum NO levels, nNOSα, and normalizing Nrf2-Phase II enzymes, inflammatory response, and mitogen-activated protein kinase (MAPK) protein expression in ovariectomized diabetic rodent model [88]. We speculate that sex hormones may be helpful in suppressing COVID-19 symptoms by attenuating impaired Nrf2-NO signaling in targeted organs.

The drugs described include several possible contenders for treatment of the disease, but more evidence is necessary before an official treatment drug is endorsed. For this to occur, further in vitro, in vivo and clinical trials are warranted to determine the possible roles of the drugs in the management of COVID-19.

8. New and Ongoing Research

Research for vaccines and drugs to fight COVID-19 infections has been a priority in most of the world's institutions. Until an effective vaccine/drug is developed or discovered, reliable and efficient testing has become one of the United States most significant needs. ACE-2 expression has been found to be higher in salivary glands when compared to the lungs. Therefore, SARS-CoV-2 can be detected in saliva earlier and even before lung lesions emerge, and patients can present as asymptomatic carriers. A possible correlation between SARS-CoV-2 infections is the association with sialadenitis. The virus can cause lysis of the acinar cells in the salivary glands leaking salivary amylase into the bloodstream, leading to chronic sialadenitis. Dentists diagnosing sialadenitis may recommend that patients are tested for COVID-19 even though they might not present with the normal symptoms [27]. Salivary testing is widely used for the diagnosis of SARC-CoV-2 RNA among COVID-19 patients across the world.

Syncope or near-syncope may be a sign of COVID-19 infection [117,142]. This is still a preliminary report, only conducted in non-U.S. patients. The variation in the prevalence of tobacco use, cardiovascular disease, and dietary patterns may be confounding factors in correlating syncope with COVID-19 infection [117,142].

Vitamin D (1,25-dihydroxycholecalciferol) deficiencies have recently been linked to worse prognoses in COVID-19 infections. Vitamin D was found to increase the production of anti-inflammatory cytokines such as defensins and cathelicidins, which in turn mediate the response of the immune system to the infection. Pro-inflammatory cytokines damage lung epithelium and induce the pneumonia-like symptoms associated with a COVID-19 infection. Vitamin D deficiency may be correlated with an increased risk of "cytokine-storm" immune activity. Nutritionists recommend that people at risk of viral infections such as influenza and/or COVID-19 consider taking 10,000 IU/d of vitamin D3. After a few weeks on this regimen, Vitamin D concentrations should be increased to about 40–60 ng/mL (100–150 nmol/L). For those confirmed COVID-19 positive, a higher dose may be recommended. Research is still ongoing on the effects of Vitamin D and randomized controlled trials and large population studies should be conducted to evaluate these recommendations [143]. Vitamin D deficiencies may also be linked to why the African American population in the US may be more susceptible to the adverse risks of COVID-19. Another innovation in the fight against COVID-19 is the use of copper (Cu). Copper has three main anti-viral properties which are: (I) it damages viral envelopes and can destroy the DNA or RNA of the viruses; (II) it generates reactive oxygen species (ROS) that can kill the virus; and (III) it interferes with proteins that operate important functions for the virus. Copper supplements were suggested to be used in combination with remdesivir (RDV), N-acetylcysteine (NAC), nitric oxide (NO) and colchicine to treat COVID-19 [144]. Also, the survivability of SARS-CoV and SARS-CoV-2 on copper surfaces is much lower than on other metal surfaces. On stainless steel, SARS-CoV-2 survived for up to three days and was undetectable after four days. However, on copper SARS-CoV-2 survived for 4 h. Using copper in hospital settings and dental offices on frequently touched metal surfaces may have an increased effect on lowering the chances of surface related infections [145].

Biomarkers are critical to determining whether interventions are favorable to relieve patients from disease progression. Specific biomarkers such as cardiac and proinflammatory cytokines are elevated in some COVID-19 patients and in AA subjects with diabetes, hypertension and cardiovascular disease (CVD) and more recently periodontal disease [146]. Some of these biomarkers include cTn1/T, BNP, and CK-MB. Elevated cTnT was detected in COVID-19 patients with CVD, and predicted an acute myocardial injury and admission to an intensive care unit (ICU) in 4 out of 5 patients [147]. AA are diagnosed and treated for diabetes, hyper-tension and CVD at higher rates than Caucasians; however, it is yet to be determined whether biomarkers in AA are altered compared to Caucasian patients.

These and many other new strategies are being developed to combat the spread and effects of COVID-19. With continued perseverance COVID-19 will become a disease that the scientific community has well under control.

In conclusion, the SARS-CoV-2 virus has had an indelible effect globally and dentistry is not excluded. New standard protocols are implemented in dental offices worldwide and until an effective vaccine or drug is produced, much of these protocols will remain in effect long-term. A good understanding of the etiology, mechanism of infection, and epidemiology of COVID-19 will help dentists treat their patients. Knowing what co-morbidities increase the risks of fatal COVID-19 outcomes will help dentists better assess what dental procedures are worth the risks of performing on COVID-19 positive patients. In addition, staying abreast of what novel drugs are created to combat the infection is important for dentists. Patients look to dentists not only for oral health advice, though that is their main task; dentists are also expected to provide patients with holistic health advice.

Information is generated everyday describing new signs and symptoms of COVID-19. Oral pathologies associated with COVID-19 are still being discovered and could be used in early diagnoses and/or onset of the disease. Research is still being done to look into saliva as a diagnostic tool for the virus. The antibodies associated with saliva and even the expression of certain proteins may be a correlated presence of the virus and can be used as an inexpensive and less invasive way to test and diagnose patients quickly and accurately.

Author Contributions: Conceptualization, P.R.G.; Writing, original draft preparation, C.J.C., B.D., N.F., J.F., J.R. and L.R.; writing, review and editing, K.B.C., C.S., J.C., C.F.-D. and P.R.G.; supervision, P.R.G. All authors have read and agreed to the published version of the manuscript.

Funding: Dental student research is supported by the HRSA-COE (D34HP00002) grant funded to the School of Dentistry, Meharry Medical College, Nashville, TN. National Institute of General Medical Sciences (NIGMS) of the National Institutes of Health (NIH) under award number- SC1GM21282 funds awarded to Pandu R. Gangula.

Acknowledgments: We thank James Tyus and Donald Odom, School of Dentistry, Meharry Medical College, Nashville, TN, USA.

Conflicts of Interest: The authors declare no conflict of interest.

References

1. Barabari, P.; Moharamzadeh, K. Novel Coronavirus (COVID-19) and Dentistry-A Comprehensive Review of Literature. *Dent. J.* **2020**, *8*, 53. [CrossRef]
2. Adhikari, S.P.; Meng, S.; Wu, Y.J.; Mao, Y.P.; Ye, R.X.; Wang, Q.Z.; Sun, C.; Sylvia, S.; Rozelle, S.; Raat, H.; et al. Epidemiology, causes, clinical manifestation and diagnosis, prevention and control of coronavirus disease (COVID-19) during the early outbreak period: A scoping review. *Infect. Dis Poverty* **2020**, *9*, 29. [CrossRef] [PubMed]
3. WHO. *Pneumonia of Unknown Cause–China*; WHO: Geneva, Switzerland, 2020.
4. Worldometer. Coronavirus Cases. Available online: https://www.worldometers.info/coronavirus/ (accessed on 4 November 2020).
5. Pereira, L.J.; Pereira, C.V.; Murata, R.M.; Pardi, V.; Pereira-Dourado, S.M. Biological and social aspects of Coronavirus Disease 2019 (COVID-19) related to oral health. *Braz. Oral Res.* **2020**, *34*, e041. [CrossRef]
6. Yu, F.; Du, L.; Ojcius, D.M.; Pan, C.; Jiang, S. Measures for diagnosing and treating infections by a novel coronavirus responsible for a pneumonia outbreak originating in Wuhan, China. *Microbes Infect.* **2020**, *22*, 74–79. [CrossRef] [PubMed]
7. Tang, S.; Mao, Y.; Jones, R.M.; Tan, Q.; Ji, J.S.; Li, N.; Shen, J.; Lv, Y.; Pan, L.; Ding, P.; et al. Aerosol transmission of SARS-CoV-2? Evidence, prevention and control. *Environ. Int.* **2020**, *144*, 106039. [CrossRef] [PubMed]
8. Herrera, D.; Serrano, J.; Roldán, S.; Sanz, M. Is the oral cavity relevant in SARS-CoV-2 pandemic? *Clin. Oral Investig.* **2020**, *24*, 2925–2930. [CrossRef] [PubMed]

9. Sampson, V.; Kamona, N.; Sampson, A. Could there be a link between oral hygiene and the severity of SARS-CoV-2 infections? *Br. Dent. J.* **2020**, *228*, 971–975. [CrossRef] [PubMed]
10. Consolo, U.; Bellini, P.; Bencivenni, D.; Iani, C.; Checchi, V. Epidemiological Aspects and Psychological Reactions to COVID-19 of Dental Practitioners in the Northern Italy Districts of Modena and Reggio Emilia. *Int. J. Environ. Res. Public Health* **2020**, *17*, 3459. [CrossRef]
11. Davies, N.G.; Klepac, P.; Liu, Y.; Prem, K.; Jit, M.; Eggo, R.M. Age-dependent effects in the transmission and control of COVID-19 epidemics. *Nat. Med.* **2020**, *26*, 1205–1211. [CrossRef]
12. Centres for Disease Control and Prevention COVID Trcaker CDC Covid Tracker. Available online: https://covid.cdc.gov/covid-data-tracker/#cases_casesinlast7days (accessed on 4 November 2020).
13. Kamate, S.K.; Sharma, S.; Thakar, S.; Srivastava, D.; Sengupta, K.; Hadi, A.J.; Chaudhary, A.; Joshi, R.; Dhanker, K. Assessing Knowledge, Attitudes and Practices of dental practitioners regarding the COVID-19 pandemic: A multinational study. *Dent. Med. Probl.* **2020**, *57*, 11–17. [CrossRef]
14. Chen, N.; Zhou, M.; Dong, X.; Qu, J.; Gong, F.; Han, Y.; Qiu, Y.; Wang, J.; Liu, Y.; Wei, Y.; et al. Epidemiological and clinical characteristics of 99 cases of 2019 novel coronavirus pneumonia in Wuhan, China: A descriptive study. *Lancet* **2020**, *395*, 507–513. [CrossRef]
15. Sohrabi, C.; Alsafi, Z.; O'Neill, N.; Khan, M.; Kerwan, A.; Al-Jabir, A.; Iosifidis, C.; Agha, R. World Health Organization declares global emergency: A review of the 2019 novel coronavirus (COVID-19). *Int. J. Surg.* **2020**, *76*, 71–76. [CrossRef]
16. Li, Q.; Guan, X.; Wu, P.; Wang, X.; Zhou, L.; Tong, Y.; Ren, R.; Leung, K.S.M.; Lau, E.H.Y.; Wong, J.Y.; et al. Early Transmission Dynamics in Wuhan, China, of Novel Coronavirus-Infected Pneumonia. *N. Engl. J. Med.* **2020**, *382*, 1199–1207. [CrossRef] [PubMed]
17. Wang, W.; Tang, J.; Wei, F. Updated understanding of the outbreak of 2019 novel coronavirus (2019-nCoV) in Wuhan, China. *J. Med. Virol.* **2020**, *92*, 441–447. [CrossRef] [PubMed]
18. Ming, W.-K.; Huang, J.; Zhang, C.J.P. Breaking down of the healthcare system: Mathematical modelling for controlling the novel coronavirus (2019-nCoV) outbreak in Wuhan, China. *bioRxiv* **2020**. [CrossRef]
19. Patel, J. Transmission routes of SARS-CoV-2. *J. Dent. Sci.* **2020**. [CrossRef]
20. Worldometer. Coronavirus (COVID-19) Mortality Rate. Available online: https://www.worldometers.info/coronavirus/ (accessed on 4 November 2020).
21. Alcendor, D.J. Racial Disparities-Associated COVID-19 Mortality among Minority Populations in the US. *J. Clin. Med.* **2020**, *9*, 2442. [CrossRef]
22. The Covid Tracking Project. Available online: https://covidtracking.com/race (accessed on 4 November 2020).
23. Kuy, S.; Tsai, R.; Bhatt, J.; Chu, Q.D.; Gandhi, P.; Gupta, R.; Gupta, R.; Hole, M.K.; Hsu, B.S.; Hughes, L.S.; et al. Focusing on Vulnerable Populations During COVID-19. *Acad. Med.* **2020**, *95*, e2–e3. [CrossRef]
24. Riad, A.; Klugar, M.; Krsek, M. COVID-19-Related Oral Manifestations: Early Disease Features? *Oral Dis.* **2020**. [CrossRef]
25. Sinjari, B.; D'Ardes, D.; Santilli, M.; Rexhepi, I.; D'Addazio, G.; Di Carlo, P.; Chiacchiaretta, P.; Caputi, S.; Cipollone, F. SARS-CoV-2 and Oral Manifestation: An Observational, Human Study. *J. Clin. Med.* **2020**, *9*, 3218. [CrossRef]
26. Dar Odeh, N.; Babkair, H.; Abu-Hammad, S.; Borzangy, S.; Abu-Hammad, A.; Abu-Hammad, O. COVID-19: Present and Future Challenges for Dental Practice. *Int. J. Environ. Res. Public Health* **2020**, *17*, 3151. [CrossRef] [PubMed]
27. Baghizadeh Fini, M. Oral saliva and COVID-19. *Oral Oncol.* **2020**, *108*, 104821. [CrossRef] [PubMed]
28. Amorim dos Santos, J.; Normando, A.G.C.; Carvalho da Silva, R.L.; De Paula, R.M.; Cembranel, A.C.; Santos-Silva, A.R.; Guerra, E.N.S. Oral mucosal lesions in a COVID-19 patient: New signs or secondary manifestations? *Int. J. Infect. Dis.* **2020**, *97*, 326–328. [CrossRef] [PubMed]
29. Brandão, T.B.; Gueiros, L.A.; Melo, T.S.; Prado-Ribeiro, A.C.; Nesrallah, A.C.F.A.; Prado, G.V.B.; Santos-Silva, A.R.; Migliorati, C.A. Oral lesions in patients with SARS-CoV-2 infection: Could the oral cavity be a target organ? *Oral Surg. Oral Med. Oral Pathol. Oral Radiol.* **2020**. [CrossRef] [PubMed]
30. Harikrishnan, P. Gustatory Dysfunction as an Early Symptom in COVID-19 Screening. *J. Craniofac. Surg.* **2020**, *6*, e656–e658. [CrossRef]
31. Dawson, P.; Rabold, E.M.; Laws, R.L.; Conners, E.E.; Charpure, R.; Yin, S.; Buono, S.A.; Dasu, T.; Bhattacharyya, S.; Westergaard, R.P.; et al. Loss of Taste and Smell as Distinguishing Symptoms of Coronavirus Disease 2019. *Clin. Infect. Dis.* **2020**. [CrossRef]
32. Zhang, H.; Zhang, Y.; Wu, J.; Li, Y.; Zhou, X.; Li, X.; Chen, H.; Guo, M.; Chen, S.; Sun, F.; et al. Risks and features of secondary infections in severe and critical ill COVID-19 patients. *Emerg. Microbes Infect.* **2020**, *9*, 1958–1964. [CrossRef]
33. Lansbury, L.; Lim, B.; Baskaran, V.; Lim, W.S. Co-infections in people with COVID-19: A systematic review and meta-analysis. *J. Infect.* **2020**, *81*, 266–275. [CrossRef]
34. Hsu, J. How covid-19 is accelerating the threat of antimicrobial resistance. *BMJ* **2020**, 369. [CrossRef]
35. Pitones-Rubio, V.; Chavez-Cortez, E.G.; Hurtado-Camarena, A.; Gonzalez-Rascon, A.; Serafin-Higuera, N. Is periodontal disease a risk factor for severe COVID-19 illness? *Med. Hypotheses* **2020**, *144*, 109969. [CrossRef]
36. Lo Giudice, R. The Severe Acute Respiratory Syndrome Coronavirus-2 (SARS CoV-2) in Dentistry. Management of Biological Risk in Dental Practice. *Int. J. Environ. Res. Public Health* **2020**, *17*, 3067. [CrossRef]
37. Kelly, N.; Nic Iomhair, A.; McKenna, G. Can oral rinses play a role in preventing transmission of Covid 19 infection? *Evid. Based Dent.* **2020**, *21*, 42–43. [CrossRef] [PubMed]

38. Shang, J.; Wan, Y.; Luo, C.; Ye, G.; Geng, Q.; Auerbach, A.; Li, F. Cell entry mechanisms of SARS-CoV-2. *Proc. Natl. Acad. Sci. USA* **2020**, *117*, 11727–11734. [CrossRef] [PubMed]
39. Yuki, K.; Fujiogi, M.; Koutsogiannaki, S. COVID-19 pathophysiology: A review. *Clin. Immunol.* **2020**, *215*, 108427. [CrossRef] [PubMed]
40. Perico, L.; Benigni, A.; Remuzzi, G. Should COVID-19 Concern Nephrologists? Why and to What Extent? The Emerging Impasse of Angiotensin Blockade. *Nephron* **2020**, *144*, 213–221. [CrossRef] [PubMed]
41. Lubel, J.; Garg, M. Renin-Angiotensin-Aldosterone System Inhibitors in Covid-19. *N. Engl. J. Med.* **2020**, *382*, e92. [CrossRef]
42. Watkins, J. Preventing a covid-19 pandemic. *BMJ* **2020**, *368*, m810. [CrossRef]
43. Hamming, I.; Timens, W.; Bulthuis, M.L.; Lely, A.T.; Navis, G.; van Goor, H. Tissue distribution of ACE2 protein, the functional receptor for SARS coronavirus. A first step in understanding SARS pathogenesis. *J. Pathol.* **2004**, *203*, 631–637. [CrossRef]
44. Olagnier, D.; Farahani, E.; Thyrsted, J.; Blay-Cadanet, J.; Herengt, A.; Idorn, M.; Hait, A.; Hernaez, B.; Knudsen, A.; Iversen, M.B.; et al. SARS-CoV2-mediated suppression of NRF2-signaling reveals potent antiviral and anti-inflammatory activity of 4-octyl-itaconate and dimethyl fumarate. *Nat. Commun.* **2020**, *11*, 4938. [CrossRef]
45. Li, X.; Sun, X.; Zhang, X.; Mao, Y.; Ji, Y.; Shi, L.; Cai, W.; Wang, P.; Wu, G.; Gan, X.; et al. Enhanced Oxidative Damage and Nrf2 Downregulation Contribute to the Aggravation of Periodontitis by Diabetes Mellitus. *Oxid. Med. Cell. Longev.* **2018**, *2018*, 1–11. [CrossRef]
46. Xu, H.; Zhong, L.; Deng, J.; Peng, J.; Dan, H.; Zeng, X.; Li, T.; Chen, Q. High expression of ACE2 receptor of 2019-nCoV on the epithelial cells of oral mucosa. *Int. J. Oral Sci.* **2020**, *12*, 8. [CrossRef]
47. Hassan, S.; Jawad, M.; Ahjel, S.; Singh, R.; Singh, J.; Awad, S.; Hadi, N. The Nrf2 Activator (DMF) and Covid-19: Is there a Possible Role? *Med. Arch.* **2020**, *74*, 134. [CrossRef]
48. Fang, Y.; Gao, F.; Liu, Z. Angiotensin-converting enzyme 2 attenuates inflammatory response and oxidative stress in hyperoxic lung injury by regulating NF-κB and Nrf2 pathways. *QJM An. Int. J. Med.* **2019**, *112*, 914–924. [CrossRef]
49. Jacobs, M.; Van Eeckhoutte, H.P.; Wijnant, S.R.A.; Janssens, W.; Joos, G.F.; Brusselle, G.G.; Bracke, K.R. Increased expression of ACE2, the SARS-CoV-2 entry receptor, in alveolar and bronchial epithelium of smokers and COPD subjects. *Eur. Respir. J.* **2020**, *56*, 2002378. [CrossRef]
50. Wysocki, J.; Lores, E.; Ye, M.; Soler, M.J.; Batlle, D. Kidney and Lung ACE2 Expression after an ACE Inhibitor or an Ang II Receptor Blocker: Implications for COVID-19. *J. Am. Soc. Nephrol.* **2020**, *31*, 1941–1943. [CrossRef]
51. Zhang, H.; Kang, Z.; Gong, H.; Xu, D.; Wang, J.; Li, Z.; Li, Z.; Cui, X.; Xiao, J.; Zhan, J.; et al. Digestive system is a potential route of COVID-19: An analysis of single-cell coexpression pattern of key proteins in viral entry process. *Gut* **2020**, *69*, 1010–1018. [CrossRef]
52. Xiao, F.; Tang, M.; Zheng, X.; Liu, Y.; Li, X.; Shan, H. Evidence for Gastrointestinal Infection of SARS-CoV-2. *Gastroenterology* **2020**, *158*, 1831–1833. [CrossRef]
53. Cuadrado, A.; Pajares, M.; Benito, C.; Jimenez-Villegas, J.; Escoll, M.; Fernandez-Gines, R.; Garcia Yague, A.J.; Lastra, D.; Manda, G.; Rojo, A.I.; et al. Can Activation of NRF2 Be a Strategy against COVID-19? *Trends Pharmacol. Sci.* **2020**, *41*, 598–610. [CrossRef]
54. Deramaudt, T.B.; Dill, C.; Bonay, M. Regulation of oxidative stress by Nrf2 in the pathophysiology of infectious diseases. *Med. Mal. Infect.* **2013**, *43*, 100–107. [CrossRef] [PubMed]
55. Chen, Y.; Guo, Y.; Pan, Y.; Zhao, Z.J. Structure analysis of the receptor binding of 2019-nCoV. *Biochem. Biophys. Res. Commun.* **2020**. [CrossRef]
56. Chiu, A.V.; Al Saigh, M.; McCulloch, C.A.; Glogauer, M. The Role of NrF2 in the Regulation of Periodontal Health and Disease. *J. Dent. Res.* **2017**, *96*, 975–983. [CrossRef] [PubMed]
57. Zhao, S.; Ghosh, A.; Lo, C.S.; Chenier, I.; Scholey, J.W.; Filep, J.G.; Ingelfinger, J.R.; Zhang, S.L.; Chan, J.S.D. Nrf2 Deficiency Upregulates Intrarenal Angiotensin-Converting Enzyme-2 and Angiotensin 1-7 Receptor Expression and Attenuates Hypertension and Nephropathy in Diabetic Mice. *Endocrinology* **2018**, *159*, 836–852. [CrossRef]
58. Bousquet, J.; Cristol, J.-P.; Czarlewski, W.; Anto, J.M.; Martineau, A.; Haahtela, T.; Fonseca, S.C.; Iaccarino, G.; Blain, H.; Fiocchi, A.; et al. Nrf2-interacting nutrients and COVID-19: Time for research to develop adaptation strategies. *Clin. Transl. Allergy* **2020**, *10*, 58. [CrossRef]
59. Sampath, C.; Srinivasan, S.; Freeman, M.L.; Gangula, P.R. Inhibition of GSK-3β restores delayed gastric emptying in obesity-induced diabetic female mice. *Am. J. Physiol. Liver Physiol.* **2020**, *319*, G481–G493. [CrossRef] [PubMed]
60. Hoffmann, M.; Kleine-Weber, H.; Schroeder, S.; Kruger, N.; Herrler, T.; Erichsen, S.; Schiergens, T.S.; Herrler, G.; Wu, N.H.; Nitsche, A.; et al. SARS-CoV-2 Cell Entry Depends on ACE2 and TMPRSS2 and Is Blocked by a Clinically Proven Protease Inhibitor. *Cell* **2020**, *181*, 271–280. [CrossRef]
61. Ozdemir, B.; Yazici, A. Could the decrease in the endothelial nitric oxide (NO) production and NO bioavailability be the crucial cause of COVID-19 related deaths? *Med. Hypotheses* **2020**, *144*, 109970. [CrossRef]
62. Green, S.J. Covid-19 accelerates endothelial dysfunction and nitric oxide deficiency. *Microbes Infect.* **2020**, *22*, 149–150. [CrossRef]
63. Akerstrom, S.; Gunalan, V.; Keng, C.T.; Tan, Y.J.; Mirazimi, A. Dual effect of nitric oxide on SARS-CoV replication: Viral RNA production and palmitoylation of the S protein are affected. *Virology* **2009**, *395*, 1–9. [CrossRef]
64. Saura, M.; Zaragoza, C.; McMillan, A.; Quick, R.A.; Hohenadl, C.; Lowenstein, J.M.; Lowenstein, C.J. An antiviral mechanism of nitric oxide: Inhibition of a viral protease. *Immunity* **1999**, *10*, 21–28. [CrossRef]

65. Mancini, L.; Quinzi, V.; Mummolo, S.; Marzo, G.; Marchetti, E. Angiotensin-Converting Enzyme 2 as a Possible Correlation between COVID-19 and Periodontal Disease. *Appl. Sci.* **2020**, *10*, 6224. [CrossRef]
66. Elisetti, N. Periodontal pocket and COVID-19: Could there be a possible link? *Med. Hypotheses* **2020**, 110355. [CrossRef]
67. Nishiga, M.; Wang, D.W.; Han, Y.; Lewis, D.B.; Wu, J.C. COVID-19 and cardiovascular disease: From basic mechanisms to clinical perspectives. *Nat. Rev. Cardiol.* **2020**, *17*, 543–558. [CrossRef]
68. Guzik, T.J.; Mohiddin, S.A.; Dimarco, A.; Patel, V.; Savvatis, K.; Marelli-Berg, F.M.; Madhur, M.S.; Tomaszewski, M.; Maffia, P.; D'Acquisto, F.; et al. COVID-19 and the cardiovascular system: Implications for risk assessment, diagnosis, and treatment options. *Cardiovasc. Res.* **2020**, *116*, 1666–1687. [CrossRef]
69. Villapol, S. Gastrointestinal symptoms associated with COVID-19: Impact on the gut microbiome. *Transl. Res.* **2020**, *226*, 57–69. [CrossRef]
70. El Moheb, M.; Naar, L.; Christensen, M.A.; Kapoen, C.; Maurer, L.R.; Farhat, M.; Kaafarani, H.M.A. Gastrointestinal Complications in Critically Ill Patients With and Without COVID-19. *JAMA* **2020**. [CrossRef]
71. Ryan, P.M.; Caplice, N. COVID-19 and relative angiotensin-converting enzyme 2 deficiency: Role in disease severity and therapeutic response. *Open Hear.* **2020**, *7*, e001302. [CrossRef]
72. Kumar, A.; Faiq, M.A.; Pareek, V.; Raza, K.; Narayan, R.K.; Prasoon, P.; Kumar, P.; Kulandhasamy, M.; Kumari, C.; Kant, K.; et al. Relevance of SARS-CoV-2 related factors ACE2 and TMPRSS2 expressions in gastrointestinal tissue with pathogenesis of digestive symptoms, diabetes-associated mortality, and disease recurrence in COVID-19 patients. *Med. Hypotheses* **2020**, *144*, 110271. [CrossRef]
73. Chen, L.; Zhao, J.; Peng, J.; Li, X.; Deng, X.; Geng, Z.; Shen, Z.; Guo, F.; Zhang, Q.; Jin, Y.; et al. Detection of 2019-nCoV in Saliva and Characterization of Oral Symptoms in COVID-19 Patients. *SSRN Electron. J.* **2020**. [CrossRef]
74. Pedrosa, M.; Da, S.; Sipert, C.R.; Nogueira, F.N. Salivary Glands, Saliva and Oral Findings in COVID-19 Infection. *Pesqui. Bras. Odontopediatria Clin. Integr.* **2020**, *20*. [CrossRef]
75. Saniasiaya, J. Xerostomia and COVID-19: Unleashing Pandora's Box. *Ear Nose Throat J.* **2020**, 014556132096035. [CrossRef]
76. Xu, J.; Li, Y.; Gan, F.; Du, Y.; Yao, Y. Salivary Glands: Potential Reservoirs for COVID-19 Asymptomatic Infection. *J. Dent. Res.* **2020**, *99*, 989. [CrossRef] [PubMed]
77. Wang, W.K.; Chen, S.Y.; Liu, I.J.; Chen, Y.C.; Chen, H.L.; Yang, C.F.; Chen, P.J.; Yeh, S.H.; Kao, C.L.; Huang, L.M.; et al. Detection of SARS-associated coronavirus in throat wash and saliva in early diagnosis. *Emerg Infect. Dis.* **2004**, *10*, 1213–1219. [CrossRef] [PubMed]
78. To, K.K.; Tsang, O.T.; Yip, C.C.; Chan, K.H.; Wu, T.C.; Chan, J.M.; Leung, W.S.; Chik, T.S.; Choi, C.Y.; Kandamby, D.H.; et al. Consistent Detection of 2019 Novel Coronavirus in Saliva. *Clin. Infect. Dis.* **2020**, *71*, 841–843. [CrossRef] [PubMed]
79. Hajifathalian, K.; Mahadev, S.; Schwartz, R.E.; Shah, S.; Sampath, K.; Schnoll-Sussman, F.; Jr, R.S.B.; Carr-Locke, D.; Cohen, D.E.; Sharaiha, R.Z. SARS-COV-2 infection (coronavirus disease 2019) for the gastrointestinal consultant. *World J. Gastroenterol.* **2020**, *26*, 1546–1553. [CrossRef] [PubMed]
80. Ferreira, C.; Viana, S.D.; Reis, F. Gut Microbiota Dysbiosis–Immune Hyperresponse–Inflammation Triad in Coronavirus Disease 2019 (COVID-19): Impact of Pharmacological and Nutraceutical Approaches. *Microorganisms* **2020**, *8*, 1514. [CrossRef]
81. Singh, R.; Chandrashekharappa, S.; Bodduluri, S.R.; Baby, B.V.; Hegde, B.; Kotla, N.G.; Hiwale, A.A.; Saiyed, T.; Patel, P.; Vijay-Kumar, M.; et al. Enhancement of the gut barrier integrity by a microbial metabolite through the Nrf2 pathway. *Nat. Commun.* **2019**, *10*, 89. [CrossRef]
82. Vázquez-Torres, A.; Bäumler, A.J. Nitrate, nitrite and nitric oxide reductases: From the last universal common ancestor to modern bacterial pathogens. *Curr. Opin. Microbiol.* **2016**, *29*, 1–8. [CrossRef]
83. Dinakaran, V.; Mandape, S.N.; Shuba, K.; Pratap, S.; Sakhare, S.S.; Tabatabai, M.A.; Smoot, D.T.; Farmer-Dixon, C.M.; Kesavalu, L.N.; Adunyah, S.E.; et al. Identification of Specific Oral and Gut Pathogens in Full Thickness Colon of Colitis Patients: Implications for Colon Motility. *Front. Microbiol.* **2018**, *9*, 3220. [CrossRef]
84. Walker, M.Y.; Pratap, S.; Southerland, J.H.; Farmer-Dixon, C.M.; Lakshmyya, K.; Gangula, P.R. Role of oral and gut microbiome in nitric oxide-mediated colon motility. *Nitric Oxide Biol. Chem.* **2018**, *73*, 81–88. [CrossRef]
85. Sampath, C.; Sprouse, J.C.; Freeman, M.L.; Gangula, P.R. Activation of Nrf2 attenuates delayed gastric emptying in obesity induced diabetic (T2DM) female mice. *Free Radic. Biol. Med.* **2019**, *135*, 132–143. [CrossRef]
86. Gangula, P.; Ravella, K.; Chukkapalli, S.; Rivera, M.; Srinivasan, S.; Hale, A.; Channon, K.; Southerland, J.; Kesavalu, L. Polybacterial Periodontal Pathogens Alter Vascular and Gut BH4/nNOS/NRF2-Phase II Enzyme Expression. *PLoS ONE* **2015**, *10*, e0129885. [CrossRef] [PubMed]
87. Al-Lami, R.A.; Urban, R.J.; Volpi, E.; Algburi, A.M.A.; Baillargeon, J. Sex Hormones and Novel Corona Virus Infectious Disease (COVID-19). *Mayo Clin. Proc.* **2020**, *95*, 1710–1714. [CrossRef] [PubMed]
88. Sprouse, J.C.; Sampath, C.; Gangula, P.R. Supplementation of 17β-Estradiol Normalizes Rapid Gastric Emptying by Restoring Impaired Nrf2 and nNOS Function in Obesity-Induced Diabetic Ovariectomized Mice. *Antioxidants* **2020**, *9*, 582. [CrossRef] [PubMed]
89. García, L.F. Immune Response, Inflammation, and the Clinical Spectrum of COVID-19. *Front. Immunol.* **2020**, *11*. [CrossRef] [PubMed]
90. Tang, Y.; Liu, J.; Zhang, D.; Xu, Z.; Ji, J.; Wen, C. Cytokine Storm in COVID-19: The Current Evidence and Treatment Strategies. *Front. Immunol.* **2020**, *11*. [CrossRef]

91. Cecchini, R.; Cecchini, A.L. SARS-CoV-2 infection pathogenesis is related to oxidative stress as a response to aggression. *Med. Hypotheses* **2020**, *143*, 110102. [CrossRef]
92. Liu, Z.; Xiao, X.; Wei, X.; Li, J.; Yang, J.; Tan, H.; Zhu, J.; Zhang, Q.; Wu, J.; Liu, L. Composition and divergence of coronavirus spike proteins and host ACE2 receptors predict potential intermediate hosts of SARS-CoV-2. *J. Med. Virol.* **2020**, *92*, 595–601. [CrossRef]
93. Furuhashi, M.; Moniwa, N.; Mita, T.; Fuseya, T.; Ishimura, S.; Ohno, K.; Shibata, S.; Tanaka, M.; Watanabe, Y.; Akasaka, H.; et al. Urinary angiotensin-converting enzyme 2 in hypertensive patients may be increased by olmesartan, an angiotensin II receptor blocker. *Am. J. Hypertens* **2015**, *28*, 15–21. [CrossRef]
94. Kwok, S.; Adam, S.; Ho, J.H.; Iqbal, Z.; Turkington, P.; Razvi, S.; Le Roux, C.W.; Soran, H.; Syed, A.A. Obesity: A critical risk factor in the COVID-19 pandemic. *Clin. Obes.* **2020**, *10*. [CrossRef]
95. Cuschieri, S.; Grech, S. Obesity population at risk of COVID-19 complications. *Glob. Health Epidemiol. Genom.* **2020**, *5*, e6. [CrossRef]
96. Yaribeygi, H.; Sathyapalan, T.; Jamialahmadi, T.; Sahebkar, A. The Impact of Diabetes Mellitus in COVID-19: A Mechanistic Review of Molecular Interactions. *J. Diabetes Res.* **2020**, *2020*, 1–9. [CrossRef]
97. Sahni, V.; Gupta, S. COVID-19 & Periodontitis: The cytokine connection. *Med. Hypotheses* **2020**, *144*, 109908. [CrossRef] [PubMed]
98. Ye, Q.; Wang, B.; Mao, J. The pathogenesis and treatment of the 'Cytokine Storm' in COVID-19. *J. Infect.* **2020**, *80*, 607–613. [CrossRef] [PubMed]
99. Daniel, R.; Gokulanathan, S.; Shanmugasundaram, N.; Lakshmigandhan, M.; Kavin, T. Diabetes and periodontal disease. *J. Pharm. Bioallied Sci.* **2012**, *4*, 280. [CrossRef] [PubMed]
100. Patel, J.; Woolley, J. Necrotizing periodontal disease: Oral manifestation of COVID-19. *Oral Dis.* **2020**, odi.13462. [CrossRef]
101. Riad, A.; Kassem, I.; Hockova, B.; Badrah, M.; Klugar, M. Halitosis in COVID-19 patients. *Spec. Care Dent.* **2020**, scd.12547. [CrossRef]
102. Peng, X.; Xu, X.; Li, Y.; Cheng, L.; Zhou, X.; Ren, B. Transmission routes of 2019-nCoV and controls in dental practice. *Int. J. Oral Sci.* **2020**, *12*, 9. [CrossRef]
103. Henrique Braz-Silva, P.; Pallos, D.; Giannecchini, S.; To, K.K. SARS-CoV-2: What can saliva tell us? *Oral Dis.* **2020**. [CrossRef]
104. Martin Carreras-Presas, C.; Amaro Sanchez, J.; Lopez-Sanchez, A.F.; Jane-Salas, E.; Somacarrera Perez, M.L. Oral vesiculobullous lesions associated with SARS-CoV-2 infection. *Oral Dis.* **2020**. [CrossRef]
105. Estrich, C.G.; Mikkelsen, M.; Morrissey, R.; Geisinger, M.L.; Ioannidou, E.; Vujicic, M.; Araujo, M.W.B. Estimating COVID-19 prevalence and infection control practices among US dentists. *J. Am. Dent. Assoc.* **2020**, *151*, 815–824. [CrossRef]
106. Bidra, A.S.; Pelletier, J.S.; Westover, J.B.; Frank, S.; Brown, S.M.; Tessema, B. Comparison of In Vitro Inactivation of SARS CoV-2 with Hydrogen Peroxide and Povidone-Iodine Oral Antiseptic Rinses. *J. Prosthodont.* **2020**, *29*, 599–603. [CrossRef]
107. Mousavi, E.S.; Kananizadeh, N.; Martinello, R.A.; Sherman, J.D. COVID-19 Outbreak and Hospital Air Quality: A Systematic Review of Evidence on Air Filtration and Recirculation. *Environ. Sci. Technol.* **2020**. [CrossRef] [PubMed]
108. Phone Advise Line Tool. Available online: https://www.cdc.gov/coronavirus/2019-ncov/hcp/phone-guide/index.html (accessed on 4 November 2020).
109. Prevention, C. For D.C. and Interim Infection Prevention and Control Guidance for Dental Settings during the Coronavirus Disease 2019 (COVID-19) Pandemic. 2020. Available online: https://www.cdc.gov/coronavirus/2019-ncov/hcp/dental-settings.html (accessed on 4 November 2020).
110. Ahmed, M.A.; Jouhar, R.; Ahmed, N.; Adnan, S.; Aftab, M.; Zafar, M.S.; Khurshid, Z. Fear and Practice Modifications among Dentists to Combat Novel Coronavirus Disease (COVID-19) Outbreak. *Int. J. Environ. Res. Public Health* **2020**, *17*, 2821. [CrossRef]
111. Vergara-Buenaventura, A.; Chavez-Tunon, M.; Castro-Ruiz, C. The Mental Health Consequences of Coronavirus Disease 2019 Pandemic in Dentistry. *Disaster Med. Public Health Prep.* **2020**, 1–4. [CrossRef] [PubMed]
112. Xiao, C. A Novel Approach of Consultation on 2019 Novel Coronavirus (COVID-19)-Related Psychological and Mental Problems: Structured Letter Therapy. *Psychiatry Investig.* **2020**, *17*, 175–176. [CrossRef] [PubMed]
113. Park, S.C.; Park, Y.C. Mental Health Care Measures in Response to the 2019 Novel Coronavirus Outbreak in Korea. *Psychiatry Investig.* **2020**, *17*, 85–86. [CrossRef]
114. Shacham, M.; Hamama-Raz, Y.; Kolerman, R.; Mijiritsky, O.; Ben-Ezra, M.; Mijiritsky, E. COVID-19 Factors and Psychological Factors Associated with Elevated Psychological Distress among Dentists and Dental Hygienists in Israel. *Int. J. Environ. Res. Public Health* **2020**, *17*, 2900. [CrossRef]
115. Ferneini, E.M. The Financial Impact of COVID-19 on Our Practice. *J. Oral Maxillofac. Surg.* **2020**, *78*, 1047–1048. [CrossRef]
116. Khader, Y.; Al Nsour, M.; Al-Batayneh, O.B.; Saadeh, R.; Bashier, H.; Alfaqih, M.; Al-Azzam, S.; AlShurman, B.A. Dentists' Awareness, Perception, and Attitude Regarding COVID-19 and Infection Control: Cross-Sectional Study Among Jordanian Dentists. *JMIR Public Health Surveill.* **2020**, *6*, e18798. [CrossRef]
117. Botros, N.; Iyer, P.; Ojcius, D.M. Is there an association between oral health and severity of COVID-19 complications? *Biomed. J.* **2020**, *43*, 325–327. [CrossRef]
118. Spicciarelli, V.; Marruganti, C.; Viviano, M.; Baldini, N.; Franciosi, G.; Tortoriello, M.; Ferrari, M.; Grandini, S. A new framework to identify dental emergencies in the COVID-19 era. *J. Oral Sci.* **2020**, *62*, 344–347. [CrossRef] [PubMed]
119. Gonzalez-Olmo, M.J.; Ortega-Martinez, A.R.; Delgado-Ramos, B.; Romero-Maroto, M.; Carrillo-Diaz, M. Perceived vulnerability to Coronavirus infection: Impact on dental practice. *Braz. Oral Res.* **2020**, *34*, e044. [CrossRef] [PubMed]

120. Woodall, T.; Ramage, M.; LaBruyere, J.T.; McLean, W.; Tak, C.R. Telemedicine Services During COVID-19: Considerations for Medically Underserved Populations. *J. Rural. Health* **2020**. [CrossRef] [PubMed]
121. Caspi, G.; Chen, J.; Liverant-Taub, S.; Shina, A.; Caspi, O. Heat Maps for Surveillance and Prevention of COVID-19 Spread in Nursing Homes and Assisted Living Facilities. *J. Am. Med. Dir. Assoc.* **2020**, *21*, 986–988.e1. [CrossRef] [PubMed]
122. Machado, R.A.; de Souza, N.L.; Oliveira, R.M.; Martelli Junior, H.; Bonan, P.R.F. Social media and telemedicine for oral diagnosis and counselling in the COVID-19 era. *Oral Oncol.* **2020**, *105*, 104685. [CrossRef] [PubMed]
123. Leonel, A.; Martelli-Junior, H.; Bonan, P.R.F.; Kowalski, L.P.; da Cruz Perez, D.E. COVID-19, head and neck cancer, and the need of training of health students and practitioners regarding to tobacco control and patient counseling. *Oral Oncol.* **2020**, *106*, 104739. [CrossRef]
124. Martinez, M.A. Compounds with Therapeutic Potential against Novel Respiratory 2019 Coronavirus. *Antimicrob. Agents Chemother.* **2020**, *64*. [CrossRef]
125. Gordon, C.J.; Tchesnokov, E.P.; Feng, J.Y.; Porter, D.P.; Gotte, M. The antiviral compound remdesivir potently inhibits RNA-dependent RNA polymerase from Middle East respiratory syndrome coronavirus. *J. Biol. Chem.* **2020**, *295*, 4773–4779. [CrossRef]
126. Holshue, M.L.; DeBolt, C.; Lindquist, S.; Lofy, K.H.; Wiesman, J.; Bruce, H.; Spitters, C.; Ericson, K.; Wilkerson, S.; Tural, A.; et al. First Case of 2019 Novel Coronavirus in the United States. *N. Engl. J. Med.* **2020**, *382*, 929–936. [CrossRef]
127. Li, G.; De Clercq, E. Therapeutic options for the 2019 novel coronavirus (2019-nCoV). *Nat. Rev. Drug Discov.* **2020**, *19*, 149–150. [CrossRef]
128. Li, H.; Zhou, Y.; Zhang, M.; Wang, H.; Zhao, Q.; Liu, J. Updated Approaches against SARS-CoV-2. *Antimicrob. Agents Chemother.* **2020**, *64*. [CrossRef] [PubMed]
129. Simsek Yavuz, S.; Unal, S. Antiviral treatment of COVID-19. *Turk. J. Med. Sci.* **2020**, *50*, 611–619. [CrossRef] [PubMed]
130. Yao, X.; Ye, F.; Zhang, M.; Cui, C.; Huang, B.; Niu, P.; Liu, X.; Zhao, L.; Dong, E.; Song, C.; et al. In Vitro Antiviral Activity and Projection of Optimized Dosing Design of Hydroxychloroquine for the Treatment of Severe Acute Respiratory Syndrome Coronavirus 2 (SARS-CoV-2). *Clin. Infect. Dis.* **2020**, *71*, 732–739. [CrossRef] [PubMed]
131. Gandhi, Z.; Mansuri, Z.; Bansod, S. Potential Interactions of Remdesivir with Pulmonary Drugs: A Covid-19 Perspective. *SN Compr. Clin. Med.* **2020**, *2*, 1707–1708. [CrossRef] [PubMed]
132. Parikh, N.; Venishetty, V.K.; Sistla, R. Simultaneous Determination of Ketoconazole, Ritonavir and Lopinavir in Solid Lipid Nanoparticles by RP-LC. *Chromatographia* **2010**, *71*, 941–946. [CrossRef]
133. Brown, R. Hydroxychloroquine and "off-label" utilization in the treatment of oral conditions. *Oral Surg. Oral Med. Oral Pathol. Oral Radiol.* **2020**, *129*, 643–644. [CrossRef]
134. Linker, R.A.; Lee, D.-H.; Ryan, S.; van Dam, A.M.; Conrad, R.; Bista, P.; Zeng, W.; Hronowsky, X.; Buko, A.; Chollate, S.; et al. Fumaric acid esters exert neuroprotective effects in neuroinflammation via activation of the Nrf2 antioxidant pathway. *Brain* **2011**, *134*, 678–692. [CrossRef]
135. Alvarez, R.A.; Berra, L.; Gladwin, M.T. Home Nitric Oxide Therapy for COVID-19. *Am. J. Respir. Crit. Care Med.* **2020**, *202*, 16–20. [CrossRef]
136. Prescott, H.C.; Rice, T.W. Corticosteroids in COVID-19 ARDS. *JAMA* **2020**, *324*, 1292. [CrossRef]
137. Mishra, G.P.; Mulani, J. Corticosteroids for COVID-19: The search for an optimum duration of therapy. *Lancet Respir. Med.* **2020**. [CrossRef]
138. Sen, S.; Sen, S.; Dutta, A.; Abhinandan, A.; Kumar, V.; Kumar Singh, A. Oral manifestation and its management in postmenopausal women: An integrated review. *Menopausal Rev.* **2020**, *19*, 101–103. [CrossRef] [PubMed]
139. Guan, X.; Guan, Y.; Shi, C.; Zhu, X.; He, Y.; Wei, Z.; Yang, J.; Hou, T. Estrogen deficiency aggravates apical periodontitis by regulating NLRP3/caspase-1/IL-1β axis. *Am. J. Transl. Res.* **2020**, *12*, 660–671. [PubMed]
140. Arias-Herrera, S.; Bascones-Ilundian, C.; Bascones-Martínez, A. Difference in the expression of inflammatory mediators in gingival crevicular fluid in postmenopausal patients with chronic periodontitis with and without menopausal hormone therapy. *Eur. J. Obstet. Gynecol. Reprod. Biol. X* **2019**, *3*, 100021. [CrossRef] [PubMed]
141. Mauvais-Jarvis, F.; Klein, S.L.; Levin, E.R. Estradiol, Progesterone, Immunomodulation, and COVID-19 Outcomes. *Endocrinology* **2020**, *161*. [CrossRef]
142. Chen, T.; Hanna, J.; Walsh, E.E.; Falsey, A.R.; Laguio-Vila, M.; Lesho, E. Syncope, Near Syncope, or Nonmechanical Falls as a Presenting Feature of COVID-19. *Ann. Emerg. Med.* **2020**, *76*, 115–117. [CrossRef]
143. Grant, W.B.; Lahore, H.; McDonnell, S.L.; Baggerly, C.A.; French, C.B.; Aliano, J.L.; Bhattoa, H.P. Evidence that Vitamin D Supplementation Could Reduce Risk of Influenza and COVID-19 Infections and Deaths. *Nutrients* **2020**, *12*, 988. [CrossRef]
144. Andreou, A.; Trantza, S.; Filippou, D.; Sipsas, N.; Tsiodras, S. COVID-19: The Potential Role of Copper and N-acetylcysteine (NAC) in a Combination of Candidate Antiviral Treatments against SARS-CoV-2. *In Vivo (Brooklyn)* **2020**, *34*, 1567–1588. [CrossRef]
145. Aboubakr, H.A.; Sharafeldin, T.A.; Goyal, S.M. Stability of SARS-CoV-2 and other coronaviruses in the environment and on common touch surfaces and the influence of climatic conditions: A review. *Transbound. Emerg. Dis.* **2020**. [CrossRef]
146. Yancy, C.W. COVID-19 and African Americans. *JAMA* **2020**, *323*, 1891–1892. [CrossRef]
147. Aboughdir, M.; Kirwin, T.; Abdul Khader, A.; Wang, B. Prognostic Value of Cardiovascular Biomarkers in COVID-19: A Review. *Viruses* **2020**, *12*, 527. [CrossRef]

Journal of
Clinical Medicine

MDPI

Review

Bio-Inspired Systems in Nonsurgical Periodontal Therapy to Reduce Contaminated Aerosol during COVID-19: A Comprehensive and Bibliometric Review

Andrea Butera [1,*], Carolina Maiorani [1], Valentino Natoli [2], Ambra Bruni [3], Carmen Coscione [4], Gaia Magliano [5], Giulia Giacobbo [6], Alessia Morelli [7], Sara Moressa [4] and Andrea Scribante [8]

1 Unit of Dental Hygiene, Section of Dentistry, Department of Clinical, Surgical, Diagnostic and Pediatric Sciences, University of Pavia, 27100 Pavia, Italy; carolina.maiorani01@universitadipavia.it
2 DDS, Private Dental Practice, 72015 Fasano, Italy; valentinonatoliodn@gmail.com
3 Free Lancer, 03100 Frosinone, Italy; ambrabruni@libero.it
4 Free Lancer, 10121 Turin, Italy; carmen.coscionedh@gmail.com (C.C.); moressa.sara@gmail.com (S.M.)
5 Free Lancer, 31100 Treviso, Italy; gaia.magliano@gmail.com
6 Free Lancer, 20019 Milan, Italy; giulia.giacobbo91@gmail.com
7 Free Lancer, 61121 Pesaro, Italy; morelli.alessia@hotmail.it
8 Unit of Orthodontics and Pediatric Dentistry, Section of Dentistry, Department of Clinical, Surgical, Diagnostic and Pediatric Sciences, University of Pavia, 27100 Pavia, Italy; andrea.scribante@unipv.it
* Correspondence: andrea.butera@unipv.it

Received: 11 November 2020; Accepted: 29 November 2020; Published: 2 December 2020

Abstract: Background: On 30 January 2020, a public health emergency of international concern was declared as a result of the new COVID-19 disease, caused by the SARS-CoV-2 virus. This virus is transmitted by air and, therefore, clinical practices with the production of contaminant aerosols are highly at risk. The purpose of this review was to assess the effectiveness of bio-inspired systems, as adjuvants to nonsurgical periodontal therapy, in order to formulate bio-inspired protocols aimed at restoring optimal condition, reducing bacteremia and aerosols generation. Methods: A comprehensive and bibliometric review of articles published in English. Research of clinical trials (RCTs) were included with participants with chronic or aggressive periodontal disease, that have compared benefits for nonsurgical periodontal therapy (NSPT). Results: Seventy-four articles have been included. For probing depth (PPD) there was a statically significant improvement in laser, probiotic, chlorhexidine groups, such as gain in clinical attachment level (CAL). Bleeding on probing (BOP) reduction was statistically significant only for probiotic and chlorhexidine groups. There were changes in microbiological and immunological parameters. Conclusions: The use of bio-inspired systems in nonsurgical periodontal treatment may be useful in reducing risk of bacteremia and aerosol generation, improving clinical, microbiological and immunological parameters, of fundamental importance in a context of global pandemic, where the reduction of bacterial load in aerosols becomes a pivotal point of clinical practice, but other clinical trials are necessary to achieve statistical validity.

Keywords: periodontitis; bio-inspired; nonsurgical periodontal therapy; dentistry; dental hygiene

1. Introduction

On 30 January 2020, a public health emergency of international importance was declared as a result of the new disease COVID-19, an infection caused by a virus never identified in humans, SARS-CoV-2. The virus belongs to the family Coronaviridae, genetically placed within the genus Betacoronavirus, with a distinct clade in the lineage B of the sub-genus Sarbecovirus as well as two non-human Sars-like strains. It is an RNA virus covered by a capsid and a peri-capsid, crossed by glycoproteic structures that give it the typical appearance of a corona; it binds to the cell thanks to the interaction of the spike protein with the cellular receptor angiotensin-convertin enzyme 2 (ACE2) [1–3]. In addition to the definition, the mode of transmission of the virus has also been configured, which occurs mainly through inhalation, ingestion and direct contact of the mucous membranes with droplets of saliva; it is also essential to remember that the virus can survive on hands, objects or surfaces that have been exposed to infected saliva [3].

In Italy, the reported cases have grown dramatically over time, leading the country to gain a prominent position in the international scenario of infected patients.

This emerging pandemic and its serious outbreak led the Italian government to promote drastic impact measures to flatten the infection curve and, in turn, prevent health systems from collapsing. In fact, the limitation of people moving away from home, the social distancing, the cessation of almost all work activities and the request to the population to use masks and protective gloves, have the aim of minimizing the likelihood of non-infected persons coming into contact with persons who have contracted the virus; some professions, however, have had to guarantee a public service, such as dentistry [4].

1.1. The Problem in Dentistry

On 15 March 2020, the New York Times published an article titled "The Workers Face the Greatest Coronavirus Risk", where an impressive scheme has described that dentists, dental hygienists, secretaries, chair assistants and laboratory technicians are among the workers most at risk of being affected by COVID-19 [5]. So, on the one hand there is a request to continue to offer a service for emergencies, and on the other hand operators must be able to work safely, while being exposed to great risk: direct contact, and contact with biological liquids and aerosols. In this regard, an article has recently been published by researchers of the Wuhan University School and Hospital of Stomatology with the aim of providing recommendations to dentists, for the management of the patient: minimize operations that can produce droplets or aerosols and use low- or high-volume vacuum cleaners to reduce them [6]. Since the viral load in saliva is very high, rinsing with antiseptic mouthrinses can only reduce the infectious amount, but is not able to eliminate virus [7]. The Regional Federation of Medical Surgeons and Dentists has also made available guidelines for patient management, where the telephone triage is mandatory with simple questions (Figure 1), to be able to frame the patient and assess the existence of an impossible performance. In addition, it is necessary to provide adequate air exchange in the operating room after each individual patient and to have adequate personal protective equipment. Among the figures working in the dental team, one of the most exposed professionals is definitely the dental hygienist, both for the close working distance, and for the use of instrumentation able to produce a large amount of aerosol [8]. In fact, ultrasonic scalers produce contaminant aerosols [9], defined as the suspension of extremely fine particles in the air, which can be liquid, solid, or a combination of both, with a diameter of 50 μm or less [10], and which may transmit pathogenic micro-organisms dangerous to health [11,12]. It can therefore be said that most dental procedures produce droplets and contaminant aerosols. This risk is related to the number of pathogens present in the aerosol/spray, and some instruments, such as rotating instruments, ultrasonic scalers and piezo tools, produce a greater amount of spray and aerosols than other instruments such as air-to-water syringes. The SARS-CoV-2 virus has a high affinity for epithelial lung cells and those of the salivary glands (large number of ACE2 receptors), and during a oral hygiene session with an infected patient, a large amount of virus is excreted to the aerosol spray, which can be inhaled by the health professional; the ACE2 expressing cells in oral tissues might provide possible routes of entry for the 2019-nCov, and thus, the oral cavity might be a potential risk route of 2019-nCov infection [13,14]. Bizzocca et al. have attributed risk scores for the dental team and patients for each procedure to be: direct contact with saliva (score 1), direct contact with blood (score 2), production of low levels of spray/aerosol via air–water syringes (score 3), the production of high levels of spray/aerosol by use of rotating, ultrasound and piezoelectric tools (score 4): "tartar scaling" has one of the most high risk (7.5), such as some surgical or endodontic procedures [15].

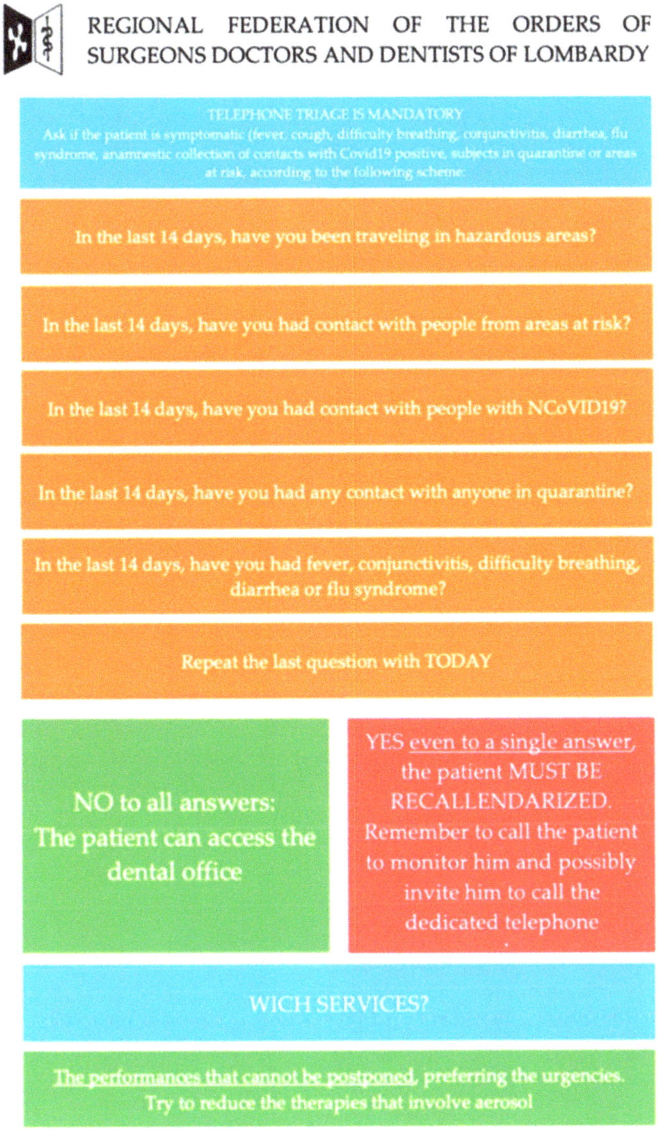

Figure 1. Telephone triage before entering the office.

Several strategies can be implemented to contain this problem, such as antiseptic pre-treatment rinsing, which helps control the infectious agents in aerosol [16,17], reducing the colonies by up to 94% [18], or the use of a rubber dam, which would seem to eliminate any contamination from blood and saliva. In fact, the latter has several limitations, as it is inapplicable in the procedures of scaling–root planning (SRP), periodontal surgery and prophylaxis routine. Reducing bacteriemia must be among the main objectives of nonsurgical periodontal therapy, regardless of the historical moment in which we are living: it is necessary to manage the production of contaminating aerosols, favoring therapies that make use of new technologies, which are increasingly minimally invasive, such as lasers, ozone and probiotics, and disinfectants with bactericidal action, such as chlorhexidine and ozone (although the latter require further studies to validate their effectiveness).

1.2. Oral Microbiota and Periodontal Disease

A well-balanced oral microbiota is essential in preventing the onset of oral cavity diseases. However, we do not always find ourselves in a state of eubiosis, and therefore in that physiological condition of functional balance in which bacteria and structures operate in a balanced manner, favoring absorption and regulation of the system. Very often, in fact, we move from a state of microbial equilibrium in which the oral microbiota produces the metabolites necessary for the human body, with positive effects for human health, and we move to a state of dysbiosis. In this particular condition, not only does the gene coding of useful molecules fail, but harmful compounds are partially metabolized by pathogenic microorganisms, also part of the microbiota. By the term of dysbiosis is meant, therefore, the pathological condition of functional imbalance of the digestive system, where the functions of the selective barrier are lost [19]. The clinical objective is to restore the symbiotic balance between bacteria and host.

Periodontal disease is a multifactorial, degenerative and irreversible disease affecting the tissues supporting the teeth: one of the main factors is undoubtedly the formation of bacterial biofilms. Its control, in fact, promotes the prevention and maintenance of good health by the oral cable [20].

Therefore, the basic periodontal treatment aims to eliminate hard and soft deposits above and below the gingiva, establishing the conditions to allow effective control of the bacterial plaque: in this sense, scaling and root planning through the use of manual and ultrasonic instrumentation, turns out to be the gold-standard procedure for debridement of root surfaces, demonstrating clinical and microbiological benefits [21]. However, traditional nonsurgical periodontal therapy has limitations: longer sessions, less comfort for the patient, excessive instrumentation (overtreatment); it is also performed in several sessions, usually one appointment for each quadrant, so there is the possibility of bacterial recolonization with consequent delay in the healing of the patient [22].

In the context of the increasing new approaches to periodontal treatment and in view of the increasing possibility of a proactive therapy, that is, a therapy able to solve clinical problems at the first symptoms or to prevent them altogether, bio-inspired protocols have been developed for the achievement of health conditions and the respect of tissues, favoring the restoration of a microbiological balance. This is made possible by the new technology available, which has enabled the introduction of different methods for the treatment of patients with periodontal disease, using the support of laser devices, ozone therapy, airflow powders based on glycine and/or erythritol, and also the use of probiotics, thus reducing the chemical–pharmacological action. From the literature, we know that the laser has been extensively studied to highlight its benefits in nonsurgical periodontal treatment. From different clinical trials, in fact, it is clear that the main effects are found in the reduction of the probing depth and in the gain of the clinical attachment with the use of a Er:YAG laser (as described in [23], after nonsurgical periodontal therapy in [24], and laser compared with SRP alone in [25]), but also Nd:YAG laser was used in cases where there was bleeding on probing, after nonsurgical periodontal therapy with ultrasonic and hand instruments [26,27]. Further improvements were found in the decrease in levels of IL-1β and TNF-α following photodynamic therapy [28]. The lasers used were used at different wavelengths, even surgically, associated with or compared to nonsurgical periodontal therapy. Additional benefits are evident with the use of ozone devices in the most significant periodontal clinical parameters, resulting in reduction of inflammatory parameters in a quarterly follow-up, such as PTX-3, IL-1β, Hs CRP [29], and bacterial count [30], especially of aggregatibacter actinomycentemcomintans (reduction of 25%) [31]. As for glycine and/or erythritol powders, on the other hand, they are more frequently used in periodontal support therapy for the removal of the subgingival biofilm, with greater comfort for the patient [32–34]. Finally, the use of probiotics showed an improvement in the epidemiological indices of reference for periodontal disease [35], as well as a reduction of the bacteria belonging to the red and orange complex of socransky and the proinflammatory cytokines [36].

Additionally, it is known from the literature that chlorhexidine is the antibacterial compound with bactericidal action most used as a support of periodontal therapy, in favor of the reduction of the pocket depth [37,38] and in the change of the subgingival microbiota [39,40]; is mainly used in the form associated with the Xanthan gel, when the latter is able to stabilize the molecule in subgingival tissues for a sufficient time [38]. On the basis of this information and available knowledge, a study was conducted to verify the effects of chlorhexidine on the oral microbiome, and it emerged that it significantly increased the abundance of Firmicutes and Proteobacteria and reduced the content of Bacteroidetes, TM7, SR1 and Fusobacteria. This shift was associated with a significant decrease in saliva pH and buffering capacity, accompanied by increased levels of lactate and saliva glucose. Lower concentrations of saliva and plasma nitrites were found after the use of chlorhexidine, followed by a tendency to increase systolic pressure. Overall, this study shows that mouthwash containing chlorhexidine is associated with an important change in the salivary microbiome, which leads to more acidic conditions and a lower availability of nitrites [41]. In addition, it is shown that a rinse with chlorhexidine prior to any dental procedure can reduce the likelihood of cross-infection, due to the presence of bacteria in the environment and the spread of aerosols [42], and the risk of bacterial infections [43], which can be induced by simple oral hygiene maneuvers, but also by more complex procedures, such as scaling and root planning [44]. In fact, periodontal disease contributes to systemic blood flow and to the migration of microorganisms, and their products, throughout the body [45,46]: bacteria have developed mechanisms to invade and adapt in host cells, escaping the host's immune response and releasing free toxins, causing transient bacteremia. This explains the relationship between oral and systemic conditions and the importance of pre-treatment rinses with antimicrobial action, from which it is reasonable to expect a positive effect on bacteremia.

In order to approach bio-inspired systems, even in this historical context, without giving up the tools now needed in daily clinical practice, it is essential to focus on the concept of bacteremia and generation of aerosols, to understand how to best manage the instrumentation, evaluating scientifically validated protocols in literature: all these protocols, aim at the reduction of bacteriemia and therefore the bacterial load present in aerosols.

A patient with altered periodontal status needs strict controls that aim at restoring biological conditions and are minimally invasive, such as the use of ultrasonic inserts that are best suited to the shape of the element taken into consideration, or diamond inserts, if forks are also involved; the aggressiveness of a manual instrumentation would lead to a the re-entry of bleeding and periodontal pockets, but also to a greater loss of tissue, that is, an increase of the gum recessions and probable loss of adherent gums. Moreover, in an environment that is increasingly being defined by the mini-invasiveness of any therapy that aims at restoring the aesthetic, also antimicrobial agents should be reviewed. Similar results to those obtainable with the irrigation of the pockets with chlorhexidine, are with the use of ozone, whether in liquid, gaseous or gel form for an immediate decontamination of the grooves and/or periodontal pockets, being a powerful natural disinfectant. Additionally, for the control of gingival inflammation and for a proper restoration of the oral microbiome, an alternative may be the use of lactobacilli-based probiotics, administering two of them daily, in such a way as to reduce the bacterial population, particularly streptococci. Another aspect to take into account during the treatment of periodontal disease is the treatment of hard tissues with bio-inspired materials. Biomimetics nanohydroxyapatite products can be recommended for the remineralization of dental enamel, allowing a more accurate retention of surfaces [47], especially during orthodontic treatment than can alter the oral environment [46] and detersion efficacy [48].

Bad oral hygiene habits can encourage the accumulation of periodontal pathogens in the oral cavity and dysbiosis can accelerate the decline of lung function: in addition, pathogenic bacteria such as treponema denticola, P. gingivalis, fusobacterium nucleatum, aggregatibacter actinomycetemcomitans and veillonella parvula, were found in the lungs of patients admitted to the ICU [49]. Their presence, can not only change the microbial composition of the respiratory system, but also promote a number of responses of cytokines, affecting the immune homeostasis of the lungs: spherical levels of IL-6 and IL-8 increase significantly in patients with pulmonary dysfunction and local inflammatory factors spread into the systemic circulation. Changes in cytokines are assumed to reflect the state of the disease to a certain extent [50].

A high bacterial and viral load in the mouth can lead to complications in systemic diseases such as cardiovascular diseases, neurodegenerative diseases and autoimmune diseases, further supporting the bond between the mouth and the body: risk factors established for COVID-19 (age, sex and comorbidity) are also strongly implicated in imbalances in the oral microbiome. In fact, diabetes, blood hypertension and heart disease are associated with a greater number of F. nucleatum, P. intermedia and P. gingivalis, favoring the progression of periodontal disease: Patients with periodontal disease increase the risk for cardiovascular disease by 25%, for high blood pressure by 20% and triple the risk for diabetes mellitus [51–54]. Epithelial sensitization and hematogenic diffusion of proinflammatory mediators such as cytokines, produced in the periodontal diseased tissue, can increase systemic inflammation and decrease airflow: this can be exacerbated by the stimulation of the liver to produce acute phase proteins, such as interleukin-6, which boost the inflammatory response of the lungs and the rest of the body. Similarly, patients with COVID-19 in severe form also express systemic inflammation and higher levels of IL-6, IL-2, IL-10, TNF and C-reactive protein [55].

2. Materials and Methods

2.1. Focus Question

Can the use of lasers, ozone, probiotics, glycine and/or erythritol, chlorhexidine in combination with nonsurgical periodontal treatment have additional beneficial effects on the clinical parameters of periodontal disease? Can these bio-inspired instruments be used to reduce the risk of bacteremia during COVID-19 disease?

2.2. Elegibility Criteria

First, we have analyzed studies in accordance with the following inclusion criteria:

Type of studies. Randomized controlled clinical trials, controlled clinical trials, prospective clinical trials, in vivo retrospective clinical trials with the approval of the Ethics Committee.

Types of participants. Participants with chronic and/or aggressive periodontal disease were considered. (1) Patients undergoing periodontal surgery or nonsurgical periodontal treatment within three months prior to the beginning of the clinical trials examined were excluded; (2) undergoing maintenance therapy or periodontal support, or (3) treatment of residual pockets, following periodontal or nonsurgical surgical therapy; (4) patients with concomitant systemic pathologies that could have affected the periodontal outcome were excluded.

Type of interventions. Clinical trials that have compared benefits for scaling and root planning in quadrant or full-mouth (SRP/FMD). The experimental group assisted by one or more laser treatments such as, diode lasers, Er:YAG laser, Nd:YAG laser, Er, Cr:YSGG laser, photobiomodulation (PBM), photodinamic therapy (PDT); ozone treatments such as, ozone gas, ozone water, ozone gel; treatments with probiotics such as Lactobacillus or Bifidobacterium; treatments with glycine airpolishing or periopolishing; treatments with erythritol airpolishing or periopolishing; chlorhexidine treatments such as, chlorhexidine mouthwash, gel, chip or varnish. One or more control groups administered a placebo or control treatment other than the experimental one.

Outcome type. Primary outcomes: plaque index (PI), blindind on probing (BOP), probing depth (PPD), and clinical attachment level (CAL). Other clinical parameters, where present, such as gingival index (GI), gingival recession (GR(REC)), gingival margin index (MGI), modified bleeding index (MBI), gingival bleeding index (GBI), sulcular bleeding index (SBI), full mouth plaque score (FMPS), visible plaque index (VPI), visible plaque index (API) and microbiological and immunological parameters have been considered.

We have included in the second phase only those studies that met all the inclusion criteria, that is to say, the analysis of the selected studies according to the exclusion criteria: (1) clinical studies where the authors have not reported at least one of the clinical parameters chosen as outcomes; (2) clinical studies where participants have undergone periodontal surgery or nonsurgical periodontal treatment during the 3 months prior to the beginning of the clinical trials examined; (3) clinical studies performed on participants with concomitant systemic pathologies that could have affected the periodontal outcome; (4) studies performed on participants in support/maintenance therapy; (5) clinical studies carried out on participants for the treatment of residual pockets, following periodontal surgical or nonsurgical therapy; (6) clinical studies where laser, ozone, probiotics, glycine, erythritol or chlorhexidine have not been used as a test group; (7) in vitro or animal clinical studies; (8) clinical trials carried out without the approval of the Ethics Committee.

The risk of bias was determined evaluating: adequate sequence generated (participants should be allocated to groups, using a true randomization sequence), allocation concealment (participants and investigators should not be able to predict allocation before participants are included in the study), blinding (participants and investigators should be unaware of the allocation to ensure that everyone gets the same amount of attention; the blindness of those who evaluate the outcomes may reduce the risk that knowledge of the intervention received, influence the measurement of outcomes), incomplete outcome data (report should describe how the outcomes have been measured in the method section) and registration of outcome (results should be reported for each outcome identified at the beginning).

2.3. Search Strategy

The review is based on the research of clinical trials (RCTs) in reference to the PICOT model (Population, Intervention, Comparison, Outcome, Timing), identified through bibliographic research in electronic databases, examining the bibliography of articles, on Pubmed (MEDLINE) and Google Scholar. Initially, all abstracts of clinical studies published from January 2010 to March 2020 were taken into consideration which evaluated the effect of the addition of laser therapy, ozone therapy, probiotics, glycine and erythritol, chlorhexidine to nonsurgical periodontal therapy in the treatment of periodontal disease.

2.4. Research

We performed the search using: "periodontal disease", "periodontitis", "nonsurgical periodontal treatment", "laser", "RCTs AND laser AND periodontal disease", "laser AND periodontitis", "laser AND nonsurgical periodontal treatment", "ozone", "RCTs AND ozone AND periodontal disease", "ozone AND periodontitis", "ozone AND nonsurgical periodontal treatment", "probiotics", "RCTs AND probiotics AND periodontal disease", "probiotics AND periodontitis", "probiotics AND nonsurgical periodontal treatment", "RCTs AND glycine AND periodontal disease", "glycine AND periodontitis", "glycine AND nonsurgical periodontal treatment", "erythritol", "RCTs AND erythritol AND periodontal disease", "erythritol AND periodontitis", "erythritol AND nonsurgical periodontal treatment", "chlorhexidine", "RCTs AND chlorhexidine AND periodontal disease", "chlorhexidine AND periodontitis", "chlorhexidine AND nonsurgical periodontal treatment". We have included patients with chronic periodontitis or aggressive periodontitis, based on the classification of periodontal diseases proposed by Armitage in 1999 and the new classification presented on 22 June 2018 on the occasion of the Europerio9.

2.5. Screening and Selection of Articles

Titles and abstracts were collected, in which were present the search keywords and the information related to the inclusion criteria to proceed with the reading in full-text. After reading in detail, the studies that met all the selection criteria were evaluated, to then extract and analyze the data collected.

2.6. Search Outcome and Evaluation

The first research outcomes were PI, BOP, PPD, CAL. Other interesting outcomes, where present, were the changes in the subgingival plate. Information was extracted from each study on (1) participants' characteristics (age and disease characteristics) and criteria for inclusion and exclusion from the clinical trial in question; (2) intervention (modality) vs. placebo or vs. no treatment or vs. comparison treatment (different from the one tested, therefore different from laser, ozone, glycine, erythritol, probiotics and chlorhexidine); (3) outcome (possible improvement of the clinical parameters examined for the treatment groups included); (4) clinical data examined (PPD, CAL, BOP, PI); (5) other clinical data (possible microbiological evaluation); (6) follow-up.

3. Results

3.1. Study Selection

A total of 458 articles on the use of minimally invasive technologies in nonsurgical periodontal treatment emerged from several researchers. Subsequently, from a first reading of the abstracts found, we eliminated: (1) articles emerged in more researches carried out; (2) review and meta-analysis; (3) articles on the treatment of mucositis and peri-implantitis; (4) articles on the treatment of gingivitis; (5) articles on the treatment of gingivitis and periodontitis in orthodontic treatment. A total of 96 studies were therefore identified (52 laser studies; 8 ozone studies; 10 airpolishing studies; 25 probiotic studies; 21 chlorhexidine studies) on nonsurgical periodontal treatment, approved by the Ethics Committee.

In a second phase, following the full-text reading, 11 clinical studies (4 inherent to the laser; 1 inherent to the ozone; 1 inherent to the airpolishing; 4 inherent to the probiotics; 1 inherent to the chlorhexidine), of which there was only the availability of reading the abstract and further 10 studies not in compliance with the eligibility criteria.

74 articles have been included (36 RCTs nonsurgical periodontal therapy (NSPT) + laser; 5 RCTs NSPT + ozone; 3 RCTs NSPT + airpolishing; 15 RCTs NSPT + probiotics; 15 RCTs NSPT + chlorhexidine; Figure 2).

3.2. Characteristics of Studies

3.2.1. NSPT and Laser

Methods. The 36 studies selected for the review were randomized clinical trials published in English. The duration of studies varied from 1 to 12 months for a total average of about 5 months (5.25), where 5.5% of studies had a follow-up of 1 month, 2.8% of 2 months, 30.6% of 3 months (these studies have some limits related to pocket depth and clinical attachment gain, because the follow-up is too short to allow the re-attachment), 50% of 6 months and 11.1% of 1 year. The 27.8% of the studies analyzed were conducted in Turkey, a further 27.8% in Brazil and India (equally distributed), 8.3% in Spain, 11.1% in Italy and China (equally distributed) and 25% in Germany, the Netherlands, Poland, Croatia, Greece, Iran, Serbia, Arabia and Thailand (equally distributed). Randomization of the studies was performed with different methods: computer-generated table, where the majority of allocation concealment was done through the use of opaque sealed envelopes, or tossing/flipping a coin; the 58.3% of clinical trials was designed in split-mouth.

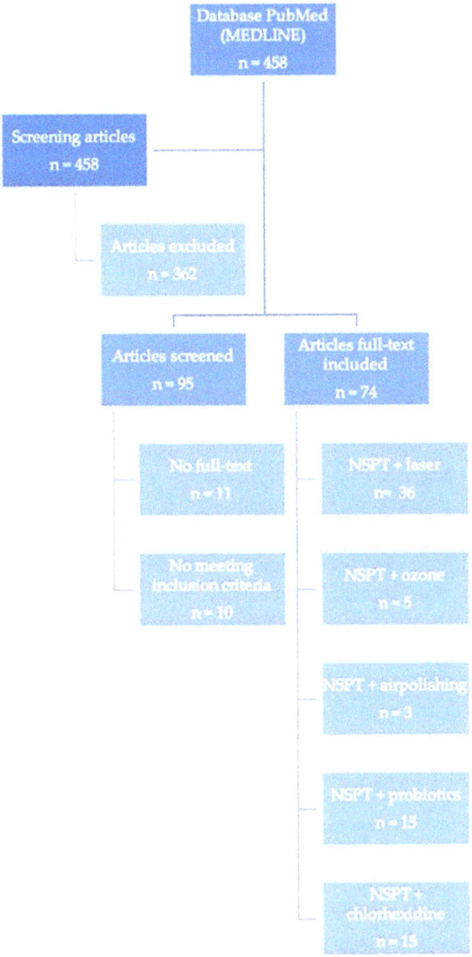

Figure 2. Articles included in the present investigation. NSPT: nonsurgical periodontal therapy.

Participants. Studies on average recruited about 31 patients (31.61), where 66.7% of studies included ≤31 patients and 33.3% of studies included >31 patients. The main inclusion criteria included: age ≥18 (100% of the studies examined), presence of at least 2 teeth with at least 1 site with PPD and bleeding on probing in each quadrant, have not undergone periodontal surgery or nonsurgical periodontal treatment within 3 months prior to the start of clinical trials, without any systemic pathology that could affect periodontal clinical parameters and patients who did not require antibiotic prophylaxis for dental treatments.

Interventions. Patients underwent nonsurgical periodontal treatment (scaling and root planning in full-mouth or in quadrants) in addition to laser therapy for the test group. The 25% of the studies used the PDT, 19.4% the diode laser, 16.7% Er:YAG laser, 16.7% used Nd:YAG laser or Er,Cr:YSGG laser (equally distributed), 13.9% the PBM, 5.6% used a combination with Er:YAG and Nd:YAG laser and 2.7% of the studies used, instead, a combination of PDT and PBM. The control group was only subjected to nonsurgical periodontal therapy. Some of the studies included used one or more test groups (eight clinical trials, 22.2% of the total studies) and one or more control groups (one clinical trial, 2.8% of the total studies). The patients have undergone scaling and root planning with ultrasonic and hand instruments: the laser was used, in most cases, immediately after nonsurgical periodontal treatment, except for some lasers (such as Er:YAG) that were used before therapy.

Primary outcomes. In most of the studies they were PPD and CAL; in one study, among the primary outcomes, was also the bacterial count; all studies have evaluated every type of adverse event. The frequency of evaluation of outcomes was variable: monthly, quarterly, half-yearly or a single final evaluation at one year.

Secondary and additional outcomes. BOP, PI (or VPI, FMPS), API GI, SBI, bleeding index (BI), GR (REC) were clinical parameters evaluated in addition to the probing depth and the loss of clinical attachment; they have not been recorded in all the studies examined. Some studies have also performed microbiological and immunological (61.1% of the total); other studies: one study evaluated the perception of the patient during treatment; one study evaluated fluctuation of periodontal somatosensory function and gingival microcirculation and two further studies evaluated the patient's halitosis.

3.2.2. NSPT and Ozone

Methods. The 5 studies selected for review were randomized clinical trials published in English. The duration of studies varied from 1 to 3 months for a total average of about 2 months (2.2), where 20% of studies had a follow-up of 1 month, 80% a follow-up of 2 and 3 months (40% each). Additionally, in these clinical trials the follow-up is too short for evaluate improvements in clinical parameters. The 60% of the studies were conducted in Turkey, while the remaining clinical trials were conducted in Japan and Poland. Randomization of studies was performed with different methods: computer-generated/randomization list or tossing a coin; the 40% of studies were designed in split-mouth.

Participants. Studies on average recruited about 32 patients (32.2), where 40% of studies included ≤32 patients, while 60% of studies included >32 patients. The main inclusion criteria included: age ≥18 (100% of the studies examined), presence of at least a 2 teeth with at least 1 site with PPD and bleeding on probing in each quadrant, have not undergone periodontal surgery or nonsurgical periodontal treatment within 3 months prior to the start of clinical trials, without any systemic pathology that could affect periodontal clinical parameters and patients who did not require antibiotic prophylaxis for dental treatments.

Interventions. Patients underwent nonsurgical periodontal treatment (scaling and root planning in full-mouth or in quadrants) in addition to ozone therapy. Most studies used ozone in gaseous form, while one study evaluated the effect of NBW3 (ozonated water nanobubbles). The patients have undergone to scaling and root planning with ultrasonic and hand instruments: ozone was used immediately after periodontal treatment.

Primary outcomes. In most of the studies they were PPD and CAL. In one study they were included as primary outcomes PPD, GI, PI and BOP (the difference between these variables was then used as secondary outcomes); all studies evaluated each type of adverse event. The frequency of evaluation of outcomes was variable: monthly or quarterly.

Secondary and additional outcomes. BOP, PI, GI, SBI, API are clinical parameters evaluated in addition to the probing depth and the loss of clinical attachment; they have not been recorded in all the studies examined. A microbiological and/or immunological evaluation was carried out in all the studies examined; one study evaluated the antioxidant status (TAS), total oxidant status (TOS), nitric oxide (NO), 8-hydroxy-2′-deoxyguanosine (8-Ohdg), myeloperoxidase (MPO), glutathione (GSH), malondialdehyde (MDA), and transforming growth factor-beta (TGF-β) and one study evaluated the MMP-1, MMP-8 and MMP-9 levels.

3.2.3. NSPT and Airpolishing

Methods. The 3 studies selected for the review were randomized clinical trials published in English. The duration of the studies varied from 1 to 6 months: 1 study had a follow-up of 1 month,

1 study had a follow-up of 3 months and the last one a follow-up of 6 months; two studies had a too short treatment period for settlement of clinical improvement acts. The three clinical trials were conducted in Korea, Turkey and China. Randomization of studies and was performed with different methods: computer-randomized or tossing a coin.

Participants. Studies have on average recruited 36 patients, where 66.7% (two studies) included ≤36 patients and 33.3% (one study only) included >36 patients. The main inclusion criteria included: age ≥18 (100% of the studies examined), presence of at least a 2 teeth with at least 1 site with PPD and bleeding on probing in each quadrant, have not undergone periodontal surgery or nonsurgical periodontal treatment within 3 months prior to the start of clinical trials, without any systemic pathology that could affect periodontal clinical parameters and patients who did not require antibiotic prophylaxis for dental treatments.

Interventions. Patients underwent nonsurgical periodontal treatment (scaling and root planning in full-mouth or in quadrants) in addition to airpolishing with glycine and/or erythritol immediately after treatment (two studies with glycine and one study with erythritol).

Primary outcomes. Studies carried out evaluated PPD, CAL, BOP; all studies evaluated each type of adverse event. The frequency of evaluation of outcomes was variable: monthly or quarterly.

Secondary and additional outcomes. PI, GI, GR are clinical parameters evaluated in addition to the probing depth and the loss of clinical attachment; they have not been recorded in all the studies examined. Two studies performed a microbiological or immunological analysis; one study only evaluated the patient's halitosis through volatile sulfur compounds (VSCs).

3.2.4. NSPT and Probiotics

Methods. The 15 studies selected for the review were randomized clinical trials in English. The duration of studies varied from 1 to 12 months for a total average of 5 months, where: 26.7% of studies had a follow-up of 1 month, 6.7% a follow-up of 2 months, 26.7% a follow-up of 3 months, 6.7% a follow-up of 9 months and 13.3% a follow-up of 1 year. In order to establish the effectiveness of therapy, it is necessary to ensure a follow-up of 3 months: so, the 33.4% of studies analyzed are insufficient to assess improvements. The portion of 26.7% of the studies were conducted in India, 20% in Turkey, 14.3% in Chile and 40% in China, Brazil, Iran, Spain, Pakistan, Arabia (equally distributed). Randomization of studies was performed using different methods: computer-based randomization and sealed opaque envelopes; one study was designed in split-mouth (for scaling and root planning (SRP) treatment).

Participants. Studies on average recruited 42 patients (42.86), where 80% of studies included ≤46 patients and 20% included >46 patients. The main inclusion criteria included: age ≥18 (100% of the studies examined), presence of at least a 2 teeth with at least 1 site with PPD and bleeding on probing in each quadrant, have not undergone periodontal surgery or nonsurgical periodontal treatment within 3 months prior to the start of clinical trials, without any systemic pathology that could affect periodontal clinical parameters and patients who did not require antibiotic prophylaxis for dental treatments.

Interventions. Patients underwent nonsurgical periodontal treatment (scaling and root planning in full-mouth or in quadrants) in addition to the administration of probiotics, mainly bifidobacteria and lactobacilli. Some of the studies included used one or more test groups (four clinical trials, 26.7% of the total studies) and one or more control groups (one clinical trial, 6.7% of the total studies). In the majority of studies probiotics were administered in lozenges (in two studies probiotics were administered in mouthwash and in one study they were administered in sachets).

Primary outcomes. In most of the studies they were PPD and CAL; all studies evaluated each type of adverse event. The frequency of evaluation of outcomes was variable: monthly, quarterly, half-yearly or a single final evaluation at one year.

Secondary and additional outcomes. BOP, PI, SBI, GI, GBI, MGI, MBI are clinical parameters evaluated in addition to the probing depth and the loss of clinical attachment; they have not been recorded in all the studies examined. Some studies have also performed microbiological and immunological (60% of the total); one study has also evaluated halitosis through ORG and BANA tests.

3.2.5. NSPT and Chlorhexidine

Methods. The 15 studies selected for the review were randomized clinical trials in English. The duration of studies varied from 1 to 12 months for a total average of 3 months (3.8), where: 20% had a follow-up of 1 month, 53.3% a follow-up of 3 months, 20% a follow-up of 6 months and 6.7% a follow-up of 1 year; 20% of studies, that have had a follow-up of 1 month, are unsuitable to provide effective results in pocket depth and in the gain of clinical attachment. 46.7% of the studies were conducted in India, 13.3% in Germany and 40% in Bosnia and Herzegovina, Iran, Italy, Arabia, Brazil, Spain (also distributed). Randomization of the studies was performed with different methods: computer-generated table, where the majority of allocation concealment was done through the use of opaque sealed envelopes, or tossing/flipping a coin; the 40% of clinical trials was designed in split-mouth.

Participants. Studies have on average recruited 36 patients (36.3), where 66.7% of studies included ≤36 patients and 33.3% included >36 participants. The main inclusion criteria included: age ≥18 (100% of the studies examined), presence of at least a 2 teeth with at least 1 site with PPD and bleeding on probing in each quadrant, have not undergone periodontal surgery or nonsurgical periodontal treatment within 3 months prior to the start of clinical trials, without any systemic pathology that could affect periodontal clinical parameters and patients who did not require antibiotic prophylaxis for dental treatments.

Interventions. Patients underwent nonsurgical periodontal treatment (scaling and root planning in full-mouth or in quadrants) in addition to rinsing or gingival irrigations with chlorhexidine after therapy (mouthwash, gel, chip or varnish). Some of the included studies used one or more test groups (60% of the total studies) and one or more control groups (13.3% of the total studies).

Primary outcomes. In most of the studies they were PPD and CAL; all studies evaluated each type of adverse event. The frequency of evaluation of outcomes was variable: monthly, quarterly, half-yearly or a single final evaluation at one year.

Secondary and additional outcomes. BOP, PI (PS), GR (REC), PBI, GI, BGI are clinical parameters evaluated in addition to the probing depth and loss of clinical attachment; they have not been recorded in all studies examined. Some studies have also performed microbiological (or analysis of plaque) and immunological (46.7% of the total); one study has also taken into analysis systemic and hematological parameters.

3.3. *Synthesis of Results*

3.3.1. PPD

PPD and Laser

The probing depth has improved in all clinical trials examined; only one study did not consider PPD as a clinical parameter. For a total of 35 studies, therefore, although there was an improvement, there were no statistically significant differences between treatment groups in 65.7% of studies; there was a higher gain in pocket depth for the test group (statistically significant difference between treatment groups) in 31.4% of studies (one study showed a greater reduction in PPD in the control group, subject to only scaling and root planning). A portion of 54.5% of these were treated with PDT or Er:YAG laser (equally distributed) and 45.5% with PBM (photobiomodulation), diode laser or Nd:YAG laser, a combination of Er:YAG and Nd:YAG or a combination of PDT and PBM, (equally distributed); there was an improvement in pockets greater than or equal to 7 mm [25,56–59] and a reduction in sites with PPD greater than 4.5 mm [60]. In some clinical trials, although there were no significant differences between treatment groups, the probing depth was significantly reduced in the test group [25,56–65].

PPD and Ozone

The probing depth has improved in all the clinical trials examined. For a total of 5 studies, therefore, although found an improvement, there were no statistically significant differences between treatment groups; one study found an improvement in the PPD parameter in favor of ozone therapy, although there were no significant differences [30].

PPD and Airpolishing

The probing depth has improved in all the clinical trials examined. For a total of 3 studies, therefore, although there was an improvement, there were no statistically significant differences between treatment groups.

PPD and Probiotics

The probing depth has improved in all the clinical trials examined. For a total of 15 studies, although there was an improvement, there were no statistically significant differences between treatment groups in 60% of studies; there was more gain in pocket depth for the test group (statistically significant difference between treatment groups) in 40% of studies. Of these 66.7% were treated with strains of lactobacilli and 33.3% with strains of bifidobacteria or a combination of lactobacilli and bifidobacteria (equally distributed). In some clinical trials, although there were no significant differences between treatment groups, the depth of the survey was reduced more in the test group for moderate and deep periodontal pockets [66–68].

PPD and Chlorhexidine

The probing depth has improved in all the clinical trials examined. For a total of 15 studies, although there was an improvement, there were no statistically significant differences between treatment groups in 53.3% of studies; there was more gain in pocket depth for the test group (statistically significant difference between treatment groups) in 46.7% of studies. Of these 57.1% was treated with chlorhexidine chip or chlorhexidine gel (equally distributed) and 42.9% was treated with chlorhexidine mouthwash, chlorhexidine varnish or a full-mouth disinfection protocol (then gingival irrigation with chlorhexidine gel, tongue brushing with chlorhexidine gel and rinsing with chlorhexidine mouthwash), equally distributed.

3.3.2. CAL

CAL and Laser

The loss of clinical attachment has improved in all the clinical trials examined; three studies have not considered CAL (RAL) as a clinical parameter. For a total of 33 studies, therefore, although there was an improvement, there were no statistically significant differences between treatment groups in 66.7% of studies; there was a higher gain in clinical attack for the test group (statistically significant difference between treatment groups) in 33.3% of studies. Of these 54.5% was treated with PDT, PBM, or a combination of Er:YAG and Nd:YAG (equally distributed) and 18.2% with Er:YAG, diode laser or a combination of PDT and PBM, equally distributed; an improvement was observed in pockets greater than 4.5 mm [58] and over 7 mm [25,58].

CAL and Ozone

The loss of clinical attachment is improved in all the clinical trials examined. For a total of 5 studies there was an improvement in follow-up, although, even in this case, there were no significant differences between treatment groups; one study found a greater gain in clinical attachment in favor of ozone therapy, without significant differences [30].

CAL and Airpolishing

The loss of clinical attachment is improved in all the clinical trials examined. For a total of 3 studies, there was therefore an improvement in follow-up, although, again, there were no significant differences between treatment groups.

CAL and Probiotics

The loss of clinical attachment has improved in all clinical trials examined. For a total of 15 studies, although there was an improvement, there were no statistically significant differences between treatment groups in 75% of studies; there was more gain in pocket depth for the test group (statistically significant difference between treatment groups) in 25% of studies. Of these 66.7% were treated with lactobacilli strains and only one study with bifidobacteria strains. In some clinical trials, although there were no significant differences between treatment groups, the gain in clinical attachment was best in the test group, for moderate or severe periodontal pockets [67].

CAL and Chlorhexidine

The loss of clinical attachment improved in all clinical trials examined; two studies did not consider CAL as a clinical parameter. For a total of 13 studies, although there was an improvement, there were no statistically significant differences between treatment groups in 69.2%; there was a higher gain in clinical attachment (statistically significant difference between treatment groups) in 23.1% of studies (one study found a greater improvement in CAL in the control group, subject to only scaling and root planning [69]).

3.3.3. BOP

BOP and Laser

Bleeding on probing improved in all clinical trials examined; 11 studies did not consider BOP. For a total of 25 studies, therefore, although there was an improvement, there were no statistically significant differences between treatment groups in 60% of studies; there was a higher gain in terms of BOP for the test group (statistically significant difference between treatment groups) in 12% of studies. Two studies have had greater improvements in bleeding at the poll for control groups [70,71].

BOP and Ozone

Bleeding on probing improved in all clinical trials examined; only one study did not consider BOP as a clinical parameter. For a total of 4 studies, there was therefore an improvement in follow-up, but there were no significant differences between treatment groups: one study reported significant improvements for bleeding on probing with the use of ozone [30].

BOP and Airpolishing

Bleeding on probing has improved in all the clinical trials examined. For a total of four studies, there was an improvement in follow-up, but there were no significant differences between treatment groups.

BOP and Probiotics

Bleeding on probing has improved in all clinical trials examined. For a total of 15 studies, although there was an improvement, there were no statistically significant differences between treatment groups in 72.7% of studies; there was a higher gain in terms of BOP for the test group (statistically significant difference between treatment groups) in 27.3% of studies (all treated with lactobacilli strains).

BOP and Chlorhexidine

Bleeding on probing has improved in all clinical trials examined; six studies did not consider BOP as a clinical parameter. For a total of 9 studies, therefore, although there was an improvement, there were no statistically significant differences between treatment groups in 66.7% of studies; there was a significant improvement for the test group (statistically significant difference between treatment groups) in 33.3% of studies.

3.3.4. PI

PI and Laser

The plaque index has improved in all the clinical trials examined; seven studies have not considered PI as a clinical parameter. For a total of 29 studies, therefore, although there was an improvement, there were no significant differences between treatment groups in 82.7% of studies; there was a greater improvement in the plaque index for the test group (statistically significant difference between treatment groups) in 13.8% of cases (one study had a better result in the control group [47]).

PI and Ozone

The plaque index has improved in all clinical trials examined; only one study did not consider PI as a clinical parameter. For a total of four studies, there was therefore an improvement in follow-up, but there were no significant differences between treatment groups.

PI and Airpolishing

The plaque index has improved in all clinical trials examined; only one study did not consider PI as a clinical parameter. For a total of two studies, there was therefore an improvement in follow-up, but there were no significant differences between treatment groups.

PI and Probiotics

The plaque index has improved in all clinical trials examined; only one study did not consider PI as a clinical parameter. For a total of 14 studies, although there was an improvement, there were no statistically significant differences between treatment groups in 71.4%; there was a greater improvement in plaque indices for the test group in 28.6% of studies (all treated with lactobacilli strains).

PI and Chlorhexidine

The plaque index has improved in all the clinical trials examined; two studies have not considered PI as a clinical parameter. For a total of 13 studies, although there was an improvement, there were no statistically significant differences between treatment groups in 46.1% of studies; there was a greater improvement in the plaque index for the test group (statistically significant difference between treatment groups) in 46.1% of studies (one study achieved a better result in SRP treatment [69]).

3.3.5. Microbiological and Immunological Analysis

Microbiological and Immunological Analysis: Laser

Improvements were found in bacterial count [72], in the number of pathogens belonging to the red complex [59] and orange [59,73], a reduction of aggregatibacter actinomycetemcomitans, porphyromonas gingivalis, prevotella intermedia, prevotella nigrescens, tannerella forsythia [24], an improvement in levels IL 1-β and TNα [26] and ratio levels of IL1-β and IL-10 [59].

Microbiological and Immunological Analysis: Ozone

There were improvements in GCF PTX-3 levels [29], an increase in TGF-β levels [73,74], a significant reduction in the number of bacteria present in subgingival plaque [30], especially prevotella intermedia [75]; one study found increased MMP levels in patients with chronic periodontitis and decreased MMP levels in patients with aggressive periodontitis [76].

Microbiological and Immunological Analysis: Airpolishing

There was an improvement in the number of bacteria present, with a difference in the relative expression of porphyromonas gingivalis [77] and a significant reduction in a quarterly follow-up of GCF [78].

Microbiological and Immunological Analysis: Probiotics

There have been improvements in bacterial count for obligatory anerobics [79], a reduction in red and orange complex bacteria [36,80], a reduction in proinflammatory cytokines [36] and an increase in TIMP-1 levels [81].

Microbiological and Immunological Analysis: Chlorhexidine

Improvements were found in anaerobic bacterial count [82], a reduction of the bacteria belonging to the red complex [83] and a reduction of capnocytophaga ssp. [84].

3.3.6. Results of Single Studies and Bias

Supplementary Tables S1–S5 (these tables reported the number of participants who completed the follow-up and were included in the analysis of the results).

Table 1 shows the risk of bias of the main articles examined. This review present a relatively low risk of bias.

Table 1. Risk of Bias.

	Adequate Sequence Generated	Allocation Concealment	Blinding	Incomplete Outcome Data	Registration Outcome
Dukić 2013	+	+	+	+	+
de Melo Soares 2019	−	+	?	+	+
Moreira 2015	+	+	+	+	+
Gündoğar 2016	+	+	+	+	+
Hayakumo 2013	−	+	?	+	+
Teughels 2013	+	+	+	+	+
Lecic 2016	−	?	?	+	+
Park 2018	−	?	?	+	+
Vivekananda 2010	?	+	+	+	+

Green symbol: Low risk of bias; Yellow symbol: Moderate risk of bias; Red symbol: Elevate risk of bias.

4. Discussion

The purpose of this review was to assess the effectiveness of minimally invasive therapies, as adjuvants to nonsurgical periodontal therapy, in order to formulate operational protocols aimed at restoring optimal conditions, respecting biological tissues, but also to the reduction of bacteremia, in an increasingly evolving historical context.

The reduction of bacteriemia is the main objective of nonsurgical periodontal therapy: this would prevent the spread of proinflammatory mediators, such as cytokines, and increase systemic inflammation; in addition, trying to reduce the bacterial load of patients, would reduce the production of highly contaminating aerosols. We must promote the use of rinse chlorhexidine or hydrogen peroxide before each dental procedure, the adoption of new therapies such as laser and ozone, the administration of probiotics, in order to minimize the use of instruments that produce aerosols, such as ultrasound and air and periopolishing systems.

4.1. Rinse Pre-Treatment

As already mentioned, it is generally believed that a preoperative antimicrobial mouthwash reduces the bacterial charge inside the oral cavity. However, as indicated by The Guidelines for the diagnosis and treatment of new coronavirus pneumonia (fifth edition), chlorhexidine is not effective to kill SARS-CoV-2 [2]. It is vulnerable to oxidation, therefore, the use of oxidizing agents containing 1% hydrogen peroxide or 0.2% iodopovidone is recommended in order to reduce the salivary load of oral microbes, including the potential transport of virus [85,86], before all dental procedures; a mouthwash based on ozonated olive oil or the use of ozonated water appliances could be useful in this respect. Ozone, in fact, seems to be effective against virus [87].

4.2. Modified Full-Mouth Disinfection and Chlorhexidine

Chlorhexidine has always been used in nonsurgical periodontal treatment due to its antimicrobial, bactericidal and bacteriostatic effect (in concentrations from 0.12% to 0.20%), high substantivity and lack of systemic toxicity [37], effective in the reduction of periodontal indexes [88,89], resulting in this way an antiseptic useful to produce benefits in patients with periodontal disease [69,82–84,88–93]; other authors, instead, argue that the use of chlorhexidine is not able to produce additional benefits to the treatment, compared to only scaling and root planning [94], having a minor role even in the long term [95].

In 1995, Quirynen introduced the "full mouth disinfection" treatment to prevent reinfection of treated sites during conventional periodontal therapy (quadrant therapy). The treatment consists of scaling and root planning performed over a period of 24 h, combined with gingival irrigation with 1% chlorhexidine gel, tongue brushing with 1% chlorhexidine gel and final rinsing with 0.2% chlorhexidine mouthwash. Then the patients follow a 2-month home protocol, continuing to brush the tongue with a 1% chlorhexidine gel and a rinse with 0.20% mouthwash, twice a day. This approach is effective in reducing microbial load, resulting in improved periodontal indices [96].

In 2014, a study conducted by the Tuscan Stomatological Institute, proposed an amendment to the Quirynen protocol, elaborating the concept of modified full-mouth disinfection, with the idea that it was more effective to get the reduction of bacterial load before the session of scaling and root planning, performing the disinfection protocol with chlorhexidine two weeks before treatment. So the first session is dedicated exclusively to the motivation and instruction of the patient in order to reduce bacteremia and recondition tissues, establishing a relationship of trust: this approach aims to reduce the bacterial load and clinical indices, thus reducing the patient's discomfort, pain and bleeding before they can proceed to the treatment itself. Then we proceed to the actual treatment in full-mouth, with consequent revaluation in order to establish a tailor-made periodontal support therapy [97]. Therefore the results of this study showed a significant reduction of bleeding, thus favoring both the patient's comfort and the operator's procedure. In addition, the classic full-mouth approach highlights that the experience perceived by the patient is a fundamental component of the overall effect in nonsurgical full-mouth periodontal therapy, with anesthesia. In fact, the negative experience of anxiety results in a greater evasion resulting in delay in oral hygiene appointments and worsening of oral health [98].

The modified full-mouth, on the other hand, supports the modern trend towards more patient-centered approaches that become a proactive part of preventive therapy. Therefore, the real advantage of the two-week preparation period is the patient's understanding of the therapy, which, acting beforehand on the clinical symptoms before treatment, allows the use of local anesthetics [97,98].

4.3. Measures for Modified Full-Mouth Disinfection

We have already seen that in this case it is the risk of pre-therapy bacteremia, which allows to avoid manual overtreatment and tissue contraction, reducing the discomfort for the patient. Furthermore, in order to reduce the contaminating aerosol, in this case, an ultrasonic ablator can be used in 'soft-mode' mode, thus reducing the width of movement of the insert, maintaining the same frequency (Figure 3).

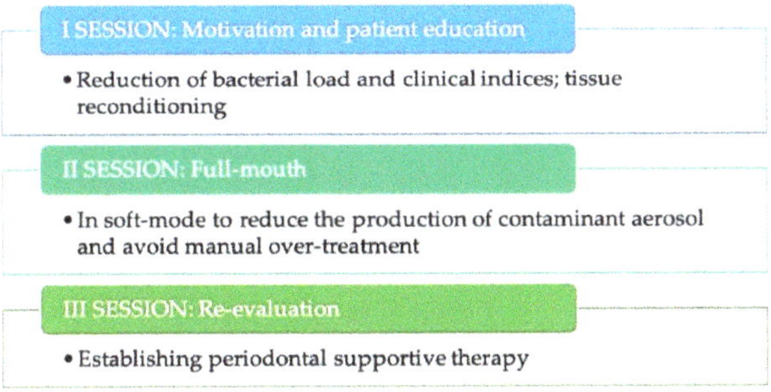

Figure 3. Sessions for modified full mout disinfection protocol.

However, as indicated by the Guidelines for the diagnosis and treatment of new coronavirus pneumonia (fifth edition), chlorhexidine, is not effective to kill SARS-CoV-2. It is vulnerable to oxidation, so it is recommended to use oxidizing agents containing 1% hydrogen peroxide or 0.2% iodopovidone, in order to reduce the salivary load of oral microbes, including the potential transport of virus [2]. So, in the light of this statement, we might consider modifying the pre- patient's home protocol treatment, for example the use of a gel based on sunflower oil ozonized 15% and rinse with a mouthwash based on ozonated olive oil.

4.4. Laser Therapy

For many years, the laser has been recommended as an additional or additional protocol in the treatment of nonsurgical periodontal disease [73], due to its ability to achieve tissue ablation effects, hemostats, bactericides and detoxifiers against periodontal pathogenic bacteria [99].

Several studies have proven the effectiveness of laser use during periodontal therapy, highlighting an improvement in depth of survey, in the gain of clinical attachment and in the reduction of gingival bleeding in moderate and severe pockets: after a single application of the 810 nm diode laser, improvements have been achieved in parameters such as PPD and CAL [56,73,100] but also in levels of IL1-β [62]; other authors, however, argue that there are no further benefits in clinical parameters with the use of a diode laser, compared to/e solo/e scaling and root planning [101]. Also photodynamic therapy produces benefits in periodontal pockets [102], in the index of gingival bleeding and in gingival inflammation [64], as well as being effective in single-rooted teeth with aggressive periodontal disease [59], as well as the PBM [61,103–105] and Er:YAG laser [23,58,106], which is also favourable for the reduction and control of the proliferation of microorganisms [24,70], and Er,Cr:YSGG [63,107]. Less significant, however, is the Nd:YAG laser if not used in combination with Er.YAG laser, thus improving clinical and microbiological parameters for moderate and severe pockets, even in areas difficult to reach [25,72].

4.5. Measures for Laser Therapy in Modified Full-Mouth Disinfection

The modified full-mouth disinfection protocol can also be revised with the use of the laser. We recommend the use of diode laser during the scaling and root planning session for about 20–30 s in each periodontal pocket (810–980 nm, 1.5 W), favoring biostimulation, decontamination and cauterization of the tissue. Use it at the end of treatment in the II session (Figure 4).

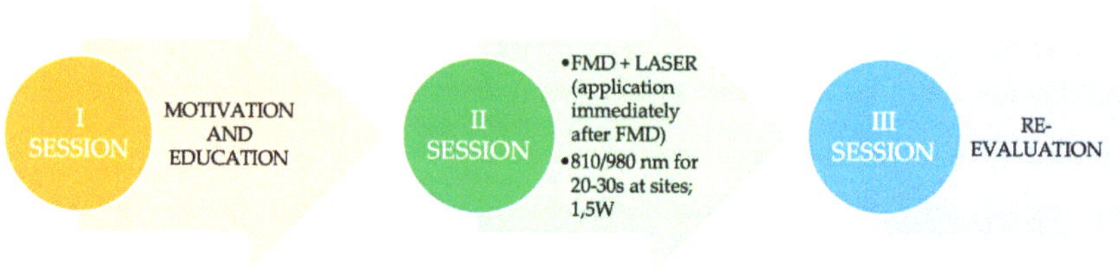

Figure 4. Laser as an adjuvant to the modified full mouth disinfection protocol. FMD: Full mouth disinfection; 1.5 W: 1.5 Watt.

4.6. Ozonetherapy

Ozone is an allotropic form of the oxygen molecule that occurs naturally in the Earth's atmosphere: in medicine, a mixture of pure oxygen and pure ozone is used in the ratio between 95% and 99.95% and between 0.05% and 5% [108–110], respectively. It is applied as a powerful disinfectant, able to control bleeding and the cleaning of wounds in soft tissues, improving healing, with the increase of the supply of local oxygen [109,111]. In addition, at a high concentration, it kills bacteria very quickly and is a thousand times more powerful than other anti-bacterial agents [108].

The antibacterial action is related to the ability to react with double lipid bonds, thus leading to the lysis of the bacterial wall and the distortion of the content of bacterial cells; entering the cell promotes the oxidation of nucleic amino acids. It also inactivates viruses by spreading through the protein coating in the nucleus, causing damage to viral nucleic acid [112]. The use of dentistry provides only the topical application in the form of gas, water or oil, with a multitude of effects: anti-microbial, analgesic, oxygenating, anti-edema, immunomodulating [113].

It is also associated in the treatment of periodontal disease, as it affects the cellular and humoral immune system by stimulating the proliferation of immunocompetent cells and the synthesis of immunoglobulins. Biologically active substances, such as interleukins, leukotrienes and prostaglandins, which are useful in reducing inflammation and wound healing, are synthesized after the application of ozone [78]. In recent years, several clinical trials have been conducted to evaluate the effectiveness of ozone therapy as an adjunct to nonsurgical periodontal therapy. It has been noted that ozone both in gaseous and aqueous form reduces the growth of aggregatibacter actinomycentemcomintans, tannerella forsythensis, treponema denticola, porphyromonas gingivalis and prevotella intermedia [114]. Recently, the antimicrobial activity against specific periodontal pathogens of ozonated water has been shown: its use has shown a significant reduction in the number of bacteria present in the subgingival plaque [30].

4.7. Measures for Ozone Therapy in Modified Full-Mouth Disinfection

The modified full-mouth disinfection protocol can also be revised with the use of ozone, given the recent studies that highlight its potential effect against SARS-CoV-2 virus. It might be useful to associate ozone therapy (gas or water) to the first motivational session, promoting home products for a continuous contribution of the active ingredient; in fact, toothpastes, gels and mouthwashes are available. Subsequently for the causal therapy can be applied both at the beginning and at the end of treatment: 3–4 close applications are desirable in order to stimulate the healing of the tissue (Figure 5).

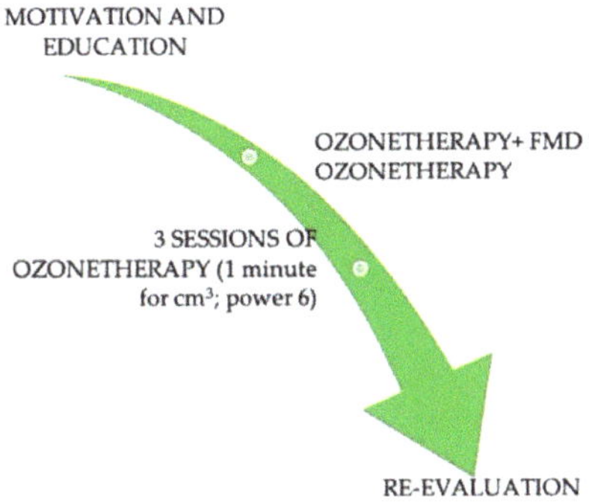

Figure 5. Ozone ad an adjuvant to the modified full mouth disinfection protocol. FMD: Full mouth disinfection.

4.8. Airpolishing

The use of airpolishing with glycine is effective in the removal of biofilm above and below gingival and is increasingly used in maintenance periodontal therapy, reducing the formation of bacterial colonies in periodontal pockets [115]: FFP2 mask respirators are critical to protect dental hygienists and dentists and their importance it has been recognized [116]. In fact in periodontal pockets from 1 to 4 mm, the airpolishing with glycine, using a classic nozzle, is more effective in the removal of the subgingival biofilm than manual or ultrasonic instruments; in pockets from 5 to 9 mm, we recommend a perio tip [117], without causing periodontal tissue damage [118]. Another powder used is erythritol, introduced later, which is also suitable for the removal of biofilm, for the size of its particles, relatively small, and for the more stable chemical properties, compared to glycine [119]; it is also effective against some periodontal bacteria, such as Porphyromonas gingivalis [120] and Aggregatibacter actinomycentemcomintans [34].

It is a therapeutic choice common in clinical practice: a good compliance of the patient and an effective initial treatment, through the use of laser and ozone therapy to reduce the bacterial charge in the periodontal pockets, minimizes its use in necessary cases.

4.9. Measures for Airpolishing

The use of a perio tip, then of inserts created specifically for a deplaquing subgingival, having a jet confined within the periodontal pocket, can help to reduce the production of aerosol contaminant. Another important consideration, to avoid greater exposure to the clinical risk of contracting the virus SARS-CoV-2, is the choice of suitable powders: glycine and erythritol, being two very fine powders. They are not instruments of choice for a supragingival deplaquing or for the removal of extrinsic spots, because they would require more time to use; in this case, it is preferable to use powders based on calcium carbonate, whose spherical particles have a particle size ranging from 45 µm to 75 µm, less abrasive than sodium bicarbonate and therefore less aggressive on the tissues (Figure 6).

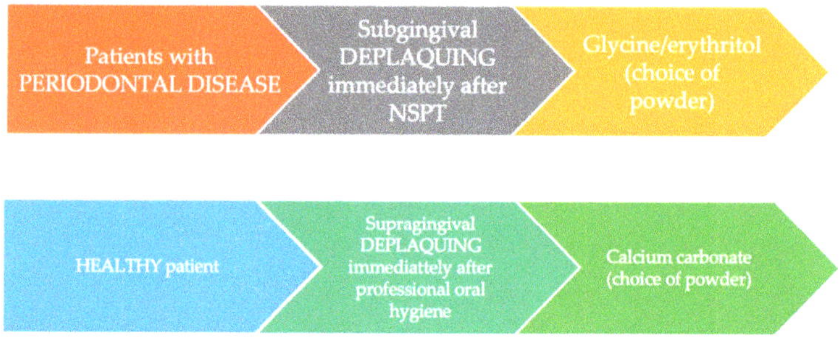

Figure 6. How to choose the type of powder, based on the oral health of the patient. NSPT: nonsurgical periodontal therapy.

4.10. Home Hygiene Advice: The Probiotic Theme

Taking up the concept of oral microbiome, to reduce the chemical–pharmacological action and maintain a proper microbiological balance within the oral cavity, probiotics or bio-inspired products based on probiotics, such as toothpastes, mouthrinses or chewable gums can be recommended. The issue of probiotics begins to make its way even more in the dental field: according to the official definition of the World Health Organization probiotics are living organisms that, administered in adequate quantities, bring a benefit to the health of the host. Currently it has been shown that they are able to provide beneficial effects to the organism through the mechanism of stabilization of the microbial flora and modulation of the immune system of the host. Bacteria capable of exerting one or more of these effects are predominantly lactobacilli or bifidobacteria.

Recent studies have highlighted the usefulness that probiotics could have for the prevention or treatment of certain diseases of the oral cavity such as caries, gingivitis and periodontitis, that are associated with a variation in the composition of the microbial flora and the activity of bacterial species as well as the reaction of the host. Several studies have proven their effectiveness in reducing anaerobic bacterial load [79] and highly virulent bacteria belonging to the red and orange complex [36,67,80], helping tissue healing, in terms of depth of survey, loss of clinical attack, gingival bleeding and plaque index.

In view of these considerations, toothpastes containing selected and tindalized probiotics are available on the market, namely Bifidobacterium and Lactobacillus, which have an antimicrobial action that allows blockage of the growth of pathogenic bacteria, but above all they are able to bind to the toxins that are released by the latter, inhibiting their action. In addition, these toothpastes also have inside them the Mastic of Chios, known for its bacterial and anti-inflammatory properties, which acts as an immunostimulant. The chewable gums, on the other hand, mentioned above, contain microrepair, therefore microcrystals of hydroxyapatite, added with three billion of selected probiotics, that is Lactobacillus reuteri, Lactobacillus salivarius and Lactobacillus plantarum, vitamin C, vitamin D3, calcium and zinc. It is recommended to use for at least 20 min once a day, preferably after a proper cleansing, and continued for 10 days. In addition, previously, dental machines, mouthwashes and gels based on olive oil or ozonated sunflower seed oil were also mentioned as a continuation of the causal therapy for a continuous release of ozone at the tissue level.

5. Conclusions

To understand human health in its entirety and to intervene in a timely manner on the disease with precise and effective bio-inspired therapies that aim not only to solve the problem in the immediate, but also to reduce or even avoid relapse, we absolutely need to know the oral microbiome. In addition, knowing in depth the stability or variability of the human microbiota will allow us to better assess the health status of each patient in a holistic sense: to periodontics, an analysis of the oral microbiome will allow to associate, beyond reasonable doubt, the presence and severity of a possible periodontal disease. Given the link of the latter with a long series of different diseases, the collaboration between the dentist and other specialist doctors will ensure more timely, accurate and calibrated care for each patient. Therefore, analyzing the available scientific literature, we can evaluate ever more minimally invasive therapies, which aim at the reduction of bacteremia and the reduction of periodontal reference indices, with advantageous results for both the operator and the patient: laser, ozone, probiotics, glycine and erythritol appear to be a valuable support for nonsurgical periodontal treatment. This concept is even more important in a global pandemic situation, where the reduction of the bacterial load present in aerosols becomes a primary outcome, in order to manage the clinical risk in public or private health environments, without necessarily abandoning the promising instruments adopted so far. Bio-inspired systems have shown improvements in clinical parameters of greater relevance, such as depth of survey, loss of clinical attack, gingival bleeding and the index of plaque, accompanied by a reduction in bacterial load and proinflammatory cytokines, but these improvements have not been statistically significant. The risk of bias of the present investigation is relatively low, but it is not absent. Additionally, some studies present more than one aspect with uncertain or high risk. Therefore, future randomized clinical studies on the topic would be welcomed.

Further studies, aimed at assessing the effectiveness of the success of nonsurgical periodontal therapy, adjuvant by the use of laser and ozone therapy, airpolishing, probiotics and chlorhexidine, on the reduction of the risk caused by the new coronavirus are probably needed. This will promote a better management of health-workers' risks of generating contaminated aerosols from patients who undergo nonsurgical periodontal therapy; limiting the chemical–pharmacological action to an initial period in order to manage and respect the biological tissues and avoiding, finally, an overtreatment.

Supplementary Materials: The following are available online at http://www.mdpi.com/2077-0383/9/12/3914/s1, Table S1: Non surgical periodontal therapy and laser, Table S2: Non surgical periodontal therapy and ozone, Table S3: Non surgical periodontal therapy and air-polishing, Table S4: Non surgical periodontal therapy and probiotics, Table S5: Non surgical periodontal therapy and chlorexidine.

Author Contributions: A.S. and A.B. (Andrea Butera), conceived the ideas; V.N., A.B. (Ambra Bruni), C.C., G.M., G.G., A.M. and S.M. searched articles; C.M. collected the data; A.B. (Andrea Butera) and C.M. led the writing. All authors have read and agreed to the published version of the manuscript.

Funding: This research received no external funding.

Conflicts of Interest: The authors declare no conflict of interest.

References

1. Spagnuolo, G.; De Vito, D.; Rengo, S.; Tatullo, M. COVID-19 Outbreak: An overview on dentistry. *Int. J. Environ. Res. Public Health* **2020**, *17*, 2094. [CrossRef]
2. Peng, X.; Xu, X.; Li, Y.; Cheng, L.; Zhou, X.; Ren, B. Transmission routes of 2019-nCoV and controls in dental practice. *Int. J. Oral Sci.* **2020**, *12*, 9. [CrossRef]
3. Available online: https://www.epicentro.iss.it/coronavirus/faq (accessed on 6 April 2020).
4. Coulthard, P. Dentistry and coronavirus (COVID-19)—Moral decision making. *Br. Dent. J.* **2020**, *228*, 503–505. [CrossRef]
5. Available online: https://www.nytimes.com/interactive/2020/03/15/business/economy/coronavirus-worker-risk.html (accessed on 22 May 2020).
6. Meng, L.; Hua, F.; Bian, Z. Coronavirus Disease 2019 (COVID-19): Emerging and future challenges for dental and oral medicine. *J. Dent. Res.* **2020**, *99*, 481–487. [CrossRef]
7. French Society of Stomatology, Maxillo-Facial Surgery and Oral Surgery (SFSCMFCO). Practitioners specialized in oral health and coronavirus disease 2019: Professional guidelines from the French society of stomatology, maxillofacial surgery and oral surgery, to form a common front against the infectious risk. *J. Stomatol. Oral Maxillofac. Surg.* **2020**, *121*, 155–158. [CrossRef]
8. Retamal-Valdes, B.; Soares, G.M.; Stewart, B.; Figueiredo, L.C.; Faveri, M.; Miller, S.; Zhang, Y.P.; Feres, M. Effectiveness of a pre-procedural mouthwash in reducing bacteria in dental aerosols: Randomized clinical trial. *Braz. Oral Res.* **2017**, *31*, e21. [CrossRef]

9. Arabaci, T.; Ciçek, Y.; Canakçi, C.F. Sonic and ultrasonic scalers in periodontal treatment: A review. *Int. J. Dent. Hyg.* **2007**, *5*, 2–12. [CrossRef] [PubMed]
10. Auplisti, G.; Needleman, I.G.; Moles, D.R.; Newman, H.N. Diamond-coated sonic tips are more efficient for open debridment of molar furcations. A comparative manikin study. *J. Clin. Periodontol.* **2000**, *27*, 302–307. [CrossRef]
11. Goldman, H.S.; Hartman, K.S.; Messite, J. *Occupational Hazards in Dentistry*; Year Book Medical Publishers: Chicago, IL, USA, 1984.
12. Rivera-Hidalgo, F.; Barnes, J.B.; Harrel, S.K. Aerosol and splatter production by focused spray standard ultrasonic inserts. *J. Periodontol.* **1999**, *70*, 473–477. [CrossRef]
13. Xu, H.; Zhong, L.; Deng, J.; Peng, J.; Dan, H.; Zeng, X.; Li, T.; Chen, Q. High exspression of ACE2 receptor of 2019-nCoV on the epithelial cells of oral mucosa. *Int. J. Oral Sci.* **2020**, *12*, 8. [CrossRef]
14. Van Doremalen, N.; Bushmaker, T.; Morris, D.H.; Holbrook, M.G.; Gamble, A.; Williamson, B.N.; Tamin, A.; Harcourt, J.L.; Thornburg, N.J.; Gerber, S.I.; et al. Aerosol and surface stability of SARS-CoV-2 as compared with SARS-CoV-1. *N. Engl. J. Med.* **2020**, *382*, 1564–1567. [CrossRef] [PubMed]
15. Bizzocca, M.E.; Campisi, G.; Lo Muzio, L. An innovative risk-scoring system of dental procedures and safety protocols in the COVID-19 era. *BMC Oral Health* **2020**, *20*, 301. [CrossRef]
16. Trenter, S.C.; Walmsley, A.D. Ultrasonic dental scaler associated hazards. *J. Clin. Periodontol.* **2003**, *30*, 95–101. [CrossRef]
17. Wirthlin, M.R.; Marshall, G.V. Evaluation of ultrasonic scaling unit waterline contamination after use of chlorine dioxide mouthrinse lavage. *J. Periodontol.* **2001**, *72*, 401–410. [CrossRef] [PubMed]
18. Fine, D.H.; Yip, J.; Furgang, D.; Barnett, M.L.; Olshan, A.M.; Vincent, J. Reducing bacteria in dental aerosols: Pre-procedural use of an antiseptic mouthrinse. *JADA* **1993**, *129*, 1241–1249. [CrossRef]
19. Available online: https://microbioma.it (accessed on 6 April 2020).
20. Christgau, M.; Manner, T.; Beur, S.; Hiller, K.A.; Schmalz, G. Periodontal healing after non-surgical therapy with a new ultrasonic device: A randomized controlled clinical trial. *J. Clin. Periodontol.* **2002**, *34*, 137–147. [CrossRef]
21. Cobbo, C.M. Clinical significance of non-surgical periodontal therapy: An evidence-based perspective of scaling and root planing. *J. Clin. Periodontol.* **2002**, *29* (Suppl. S2), 6–16. [CrossRef]
22. Quirynen, M.; De Soete, M.; Dierickx, K.; Van Steenberghe, D. The intra-oral translocation of periodontopathogens jeopardises the outcome of periodontal therapy. A review of the literature. *J. Clin. Periodontol.* **2001**, *28*, 499–507. [CrossRef]
23. Zhou, X.; Lin, M.; Zhang, D.; Song, Y.; Wang, Z. Efficacy of Er:YAG laser on periodontitis as an adjunctive non-surgical treatment: A split-mouth randomized controlled study. *J. Clin. Periodontol.* **2019**, *46*, 539–547. [CrossRef]
24. Yilmaz, S.; Algan, S.; Gursoy, H.; Noyan, U.; Kuru, B.E.; Kadir, T. Evaluation of the clinical and antimicrobial effects of the Er:YAG laser or topical gaseous ozone as adjuncts to initial periodontal therapy. *Photomed. Laser Surg.* **2013**, *31*, 293–298. [CrossRef]
25. Sağlam, M.; Köseoğlu, S.; Taşdemir, I.; Erbak Yılmaz, H.; Savran, L.; Sütçü, R. Combined application of Er:YAG and Nd:YAG lasers in treatment of chronic periodontitis. A split-mouth, single-blind, randomized controlled trial. *J. Periodontal. Res.* **2017**, *52*, 853–862. [CrossRef]
26. Abduljabbar, T.; Vohra, F.; Kellesarian, S.V.; Javed, F. Efficacy of scaling and root planning with and without adjunct Nd:YAG laser therapy on clinical periodontal parameters and gingival crevicular fluid interleukin 1-beta and tumor necrosis factor-alpha levels among patients with periodontal disease: A prospective randomized split-mouth clinical study. *J. Photochem. Photobiol. B* **2017**, *169*, 70–74.
27. Gou, H.; Fan, R.; Chen, X.; Li, L.; Wang, X.Q.; Xu, Y.; Svensson, P.; Wang, K.L. Adjunctive effects of laser therapy on somatosensory function and vasomotor regulation of periodontal tissues in patients with periodontitis- a randomized controlled clinical trial. *J. Periodontol.* **2020**, *91*, 1307–1317. [CrossRef]
28. Talebi, J.M.; Taliee, R.; Mojahedi, M.; Meymandi, M.; Torshabi, M. Microbiological efficacy of photodynamic therapy as an adjunct to non-surgical periodontal treatment: A clinical trial. *Lasers Med. Sci.* **2016**, *7*, 126–130. [CrossRef]
29. Tasdemir, Z.; Oskaybas, M.N.; Alkan, A.B.; Cakmak, O. The effects of ozone therapy on periodontal therapy: A randomized placebo-controlled clinical trial. *Oral Dis.* **2019**, *25*, 1195–1202. [CrossRef]

30. Hayakumo, S.; Arakawa, S.; Mano, Y.; Izumi, Y. Clinical and microbiological effects of ozone nano-bubble water irrigation as an adjunct to mechanical subgingival debridement in periodontitis patients in a randomized controlled trial. *Clin. Oral Investig.* **2013**, *17*, 379–388. [CrossRef]
31. Kshitish, D.; Laxman, V.K. The use of ozonated water and 0.2% chlorhexidine in the treatment of periodontitis patients: A clinical and microbiologic study. *Indian J. Dent. Res.* **2010**, *21*, 341–348.
32. Lu, H.; He, L.; Zhao, Y.; Meng, H. The effect of supragingival glycine air polishing on periodontitis during maintenance therapy: A randomized controlled trial. *PeerJ* **2018**, *6*, e437. [CrossRef]
33. Wennström, J.L.; Dahlén, G. Ramberg, Subgingival debridement of periodontal pockets by air polishing in comparison with ultrasonic instrumentation during maintenance therapy. *J. Clin. Periodontol.* **2011**, *38*, 820–827. [CrossRef]
34. Müller, N.; Moëne, R.; Cancela, J.A.; Mombelli, A. Subgingival air-polishing with erythritol during periodontal maintenance: Randomized clinical trial of twelve months. *J. Clin. Periodontol.* **2014**, *41*, 883–889. [CrossRef]
35. Pelekos, G.; Ho, S.N.; Acharya, A.; Leung, W.K.; McGrath, C. A double-blind, paralleled-arm, placebo-controlled and randomized clinical trial of the effectiveness of probiotics as an adjunct in periodontal care. *J. Clin. Periodontol.* **2019**, *46*, 1217–1227. [CrossRef]
36. Invernici, M.M.; Salvador, S.L.; Silva, P.H.F.; Soares, M.S.M.; Casarin, R.; Palioto, D.B.; Souza, S.L.S.; Taba, M., Jr.; Novaes, A.B., Jr.; Furlaneto, F.A.C.; et al. Effects of Bifidobacterium probiotic on the treatment of chronic periodontitis: A randomized clinical trial. *J. Clin. Periodontol.* **2018**, *45*, 1198–1210. [CrossRef]
37. De Costa, F.N.L.; Amaral, C.D.S.F.; Barbirato, D.D.S.; Leão, A.T.T.; Fogacci, M.F. Chlorhexidine mouthwash as an adjunct to mechanical therapy in chronic periodontitis: A meta-analysis. *J. Am. Dent. Assoc.* **2017**, *148*, 308–318. [CrossRef]
38. Zhao, H.; Hu, J.; Zhao, L. Adjunctive subgingival application of chlorhexidine gel in nonsurgical periodontal treatment for chronic periodontitis: A systematic review and meta-analysis. *BMC Oral Health* **2020**, *20*, 34. [CrossRef]
39. Paolantonio, M.; D'Angelo, M.; Grassi, R.F.; Perinetti, G.; Piccolomini, R.; Pizzo, G.; Annunziata, M.; D'Archivio, D.; D'Ercole, S.; Nardi, G.; et al. Clinical and microbiologic effects of subgingival controlled-release delivery of chlorhexidine chip in the treatment of periodontitis: A multicenter study. *J. Clin. Periodontol.* **2008**, *79*, 271–282. [CrossRef]
40. Manthena, S.; Ramesh, A.; Srikanth, A.; Rao, R.M.V.; Preethi, L.P.; Pallavi, S.Y. Comparative evaluation of subgingivally delivered chlorhexidine varnish and chlorhexidine gel in reducing microbial count after mechanical periodontal therapy. *J. Basic Clin. Pharm.* **2014**, *6*, 24–28. [CrossRef]
41. Bescos, R.; Ashworth, A.; Cutler, C.; Brookes, Z.L.; Belfield, L.; Rodiles, A.; Casas-Agustench, P.; Farnham, G.; Liddle, L.; Burleigh, M.; et al. Effects of Chlorhexidine mouthwash on the oral microbiome. *Sci. Rep.* **2020**, *10*, 5254. [CrossRef]
42. Devker, N.R.; Mohitey, J.; Vibhute, A.; Chouhan, V.S.; Chavan, P.; Malagi, S.; Joseph, R. A study to evaluate and compare the efficacy of preprocedural mouthrinsing and high volume evacuator attachment alone and in combination in reducing the amount of viable aerosols produced during ultrasonic scaling procedure. *J. Contemp. Dent. Pract.* **2012**, *13*, 681–689.
43. Tomás, I.; Alvarez, M.; Limeres, J.; Tomás, M.; Medina, J.; Otero, J.L.; Diz, P. Effect of a chlorhexidine mouthwash on the risk of postextraction bacteremia. *Infect. Control. Hosp. Epidemiol.* **2007**, *28*, 577–582. [CrossRef]
44. Horliana, A.C.; Chambrone, L.; Foz, A.M.; Artese, H.P.C.; de Sousa Rabelo, M.; Pannuti, C.M.; Romito, G.A. Dissemination of periodontal pathogens in the bloodstream after periodontal procedures: A systematic review. *PLoS ONE* **2014**, *9*, e98271. [CrossRef]
45. Kinane, D.F.; Riggio, M.P.; Walker, K.F.; MacKenzie, D.; Shearer, B. Bacteraemia following periodontal procedures. *J. Clin. Periodontol.* **2005**, *32*, 708–713. [CrossRef]
46. Sfondrini, M.F.; Debiaggi, M.; Zara, F.; Brerra, R.; Comelli, M.; Bianchi, M.; Pollone, S.R.; Scribante, A. Influence of lingual bracket position on microbial and periodontal parameters in vivo. *J. Appl. Oral Sci.* **2012**, *20*, 357–361. [CrossRef]
47. Scribante, A.; Dermenaki Farahani, M.R.; Marino, G.; Matera, C.; Rodriguez y Baena, R.; Lanteri, V.; Butera, A. Biomimetic Effect of Nano-Hydroxyapatite in Demineralized Enamel before Orthodontic Bonding of Brackets and Attachments: Visual, Adhesion Strength, and Hardness in In Vitro Tests. *BioMed Res. Int.* **2020**, *2020*, 6747498. [CrossRef]

48. Scribante, A.; Sfondrini, M.F.; Collesano, V.; Tovt, G.; Bernardinelli, L.; Gandini, P. Dental Hygiene and Orthodontics: Effect of Ultrasonic Instrumentation on Bonding Efficacy of Different Lingual Orthodontic Brackets. *BioMed Res. Int.* **2017**, *2017*, 3714651. [CrossRef]
49. Kumar, P.S. From focal sepsis to periodontal medicine: A century of exploring the role of the oral microbiome in systemic disease. *J. Physiol.* **2017**, *595*, 465–476. [CrossRef]
50. Olsen, I.; Yamazaki, K. Can oral bacteria affect the microbiome of the gut? *J. Oral Microbiol.* **2019**, *11*, 1586422. [CrossRef]
51. Takahashi, K.; Nishimura, F.; Kurihara, M.; Ywamoto, Y.; Takashiba, S.; Miyata, T.; Murayama, Y. Subgingival microflora and antibody responses against periodontal bacteria of young Japanese patients with type 1 diabetes mellitus. *J. Int. Acad. Periodontol.* **2001**, *3*, 104–111.
52. Paizan, M.L.M.; Vilela-Martin, J.F. Is there an Association between Periodontitis and Hypertension? *Curr. Cardiol. Rev.* **2014**, *10*, 355–361. [CrossRef]
53. Presha, P.M.; Alba, A.L. Periodontitis and diabetes: A two-way relationship. *Diabetologia* **2012**, *55*, 21–31. [CrossRef]
54. Aguiler, E.M.; Suva, J.; Buti, J.; Czesnikiewicz-Guzik, M.; Barbosa Ribeiro, A.; Orlandi, M.; Guzik, T.J.; Hingorani, A.D.; Nart, J.; D'Aiuto, F. Periodontitis is associated with hypertension: A systematic review and meta-analysis. *Cardiovasc. Res.* **2020**, *116*, 28–39. [CrossRef]
55. Sampson, V.; Kamona, N.; Sampson, A. Could there be a link between oral hygiene and the severity of SARS-CoV-2 infections? *Br. Dent. J.* **2020**, *228*, 971–975. [CrossRef]
56. Dukić, W.; Bago, I.; Aurer, A.; Roguljić, M. Clinical effectiveness of diode laser therapy as an adjunct to non-surgical periodontal treatment: A randomized clinical study. *J. Periodontol.* **2013**, *84*, 1111–1117. [CrossRef]
57. De Melo Soares, M.S.; D'Almeida Borges, C.; de Mendonça Invernici, M.; Frantz, F.G.; de Figueiredo, L.C.; de Souza, S.L.S.; Taba, M., Jr.; Messora, M.R.; Novaes, A.B., Jr. Antimicrobial photodynamic therapy as adjunct to non-surgical periodontal treatment in smokers: A randomized clinical trial. *Clin. Oral Investig.* **2019**, *23*, 3173–3182. [CrossRef]
58. Zengin Celik, T.; Saglam, E.; Ercan, C.; Akbas, F.; Nazaroglu, K.; Tunali, M. Clinical and microbiological effects of the se of erbium: Yttrium-aluminum-garnet laser on chronic periodontitis in addition to nonsurgical periodontal treatment: A randomized clinical trial-6 months follow-up. *Photomed. Laser Surg.* **2019**, *37*, 182–190. [CrossRef]
59. Moreira, A.L.; Novaes, A.B., Jr.; Grisi, M.F.; Taba, M., Jr.; Souza, S.L.; Palioto, D.B.; de Oliveira, P.G.; Casati, M.Z.; Casarin, R.C.; Messora, M.R. Antimicrobial photodynamic therapy as an adjunct to non-surgical treatment of aggressive periodontitis: A split-mouth randomized controlled trial. *J. Periodontol.* **2015**, *86*, 376–386. [CrossRef]
60. Sanz-Sánchez, I.; Ortiz-Vigón, A.; Matos, R.; Herrera, D.; Sanz, M. Clinical efficacy of subgingival debridement with adjunctive erbium:yttrium-aluminum-garnet lasertreatment in patients with chronic periodontitis: A randomized clinical trial. *J. Periodontol.* **2015**, *86*, 527–535. [CrossRef]
61. Gündoğar, H.; Şenyurt, S.Z.; Erciyas, K.; Yalım, M.; Üstün, K. The effect of low-level laser therapy on non-surgical periodontal treatment: A randomized controlled, single-blind, split-mouth clinical trial. *Lasers Med. Sci.* **2016**, *31*, 1767–1773. [CrossRef]
62. Üstün, K.; Erciyas, K.; Sezer, U.; Şenyurt, S.Z.; Gündoğar, H.; Üstün, Ö.; Öztuzcu, S. Clinical and biochemical effects of 810 nm diode laser as an adjunct to periodontal therapy: A randomized split-mouth clinical trial. *Photomed. Laser Surg.* **2014**, *32*, 61–66. [CrossRef]
63. Dereci, Ö.; Hatipoğlu, M.; Sindel, A.; Tozoğlu, S.; Üstün, K. The efficacy of Er,Cr:YSGG laser supported periodontal therapy on the reduction of peridodontal disease related oral malodor: A randomized clinical study. *Head Face Med.* **2016**, *12*, 20. [CrossRef]
64. Bundidpun, P.; Srisuwantha, R.; Laosrisin, N. Clinical effects of photodynamic therapy as an adjunct to full-mouth ultrasonic scaling and root planing in treatment of chronic periodontitis. *Laser Ther.* **2018**, *27*, 33–39. [CrossRef]
65. Jose, K.A.; Ambooken, M.; Mathew, J.J.; Issac, A.V.; Kunju, A.P.; Parameshwaran, R.A. Management of chronic periodontitis using chlorhexidine chip and diode laser-a clinical study. *J. Clin. Diagn. Res.* **2016**, *10*, ZC76–ZC80. [CrossRef]

66. Morales, A.; Carvajal, P.; Silva, N.; Hernandez, M.; Godoy, C.; Rodriguez, G.; Cabello, R.; Garcia-Sesnich, J.; Hoare, A.; Diaz, P.I.; et al. Clinical effects of lactobacillus rhamnosus in non-surgical treatment of chronic periodontitis: A randomized placebo-controlled trial with 1-year follow-up. *J. Periodontol.* **2016**, *87*, 944–952. [CrossRef]
67. Teughels, W.; Durukan, A.; Ozcelik, O.; Quirynen, M.; Haytac, M.C. Clinical and microbiological effects of lactobacillus reuteri probiotics in the treatment of chronic periodontitis: A randomized placebo-controlled study. *J. Periodontol.* **2013**, *40*, 1025–1035. [CrossRef]
68. Penala, S.; Kalakonda, B.; Pathakota, K.R.; Jayakumar, A.; Koppolu, P.; Lakshmi, B.V.; Pandey, R.; Mishra, A. Efficacy of local use of probiotics as an adjunct to scaling and root planing in chronic periodontitis and halitosis: A randomized controlled trial. *J. Res. Pharm. Pract.* **2016**, *5*, 86–93. [CrossRef]
69. Lecic, J.; Cakic, S.; Janjic Pavlovic, O.; Cicmil, A.; Vukotic, O.; Petrovic, V.; Cicmil, S. Different methods for subgingival application of chlorhexidine in the treatment of patients with chronic periodontitis. *Acta Odontol. Scand.* **2016**, *74*, 502–507. [CrossRef]
70. Lopes, B.M.; Theodoro, L.H.; Melo, R.F.; Thompson, G.M.; Marcantonio, R.A. Clinical and microbiologic follow-up evaluations after non-surgical periodontal treatment with erbium:YAG laser and scaling and root planning. *J. Periodontol.* **2010**, *81*, 682–691. [CrossRef]
71. Chitsazi, M.T.; Shirmohammadi, A.; Pourabbas, R.; Abolfazli, N.; Farhoudi, I.; Daghig Azar, B.; Farhadi, F. Clinical and microbiological effects of photodynamic therapy associated with non-surgical treatment in aggressive periodontitis. *J. Dent. Res. Dent. Clin. Dent. Prospect.* **2014**, *8*, 153–159.
72. Grzech-Leśniak, K.; Sculean, A.; Gašpirc, B. Laser reduction of specific microorganisms in the periodontal pocket using Er:YAG and Nd:YAG lasers: A randomized controlled clinical study. *Lasers Med. Sci.* **2018**, *33*, 1461–1470. [CrossRef]
73. Matarese, G.; Ramaglia, L.; Cicciù, M.; Cordasco, G.; Isola, G. The effects of diode laser therapy as an adjunct to scaling and root planing in the treatment of aggressive periodontitis: A 1-year randomized controlled clinical trial. *Photomed. Laser Surg.* **2017**, *35*, 702–709. [CrossRef]
74. Seydanur Dengizek, E.; Serkan, D.; Abubekir, E.; Bay, K.; Otlu, O.; Arife, C. Evaluating clinical and laboratory effects of ozone in non-surgical periodontal treatment: A randomized controlled trial. *J. Appl. Oral Sci.* **2019**, *27*, e20180108. [CrossRef]
75. Uraz, A.; Karaduman, B.; Isler, S.Ç.; Gönen, S.; Çetiner, D. Ozone application as adjunctive therapy in chronic periodontitis: Clinical, microbiological and biochemical aspects. *J. Dent. Sci.* **2019**, *14*, 27–37. [CrossRef] [PubMed]
76. Skurska, A.; Pietruska, M.D.; Paniczko-Drężek, A.; Dolińska, E.; Zelazowska-Rutkowska, B.; Zak, J.; Pietruski, J.; Milewski, R.; Wysocka, J. Evaluation of the influence of ozonotherapy on the clinical parameters and MMP levels in patients with chronic and aggressive periodontitis. *Adv. Med. Sci.* **2010**, *55*, 297–307. [CrossRef]
77. Park, E.J.; Kwon, E.Y.; Kim, H.J.; Lee, J.Y.; Choi, J.; Joo, J.Y. Clinical and microbiological effects of the supplementary use of an erythritol powder air-polishing device in non-surgical periodontal therapy: A randomized clinical trial. *J. Periodontal. Implant. Sci.* **2018**, *48*, 295–304. [CrossRef]
78. Tsang, Y.C.; Corbet, E.F.; Jin, L.J. Subgingival glycine powder air-polishing as an additional approach to nonsurgical periodontal therapy in subjects with untreated chronic periodontitis. *J. Periodontal. Res.* **2018**, *53*, 440–445. [CrossRef] [PubMed]
79. Tekce, M.; Ince, G.; Gursoy, H.; Dirikan Ipci, S.; Cakar, G.; Kadir, T.; Yılmaz, S. Clinical and microbiological effects of probiotic lozenges in the treatment of chronic periodontitis: A 1-year follow-up study. *J. Clin. Periodontol.* **2015**, *42*, 363–372. [CrossRef]
80. Vivekananda, M.R.; Vandana, K.L.; Bhat, K.G. Effect of the probiotic *Lactobacilli reuteri* (Prodentis) in the management of periodontal disease: A preliminary randomized clinical trial. *J. Oral Microbiol.* **2010**, *2*, 5344. [CrossRef]
81. İnce, G.; Gürsoy, H.; İpçi, Ş.D.; Cakar, G.; Emekli-Alturfan, E.; Yılmaz, S. Clinical and biochemical evaluation of lozenges containing lactobacillus reuteri as an adjunct to non-surgical periodontal therapy in chronic periodontitis. *J. Periodontol.* **2015**, *86*, 746–754. [CrossRef]
82. John, P.; Lazarus, F.; George, J.P.; Selvam, A.; Prabhuji, M.L. Adjunctive effects of a piscean collagen-based controlled-release chlorhexidine chip in the treatment of chronic periodontitis: A clinical and microbiological study. *J. Clin. Diagn. Res.* **2015**, *9*, ZC70–ZC74. [CrossRef]

83. Gonzales, J.R.; Harnack, L.; Schmitt-Corsitto, G.; Boedeker, R.H.; Chakraborty, T.; Domann, E.; Meyle, J. A novel approach to the use of subgingival controlled-release chlorhexidine delivery in chronic periodontitis: A randomized clinical trial. *J. Periodontol.* **2011**, *82*, 1131–1139. [CrossRef]
84. García-Gargallo, M.; Zurlohe, M.; Montero, E.; Alonso, B.; Serrano, J.; Sanz, M.; Herrera, D. Evaluation of new chlorhexidine- and cetylpyridinium chloride-based mouthrinse formulations adjunctive to scaling and root planing: Pilot study. *Int. J. Dent. Hyg.* **2017**, *15*, 269–279. [CrossRef]
85. Kanagalingam, J.; Feliciano, R.; Hah, J.H.; Labib, H.; Le, T.A.; Lin, J.C. Practical use of povidone-iodine antiseptic in the maintenance of oral health and in the prevention and treatment of common oropharyngeal infections. *Int. J. Clin. Pract.* **2015**, *60*, 1247–1256. [CrossRef]
86. Kim, S.Y.; Noh, K.P.; Kim, H.K.; Kim, S.G.; Kook, J.K.; Park, S.N. Salivary bacterial counts after application of povidone-iodine and chlorhexidine. *J. Korean Assoc. Oral Maxillofac. Surg.* **2009**, *35*, 312–510.
87. Ricevuti, G.; Franzini, M.; Valdenassi, L. Oxygen-ozone immunoceutical therapy in COVID-19 outbreak: Facts and figures. *Ozone Ther.* **2020**, *5*, 9014. [CrossRef]
88. Anand, V.; Govila, V.; Gulati, M.; Anand, B.; Jhingaran, R.; Rastogi, P. Chlorhexidine-thymol varnish as an adjunct to scaling and root planing: A clinical observation. *J. Oral Biol. Craniofac. Res.* **2012**, *2*, 83–89. [CrossRef]
89. Singh, A.; Sridhar, R.; Shrihatti, R.; Mandloy, A. Evaluation of turmeric chip compared with chlorhexidine chip as a local drug delivery agent in the treatment of chronic periodontitis: A split mouth randomized controlled clinical trial. *J. Altern. Complement. Med.* **2018**, *24*, 76–84. [CrossRef] [PubMed]
90. Jain, M.; Dave, D.; Jain, P.; Manohar, B.; Yadav, B.; Shetty, N. Efficacy of xanthan based chlorhexidine gel as an adjunct to scaling and root planing in treatment of the chronic periodontitis. *J. Indian Soc. Periodontol.* **2013**, *17*, 439–443. [CrossRef]
91. Chitsazi, M.T.; Kashefimehr, A.; Pourabbas, R.; Shirmohammadi, A.; Ghasemi Barghi, V.; Daghigh Azar, B. Efficacy of subgingival application of xanthan-based chlorhexidine gel adjunctive to full-mouth root planing assessed by Real-time PCR: A microbiologic and clinical study. *J. Dent. Res. Dent. Clin. Dent. Prospect.* **2013**, *7*, 95–101.
92. Calderini, A.; Pantaleo, G.; Rossi, A.; Gazzolo, D.; Polizzi, E. Adjunctive effect of chlorhexidine antiseptics in mechanical periodontal treatment: First results of a preliminary case series. *Int. J. Dent. Hyg.* **2013**, *11*, 180–185. [CrossRef]
93. Fonseca, D.C.; Cortelli, J.R.; Cortelli, S.C.; Miranda Cota, L.O.; Machado Costa, L.C.; Moreira Castro, M.V.; Oliveira Azevedo, A.M.; Costa, F.O. Clinical and microbiologic evaluation of scaling and root planing per quadrant and one-stage full-mouth disinfection associated with azithromycin or chlorhexidine: A clinical randomized controlled trial. *J. Periodontol.* **2015**, *86*, 1340–1351. [CrossRef]
94. Medaiah, S.; Srinivas, M.; Melath, A.; Girish, S.; Polepalle, T.; Dasari, A.B. Chlorhexidine chip in the treatment of chronic periodontitis—A clinical study. *J. Clin. Diagn. Res.* **2014**, *8*, ZC22–ZC25.
95. Krück, C.; Eick, S.; Knöfler, G.U.; Purschwitz, R.E.; Jentsch, H.F. Clinical and microbiologic results 12 months after scaling and root planing with different irrigation solutions in patients with moderate chronic periodontitis: A pilot randomized trial. *J. Periodontol.* **2012**, *83*, 312–320. [CrossRef]
96. Quirynen, M.; Bollen, C.M.; Vandekerckhove, B.N.; Dekeyser, C.; Papaioannou, W.; Eyssen, H. Full- vs. partial-mouth disinfection in the treatment of periodontal infections: Short-term clinical and microbiological observations. *J. Dent. Res.* **1995**, *74*, 1459–1467. [CrossRef]
97. Genovesi, A.M.; Marconcini, S.; Ricci, M.; Marchisio, O.; Covani, F.; Covani, U. Evaluation of a decontamination protocol prior to a full-mouth disinfection procedure: A randomized clinical study. *J. Dent. Oral Hyg.* **2014**, *6*, 77–84.
98. Marconcini, S.; Goulding, M.; Oldoini, G.; Attanasio, C.; Giammarinaro, E.; Genovesi, A. Clinical and patient-centered outcomes post non-surgical periodontal therapy with the use of a non-injectable anesthetic product: A randomized clinical study. *J. Investig. Clin. Dent.* **2019**, *10*, e12446. [CrossRef]
99. Schwarz, F.; Aoki, A.; Becker, J.; Sculean, A. Laser application in non-surgical periodontal therapy: A systematic review. *J. Clin. Periodontol.* **2008**, *35* (Suppl. S8), 29–44. [CrossRef]
100. Manjunath, S.; Singla, D.; Singh, R. Clinical and microbiological evaluation of the synergistic effects of diode laser with nonsurgical periodontal therapy: A randomized clinical trial. *J. Indian Soc. Periodontol.* **2020**, *24*, 145–149.

101. Euzebio Alves, V.T.; de Andrade, A.K.; Toaliar, J.M.; Conde, M.C.; Zezell, D.M.; Cai, S.; Pannuti, C.M.; De Micheli, G. Clinical and microbiological evaluation of high intensity diode laser adjutant to non-surgical periodontal treatment: A 6-month clinical trial. *Clin. Oral Investig.* **2013**, *17*, 87–95. [CrossRef]
102. Berakdar, M.; Callaway, A.; Eddin, M.F.; Ross, A.; Willershausen, B. Comparison between scaling-root-planing (SRP) and SRP/photodynamic therapy: Six-month study. *Head Face Med.* **2012**, *8*, 12. [CrossRef]
103. Mishra, A.; Shergill, N. The effect of low-level laser therapy on nonsurgical periodontal therapy: A clinico-biochemical study. *J. Dent. Lasers* **2018**, *12*, 14–17. [CrossRef]
104. Aykol, G.; Baser, U.; Maden, I.; Kazak, Z.; Onan, U.; Tanrikulu-Kucuk, S.; Ademoglu, E.; Issever, H.; Yalcin, F. The effect of low-level laser therapy as an adjunct to non-surgical periodontal treatment. *J. Periodontol.* **2011**, *82*, 481–488. [CrossRef]
105. Petrović, M.S.; Kannosh, I.Y.; Milašin, J.M. Clinical, microbiological and cytomorphometric evaluation of low-level laser therapy as an adjunct to periodontal therapy in patients with chronic periodontitis. *J. Int. Dent. Hyg.* **2018**, *16*, e120–e127. [CrossRef]
106. Sanz-Sánchez, I.; Ortiz-Vigón, A.; Herrera, D.; Sanz, M. Microbiological effects and recolonization patterns after adjunctive subgingival debridement with Er:YAG laser. *Clin. Oral Investig.* **2016**, *20*, 1253–1261. [CrossRef]
107. Üstun, K.; Hatipoglu, M.; Daltaban, O.; Felek, R.; Firat, M.Z. Clinical and biochemical effects of erbium, chromium: Yttrium, scandium, gallium, garnet laser treatment as a complement to periodontal treatment. *Niger J. Clin. Pract.* **2018**, *21*, 1150–1157.
108. Gupta, G.; Mansi, B. Ozone therapy in periodontics. *Med. J. Life* **2012**, *5*, 59–67.
109. Srikanth, A.; Sathish, M.; Sri Harsha, A.V. Application of ozone in the treatment of periodontal disease. *J. Pharm. Bioallied Sci.* **2013**, *5* (Suppl. S1), S89–S94. [CrossRef]
110. Elvis, A.M.; Ekta, J.S. Ozone therapy: A clinical review. *J. Nat. Sci. Biol. Med.* **2011**, *2*, 66–70. [CrossRef]
111. Mollica, P.; Harris, R. Integrating Oxygen/Ozone Therapy into Your Practice. Available online: www.acimd.net (accessed on 13 January 2010).
112. Gandhi, K.K.; Cappetta, E.G.; Pavaskar, R. Effectiveness of the adjunctive use of ozone and chlorhexidine in patients with chronic periodontitis. *BDJ Open* **2019**, *5*, 17. [CrossRef]
113. Suh, Y.; Patel, S.; Kaitlyn, R.; Gandhi, J.; Joshi, G.; Smith, N.L.; Khan, S.A. Clinical utility of ozone therapy in dental and oral medicine. *Med. Gas. Res.* **2019**, *9*, 163–167.
114. Bezrukova, I.V.; Petrukhina, N.B.; Voinov, P.A. Experience in medical ozone use for root canal treatment. *Stomatologiia* **2005**, *84*, 20–22.
115. Petersilka, G.J.; Steinmann, D.; Häberlein, I.; Heinecke, A.; Flemmig, T.F. Subgingival plaque removal in buccal and lingual sites using a novel low abrasive air-polishing powder. *J. Clin. Periodontol.* **2003**, *30*, 328–333. [CrossRef]
116. Farronato, M.; Boccalari, E.; Del Rosso, E.; Lanteri, V.; Mulder, R.; Maspero, C. A Scoping Review of Respirator Literature and a Survey among Dental Professionals. *Int. J. Environ. Res. Public Health* **2020**, *17*, 5968. [CrossRef]
117. Cobb, C.M.; Daubert, D.M.; Davis, K. Consensus conference findings on supragingival and subgingival air polishing. *Compend. Contin. Educ. Dent.* **2017**, *38*, e1–e4.
118. Ng, E.; Byun, R.; Spahr, A.; Divnic-Resnik, T. The efficacy of air polishing devices in supportive periodontal therapy: A systematic review and meta-analysis. *Quintessence Int.* **2018**, *49*, 453–467. [PubMed]
119. Hägi, T.T.; Hofmänner, P.; Salvi, G.E.; Ramseier, C.A.; Sculean, A. Clinical outcomes following subgingival application of a novel erythritol powder by means of air polishing in supportive periodontal therapy: A randomized, controlled clinical study. *Quintessence Int.* **2013**, *44*, 753–761.
120. Hashino, E.; Kuboniwa, M.; Alghamdi, S.A.; Yamaguchi, M.; Yamamoto, R.; Cho, H.; Amano, A. Erythritol alters microstructure and metabolomic profiles of biofilm composed of *Streptococcus gordonii* and *Porphyromonas gingivalis*. *Mol. Oral Microbiol.* **2013**, *28*, 435–451. [CrossRef]

Publisher's Note: MDPI stays neutral with regard to jurisdictional claims in published maps and institutional affiliations.

Journal of
Clinical Medicine

MDPI

Article

Psychological Functioning of Patients Undergoing Oral Surgery Procedures during the Regime Related with SARS-CoV-2 Pandemic

Dorota Pylińska-Dąbrowska [1,*,†], Anna Starzyńska [1,*,†], Wiesław Jerzy Cubała [2], Karolina Ragin [1], Daniela Alterio [3] and Barbara Alicja Jereczek-Fossa [3,4]

1 Oral Surgery Department, Medical University of Gdańsk, 80-211 Gdańsk, Poland; karolina.ragin@gumed.edu.pl
2 Department of Adult Psychiatry, Medical University of Gdańsk, 80-211 Gdańsk, Poland; wieslaw.cubala@gumed.edu.pl
3 Department of Oncology and Hemato-Oncology, University of Milan, 20122 Milano, Italy; daniela.alterio@ieo.it (D.A.); barbara.jereczek@ieo.it (B.A.J.-F.)
4 Division of Radiotherapy, IEO European Institute of Oncology, IRCCS, 20141 Milan, Italy
* Correspondence: 37670@gumed.edu.pl (D.P.-D.); ast@gumed.edu.pl (A.S.)
† These authors contributed equally to this work.

Received: 6 September 2020; Accepted: 15 October 2020; Published: 18 October 2020

Abstract: The coronavirus pandemic has become a huge global challenge medically, economically and psychologically. The COVID-19 pandemic shows that the population can experience general psychological distress. The sanitary regime in dental offices and lack of vaccine for coronavirus may have an impact on the level of dental anxiety among patients undergoing oral surgery procedures. A clinical study was conducted between November 2019 and September 2020. A total of 175 patients ($n = 175$) were enrolled in the research. The aim of the study was to assess the attitude of patients towards the new situation related to the reduced availability of dental offices providing oral surgery procedures. The level of anxiety associated with surgical intervention was measured using a self-made COVID-19 questionnaire and the MDAS scale. The ED-5Q questionnaire and EQ-VAS scale were also used in this research. The study showed that 21.9% of respondents presented with increased anxiety about a dental visit compared with the time before the pandemic. This epidemiological situation has led to an overwhelming increase in moderate dental anxiety (M: 11.4) among patients undergoing oral surgery procedures. The quality of patients' health (EQ-VAS) related to the impact of the coronavirus pandemic and the quarantine decreased by 10 percentage points. Oral surgeons should be prepared for more anxious patients in dental offices during the pandemic.

Keywords: dental anxiety; pandemic; dentistry; oral surgery; dental care; SARS-CoV-2; COVID-19

1. Introduction

The outbreak of the coronavirus pandemic (SARS-CoV-2), which started in December 2019 in Wuhan, China, has become a huge global challenge medically, economically and psychologically [1]. On the 30 January 2020, the World Health Organization (WHO) declared the COVID-19 outbreak a global health emergency. At the end of September 2020, the WHO reported that more than 23 million people had been infected worldwide and 800,000 deaths had been caused by the SARS-CoV-2 infection [2,3]. The number of infected people around the world is still rising. The limited knowledge of COVID-19 and overwhelming news delivery may lead to anxiety and fear in the public.

Three main mechanisms of dental anxiety are hypothesized. One of them is based on patients' own experiences (mostly traumatic experiences from the past) and the other two result from external factors, such as negative-biased information and observations of negative behavior during dental treatment [4–6]. In time, it may transpire that we will also have to deal with another mechanism linked to the difficulty in finding a dental office which provides surgical services during pandemic lockdown and in accordance with the pandemic-related regime. These are factors we did not have to consider in this study. Depending on the examined population and the assessment tools, 2.5–20% of people experience dental anxiety [7,8].

The population at large may experience disappointment, stress and irritability when in isolation [9]. Psychologists from China examined the general population during the initial stage of the COVID-19 pandemic. They found that 53.8% of the respondents rated the psychological impact of the outbreak as moderate or severe, 16.5% reported moderate to severe depressive symptoms, and 28.8% reported moderate to severe anxiety symptoms [10]. Another study, which included more than 50,000 people in China during the coronavirus pandemic, showed that about 35% of people experienced psychological distress [11].

Peloso et al. reported that the pandemic has a considerable impact on dental appointments and anxiety in patients. There was an association between patients' attitudes towards the pandemic and their enthusiasm to attend a dental appointment. The author reported that at the beginning of the pandemic 28.6% of interviewees reported experiencing anxiety. Their concerns were associated with the risk of getting infected and transmitting the disease to family members [9].

There are some studies on the psychological influence of the COVID-19 pandemic on patients in different medical sectors [11–13] yet, there are no studies on patients undergoing oral surgery procedures in outpatient dental surgeries [5]. Assessing the severity of anxiety in this group of patients may contribute to the optimization of the treatment process [12].

The aim of this study was to compare the psychological functioning of patients undergoing dental surgery procedures before and after the outbreak of the pandemic.

2. Experimental Section

This study was approved by the Independent Research Ethics Committee of the Medical University in Gdańsk, Poland (NKBBN/366/2016).

A clinical study involving 175 (n = 175) patients was carried out. The patients were divided into three groups: those undergoing a surgery before the outbreak of the pandemic, those during the most severe restrictions after the COVID-19 outbreak, and those after the lifting of the most severe restrictions. The patients were consecutively recruited at the Department of Oral Surgery at the Medical University of Gdańsk. The patients' visits took place at the Oral Surgery Department from November 2019 to September 2020. In 47 instances, the procedures were performed before the SARS-CoV-2 reached Poland (first confirmed case–4 March 2020). At the time, planned surgeries were performed. Patients were given routine verbal information on the course of treatment and the post-operative indications. All verbal information was standardized and presented by the same dental surgeon. During the time of pandemic restrictions 128 (n = 128) patients were treated. They received the same verbal information as the group treated before the pandemic and the procedures were performed by the same dentist. This group was divided into two subgroups. The patients from the first subgroup (n = 57) underwent the surgeries at the time of the most severe restrictions-between 4 March 2020 and 31 May 2020. The second subgroup (n = 71) was admitted after the most severe restrictions were lifted in Poland (31 May 2020) [2].

All examined patients (175) filled in a questionnaire on their sex, age, place of residence and presence or lack of symptoms related to COVID-19. The procedures to which the patients were subjected included tooth extractions, surgical tooth extractions, abscess drainage and drain removals (Table 1). All patients gave their written informed consent for the study. Fear of coronavirus in the group operated on after the outbreak was measured using a custom-built questionnaire consisting of ten statements about COVID-19 (Table 2). A Likert scale with five sorted categories from 1 (definitely no) to 5 (definitely yes) was used here. Patients undergoing surgery before the outbreak of the pandemic did not answer questions about COVID-19. Questionnaires related to the EuroQol 5D

Quality of Life Self-esteem, which consists of two parts-EQ-5D (Five Questions of EuroQol 5D Quality of Life Self-esteem Questionnaire) and EQ-VAS (Visual Analogue Scale of EuroQol 5D Quality of Life Self-esteem Questionnaire), and the MDAS (Modified Dental Anxiety Scale) were completed by all 175 patients [14–18]. The participants had a doctor's help if they had any doubts regarding questions or answers. Patients older than 18 years of age who agreed to participate in the study were considered eligible.

2.1. MDAS: Modified Dental Anxiety Scale

The answers are: calm (1 point), a bit nervous (2 points), nervous (3 points), very nervous (4 points), and extremely nervous (5 points). Points are added up, and the results range between 5 and 25 points. A score of 5 indicates no anxiety, 6–10 a low level of anxiety, 11–14 a moderate level of anxiety and 14–18 a high level of anxiety. A result of more than 19 points indicates an extraordinarily strong level of anxiety, entitling the patient to be included in the group of people suffering from dentophobia. The use of the MDAS questionnaire with each patient before the commencement of dental treatment allows for a simple and objective assessment of the occurrence and severity of anxiety [14–17].

2.2. ED-5Q and EQ-VAS

The ED-5Q questionnaire describes function and quality of life in five dimensions: mobility, self-care, usual activities, pain or discomfort, and anxiety or depression. The EQ-VAS is a visual analogue scale on which the patient is assessing their health on a scale from 0 (worst imaginable health condition) to 100 (best imaginable health condition) [18].

2.3. Statistical Analysis

The collected data were subjected to statistical analysis using the STATISTICA 13.1 (StatSoft Inc., Tulsa, OK, USA, serial number JPZ0097539310ARACD-1) licensed by the Medical University of Gdańsk. The quantitative statistical analysis included the chi-square test. For this purpose, the following parameters have been calculated: values mean (M), median (Me), standard deviations (SD), minimum (MIN) and maximum (MAX) values. The Mantel–Haenszel test has also been used. In addition, in several cases where groups had insignificant numbers, Fisher's exact test was used. Additionally, the non-parametric Mann–Whitney test and the non-parametric Kruskal–Wallis test, supplemented by post-hoc tests, were implemented. The test results were considered significant when $p < 0.05$. Cronbach's alpha test for the COVID-19 questionnaire was 0.787, for the MDAS was 0.899 and for the ED-5Q was 0.558. The power calculation for the MDAS was −0.03, for the ED-5Q it was −0.18 and for the EQ-VAS it was 0.2.

Table 1. Characteristics of all 175 patients completing the questionnaire, divided into three groups according to the time of admission. N-number of patients; (%)-per cent of respondents; M-mean, SD-standard deviation; t-value of the Student's *t*-test; df-degrees of freedom; *p*-level of statistical significance.

		Overall Population Characteristics (N)/(%)	Before Pandemic Population Characteristics (N)/(%)	During Pandemic with High Restrictions Population Characteristics (N)/(%)	During Pandemic When the High Restrictions Were Lifted Population Characteristics (N)/(%)	χ^2	df	*p*-Value
Group		175 (100.0)	47 (26.9)	57 (32.55)	71 (40.55)			
Age	18-35	89 (50.9)	30 (33.7)	24 (27.0)	35 (39.3)	7.089563	4	0.13123
	36-55	51 (29.1)	13 (25.5)	18 (35.3)	20 (39.2)			
	56-85	35 (20.0)	4 (11.4)	15 (42.9)	16 (45.7)			
Sex	Female	108 (61.7)	29 (26.8)	30 (27.8)	49 (45.4)	3.591385	2	0.16601
	Male	67 (38.3)	18 (26.9)	27 (40.3)	22 (32.8)			
Place of residence	<10.000	45 (25.7)	13 (28.9)	16 (35.55)	16 (35.55)	13.59576 Fi = 0.28	6	0.03449
	10.000–50.000	28 (16.0)	4 (14.3)	5 (17.9)	19 (67.8)			
	50.000–100.000	30 (17.1)	12 (40.0)	11 (36.7)	7 (23.3)			
	>100.000	72 (41.1)	18 (25.0)	25 (34.7)	29 (40.3)			
Type of performed surgery	Tooth extraction	121 (69.1)	21 (17.36)	47 (38.84)	53 (43.80)	18.92567 Fi = 0.33	2	0.00008
	Surgical tooth extraction	54 (30.9)	26 (48.15)	10 (18.52)	18 (33.33)			
	Others	0	0	0	5 (38.5)			
Amount of removed teeth	One	146 (75.4)	46 (31.50)	44 (30.14)	56 (38.36)	9.761003 Fi = 0.24	2	0.00759
	More than one	29 (16.6)	1 (3.45)	13 (44.83)	15 (51.72)			
Comorbidities	None	117 (66.9)	31 (26.5)	38 (32.5)	48 (41.0)	4.412333	6	0.62106
	One	41 (23.4)	14 (34.1)	13 (31.7)	14 (34.2)			
	Two	16 (9.1)	2 (12.5)	6 (37.5)	8 (50.0)			
	More than two	1 (0.6)	0 (0.0)	0 (0.0)	1 (100.0)			

Table 2. Results of the COVID-19 questionnaire in patients treated after the outbreak of SARS-CoV-2 according to the time of admittance. N-number of patients; (%)-per cent of respondents; M-mean, SD-standard deviation; t-value of the Student's t-test; df-degrees of freedom; p-level of statistical significance.

COVID-19 Questionnaire	Number of Patients Who Chose the Affirmative Answer (N)/(%) in the Group of 128 Patients, (M/SD)	Number of Patients Who Chose the Affirmative Answer (N)/(%) in the Group of 57 Patients, during Severe Restrictions, (M/SD)	Number of Patients Who Chose the Affirmative Answer (N)/(%) in the Group of 71 Patients, When the Restrictions Were Lifted, (M/SD)	χ^2	df	p-Value
1. I am concerned about the outbreak of the coronavirus pandemic.	45 (35.2) (2.78/1.23)	21 (36.8) (2.86/1.23)	24 (33.8) (2.72/1.23)	0.1281139	1	0.72040
2. I take precautions to prevent infection, e.g., washing hands, avoiding touching door handles, avoiding contact with people	109 (85.2) (4.27/1.08)	48 (84.2) (4.32/0.95)	61 (85.9) (4.24/1.19)	0.0531619	1	0.81765
3. I follow all the Coronavirus news.	64 (50) (3.04/1.36)	26 (45.6) (3.05/1.30)	38 (53.5) (3.03/1.41)	0.2846553	1	0.59367
4. I have acquired supplies to prepare for the potential consequences of a pandemic.	43 (33.6) (2.63/1.37)	18 (31.6) (2.540/1.36)	25 (35.2) (2.70/1.39)	0.1869924	1	0.66543
5. I believe that this virus is much more dangerous than the seasonal flu.	65 (50.8) (3.32/1.32)	25 (43.9) (3.23/1.28)	40 (56.3) (3.39/1.35)	1.969725	1	0.16048
6. I am concerned that friends or family will be infected.	76 (59.4) (3.47/1.32)	39 (68.4) (3.74/1.22)	37 (52.1) (3.25/1.36)	3.486163	1	0.06188
7. I feel safe in a dentist's office when I see a high level of medical staff protection.	107 (83.6) (4.19/1.11)	49 (86.0) (4.32/0.87)	58 (81.7) (4.08/1.27)	0.4212752	1	0.51630
8. Before going to the dentist's appointment, I tried to cope with pain using home methods.	88 (68.9) (3.65/1.39)	46 (80.7) (3.98/1.17)	42 (59.2) (3.39/1.49)	4.973704	1	0.02574
9. Due to the current situation, related to the coronavirus, a dental visit makes me feel more anxious than before.	28 (21.9) (2.31/1.19)	14 (24.6) (2.32/1.31)	14 (19.7) (2.31/1.10)	0.4339412	1	0.51006
10. I believe that it is necessary to provide medicals with overalls, masks and helmets during a pandemic.	112 (87.5) (4.39/0.93)	46 (80.1) (4.32/1.05)	66 (93.0) (4.46/0.82)	4.342123	1	0.03718

3. Results

3.1. COVID-19 Questionnaire Results

In total, 128 patients completed the COVID-19 questionnaire. Patients undergoing surgeries before the outbreak of the pandemic did not answer these questions. Summary results for affirmative answers are shown in Table 2. Statistical analyses for all the respondents are shown in Tables 3 and 4. In total, 35.2% of respondents were concerned about the outbreak of the coronavirus pandemic. Half of the examined patients followed all of the news on coronavirus. A total of 50.8% of those surveyed believed that this virus is much more dangerous than seasonal flu. Every sixth respondent was concerned that friends or family would be infected. In total, 83.6% of the examined patients felt safe in a dentist's office, when they saw a high level of medical staff protection. Every fifth (21.9%) respondent reported that a dental visit made them feel more anxious than before the pandemic.

Table 3. Statistical analysis of the COVID-19 questionnaire in all patients treated after the outbreak of the SARS-CoV-2 pandemic. N—number of patients; M–mean; SD—standard deviation.

COVID	N	Mean	Median	Minimum	Maximum	SD	Skewnes	Kurtosis
Q1	128	2.781250	3.000000	1.000000	5.000000	1.229157	0.16910	−1.13026
Q2	128	4.273438	5.000000	1.000000	5.000000	1.084717	−1.76863	2.60379
Q3	128	3.039063	3.500000	1.000000	5.000000	1.359726	−0.16712	−1.35985
Q4	128	2.632813	2.000000	1.000000	5.000000	1.373948	0.37449	−1.21185
Q5	128	3.320313	4.000000	1.000000	5.000000	1.315765	−0.35988	−0.99105
Q6	128	3.468750	4.000000	1.000000	5.000000	1.315788	−0.47889	−1.01309
Q7	128	4.187500	4.500000	0.000000	5.000000	1.113624	−1.76906	2.96985
Q8	128	3.656250	4.000000	1.000000	5.000000	1.388578	−0.84930	−0.58150
Q9	128	2.312500	2.000000	1.000000	5.000000	1.195464	0.58027	−0.77846
Q10	128	4.398437	5.000000	1.000000	5.000000	0.933538	−1.94076	3.98116

Table 4. Comparison of patients operated on during severe restrictions with patients operated on after the lifting of restrictions in terms of the total score from the COVID-19 questionnaire. N-number of patients; M-mean; SD-standard deviation; t-value of the Student's *t*-test; df-degrees of freedom; *p*-level of statistical significance.

COVID-19	During Severe Restrictions			After Lifting the Restrictions			*t*-Test		
	N	*M*	*SD*	*N*	*M*	*SD*	*t*	*df*	*p*-Value
Total Score	57	34.67	6.71	71	33.59	7.67	0.83	126	0.407

Comparing patients undergoing surgeries at the time of high restrictions with patients operated on after these restrictions were lifted, statistical significance ($p < 0.05$) was found in questions 8 and 10. Statistical analyses according to the time of admittance are shown in Table 5. A total of 80.7% of patients from the first group admitted that they had tried to cope with pain using home methods before going to a dental appointment, while in the second group the percentage was almost 59.2%. Every seventh respondent operated on at the time of high restrictions expressed concern that friends or family would be infected by SARS-CoV-2, while only every fifth patient gave the same statement after the highest restrictions were lifted (Table 2).

Table 5. Statistical analysis of COVID-19 questionnaire results in patients treated after the SARS-CoV-2 pandemic according to the time of admittance. N-number of patients; R-average rank; *p*-level of statistical significance.

COVID-19	During Severe Restrictions			After the Restrictions Were Lifted			Statistical Analysis	
	N	*R*	*Me*	*N*	*R*	*Me*	*Z*	*p*-Value
Q1	57	66.82	68.99	71	62.64	66.07	0.63	0.528
Q2	57	63.96	68.00	71	64.93	65.19	−0.14	0.886
Q3	57	65.07	3.00	71	64.04	3.00	0.15	0.878
Q4	57	62.20	4.00	71	66.35	4.00	−0.63	0.532
Q5	57	61.50	4.00	71	66.91	3.00	−0.82	0.414
Q6	57	71.66	1.00	71	58.75	1.00	1.95	0.051
Q7	57	66.12	4.00	71	63.20	4.00	0.44	0.659
Q8	57	72.36	1.64	71	58.19	1.71	2.15	0.032
Q9	57	63.33	0.00	71	65.44	0.00	−0.32	0.752
Q10	57	63.52	0.00	71	65.29	0.00	−0.27	0.790

3.2. MDAS Results

Of all surveyed, 10.1% did not report any anxiety related to the dental visit. Low levels of anxiety were reported by 39.1% of patients. A moderate level of anxiety was reported in 21.1% cases. Every fifth respondent showed a high level of dental anxiety and 8.6% of patients were extremely anxious. There were no statistically significant differences for different sex or age group categories. The average result of MDAS was 11.4, which means that the examined group is characterized by a moderate level of anxiety (Table 6).

Table 6. Statistical results of MDAS, ED-5Q and EQ-VAS questionnaire according to the time of admittance. N-number of patients; M–mean; SD-standard deviation; H-the Kruskal-Wallis H test; *p*-level of statistical significance.

Result	Group	*N*	*M*	*Me*	*Min*	*Max*	*SD*	*Skewnes*	*Kurtosis*
MDAS	Before pandemic	47	11.17	10.00	5.00	24.00	5.02	0.52	−0.54
	During severe restrictions	57	11.42	10.00	5.00	25.00	5.35	0.79	0.00
	After lifting the restrictions	71	11.61	11.00	5.00	23.00	4.66	0.35	−0.83
		H(2.175) = 0.48; *p* = 0.787							
ED-5Q	Before pandemic	47	6.70	6.00	5.00	13.00	1.92	1.48	2.27
	During severe restrictions	57	7.54	7.00	5.00	19.00	2.41	2.15	8.08
	After lifting the restrictions	71	7.51	7.00	5.00	16.00	2.24	1.29	2.41
		H(2.175) = 6.11; *p* = 0.047							
EQ-VAS	Before pandemic	47	82.79	85.00	40.00	100.00	14.49	−1.27	1.381
	During severe restrictions	57	72.68	80.00	20.00	100.00	18.91	−0.871	0.420
	After lifting the restrictions	71	77.63	80.00	30.00	100.00	16.26	−0.706	−0.047
		H(2.175) = 8.85; *p* = 0.0119							

The number of low or moderate anxiety responses according to the MDAS scale was highest in the group of patients operated on after the outbreak of the pandemic. The results show that, after the introduction of restrictions related to the pandemic, the number of patients reporting medium, high or extreme levels of anxiety increased. There was no correlation found between the groups in terms of place of residence, type of procedure, history of anxiety or the time of admittance.

3.3. ED-5Q Results

The subjects whose treatment was carried out during the pandemic were characterized by a significantly higher incidence of signaling somatic symptoms and helplessness resulting from being ill (U = 2.286.500; $p < 0.05$). At the same time, the respondents operated on after the outbreak of the pandemic assessed the quality of their health significantly more negatively than those operated on before the introduction of the severe restrictions related to COVID-19 (U = 2227.500; $p < 0.01$). It was determined that there were significant differences between the three groups. Therefore, the multiple comparison procedure was performed using the *Z*-test. The *H* test showed differences between the groups, but the *Z*-test did not confirm these differences. The mean ranks (R) show that in the pre-pandemic group the ED-5Q score was lower than that of the patients undergoing surgery after the outbreak of the pandemic (Table 6).

3.4. EQ-VAS Results

The respondents operated on after the outbreak of the pandemic considered their health to be significantly worse when compared with those operated on before the introduction of restrictions related to COVID-19 (U = 2227.500; $p < 0.01$). The quality of patients' health (EQ-VAS) related to the impact of the coronavirus pandemic was approximately 72, which was 10 points less than before the pandemic (Table 6).

3.5. Results and Comorbidities

For all the respondents, a relationship between the number of comorbidities and ED-5Q was found. The results were analyzed according to the types of restrictions effective at the time. The strongest relationship between ED-5Q and the number of diseases was found in the group of patients who underwent treatment after the lifting of the most severe restrictions (Table 7). The more comorbidities the examined patients had, the more somatic symptoms resulting from being ill they reported.

Table 7. Questionnaire results and comorbidities according to the time of admittance. N-group size; R-value of Spearman's *R* test; *p*-level of statistical significance.

Comorbidities	All Respondents			Before the Pandemic			During Severe Restrictions			After Lifting the Restrictions		
	N	R	*p*-Value	N	R	*p*-Value	N	R	*p*-Value	N	R	*p*-Value
MDAS	175	0.063	0.4	47	0.116	0.433	57	0.011	0.929	71	0.071	0.556
Q1	128	0.22	0.012	0	0	0	57	0.258	0.051	71	0.187	0.117
Q2	128	−0.061	0.488	0	0	0	57	−0.019	0.884	71	−0.09	0.45
Q3	128	0.121	0.17	0	0	0	57	0.256	0.054	71	0.026	0.826
Q4	128	0.108	0.221	0	0	0	57	0.024	0.855	71	0.177	0.137
Q5	128	0.192	0.029	0	0	0	57	0.285	0.031	71	0.127	0.288
Q6	128	0.106	0.23	0	0	0	57	0.203	0.128	71	0.032	0.79
Q7	128	0.04	0.648	0	0	0	57	0.252	0.058	71	−0.11	0.359
Q8	128	−0.052	0.558	0	0	0	57	−0.242	0.068	71	0.076	0.527
Q9	128	−0.054	0.54	0	0	0	57	−0.004	0.974	71	−0.08	0.504
Q10	128	−0.071	0.409	0	0	0	57	0.093	0.487	71	−0.214	0.072
COVID-19 Total Score	128	0.155	0.08	47	0	0	57	0.203	0.129	71	0.111	0.354
ED-5Q	175	0.234	0.002	47	0.163	0.272	57	0.156	0.245	71	0.327	0.005
EQ-VAS	175	−0.09	0.235	47	0.006	0.96	57	−0.051	0.702	71	−0.181	0.13

4. Discussion

The current pandemic situation is causing mental-health problems, such as distress, anxiety and depression, both in medical workers and in patients. Due to the nature of dental procedures, during which water-air spray is generated, the risk of coronavirus infection is considered to be very high.

The small distance between the doctor and the patient during dental procedures also increases the risk of infection [5,6,19]. Increased levels of anxiety can lead to negligence in attending regular visits and emergency dental appointments, resulting in poor oral health [19–25]. There was a significant association between patients' feelings and their willingness to visit the dentist. Patients who regularly visited the dentist before the pandemic are more likely to visit the dental office during the time of COVID-19-related restrictions [11,12].

The patients whose treatments were carried out during the pandemic were characterized by a significantly higher level of ED-5Q index. Our study shows that respondents operated on after the outbreak of the pandemic assessed the quality of their health as significantly worse than those operated on earlier. There is no other published study that compares the quality of surgical patients' health before and during the pandemic using the EQ-VAS questionnaire; therefore, there is no published data with which to compare our results.

Torales et al. observed an increased percentage of people with anxiety, depression, fear and sleep problems during the COVID-19 pandemic, both in the healthy population and in people with the previously mentioned symptoms [26]. A study from China showed that 53% of people experienced feelings of anxiety and fear about the spreading pandemic [27,28]. The COVID-19 pandemic has exacerbated anxiety levels in many people. Our study shows that low, moderate and high levels of anxiety increased after the outbreak of SARS-CoV-2. The results of our study also show that the pandemic has an impact on the psychological functioning of patients.

Our study shows that the more comorbidities the examined patients have, the more somatic and invalidating symptoms resulting from being ill they reported. Public Health England suggest that patients with comorbidities such as cardiovascular diseases, diabetes, chronic respiratory diseases, hypertension and neoplastic diseases have a higher mortality rate than patients without comorbidities [29].

Although the present study reports on the important issue of oral surgery healthcare during the pandemic, the study limitations must be emphasized. The results represented a single-center experience and were obtained from a small population size. Moreover, dental anxiety is multifactorial, and this research did not explore the effects of personal traits and family-related issues, including socioeconomic status and the level of education of patients [30,31]. The study was not designed to delve into explaining the exact reasons for the observed anxiety levels in examined patients. After the outbreak of the pandemic, only patients with dental emergencies were admitted to the clinic, whereas before the outbreak, planned surgeries were performed. The reason for admittance may also be of importance when assessing anxiety levels in patients, which suggests a possible bias.

5. Conclusions

As the COVID-19 pandemic continues to spread, our findings will provide vital guidance for the development of a psychological support strategy for dental surgery patients. It is important to prepare medical staff for the necessity of a special approach towards patients during times of wide-spread coronavirus transmission. The conducted research clearly shows that the number of patients signaling anxiety related to a surgical visit has increased. The study was conducted preliminarily, before the peak of transmission occurred in Poland. Dentists do not usually screen the patients for dental anxiety. The practitioners who are interested in treating patients with dental anxiety should use a screening method to evaluate their patients' level of anxiety before the procedure. These data will help to perform oral surgery more efficiently, without burdening patients with additional anxiety. Good communication with a trusted dentist, continuity of treatment and regular dental visits, and exposure to a dental environment are the best methods for managing dental fear.

Author Contributions: Conceptualization, D.P.-D., A.S., K.R.; methodology, D.P.-D., A.S.; software, D.P.-D., A.S., K.R.; validation, D.P.-D., W.J.C., A.S.; formal analysis, D.P.-D., A.S., W.J.C.; investigation, D.P.-D., A.S.; resources, D.P.-D., A.S., K.R.; data curation, D.P.-D., A.S.; writing—original draft preparation, D.P.-D.; writing—review and editing, D.P.-D., A.S., B.A.J.-F., D.A., W.J.C., K.R.; visualization, D.P.-D., A.S., B.A.J.-F., D.A., W.J.C., K.R.;

supervision, D.P.-D., A.S., W.J.C., B.A.J.-F., D.A.; project administration, D.P.-D., A.S., W.J.C., funding acquisition, D.P.-D., W.J.C., A.S. All authors have read and agreed to the published version of the manuscript.

Funding: This research received no external funding.

Acknowledgments: The authors would like to thank all of the dentists, residents and assistants of the Oral Surgery Department at the Medical University of Gdańsk, for their help and advice.

Conflicts of Interest: The authors declare no conflict of interest.

References

1. Davenne, E.; Giot, J.B.; Huynen, P. Coronavirus et COVID-19: Coronavirus and COVID-19: Focus on a galloping pandemic. *Rev. Med. Liege* **2020**, *75*, 218–225. [PubMed]
2. World Health Organization. Statement on the Second Meeting of the International Health Regulations (2005) Emergency Committee Regarding the Outbreak of Novel Coronavirus (2019-nCoV). Available online: https://wwwwhoint/news-room/detail/30-01-2020-statement-on-the-second-meeting-of-the-international-health-regulations-(2005)-emergency-committee-regarding-the-outbreak-of-novel-coronavirus-(2019-ncov) (accessed on 30 January 2020).
3. World Health Organisation. Available online: https://www.who.int/docs/default-source/coronaviruse/situation-reports/20200801-covid-19-sitrep-194.pdf?sfvrsn=401287f3_2 (accessed on 7 May 2020).
4. Lin, C.Y. Social reaction toward the 2019 novel coronavirus (COVID-19). *Soc. Health Behav.* **2020**, *3*, 1–2. [CrossRef]
5. Leutgeb, V.; Übel, S.; Schienle, A. Can you read my pokerface? A study on sex differences in dentophobia. *Eur. J. Oral Sci.* **2013**, *121*, 465–470. [CrossRef] [PubMed]
6. Rodríguez Vázquez, L.M.; Rubiños López, E.; Varela Centelles, A.; Blanco Otero, A.I.; Varela Otero, F.; Varela Centelles, P. Stress amongst primary dental care patients. *Med. Oral Patol. Oral Cir. Bucal* **2008**, *13*, 253–256.
7. Quteish Taani, D.S. Dental fear among a young adult Saudian population. *Int. Dent. J.* **2001**, *51*, 62–66. [CrossRef] [PubMed]
8. Vassend, O. Anxiety, pain and discomfort associated with dental treatment. *Behav. Res. Ther.* **1993**, *31*, 659–666. [CrossRef]
9. Peloso, R.M.; Pini, N.I.P.; Sunfeld, N.; Mori, D.; Oliveira, A.A.; Valarelli, R.C.G. How does the quarantine resulting from COVID-19 impact dental appointments and patient anxiety levels? *Braz. Oral Res.* **2020**, *34*, e84. [CrossRef] [PubMed]
10. Wang, J.; Du, G. COVID-19 may transmit through aerosol. *Ir. J. Med. Sci.* **2020**, *189*, 1–2. [CrossRef]
11. Wang, C.; Pan, R.; Wan, X.; Tan, Y.; Xu, L.; Ho, C.S.; Ho, R.C. Immediate psychological responses and associated factors during the initial stage of the 2019 coronavirus disease (COVID-19) epidemic among the general population in China. *Int. J. Environ. Res. Public Health* **2020**, *17*, 1729. [CrossRef]
12. Armfield, J.M.; Heaton, L.J. Management of fear and anxiety in the dental clinic: A review. *Aust. Dent. J.* **2013**, *58*, 390–531. [CrossRef]
13. Cotrin, P.P.; Peloso, R.M.; Oliveira, R.C.; Oliveira, R.C.G.; Pini, P.; Valarelli, F.P.; Salvatore Freitas, K.M. Impact of coronavirus pandemic in appointments and anxiety/concerns of patients regarding orthodontic treatment. *Orthod. Craniofac. Res.* **2020**. [CrossRef]
14. Bonafé, F.S.S.; Campos, J.A.D.B. Validation and invariance of the Dental Anxiety Scale in a Brazilian sample. *Braz. Oral Res.* **2016**, *30*, 138. [CrossRef] [PubMed]
15. Humphris, G.M.; Morrison, T.; Lindsay, S.J. The Modified Dental Anxiety Scale: Validation and United Kingdom norms. *Community Dent. Health* **1995**, *12*, 143–150. [PubMed]
16. Corah, N.L. Development of a dental anxiety scale. *J. Dent. Res.* **1969**, *48*, 596. [CrossRef] [PubMed]
17. Humphris, G.; Freeman, R.; Campbell, J.; Tuutti, H.; D'Souza, V. Further evidence for the reliability and validity of the Modified Dental Anxiety Scale. *Int. Dent. J.* **2000**, *50*, 367–370. [CrossRef]
18. Balestroni, G.; Bertolotti, G. EuroQol-5D (EQ-5D): An instrument for measuring quality of life. *Monaldi Arch. Chest Dis.* **2012**, *78*, 155–159. [CrossRef]
19. Dave, M.; Seoudi, N.; Coulthard, P. Urgent dental care for patients during the COVID-19 pandemic. *Lancet* **2020**, *395*, 1257. [CrossRef]
20. Quteish Taani, D.S. Dental anxiety and regularity of dental attendance in younger adults. *J. Oral Rehabil.* **2002**, *29*, 604–608. [CrossRef]

21. Erten, H.; Akarslan, Z.Z.; Bodrumlu, E. Dental fear and anxiety levels of patients attending a dental clinic. *Quintessence Int.* **2006**, *37*, 304–310.
22. Armfield, J.M.; Spencer, A.J.; Stewart, J.F. Dental fear in Australia: Who's afraid of the dentist? *Aust. Dent. J.* **2006**, *51*, 78–85. [CrossRef]
23. Arslan, S.; Erta, E.; Ülker, M. The relationship between dental fear and sociodemographic variables. *Erciyes Med. J.* **2011**, *33*, 295–300.
24. Humphris, G.M.; Dyer, T.A.; Robinson, P.G. The modified dental anxiety scale: UK general public population norms in 2008 with further psychometrics and effects of age. *BMC Oral Health* **2009**, *9*, 20. [CrossRef] [PubMed]
25. Ahmad, M.F.; Narwani, H.; Shuhaila, A. An evaluation of quality of life in women with endometriosis who underwent primary surgery: A 6-month follow up in Sabah Women & Children Hospital, Sabah, Malaysia. *J. Obstet. Gynaecol.* **2017**, *37*, 906–911. [CrossRef]
26. Torales, J.; O'Higgins, M.; Castaldelli-Maia, J.M.; Ventriglio, A. The outbreak of COVID-19 coronavirus and its impact on global mental health. *Int. J. Soc. Psychiatry* **2020**. [CrossRef] [PubMed]
27. Zhang, Y.; Ma, Z.F. Impact of the COVID-19 pandemic on mental health and quality of life among local residents in Liaoning Province, China: A cross-sectional study. *Int. J. Environ. Res. Public Health* **2020**, *17*, 2381. [CrossRef] [PubMed]
28. Egbor, P.E.; Akpata, O. An evaluation of the sociodemographic determinants of dental anxiety in patients scheduled for intra-alveolar extraction. *Libyan J. Med.* **2014**, *9*. [CrossRef]
29. Public Health England. Disparities in the Risk and Outcomes of COVID-19. 2020. Available online: https://assets.publishing.service.gov.uk/government/uploads/system/uploads/attachment_data/file/891116/disparities_review.pdf (accessed on 1 August 2020).
30. Everts, J. Announcing Swine Flu and the Interpretation of Pandemic Anxiety. *Antipode* **2013**, *45*, 809–825. [CrossRef]
31. Fu, W.; Wang, C.; Zou, L.; Guo, Y.; Lu, Z.; Yan, S. Psychological health, sleep quality, and coping styles to stress facing the COVID-19 in Wuhan, China. *Transl. Psychiatry* **2020**, *10*, 225. [CrossRef]

Journal of
Clinical Medicine

MDPI

Article

Temporomandibular Disorders and Bruxism Outbreak as a Possible Factor of Orofacial Pain Worsening during the COVID-19 Pandemic—Concomitant Research in Two Countries

Alona Emodi-Perlman [1,†], Ilana Eli [1,†], Joanna Smardz [2], Nir Uziel [1], Gniewko Wieckiewicz [3], Efrat Gilon [1], Natalia Grychowska [4] and Mieszko Wieckiewicz [2,*]

1 Section of Dental Education, Department of Oral Rehabilitation, The Maurice and Gabriela Goldshleger School of Dental Medicine, Tel Aviv University, Tel Aviv 6139001, Israel; dr.emodi@gmail.com (A.E.-P.); elilana@tauex.tau.ac.il (I.E.); niruziel@gmail.com (N.U.); gilon.efrat@gmail.com (E.G.)
2 Department of Experimental Dentistry, Wroclaw Medical University, 50-425 Wroclaw, Poland; joannasmardz1@gmail.com
3 Department and Clinic of Psychiatry, Medical University of Silesia, 42-612 Tarnowskie Gory, Poland; gniewkowieckiewicz@gmail.com
4 Department of Prosthetic Dentistry, Wroclaw Medical University, 50-425 Wroclaw, Poland; natgrychowska@gmail.com
* Correspondence: m.wieckiewicz@onet.pl
† Equal contribution.

Received: 23 August 2020; Accepted: 27 September 2020; Published: 12 October 2020

Abstract: Background: In late December 2019, a new pandemic caused by the SARS-CoV-2 (Severe Acute Respiratory Syndrome Coronavirus 2) infection began to spread around the world. The new situation gave rise to severe health threats, economic uncertainty, and social isolation, causing potential deleterious effects on people's physical and mental health. These effects are capable of influencing oral and maxillofacial conditions, such as temporomandibular disorders (TMD) and bruxism, which could further aggravate the orofacial pain. Two concomitant studies aimed to evaluate the effect of the current pandemic on the possible prevalence and worsening of TMD and bruxism symptoms among subjects selected from two culturally different countries: Israel and Poland. Materials and Methods: Studies were conducted as cross-sectional online surveys using similar anonymous questionnaires during the lockdown practiced in both countries. The authors obtained 700 complete responses from Israel and 1092 from Poland. In the first step, data concerning TMDs and bruxism were compared between the two countries. In the second step, univariate analyses (Chi^2) were performed to investigate the effects of anxiety, depression, and personal concerns of the Coronavirus pandemic, on the symptoms of TMD, and bruxism symptoms and their possible aggravation. Finally, multivariate analyses (logistic regression models) were carried out to identify the study variables that had a predictive value on TMD, bruxism, and symptom aggravation in the two countries. Results: The results showed that the Coronavirus pandemic has caused significant adverse effects on the psychoemotional status of both Israeli and Polish populations, resulting in the intensification of their bruxism and TMD symptoms. Conclusions: The aggravation of the psychoemotional status caused by the Coronavirus pandemic can result in bruxism and TMD symptoms intensification and thus lead to increased orofacial pain.

Keywords: COVID-19; SARS-CoV-2; coronavirus pandemic; temporomandibular disorders; bruxism; orofacial pain

1. Introduction

Temporomandibular disorders (TMD) are a group of conditions that cause pain and dysfunction of the masticatory muscles, the temporomandibular joints (TMJs), and associated structures. The most common features of TMD are regional pain, limited jaw movements, and acoustic sounds from TMJs during motions [1]. The prevalence of TMD in the general population is estimated at about 10–15% [2–4], and these conditions affect women more frequently than men. Psychosocial factors, such as anxiety, stress, depression, coping strategies, and catastrophizing, may influence the onset of pain, as well as precipitate or prolong the TMD pain [5–8]. The International Association for the Study of Pain (IASP) reported that TMD-related facial pain occurs in 9–13% of the general population, while only 4–7% seek treatment. The TMD-related pain may also affect the daily activities, physical and psychosocial functioning, and quality of life of the affected individuals [9].

Bruxism is a repetitive jaw muscle activity characterized by clenching or grinding of the teeth, and/or bracing or thrusting of the mandible [10]. It can act as a potential risk factor for several negative consequences of health such as masticatory muscle pain, oral mucosa damage, mechanical tooth wear, and failures of prosthodontic constructions [11–13]. This condition is divided into sleep bruxism (SB) awake bruxism (AB). The prevalence of SB is estimated at about 16% among young adults and at 3–8% among adults, while the prevalence of AB in the general population is estimated at about 22–30%. Both forms of bruxism men and women equally [14].

Psychosocial factors, such as stress and anxiety, have been indicated as associated with both SB and AB [15–20]. However, the latest research showed that self-reported perceived stress was not correlated with the intensity of SB [21].

In late December 2019, a new unfamiliar and threatening pandemic called COVID-19 (Coronavirus 2019 disease), which is caused by the SARS-CoV-2 (Severe Acute Respiratory Syndrome Coronavirus 2) infection, began to spread around the world. Due to almost complete uncertainty about the ways of virus spread [22] and the appropriate modes of treatment, insufficient availability of health services, and no existing vaccine or efficient drug for treatment, most countries adopted the policies of social distancing and partial to total lockdown.

The situation continued, and within weeks, routine life was drastically altered. This gave rise to severe health threats, economic uncertainty, and social isolation, causing potential deleterious effects on the physical and mental health of the people. The common psychological responses of individuals to the Coronavirus pandemic included stress, anxiety, and depression [22]. All these are capable of influencing the oral and maxillofacial syndromes, such as TMD and bruxism, which could further aggravate the orofacial pain [23].

Studies aimed to: (i) evaluate the effect of the current Coronavirus pandemic on the possible prevalence and worsening of TMD and bruxism symptoms, among subjects selected from two culturally different countries: Israel and Poland; and (ii) to define the predictors of TMD and bruxism during the lock down periods, in the above countries.

2. Materials and Methods

Studies were conducted as cross-sectional online surveys using anonymous questionnaires. The final questionnaire was compiled from tools commonly used with regard to TMD, bruxism, anxiety and depression (3Q/TMD, possible/probable bruxism, and Patient Health Questionnaie-4, as detailed below), and specific questions referring to demographics, concerns specific to the Coronavirus, media consumption, etc. The latter were agreed upon, and tested for content validity, by a group of subject matter experts (SMEs). The group consisted of four dentists (AE-P, IE, NU, and EG) who work at the Tel Aviv University School of Dental Medicine and have vast clinical and academic experience in working with patients suffering from TMD and bruxism. Each SME proposed questions for the study and, following discussions, the final questions were agreed upon. The questionnaire was compiled in Hebrew and translated to Polish by the Polish group. The surveys were carried out one month after the start of the total lockdown periods in each of the countries.

2.1. Population

The questionnaire was distributed through the internet (in Hebrew in Israel, in Polish in Poland).

In Israel, the study questionnaire was posted on SurveyGizmo (https:www.mysurveygizmo.com/s3) and distributed through mailing lists of dental clinics and social media (e.g., Facebook and WhatsApp).

In Poland, the questionnaire was posted on Reddit, an American social news aggregation platform that allows the users to interact on community-created discussion forums, and on r/Polska sub-reddit.

In both countries, the responses were given anonymously by the participants.

Studies were conducted in full accordance with the World Medical Association Declaration of Helsinki. In Israel, all the study procedures were approved by the Ethics Committee of the Tel Aviv University in Israel (ID: 0001332-1). In Poland the Bioethical Committee of the Wroclaw Medical University approved the study protocol (ID: KB-302/2020). Informed consent was obtained from all the subjects as required.

2.2. Instruments

The following data were collected from the participants:

1. Demographic and general information: This included the consent to participate in the study, age, gender, and conjugal status (with partner and children, with partner but no children, with children but no partner, with roommate, alone).
2. Concerns specific to the Coronavirus: These included worries about the risk of being contaminated (yes/no), and about the financial aspects, physical health, mental health, and relationship with relatives and friends (ranging from 1—not at all to 5—very worried).
3. TMD screening: The 3Q/TMD questionnaire, which is a reliable and acceptable tool for screening the TMD conditions, was used for collecting data [24,25]. The questionnaire has an excellent negative predictive value and is regarded as a valid tool for screening [24,25]. It asks about the existence of pain in the temple, face, and jaw during mouth opening or chewing, and whether there is an experience of jaw locking. A positive response to one of these confirms the presence of TMDs.
4. Possible/probable AB: An accepted way to assess possible AB and/or SB is the use of a self-report questionnaire [12,17,26]. The questions are related to awareness (by self or being told by others) of grinding, clenching, and holding the teeth together and/or tightening the masticatory muscles during the day (scale ranging from 0—never to 4—all the time). A positive answer to one of these (either than "never") confirms the presence of "possible AB". An additional positive response to the question that refers to "being told by a dentist that you clench/grind your teeth" confirms the presence of "probable AB" [10,27].
5. Possible/probable SB: It is assessed through the question, "Do you know or have been told that you clench or grind your teeth while you sleep?" A scale ranging from 0 (never) to 4 (4–7 nights/week) is used for this assessment. Any score above 0 (never) confirms the presence of "possible SB". An additional positive response to the question that refers to "being told by a dentist that you clench/grind your teeth" confirms the presence of "probable SB" [10,27].
6. Possible aggravation of symptoms associated with TMDs and bruxism ("since the beginning of the Coronavirus confinement do you feel any changes in ... etc."). The evaluated symptoms referred to: (i) pain in temple, face, jaw or jaw joint, pain at mouth opening or chewing and jaw locking (for TMD); (ii) headache during the day in the temple area, exacerbation in pain levels during the day and change in the temple pain upon functioning (for TMD and AB); and (iii) difficulties in mouth opening upon awaking, jaw and/or muscle stiffness upon awaking and temple headache that is reduced after some time (for SB) [28]. The scores were as follows: no change, slight aggravation, significant aggravation, and improvement.

7. Anxiety and depression: The Patient Health Questionnaire-4, a brief screening tool, is used for assessing anxiety and depression [29]. The total score of this questionnaire ranges from 0 to 12, and the conditions are usually evaluated using the following cut-off scores: 0–2, normal; 3–5, mild; 6–8, moderate; 9–12 severe [29]. The questionnaire also allows performing a separate evaluation for anxiety and depression.
8. Media consumption: Report of news consumption concerning the Coronavirus pandemic through television, internet, and/or social media was also assessed (scale ranging from 1—not at all to 4—all reports/all the time).

All questions were formulated in a first person voice (referring to self), and referred to the last 30 days, namely, to the period of the lock down.

The surveys were open to anyone who entered the SurveyGizmo (https:www.mysurveygizmo.com/s3) site and/or the Facebook and/or WhatsApp apps (in Israel) or the r/Polska sub-reddit in Poland.

In Israel, complete lock down was imposed on 19 March 2020. Data were collected from 16 April (namely, four weeks after the beginning of the complete lock down) to 20 May 2020. In Poland, complete lock down was imposed on 31 March 2020. Data were collected from 29 April (four weeks after the beginning of the lockdown) to 3 May 2020.

2.3. Statistical Analysis of Data

Data analysis was performed using STATISTICA PL Version 12 software (Tulsa, OK, USA), with the level of significance set at $p < 0.05$. In the first step, the data concerning TMDs, AB, and SB were compared between the two countries (descriptive analyses). In the second step, univariate analyses (Chi^2) were performed to investigate the effects of anxiety, depression, and personal concerns of the Coronavirus pandemic (being contaminated, being influenced financially, experiencing negative effects on physical and/or mental health and on the relationship with relatives and friends) on the symptoms of TMDs, SB, and AB and their possible aggravation. Finally, multivariate analyses (logistic regression models—binomial logit models) were carried out to identify the study variables that had a predictive value on the symptoms of TMDs, AB, and SB and their aggravation.

3. Results

In Israel, a total of 867 subjects responded to the questionnaire, out of whom 80.74% ($N = 700$) fully completed it. In Poland, a total of 1096 subjects responded to the questionnaire, of which 99.63% ($N = 1092$) fully completed it.

The age groups of participants were defined according to "young adults" (age of 18–35 years) and "adults" (36–56 years old) as accepted in the literature [30]. Some significant differences existed between the two populations with regard to gender and age groups (Tables 1 and 2).

Table 1. Gender of study populations.

Gender	Percent Israel	Count	Percent Poland	Count
Male	33.6%	235	41.6%	454
Female	66.4%	465	58.4%	638
Total	100%	700	100%	1092

The Polish population had more females ($p < 0.05$), and the participants were significantly younger compared to their Israeli counterparts ($p < 0.05$).

Due to these significant differences in age and gender between the studied populations, comparisons were carried out separately for males and females, categorized into predefined age groups.

Table 2. Age of study populations.

Age	Israel			Poland		
	Female N (%)	Male N (%)	Total	Female N (%)	Male N (%)	Total
18–35	142 (30.5)	61 (26.0)	203	443 (69.4)	385 (84.8)	828
36–55	185 (39.8)	98 (41.7)	283	171 (26.8)	63 (13.9)	234
>56	127 (27.3)	73 (31.1)	200	24 (3.8)	6 (1.3)	30
N/A	11 (2.4)	3 (1.3)	14	0	0	0
Total	465	235	700	638	454	1092

3.1. Descriptive Analyses—TMDs, Possible/Probable AB, and Possible/Probable SB

1. TMD screening: The results showed that the odds of occurrence of TMDs among the Polish young adult and adult age groups (18–35 years and 36–55 years) were significantly higher for both males and females as compared to the Israeli groups (odds ratios ranged from 3.04 to 5.37). However, no such differences were observed for the elderly group (>56 years) between the populations (Table 3).

Table 3. Temporomandibular disorders (TMD) distribution.

		TMD Positive		TMD Negative		p *	OR (95% CI) #
Age	Gender	Israel	Poland	Israel	Poland		
18–35	Male N (%)	7 ((1.6)	158 (35.4)	54 (12.1)	227 (50.9)	0.0000	5.37 (2.38, 12.11)
	Female N (%)	48 (8.2)	280 (47.8)	94 (16.1)	163 (27.9)	0.0000	3.36 (2.26, 5.00)
36–55	Male N (%)	13 (8.1)	20 (12.4)	85 (52.8)	43 (26.7)	0.005	3.04 (1.38, 6.69)
	Female N (%)	47 (13.2)	105 (29.5)	138 (38.8)	66 (18.5)	0.0000	4.67 (2.9, 7.34)
>56	Male N (%)	10 (12.7)	1 (1.3)	63 (79.7)	5 (6.3)	>0.05	1.26 (0.13, 11.93)
	Female N (%)	25 (16.6)	12 (7.9)	102 (67.6)	12 (7.9)	0.003	4.08 (1.64, 10.16)
N/A		2	0	12	0	----	----
Total		152	576	548	516		

* Comparison of countries in regard to TMD positive/TMD negative in particular age and gender groups (Chi^2).
\# OR comparing Poland versus Israel in regard to TMD positive in particular age and gender groups.

2. Possible/probable AB: Similar results were found for possible/probable AB. The odds of occurrence of these conditions among the Polish participants were significantly higher in general than among the Israeli participants (except the young and elder males), with the odds ratios ranging between 2.51 and 6.41 (Table 4).

Table 4. Awake bruxism (AB) distribution.

		Probable AB (I)		Possible AB (II)		AB Negative (III)		p *	OR (95% CI) #
Age	Gender	Israel	Poland	Israel	Poland	Israel	Poland		
18–35	Male N (%)	8 (1.8)	71 (15.9)	21 (4.7)	138 (30.9)	32 (7.2)	176 (39.5)	>0.05	1.31 (0.76, 2.25)
	Female N (%)	40 (6.8)	187 (32.0)	38 (6.5)	151 (25.8)	64 (10.9)	105 (17.9)	0.0000	2.64 (1.78, 3.93)
36–55	Male N (%)	19 (11.8)	17 (10.6)	15 (9.3)	19 (11.8)	64 (39.7)	27 (16.8)	0.015	2.51 (1.31, 4.81)
	Female N (%)	46 (12.9)	94 (26.4)	38 (10.7)	50 (14.0)	101 (28.4)	27 (7.6)	0.0000	6.41 (3.88, 10.60)
>56	Male N (%)	8 (10.1)	0	4 (5.1)	1 (1.3)	61 (72.2)	5 (6.3)	>0.05	1.02 (0.11, 9.50)
	Female N (%)	30 (19.9)	9 (6.0)	9 (6.0)	6 (4.0)	88 (58.3)	9 (6.0)	0.007	3.76 (1.52, 9.33)
N/A		2	0	0	0	12	0	----	----
Total		153	378	125	365	422	349		

* Comparison of countries in regard to Possible/Probable AB/AB negative in particular age and gender groups (Chi^2). # OR comparing Poland versus Israel in regard to AB positive (Possible and Probable AB) in particular age and gender groups.

3. Possible/probable SB: The findings for possible/probable SB were also consistent. The odds of occurrence of these conditions among the Polish subjects (except for males in the two higher age

groups) were similar to those of the Israeli subjects, with the odds ratios ranging from 1.4 to 3.99 (Table 5).

Table 5. Sleep bruxism (SB) distribution.

		Probable SB (I)		Possible SB (II)		SB Negative (III)		p *	OR (95% CI) #
Age	Gender	Israel	Poland	Israel	Poland	Israel	Poland		
18–35	Male N (%)	8 (1.8)	61 (13.7)	9 (2.0)	74 (16.6)	44 (9.8)	250 (56.0)	0.008	1.40 (0.77, 2.54)
	Female N (%)	34 (5.8)	182 (31.1)	21 (3.6)	90 (15.4)	87 (14.9)	171 (29.2)	0.0000	2.52 (1.71, 3.71)
36–55	Male N (%)	22 (13.7)	16 (9.9)	9 (5.6)	7 (4.4)	67 (41.6)	40 (24.8)	>0.05	1.24 (0.64, 2.42)
	Female N (%)	50 (10.7)	84 (23.6)	23 (6.5)	21 (5.9)	112 (31.5)	66 (18.5)	0.0000	2.44 (1.59, 3.74)
>56	Male N (%)	6 (7.6)	0	4 (5.1)	1 (1.3)	63 (79.8)	5 (6.3)	>0.05	1.26 (0.13, 11.93)
	Female N (%)	29 (19.2)	8 (5.3)	4 (2.7)	6 (4.0)	94 (62.2)	10 (6.6)	0.0008	3.99 (1.62, 9.84)
N/A		3	0	0	0	11	0	----	----
Total		152	351	70	199	478	542		

* Comparison of countries in regard to Possible/Probable SB/SB negative in particular age and gender groups (Chi^2).
# OR comparing Poland versus Israel in regard to SB positive (Possible and Probable SB) in particular age and gender groups.

3.2. Aggravation of AB, SB and TMD Symptoms

Almost half (48.8%) of the Poles reported experiencing at least once a week pain in temple, face, jaw or jaw joint during the past 30 days, namely, since the beginning of the lockdown. A total of 247 individuals (22.6%) declared pain during mouth opening or chewing and 101 (9.2%) jaw locking or getting stuck at least once a week. Among the Israelis, the numbers were 166 (23.7%), 91 (13.0%), and 35 (5.0%), respectively.

Among the Polish responders, 372 (34%) reported TMD symptoms aggravation, 372 (34%) AB aggravation, and 311 (28%) SB aggravation. Among the Israeli responders, 107 (15%) reported TMD symptoms aggravation, 111 (16%) AB symptom aggravation, and 94 (13%) SB symptom aggravation.

Both in Israel and in Poland, females reported more symptoms of TMD, AB, SB and symptom aggravation, than males (Chi^2, $p < 0.05$ for all). However, further logistic regression analyses, performed among Israeli population (see below), rejected gender as a predictor of SB. Distributions of TMD, AB, SB among males and females in Poland and in Israel are presented in Tables 3–5.

3.3. The Effect of Conjugal Status

Significant relationships were observed between subjects' conjugal status and TMD aggravation, AB aggravation and SB aggravation among the Polish responders (Chi^2, $p < 0.05$, for all). Respondents living with a roommate or sharing apartment with a partner, reported more TMD and AB aggravation than those living with a spouse without children (Chi^2, $p < 0.001$ for both). They also reported higher SB symptom aggravation than those with children but with no partner or spouse ($p < 0.001$).

In Israel, no differences in TMD, AB. and SB symptom aggravation were observed among subjects with different conjugal status.

3.4. The Effect of Demographic Data on Anxiety and Depression

In Poland, anxiety was more frequent among females than males (Chi^2, $p < 0.05$). Additionally, a significant relationship was found between subjects' conjugal status and depression ($p < 0.05$). Depression was more often among respondents living with a roommate or sharing an apartment with a partner than among responders living with spouse and children ($p < 0.001$). There were no significant relationships between gender and depression or age and depression, between age and anxiety and between conjugal status and anxiety.

In the Israel, anxiety and depression were more frequent among females than males (Chi^2, $p < 0.05$). No relationships between conjugal status and depression or anxiety, and between age and depression were detected. Anxiety was more frequent among young adults (18–35 years) than among the elderly group (>56 years) (Chi^2, $p < 0.001$).

3.5. Effect of Anxiety, Depression, and Personal Concerns on TMD, SB, and AB (Chi^2)

1. TMD: The presence of anxiety, depression, or personal concerns significantly increased the odds of occurrence of TMDs among both populations. The odds ratio ranged between 1.32 (concerns of being contaminated by the virus) and 2.75 (anxiety) for the Polish subjects, while it ranged between 1.46 (concerns about personal finances due to the pandemic) and 6.4 (anxiety) for the Israeli population.

2. Possible/probable AB: The presence of anxiety, depression, and personal concerns significantly increased the odds of occurrence of possible/probable AB among both populations. The odds ratios ranged from 1.45 (concerns of being affected financially, for Polish subjects) to 2.85 (anxiety, for Israeli subjects).

3. Possible/probable SB: Mixed results were observed for possible/probable SB. In Poland the odds ratios ranged from 1.34 (concerns of being affected mentally) to 1.84 (anxiety). No effect was observed for the concerns regarding personal finances or depression. Among the Israeli subjects, the odds ratios ranged from 1.38 (worries of being affected financially) to 2.27 (anxiety). No effect was observed for worries of being contaminated by the virus.

3.6. Effect of Anxiety, Depression, and Personal Concerns on the Possible Aggravation of TMD, SB, and AB Symptoms (Chi^2)

1. Aggravation of TMD symptoms: Anxiety, depression, and personal concerns significantly increased the odds of aggravation of TMD symptoms in both populations. The odds ratios ranged from 1.58 (concerns regarding personal finances, for Polish subjects) to 3.03 (anxiety, for Polish subjects).

2. Aggravation of possible/probable AB symptoms: The obtained results were similar with regard to the aggravation of AB symptoms. The odds ratios ranged from 1.36 (concerns regarding personal finances, for Polish subjects) to 3.95 (anxiety, for Israeli subjects).

3. Aggravation of possible/probable SB symptoms: Similar results were observed for the aggravation of SB symptoms. The odds ratios ranged from 1.60 (concerns regarding personal finances, for Polish subjects) to 3.32 (anxiety, for Israeli subjects).

3.7. Multivariate Analyses (Logistic Regression)

1. TMD: The best predictors of TMD in Poland were female gender, anxiety, and personal concerns (worries of being contaminated by the virus and about the pandemic's effect on mental health) (Table 6). Aggravation of TMD was best predicted by female gender, worries of being contaminated, use of social media to look for information about the pandemic, and worries about the pandemic's effect on mental health (Table 7).

Table 6. Prediction of temporomandibular disorders (TMD) in Poland.

Effect	Predictor	Estimate	S.E.	Wald	df	OR (95% CI)	p
Gender	Female	0.384	0.065	34.516	1	2.16 (1.67, 2.78)	0.0000
Risk of contamination *	Yes	0.237	0.065	13.526	1	1.61 (1.25, 2.07)	0.0002
Anxiety	Yes	0.372	0.082	20.505	1	2.10 (1.53, 2.90)	0.0000
Mental health **	II	0.160	0.069	5.354	1	1.38 (1.05, 1.80)	0.0207

Link function: Logit. * Feeling at high risk of being contaminated (yes/no). ** Worries about the effect of the Coronavirus on mental health (not at all/a little worried (I) versus somewhat worried/worried/very worried (II)).

On the other hand, the only significant predictor of TMDs in Israel was anxiety (Estimate: 0.917, S.E.: 0.107, Wald: 73.922, df: 1, odds ratio 6.25, 95% confidence interval 4.11–9.49).

The best predictors of TMD aggravation in Israel were female gender, concerns about the pandemic's effect on the relationship with family and friends, and anxiety (Table 8).

Table 7. Prediction of temporomandibular disorders (TMD) aggravation in Poland.

Effect	Predictor	Estimate	S.E.	Wald	df	OR (95% CI)	*p*
Gender	Female	0.321	0.072	19.715	1	1.90 (1.43, 2.52)	0.0000
Risk of contamination *	Yes	0.218	0.069	10.150	1	1.55 (1.18, 2.03)	0.0014
Social media **	II	0.249	0.069	12.929	1	1.65 (1.25, 2.16)	0.0003
Anxiety	Yes	0.389	0.08	23.579	1	2.18 (1.59, 2.98)	0.0000
Mental health ***	II	0.224	0.073	9.372	1	1.57 (1.18, 2.09)	0.0022

Link function: Logit. * Feeling at high risk of being contaminated (yes/no). ** How often connecting to social media to check for news regarding the pandemic (not checking at all/checking once a day (I) versus checking several times a day/checking all the time (II)). *** Worries about the effect of the Coronavirus on mental health (not at all/a little worried (I) versus somewhat worried/worried/very worried (II)).

Table 8. Prediction of temporomandibular disorders (TMD) aggravation in Israel.

Effect	Predictor	Estimate	S.E.	Wald	df	OR (95% CI)	*p*
Gender	Female	0.255	0.127	4.041	1	1.66 (1.01, 2.74)	0.0444
Relations *	II	0.375	0.112	11.155	1	2.12 (1.36, 3.29)	0.0008
Anxiety	Yes	0.351	0.123	8.184	1	2.02 (1.25, 3.26)	0.0042

Link function: Logit. * Worries regarding the effect of the Coronavirus pandemic on relations with relatives and friends (not at all/a little worried (I) versus somewhat worried/worried/very worried (II).

2. Possible/probable AB: In Poland, the best predictors of possible/probable AB were female gender, concerns of being contaminated by the virus, and concerns about the pandemic's effect on mental health (Table 9). The aggravation of AB was best predicted by concerns about being contaminated by the virus, anxiety, concerns of the pandemic's effect on physical and/or mental health, and use of social media for obtaining information about the pandemic (Table 10).

Table 9. Prediction of awake bruxism (AB) in Poland.

Effect	Predictor	Estimate	S.E.	Wald	df	OR (95% CI)	*p*
Gender	Female	0.472	0.069	46.245	1	2.57 (1.96, 3.37)	0.0000
Risk of contamination *	Yes	0.212	0.070	9.089	1	1.53 (1.16, 2.01)	0.0026
Mental health **	II	0.249	0.075	11.041	1	1.64 (1.23, 2.21)	0.0009
Anxiety	Yes	0.334	0.095	12.215	1	1.95 (1.34, 2.83)	0.0005

Link function: Logit. * Feeling at high risk of being contaminated (yes/no). ** Worries about the effect of the Coronavirus on mental health (not at all/a little worried (I) versus somewhat worried/worried/very worried (II).

Table 10. Prediction of awake bruxism (AB) aggravation in Poland.

Effect	Predictor	Estimate	S.E.	Wald	df	OR (95% CI)	*p*
Gender	Female	0.349	0.074	22.300	1	2.01 (1.50, 2.69)	0.0000
Risk of contamination *	Yes	0.208	0.071	8.615	1	1.51 (1.15, 2.00)	0.0033
Anxiety	Yes	0.461	0.081	32.200	1	2.51 (1.82, 3.46)	0.0000
Physical health **	II	0.217	0.075	8.371	1	1.54 (1.15, 2.07)	0.0038
Mental health ***	II	0.260	0.076	11.781	1	1.68 (1.25, 2.26)	0.0006
Social media ****	II	0.241	0.071	11.516	1	1.62 (1.23, 2.14)	0.0007

Link function: Logit. * Feeling at high risk of being contaminated (yes/no). ** Worries about the effect of the Coronavirus on one's physical health (not at all/a little worried (I) versus somewhat worried/worried/very worried (II)). *** Worries about the effect of the Coronavirus on one's mental health (not at all/a little worried (I) versus somewhat worried/worried/very worried (II)). **** How often connecting to social media to check for news regarding the pandemic (not checking at all/checking once a day (I) versus checking several times a day/checking all the time (II).

In Israel, the best predictors of possible/probable AB were female gender, depression, concerns regarding personal finances, and anxiety (Table 11). The aggravation of AB was best predicted by female gender, concerns about the pandemic's effect on the relationship with relatives and friends and on mental health, and anxiety (Table 12).

Table 11. Prediction of awake bruxism (AB) in Israel.

Effect	Predictor	Estimate	S.E.	Wald	df	OR (95% CI)	p
Gender	Female	0.175	0.088	3.946	1	1.42 (1.00, 2.00)	0.0470
Depression	Yes	0.202	0.101	4.000	1	1.50 (1.01, 2.23)	0.0455
Finances *	II	0.233	0.081	8.283	1	1.59 (1.16, 2.19)	0.0040
Anxiety	Yes	0.383	0.109	12.472	1	2.15 (1.41, 3.30)	0.0004

Link function: Logit. * Worries about finances (not at al/a little worried (I) versus somewhat worried/worried/very worried (II)).

Table 12. Prediction of awake bruxism (AB) aggravation in Israel.

Effect	Predictor	Estimate	S.E.	Wald	df	OR (95% CI)	p
Gender	Female	0.333	0.134	6.208	1	1.95 (1.15, 3.29)	0.0127
Relations *	II	0.250	0.123	4.156	1	1.65 (1.02, 2.67)	0.0417
Anxiety	Yes	0.445	0.131	11.522	1	2.44 (1.46, 4.08)	0.0007
Mental health **	II	0.292	0.134	4.737	1	1.79 (1.06, 3.04)	0.0295

Link function: Logit. * Worries regarding the effect of the Coronavirus pandemic on relations with relatives and friends (not at all/a little worried (I) versus somewhat worried/worried/very worried (II)). ** Worries about the effect of the Coronavirus on one's mental health (not at all/a little worried versus somewhat worried/worried/very worried).

3. Possible/probable SB: In Poland, the best predictors of possible/probable SB were female gender, worries of being contaminated by the virus, and anxiety (Table 13). The aggravation of SB was best predicted by female gender, worries of being contaminated by the virus, anxiety, use of social media, and concerns of the pandemic's effect on mental health (Table 14).

Table 13. Prediction of sleep bruxism (SB) in Poland.

Effect	Predictor	Estimate	S.E.	Wald	df	OR (95% CI)	p
Gender	Female	0.485	0.065	55.413	1	2.64 (2.04, 3.41)	0.0000
Risk of contamination *	Yes	0.198	0.064	9.646	1	1.49 (1.16, 1.91)	0.0019
Anxiety	Yes	0.225	0.074	9.341	1	1.57 (1.18, 2.09)	0.0022

Link function: Logit. * Feeling at high risk of being contaminated (yes/no).

Table 14. Prediction of sleep bruxism (SB) aggravation in Poland.

Effect	Predictor	Estimate	S.E.	Wald	df	OR (95% CI)	p
Gender	Female	0.329	0.077	18.030	1	1.93 (1.42, 2.61)	0.0000
Risk of contamination *	Yes	0.301	0.072	17.302	1	1.83 (1.38, 2.43)	0.0000
Anxiety	Yes	0.405	0.083	24.071	1	2.25 (1.63, 3.11)	0.0000
Social media **	II	0.230	0.073	10.026	1	1.58 (1.19, 2.11)	0.0015
Mental health ***	II	0.245	0.078	9.939	1	1.63 (1.20, 2.21)	0.0016

Link function: Logit. * Feeling at high risk of being contaminated (yes/no). ** How often connecting to social media to check for news regarding the pandemic (not checking at all/checking once a day (I) versus checking several times a day/checking all the time (II)). *** Worries about the effect of the Coronavirus on one's mental health (not at all/a little worried (I) versus somewhat worried/worried/very worried (II).

In Israel, possible/probable SB was best predicted by anxiety and concerns regarding the pandemic's effect on the relationship with relatives and friends (Table 15). The aggravation of SB was best predicted by female gender, anxiety, and concerns about mental health (Table 16).

Table 15. Prediction of sleep bruxism (SB) in Israel.

Effect	Predictor	Estimate	S.E.	Wald	df	OR (95% CI)	p
Anxiety	Yes	0.323	0.103	9.762	1	1.91 (1.27, 2.86)	0.0018
Relations *	II	0.359	0.091	15.516	1	2.05 (1.43, 2.92)	0.0001

Link function: Logit. * Worries regarding the effect of the Coronavirus pandemic on relations with relatives and friends (not at all/a little worried (I) versus somewhat worried/worried/very worried (II)).

Table 16. Prediction of sleep bruxism (SB) aggravation in Israel.

Effect	Predictor	Estimate	S.E.	Wald	df	OR (95% CI)	p
Gender	Female	0.419	0.147	8.160	1	2.31 (1.30, 4.11)	0.0043
Anxiety	Yes	0.358	0.139	6.665	1	2.05 (1.19, 3.53)	0.0098
Mental health *	II	0.346	0.131	6.971	1	2.00 (1.20, 3.34)	0.0083

Link function: Logit. * Worries about the effect of the Coronavirus on one's mental health (not at all/a little worried (I) versus somewhat worried/worried/very worried (II))

4. Discussion

The two studies, carried out in two different countries, used similar tools and collected data at similar points in time, as far as the pandemic progression and lock down periods are concerned. In Israel, data collection started four weeks after the beginning of a total lockdown in the country. Schools, kindergartens, and universities were closed. Leaving home for a distance more than 100 m was prohibited, except for emergency, buying basic products, or work in vital posts (specifically defined by the government). All nonemergency medical and dental treatments were stopped. Shops, restaurants, and most public places were shut down. Personal contact with family members not cohabitating in the same home and/or with friends was forbidden. Similarly, in Poland, data collection started four weeks after the beginning of a total lockdown in the country, when the country was practicing an almost complete lockdown with similar regulations as mentioned above for Israel (with minor exceptions, e.g., there were no limitations on the distance of leaving home). Although the studied populations in Poland and in Israel were not similar, age- and/or gender-wise, the similarity in research tools and in the point in time allows us to evaluate some interesting differences between the two societies.

The first emerging finding of the two studies is that significant differences existed in the odds of occurrence of bruxism (AB and SB) and TMD between the Polish and Israeli populations during the lock down periods in the two countries. Except in a few cases (higher age group), the odds in Poland were found to be higher by several hundred percent than those in Israel.

In the general population, the prevalence of bruxism is estimated at 8–31% and tends to decrease with age [31]. SB prevalence is about 16% among young adults and 3–8% among adults, while the AB prevalence in the general population is 22–30% [14]. Even the reported prevalence of bruxing activities has a large range (2.7–57.3% for AB, 4.1–59.2% for SB) [26]. When considering TMD, it is believed that about 75% of the general population may experience at least one TMD-associated sign during their lifetime and about 33% have at least one TMD symptom at each time [32]. The differences origin mostly in different modes of measuring.

Regretfully, accurate data on possible differences in pre-pandemic occurrence of bruxism in the Polish versus Israeli populations are not available. However, some studies from Poland and from Israel suggest that the occurrence of TMD in the Polish population may differ from that in the Israeli population. Wieckiewicz et al. reported that 54% of Polish university students present TMD symptoms [33]. In another study, the same group of authors reported that 56% of participants were diagnosed with pain-related TMD after a clinical examination [34]. In Israel, Winocur et al. reported that 37% of individuals had at least one TMD symptom [35]. Thus, the differences between countries, observed in the present study, may be due to several reasons. First, the higher findings of TMD in the Polish populations may have been there before the pandemic [33–35]. Possibly, the increase in anxiety/depression in both countries affected TMD and bruxism in both countries in a proportional manner. Additionally, the differences in the demographic properties of populations were significant, a fact that might have affected the results.

As both bruxism and TMD can be caused and intensified by psychologic factors [8,31], the differences in their prevalence during the pandemic could have resulted from the psychological differences between the participants. These, in turn, may result from ethnic, socioeconomic, political, and cultural differences between the Polish and Israeli societies [36,37]. These factors could have potentially modulated the psychoemotional status of the participants, influenced their coping strategies during the Coronavirus pandemic, and in turn increased the prevalence of both bruxism and TMD in Poland. However, this issue needs a further study focused on differentiating between the populations.

It should also be emphasized that TMDs are closely associated with orofacial pain. The IASP reported that TMD-related facial pain occurs in 9–13% of the general population. As TMD-related pain can affect the daily activities, physical and psychosocial functioning, and quality of life of the affected individuals, such a relationship could play an important role during the COVID-19 pandemic [9]. Increased psychosocial distress during the pandemic can exacerbate the TMD symptoms, including those associated with orofacial pain, which in turn may further negatively affect the patients' psychoemotional status.

When the effects of anxiety, depression, and personal concerns on TMD, SB, and AB, and the aggravation of their symptoms (pain in temple, face or jaw, pain when opening mouth, sticking of jaw, headache, difficulty in mouth upon awaking, and stiffness in jaw upon awaking, etc.) were analyzed, some similarities were observed between the countries. Although the odds of occurrence of TMD, SB, and AB in Poland were by far higher than in Israel, the effects of emotional factors and of personal concerns on the associated symptoms and their aggravation were found to be similar in both countries. Anxiety, depression, and worries regarding finances, health and relationships significantly increased the odds of occurrence of bruxism and TMD in both the Polish and Israeli societies (with some minor exceptions).

Apparently, anxiety, depression, and personal worries evoked by the Coronavirus pandemic increased the prevalence of TMD and bruxism. This is in line with the literature results, that anxiety, stress, depression, coping strategies, and catastrophizing may precipitate or prolong the TMD pain [2–8], and that psychosocial factors are associated with both forms of bruxism [13,14,16–20]. When the pandemic situation kept changing rapidly from day to day, uncertainty and worries about the present and future were common and unavoidable [38,39]. Moreover, subjects had to stay home and many were unemployed, with the media constantly broadcasting apocalyptic news. Under such conditions, a significant increase in the odds of occurrence of TMD, SB, and AB is not surprising.

The one prominent difference was observed between the studied populations. The studies show that unlike the Polish participants, the worry of being contaminated by the virus did not increase the odds of occurrence of AB and SB, or aggravate the symptoms of the conditions (TMD, SB, and AB) among the Israeli subjects. This may be explained by the advanced and generally good public health services available in Israel. All the Israeli citizens have governmental health insurance and are entitled to all the necessary health services with no extra costs (besides a mandatory monthly fee). Furthermore, hospitals are considered to meet high medical standards, and medical personnel are required to be well trained. In Poland, citizens' trust in national healthcare system is limited [40].

Logistic regression models used in this study for identifying the variables that can serve as significant predictors of TMD, SB, AB, and/or the aggravation of their symptoms, showed that female gender was significant in most of the calculations. In Poland, female gender played a significant role in predicting the presence of TMD, AB, and SB, as well as the symptom aggravation, while in Israel this factor played a significant role in predicting the presence of AB (but not TMD or SB) and the aggravation of TMD, SB, and AB symptoms.

The role of gender is expected because most of the TMD patients worldwide are women [1]. In spite of the differences between the two countries, results showed that women in both places are highly vulnerable to the effects of unexpected prolonged stress situations. Aggravation of chronic pain symptoms such as TMD and symptoms associated with bruxism may be only some of the negative consequences that affect women more severely than men [41,42].

Additional factors that were consistently identified as significantly predicting the TMD, AB, and SB (and/or the symptom aggravation) in the present studies were anxiety, worries of being contaminated by the virus, and concerns about the pandemic's effect on physical or mental health (to slightly different extents in the two countries). In some instances, two additional factors were identified in the regression analyses: worries that the pandemic will affect the relationship with relatives and friends (in Israel) and the use of social media (but not TV or internet) for checking news regarding the pandemic (in Poland).

In Israel, close family ties and long-term friendships are very common in the society [43]. Apparently, the social distancing period, which prevented face-to-face meetings, took its toll on Israeli society. The fact that the use of social media affected, in some cases, the Polish, but not the Israeli, participants, may be explained by the younger age of the former. Another explanation may be that the Israeli society is constantly exposed to security tension and alerts making it more resilient [44]. The Israeli public extensively check the news at all times, and the Coronavirus crisis is no different from many other emergencies experienced by these people.

In a recent study, Varshney et al. reported that during the initial stages of the Coronavirus pandemic in India, almost one-third of the respondents manifested a significant psychological impact [45]. The factors that predicted a higher psychological impact were young age, female gender, and the presence of a physical comorbidity. The authors of the study also showed that males faced a lesser psychological impact as compared to females [45]. Thus, in spite of the differences between countries and cultures, many of the basic factors affecting the public are similar.

Several limitations of the studies should be pointed out. No inclusion and/or exclusion criteria were specified and the study samples were not predetermined. The significant differences in demographic variables might have been a reason for some of the detected differences, especially in view of the fact that gender (but not age) came out as a predictive factor in most of the models calculated for TMD, bruxism, and symptom aggravation, in both countries. Moreover, the studies were performed during a specific point in time at the first phase of the pandemic and may be indicative of the immediate stress evoked by the sudden health risk and changes in life style. Additionally, possible confounders that could have influenced the results were not under control.

Further longitudinal studies are needed to evaluate the pandemic's possible long-term mental and physical consequences. Multifactorial and multicultural research should be performed to identify the risk groups and counteract the aggravation of emotional and physical effects in the case of future global crises.

5. Conclusions

The coronavirus pandemic has caused significant adverse effects on the psychoemotional status of both Israeli and Polish populations, resulting in the intensification of their bruxism and TMD symptoms and thus leading to increased orofacial pain.

Author Contributions: A.E.-P., I.E., and M.W. contributed to study conception and design. A.E.-P., I.E., G.W., N.U., and E.G. collected the data. A.E.-P., I.E., N.G., and J.S. were involved in data analysis and interpretation. A.E.-P., I.E., M.W., and J.S. drafted the article. A.E.-P., I.E. and M.W. critically revised the article. All authors have read and agreed to the published version of the manuscript.

Funding: This research received no external funding.

Conflicts of Interest: The authors declare no conflict of interest.

References

1. LeResche, L. Epidemiology of Temporomandibular Disorders: Implications for the Investigation of Etiologic Factors. *Crit. Rev. Oral Biol. Med.* **1997**, *8*, 291–305. [CrossRef]
2. Drangsholt, M. Temporomandibular Pain. In *Epidemiology of Pain*; Crombie, I.H., Croft, P.R., Linton, S.J., LeResche, L., Von Korff, M., Eds.; IASP Press: Seattle, DC, USA, 1999; pp. 203–234.
3. Macfarlane, T.V.; Glenny, A.-M.; Worthington, H.V. Systematic review of population-based epidemiological studies of oro-facial pain. *J. Dent.* **2001**, *29*, 451–467. [CrossRef]
4. Nilsson, I.M.; List, T.; Drangsholt, M. Prevalence of temporomandibular pain and subsequent dental treatment in Swedish adolescents. *J. Oral Facial Pain* **2005**, *19*, 144–150.
5. Berger, M.; Oleszek-Listopad, J.; Marczak, M.; Szymanska, J. Psychological aspects of temporomandibular disorders—Literature review. *Curr. Issues Pharm. Med. Sci.* **2015**, *28*, 55–59. [CrossRef]

6. de Leeuw, R.; Klasser, G.D. Differential diagnosis and management of TMDs. In *Orofacial Pain: Guidelines for Assessment, Diagnosis, and Management/American Academy of Orofacial Pain*, 6th ed.; De Leeuw, R., Klasser, G.D., Eds.; Quintessence Publishing Co. Inc.: Hanover Park, Germany, 2018; pp. 143–207.
7. Lajnert, V.; Francisković, T.; Grzić, R.; Pavičić, D.K.; Bakarbić, D.; Buković, D.; Celebić, A.; Braut, V.; Fugosić, V. Depression, somatization and anxiety in female patients with temporomandibular disorders (TMD). *Coll. Antropol.* **2010**, *34*, 1415–1419. [PubMed]
8. Wieckiewicz, M.; Zietek, M.; Smardz, J.; Zenczak-Wieckiewicz, D.; Grychowska, N. Mental Status as a Common Factor for Masticatory Muscle Pain: A Systematic Review. *Front. Psychol.* **2017**, *8*. [CrossRef]
9. International Association for the Study of Pain. Temporomandibular Didorders. Orofacial Pain Fact Sheets 2016. Available online: URL:https://s3.amazonaws.com/rdcms-iasp/files/production/public/Content/ContentFolders/GlobalYearAgainstPain2/20132014OrofacialPain/FactSheets/Temporomandibular_Disorders_2016.pdf (accessed on 5 July 2020).
10. Lobbezoo, F.; Ahlberg, J.; Raphael, K.G.; Wetselaar, P.; Glaros, A.G.; Kato, T.; Santiago, V.; Winocur, E.; De Laat, A.; De Leeuw, R.; et al. International consensus on the assessment of bruxism: Report of a work in progress. *J. Oral Rehabil.* **2018**, *45*, 837–844. [CrossRef]
11. Emodi Perlman, A.; Lobbezoo, F.; Zar, A.; Rubin, P.F.; Van Selms, M.K.A.; Winocur, E. Self-Reported bruxism and associated factors in Israeli adolescents. *J. Oral Rehabil.* **2016**, *43*, 443–450. [CrossRef]
12. Van Selms, M.K.; Visscher, C.M.; Naeije, M.; Lobbezoo, F. Bruxism and associated factors among Dutch adolescents. *Commun. Dent. Oral Epidemiol.* **2012**, *41*, 353–363. [CrossRef]
13. Winocur, E.; Messer, T.; Eli, I.; Emodi-Perlman, A.; Kedem, R.; Reiter, S.; Friedman-Rubin, P. Awake and Sleep Bruxism Among Israeli Adolescents. *Front. Neurol.* **2019**, *10*. [CrossRef]
14. Manfredini, D.; Colonna, A.; Bracci, A.; Lobbezoo, F. Bruxism: A summary of current knowledge on aetiology, assessment and management. *Oral Surg.* **2019**. [CrossRef]
15. Lobbezoo, F.; Lavigne, G.J.; Tanguay, R.; Montplaisir, J.Y. The effect of the catecholamine precursor L-Dopa on sleep bruxism: A controlled clinical trial. *Mov. Disord.* **1997**, *12*, 73–78. [CrossRef] [PubMed]
16. Manfredini, D.; Arreghini, A.; Lombardo, L.; Visentin, A.; Cerea, S.; Castroflorio, T.; Siciliani, G. Assessment of Anxiety and Coping Features in Bruxers: A Portable Electromyographic and Electrocardiographic Study. *J. Oral Facial Pain Headache* **2016**, *30*, 249–254. [CrossRef] [PubMed]
17. Manfredini, D.; Fabbri, A.; Peretta, R.; Nardini, L.G.; Lobbezoo, F. Influence of psychological symptoms on home-recorded sleep-time masticatory muscle activity in healthy subjects. *J. Oral Rehabil.* **2011**, *38*, 902–911. [CrossRef]
18. Manfredini, D.; Lobbezoo, F. Role of psychosocial factors in the etiology of bruxism. *J. Oral Facial Pain* **2009**, *23*, 153–166.
19. Pierce, C.J.; Chrisman, K.; Bennett, M.E.; Close, J.M. Stress, anticipatory stress, and psychologic measures related to sleep bruxism. *J. Oral Facial Pain* **1995**, *9*, 51–56.
20. Winocur, E.; Uziel, N.; Lisha, T.; Goldsmith, C.; Eli, I. Self-reported Bruxism—Associations with perceived stress, motivation for control, dental anxiety and gagging*. *J. Oral Rehabil.* **2010**, *38*, 3–11. [CrossRef]
21. Smardz, J.; Martynowicz, H.; Wojakowska, A.; Michalek, M.; Mazur, G.; Wieckiewicz, M. Correlation between Sleep Bruxism, Stress, and Depression-A Polysomnographic Study. *J. Clin. Med.* **2019**, *8*, 1344. [CrossRef]
22. Wang, C.; Pan, R.; Wan, X.; Tan, Y.; Xu, L.; Ho, C.S.H.; Ho, R.C. Immediate Psychological Responses and Associated Factors during the Initial Stage of the 2019 Coronavirus Disease (COVID-19) Epidemic among the General Population in China. *Int. J. Environ. Res. Public Health* **2020**, *17*, 1729. [CrossRef]
23. Almeida-Leite, C.M.; Barbosa, J.S.; Conti, P.C.R. How psychosocial and economic impacts of COVID-19 pandemic can interfere on bruxism and temporomandibular disorders? *J. Appl. Oral Sci.* **2020**, *28*, e20200263. [CrossRef]
24. Lövgren, A.; Parvaneh, H.; Lobbezoo, F.; Häggman-Henrikson, B.; Wänman, A.; Visscher, C.M. Diagnostic accuracy of three screening questions (3Q/TMD) in relation to the DC/TMD in a specialized orofacial pain clinic. *Acta Odontol. Scand.* **2018**, *76*, 380–386. [CrossRef] [PubMed]
25. Lövgren, A.; Marklund, S.; Visscher, C.M.; Lobbezoo, F.; Häggman-Henrikson, B.; Wänman, A. Outcome of three screening questions for temporomandibular disorders (3Q/TMD) on clinical decision-making. *J. Oral Rehabil.* **2017**, *44*, 573–579. [CrossRef] [PubMed]
26. Manfredini, D.; Winocur, E.; Guarda-Nardini, L.; Paesani, D.; Lobbezoo, F. Epidemiology of bruxism in adults: A systematic review of the literature. *J. Oral Facial Pain* **2013**, *27*, 99–110. [CrossRef] [PubMed]

27. Lobbezoo, F.; Ahlberg, J.; Glaros, A.G.; Kato, T.; Koyano, K.; Lavigne, G.J.; De Leeuw, R.; Manfredini, D.; Svensson, P.; Winocur, E. Bruxism defined and graded: An international consensus. *J. Oral Rehabil.* **2012**, *40*, 2–4. [CrossRef] [PubMed]
28. Yap, A.; Chua, A.P. Sleep bruxism: Current knowledge and contemporary management. *J. Conserv. Dent.* **2016**, *19*, 383–389. [CrossRef]
29. Stanhope, J. Patient Health Questionnaire-4. *Occup. Med.* **2016**, *66*, 760–761. [CrossRef]
30. Petry, N.M. A comparison of young, middle-aged, and older adult treatment-seeking pathological gamblers. *Gerontologist* **2002**, *42*, 92–99. [CrossRef]
31. Manfredini, D.; Serra-Negra, J.; Carboncini, F.; Lobbezoo, F. Current Concepts of Bruxism. *Int. J. Prosthodont.* **2017**, *30*, 437–438. [CrossRef]
32. Wright, E.F. *Manual of Temporomandibular Disorders*, 3rd ed.; Wiley-Blackwell: Ames, IA, USA, 2013; pp. 1–15.
33. Wieckiewicz, M.; Grychowska, N.; Wojciechowski, K.; Pelc, A.; Augustyniak, M.; Sleboda, A.; Ziętek, M. Prevalence and Correlation between TMD Based on RDC/TMD Diagnoses, Oral Parafunctions and Psychoemotional Stress in Polish University Students. *BioMed Res. Int.* **2014**, *2014*, 472346. [CrossRef]
34. Wieckiewicz, M.; Grychowska, N.; Nahajowski, M.; Hnitecka, S.; Kempiak, K.; Charemska, K.; Balicz, A.; Chirkowska, A.; Zietek, M.; Winocur, E. Prevalence and Overlaps of Headaches and Pain-Related Temporomandibular Disorders Among the Polish Urban Population. *J. Oral Facial Pain Headache* **2020**, *34*, 31–39. [CrossRef]
35. Winocur, E.; Reiter, S.; Livine, S.; Goldsmith, C.; Littner, D. The prevalence of symptoms related to TMD and their relationship to psychological status: A gender comparison among a non-TMD patient adult population in Israel. *J. Craniomandubular Funct.* **2010**, *2*, 39–50.
36. Elran, M.; Even, S. Civilian Resilience in Israel and the COVID-19 Pandemic: Analysis of a CBS Survey. *INSS Insight*, 17 May 2020. Available online: https://www.inss.org.il/publication/coronavirus-survey/ (accessed on 5 September 2020).
37. Maciaszek, J.; Ciulkowicz, M.; Misiak, B.; Szczesniak, D.; Luc, D.; Wieczorek, T.; Fila-Witecka, K.; Gawlowski, P.; Rymaszewska, J. Mental Health of Medical and Non-Medical Professionals during the Peak of the COVID-19 Pandemic: A Cross-Sectional Nationwide Study. *J. Clin. Med.* **2020**, *9*, 2527. [CrossRef] [PubMed]
38. Wang, C.; Pan, R.; Wan, X.; Tan, Y.; Xu, L.; McIntyre, R.S.; Choo, F.N.; Tran, B.; Ho, R.C.; Sharma, V.K.; et al. A longitudinal study on the mental health of general population during the COVID-19 epidemic in China. *Brain Behav. Immun.* **2020**, *87*, 40–48. [CrossRef] [PubMed]
39. World Health Organization. Mental Health and Psychosocial Considerations during the COVID-19 Outbreak, 18 March 2020. Available online: https://apps.who.int/iris/handle/10665/License:CCBY-NC-SA3.0IGO (accessed on 10 April 2020).
40. Polak, P.; Świątkiewicz-Mośny, M.; Wagner, A. Much Ado about nothing? The responsiveness of the healthcare system in Poland through patients' eyes. *Health Policy* **2019**, *123*, 1259–1266. [CrossRef] [PubMed]
41. Moyser, M. Gender Differences in Mental Health during the COVID-19 Pandemic. Available online: https://www150.statcan.gc.ca/n1/en/pub/45-28-0001/2020001/article/00047-eng.pdf?st=NP3Kgs7n (accessed on 9 July 2020).
42. Song, K.; Xu, R.; Stratton, T.D.; Kavcic, V.; Luo, D.; Hou, F.; Bi, F.; Jiao, R.; Yan, S.; Jiang, Y. Sex differences and Psychological Stress: Responses to the COVID-19 epidemic in China. *MedRxiv* **2020**. [CrossRef]
43. Lavee, Y.; Katz, R. The Family in Israel: Between Tradition and Modernity. *Marriage Fam. Rev.* **2003**, *35*, 193–217. [CrossRef]

44. Gal, R. Social Resilience in Times of Protracted Crises: An Israeli Case Study. *Armed Forces Soc.* **2013**, *40*, 452–475. [CrossRef]
45. Varshney, M.; Parel, J.T.; Raizada, N.; Sarin, S.K. Initial psychological impact of COVID-19 and its correlates in Indian Community: An online (FEEL-COVID) survey. *PLoS ONE* **2020**, *15*, e0233874. [CrossRef]

Journal of
Clinical Medicine

MDPI

Article

SARS-CoV-2 and Oral Manifestation: An Observational, Human Study

Bruna Sinjari [1,2,*], Damiano D'Ardes [3,†], Manlio Santilli [1,2,†], Imena Rexhepi [1,2], Gianmaria D'Addazio [1,2], Piero Di Carlo [4,5], Piero Chiacchiaretta [6], Sergio Caputi [1,2,‡] and Francesco Cipollone [3,‡]

1 Department of Medical, Oral and Biotechnological Sciences, University "G. d'Annunzio" Chieti-Pescara, 66100 Chieti, Italy; manlio.santilli@alumni.unich.it (M.S.); imena.rexhepi@gmail.com (I.R.); gianmariad@gmail.com (G.D.); scaputi@unich.it (S.C.)
2 Electron Microscopy Laboratory, University "G. d'Annunzio" Chieti-Pescara, 66100 Chieti, Italy
3 Clinica Medica Institute, Department of Medicine and Aging Sciences, University "Gabriele d'Annunzio", Chieti-Pescara, 66100 Chieti, Italy; damianomatrix89@msn.com (D.D.); francesco.cipollone@unich.it (F.C.)
4 CAST, Center of Advanced studies and Technologies, University "G. d'Annunzio" Chieti-Pescara, 66100 Chieti, Italy; piero.dicarlo@unich.it
5 Department of Psychological, Health & Territorial Sciences, University "G. d'Annunzio" Chieti-Pescara, 66100 Chieti, Italy
6 Department of Neuroscience, Imaging and Clinical Sciences, University "G. d'Annunzio" Chieti-Pescara, 66100 Chieti, Italy; piero.chiacchiaretta@gmail.com
* Correspondence: b.sinjari@unich.it; Tel.: +39-392-27471479; Fax: +39-0871-3554070
† These authors contribute equally to the study as Co-authors.
‡ These authors contribute equally to the study as Co-senior author.

Received: 15 September 2020; Accepted: 3 October 2020; Published: 7 October 2020

Abstract: The correlation between SARS-CoV-2 and oral manifestations is still controversial. The aim of this observational study was to determine the oral manifestation of the hospitalized patients for COVID-19. A total of 20 patients met the inclusion criteria and gave their signed informed consent. A questionnaire of 32 questions regarding the oral and systemic health condition was administrated to these patients during the convalescence. A descriptive statistic was performed. Data were analysed through the use of χ^2 test, to assess the statistical significance. A statistically significant increase of about 30% of reporting xerostomia during hospitalization was observed ($p = 0.02$). Meanwhile, a decrease of oral hygiene was observed during the hospitalization, even if a non-statistically significant difference was shown between the two study time points (before and after hospitalization). During the hospitalization period, 25% of patients reported impaired taste, 15% burning sensation, and 20% difficulty in swallowing. An interesting result was that among the systemic conditions, hypertension was observed in 39% of patients and mostly in female patients (62.5%). Further studies are necessary to better understand the symptoms of this new virus in order to faster detect its presence in humans. Probably, a multidisciplinary team following the COVID-19 patients could be of key importance in treating this disease.

Keywords: SARS-CoV-2; COVID-19; oral manifestation; xerostomia; dysgeusia

1. Introduction

The SARS-CoV-2 (Severe Acute Respiratory Syndrome-CoronaVirus 2) is the seventh coronavirus known to infect humans [1,2]. Specifically, it belongs to the family of *Coronaviridae*, of the order *Nidovirales*, comprising large, single, plus-stranded RNA as their genome [3,4]. The new coronavirus SARS-CoV-2 has, like other coronaviruses, with high probability, a zoonotic origin [5]. Among these, α-CoV and β-CoV tend to infect the respiratory, gastrointestinal, and central nervous systems [6].

By studying nucleotide sequences thoroughly, SARS-CoV-2 has been seen to be part of β-CoV with a 79% similarity to the SARS-CoV virus already described in the past decades [7].

The main transmission routes described are direct, as caused by coughing, sneezing, droplets of saliva expelled during the phonation, or indirect by contact with the main body mucous membranes such as oral, ocular, and nasal [8–11]. Public awareness of the spread of microorganisms and infectious diseases in the dental office among the dentist, auxiliaries, and laboratory personnel has increased significantly [12]. Therefore, several scientific dental societies have produced recommendations on dental activity, specifically for the management of acute dental infections [13]. A recent paper demonstrated, through a survey, that during lockdown period endodontic urgency resulted predominant [14], thus increasing the probability of being infected if measures are not respected through the high aerosol generation during the dental procedures. All over the world, the evolution of the disease diffusion, which today counts high numbers, is being monitored. Specifically, to date, the numbers of infected people still result in a constant increase. The numbers registered by the Center for Systems Science and Engineering (CSSE) at Johns Hopkins University are 33,082,994 infected worldwide and 997,799 deaths (updated to 28 September 2020). On the other hand, cases of recovered patients are also increasing all over the world [7]. These high numbers justify the declared state of pandemic and are undoubtedly attributable to the ease of human infection of the virus itself.

The main symptoms of COVID-19 are fever, tiredness, and dry cough. Some patients may experience soreness and muscle pain, nasal congestion, runny nose, sore throat, or diarrhea, but in severe cases, the infection can cause pneumonia, severe acute respiratory syndrome, kidney failure, and even death [8]. Moreover, the possible asymptomaticity in infected patients is very important and should absolutely not be underestimated [9].

Although there are many studies in the literature on clinical signs in positive SARS-CoV-2 patients, the majority of them have not verified the oral health status of the patients [15].

Possible oral-related symptoms include: hypogeusia, xerostomia, and chemosensory alterations [16]. In fact, xerostomia has been found mainly among COVID-19 patients, due to the neuroinvasive and neurotropic potential of SARS-CoV-2. It was reported that angiotensin-converting enzyme 2 (ACE2)-positive epithelial cells of the salivary gland are an early target of SARS-CoV-2 in rhesus macaques, and these findings suggest that oral manifestations may appear due to impediment of salivary flow in COVID-19-affected patients [17]. In fact, a cross-sectional survey of 108 patients with confirmed SARS-CoV-2 in China observed that 46% of them reported dry mouth, among other symptoms [17,18].

In literature, several cases of oral manifestations apparently related to SARS-CoV-2 have been described [19–21]. The importance of good oral hygiene could be an interesting aspect to evaluate a hypothetical relationship between SARS-CoV-2 and oral manifestations. Badran et al. hypothesized that periodontal pocket could be a reservoir for this virus [22]. Periodontopathic bacteria, involved in several process like inflammation, bacteraemia, pneumonia, are also present in the metagenome of positive SARS-CoV-2 patients [23]. Several authors described case reports of SARS-CoV-2-positive patients with oral manifestations potentially compatible with this type of coronavirus [19–21]. Moreover, a key factor in the damage of the respiratory system and other organs could be related to the distribution of ACE2 receptors in the human system [24]. Therefore, cells with ACE2 receptor distribution may become host cells for the virus and further cause inflammatory reactions in related organs and tissues, such as the tongue mucosa and salivary glands [25]. It has also been demonstrated that COVID-19 acute infection, along with associated therapeutic measures, could probably contribute to adverse outcomes concerning oral health. In fact, Dziedzic and Wojtyczka, in 2020, showed that it can lead to various opportunistic fungal infections, unspecific oral ulcerations, recurrent oral herpes simplex virus (HSV-1) infection, dysgeusia, fixed drug eruptions, xerostomia linked to decreased salivary flow, ulcerations and gingivitis as a result of the impaired immune system and/or susceptible oral mucosa [26].

It is not clear if the abovementioned manifestations derive from the viral infection, or they could be caused by some systemic deteriorations, based on potential negative reactions to treatments or even possible opportunistic infections [27]. Furthermore, some reports affirm that the oral cavity represents the main channel for infection, considering also several consequences for the dental practice and the role of saliva in identifying COVID-19 [24,25]. One of the latest studies links a higher risk of getting COVID-19 to hyposalivation as well as to taste loss [28].

Although, despite the probable relationship between oral cavity and SARS-CoV-2, to date, there are also many variables that could influence the presence of the oral manifestations. In fact, most patients take a large number of drugs that may produce the oral manifestations, thus the need in evaluating in an observational study the oral manifestation of COVID-19 hospitalized patients.

Based on the hypothesis that oral manifestations could be an initial pattern typical of this virus, the aim of this study was to better understand the relationship between these manifestations and SARS-CoV-2.

2. Experimental Section

2.1. Study Design and Sample Selection

A total of 20 patients were enrolled in this observational study conducted in a period of one month (from May 2020 to June 2020). The survey was completed by 20 patients who met, during the described period, the inclusion and exclusion criteria. The average age of the participants was 69.2 years. Of these, 55% were male (aged between 44 and 91 years) and 45% female (aged between 35 and 85 years).

A specific anamnestic questionnaire of 32 questions (Appendix A) was submitted to these patients affected by SARS-CoV-2 and hospitalized in "Policlinico 'SS. Annunziata' - Chieti, Italy" with the aim to collect information related to health status, oral hygiene habits, and symptoms in the oral cavity before and during the disease manifestation. In addition, a series of questions were also addressed to the Unit of Internal Medicine of the hospital to better know the clinical condition of these patients. This observational study was administered through a printing questionnaire and, prior to completion, the patients gave their informed consent signed to the doctor working in the Unit of Internal Medicine at the "Policlinico 'SS. Annunziata'" hospital. The patients were free to participate or not (based in a volunteer way) in this observational study. The inclusion criteria were patients of both sex and of any age hospitalized for COVID-19 at the abovementioned hospital able to give their consent to participate in the study. The exclusion criteria were patients of both sex and any age hospitalized for COVID-19 at the Internal Medicine department of the SS Annunziata hospital in Chieti in need of intensive care and/or who were unable to give their consent to participate in the study or who were unable to intend or to want. The methodology adopted for the creation of the questionnaires allowed us to use both quantitative and qualitative variables, differently distributed. All the questionnaires were given to the patients during the doctor routine visits in that department. Then, all the papers were collected in a separate box with all the recommendations to reduce the contagion. The data were analysed after a period of rest from their collection.

2.2. Ethical Consideration

The study protocol was approved by the Ethical Committee of the "G. Annunzio University" of Chieti and Pescara: No. 1687 of 22 April 2020. Participants provided their informed consent in accordance with the EU General Data Protection Regulation GDPR (UE) n. 2016/679 and following the Declaration of Helsinki before beginning the completion of the questionnaire. Data collection took place in the time period from 8 May to 1 June 2020.

2.3. Statistical Analysis

Some of the answers were codified as dichotomous variables, namely as Yes/No responses, or in general as categorical variables, when a multiple-choice selection was requested. Given the nature of our survey we computed descriptive statistics for most of the questions. For each question, we computed the percentage of the respondents that gave a particular answer with respect to the number of total responses to the question. Answers obtained prior and during the disease manifestation were compared through the use of χ^2 test, to assess the statistical significance. All statistical comparisons were conducted with a significance level of $p < 0.05$. Statistical analyses were performed using the GraphPad version 8 (GraphPad Software 2365 Northsides, Dr. Suite 560 San Diego, CA, USA) statistical software.

3. Results

The results demonstrated that most of the patients (65%) had more than 20 teeth and used to go to the dentist routinely. Moreover, the majority of participants (90%) were nonsmokers. The 40% of them reported that they brushed their teeth three times a day, before hospitalization, but most of them (70%) did not use dental floss. The patients also reported that during the hospitalization period, the attention to oral hygiene decreased. In fact, the number of patients who did not brush their teeth at all increased during the hospitalization, and the number of those who regularly brush three times a day decreased, as shown in Figure 1. However, the difference between the groups was not statistically significant ($p = 0.20$). Regarding the presence of oral manifestations (i.e., xerostomia), none of the patients reported xerostomia before contracting the virus, whilst during hospitalization the percentage increased to 30%. The difference between the two study time points was statistically significant ($p = 0.02$), as shown in Figure 2. In addition, during the hospitalization period, 25% of patients reported impaired taste, 15% burning sensation, and 20% difficulty in swallowing. Finally, by comparing these data and the onset of some manifestations between sex and age, no statistically significant results emerged, although a trend in some of these was detectable (please see Appendix B). Among the latter's, the presence of hypertension was found in 40% of patients, mostly in female patients (62.5%), as shown in Figure 3. Furthermore, an interesting data aspect was that the burning sensation of the mouth was present only in female patients. In addition, 15% of patients were affected by diabetes, 15% by obesity, and 25% presented thyroid disorders such as hypothyroidism or hyperthyroidism. Of note, 95% of the patients were given the following drugs: lopinavir/ritonavir and/or hydroxychloroquine, in combination with other specific drugs for the various systemic pathologies they presented.

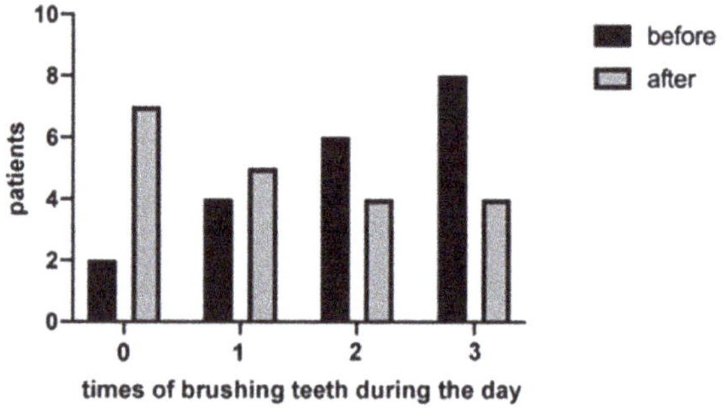

Figure 1. The graphic represents the times the patients used to brush their teeth before and after hospitalization. No statistical significance ($p = 0.20$) was shown between these two time points of the study.

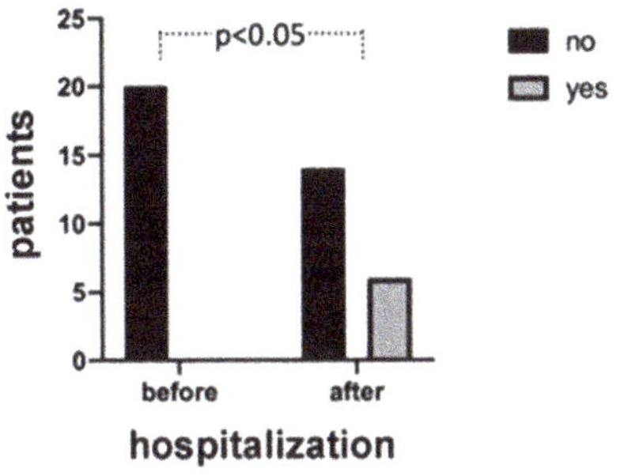

Figure 2. The xerostomia manifestation before and after hospitalization of the patients. A statistical difference was shown between the study time points ($p = 0.02$).

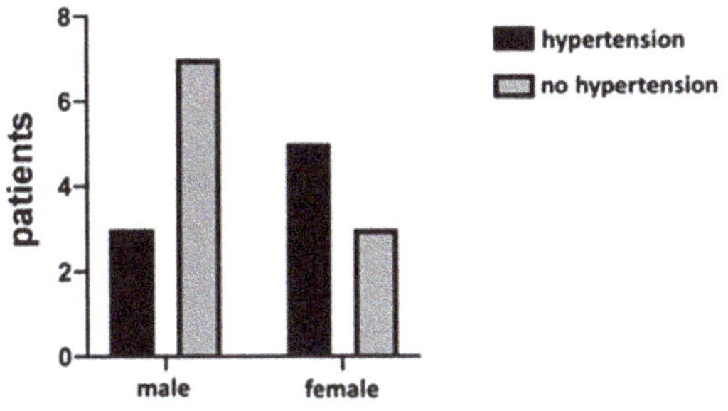

Figure 3. The graph shows the presence of hypertension between males and females. No statistical significance ($p = 0.34$) was shown between the sexes on the presence of hypertension.

4. Discussion

The aim of this observational study was to better understand the relationship between SARS-CoV-2 and oral manifestations before and during the hospitalization. Several clinicians have observed many extrapulmonary manifestations of COVID-19. In fact, the recent literature suggests that the hematologic, cardiovascular, renal, gastrointestinal and hepatobiliary, endocrinologic, neurologic, ophthalmologic, and dermatologic systems can all be implicated [29,30]. On the other hand, numerous studies have drawn attention to the oral cavity as the main route of infection [28].

Although recent evidence suggests a relevant role of the oral cavity and its mucosae in the transmission and in the pathogenicity of SARS-CoV-2, as the entrance to the body of the virus, its protective or aggravating element for the infection and progression of the virus is still controversial [28]. It has been demonstrated that there is an association between periodontitis and a higher risk of increased gravity of COVID-19 in periodontopathic patients [31]. Most of the individuals (65%) in our sample had more than 20 teeth and they used to go to the dentist for control visits, demonstrating the importance given to the oral health condition. Moreover, about 14 out of 20 of the patients with COVID-19 diagnosis had performed extractions due to periodontitis.

In addition, regarding the presence of xerostomia, only 30% of the patients developed this symptom during the period of hospitalization. These data are relevant because xerostomia has also been found in a relatively high proportion of COVID-19 patients from Chinese researchers [32]. On the other hand, these results should be carefully discussed. In fact, it has been shown that xerostomia can also be induced by different drug therapies such as: antidepressants, antipsychotics, anticholinergics, antihypertensives, antihistamines, and sedatives [33]. Furthermore, there is strong evidence that xerostomia is very common in diabetic patients and may be present in >50% of cases, and recently it was reported that the use of artificial saliva spray was shown to be effective in the treatment of xerostomia in type 1 and type 2 diabetes [34,35]. However, in our study, only 15% of patients were affected by diabetes (not specified if type 1 or type 2).

In fact, 56% of the patients enrolled in our study had these kinds of therapies, but only 5% of them manifested xerostomia during hospitalization. These data deserve attention, because the symptom of xerostomia was manifested by patients affected by COVID-19 and enrolled in our study in 30% of cases, regardless of the drug therapy followed prior to admission. Therefore, this oral manifestation can probably be linked to the disease itself. Indeed, it has been demonstrated that the salivary glands are a reservoir of the virus, thus the contagion of people by way of saliva droplets [36].

Interestingly, the SARS-CoV-2 infection has been shown to be more severe in individuals over 50 years old and with the presence of associated comorbidities such as diabetes, cardiovascular problems, and diseases involving the nervous system. These disorders have been associated with hyposalivation; in our case 15% of patients were affected by diabetes, 15% by obesity, 39% by hypertension, and 25% presented thyroid disorders such as hypothyroidism or hyperthyroidism, but none of them, before being hospitalized, reported having xerostomia. Therefore, the onset of this symptom can be associated with the drug therapy administered for the treatment of COVID-19 and also with the infectious and inflammatory processes activated by the virus itself. Regarding other symptoms such as altered taste, 25% of the participants said they had dysgeusia. This is a very important finding and in line with recent publications on this topic, which attest to 33% the frequency of COVID-19 patients who report having this symptom [37]. Indeed, dysgeusia can be described as one of the early symptoms of COVID-19 infection. Clinically, these data may allow easier identification of pre-symptomatic or asymptomatic patients. Moreover, the diagnosis of this oral manifestation may significantly reduce disease transmission, especially when diagnostic tests are not readily available and/or unpredictable [38].

Focusing on the patient's systemic conditions, it appears significant that most of the patients hospitalized for COVID-19 had previous systemic conditions such as hypertension, heart disease, oncological pathologies, pathologies affecting the thyroid gland, diabetes, and pathologies affecting the respiratory system. Furthermore, only one patient in his medical history did not report any previous pathology. In addition, it should be noted that, in a recent study on 5700 patients, the most common comorbidities were hypertension in 56.6% of cases, obesity in 41.7%, and diabetes in 33.8% of patients with diagnosis of COVID-19 [39]. Our results are in agreement with these data. In fact, about 39% of our patients had hypertension. It is almost known that such pathologies are aggravated by factors such as smoking. An interesting result that emerged from our study is that approximately 90% of the participants were nonsmokers. In the literature, there are several studies that analysed the relationship between COVID-19 and smoking. According to the World Health Organization (WHO), no studies examined tobacco use and the risk of infection or the risk of hospitalization with COVID-19 among smokers [40]. In fact, the majority of the studies in the literature are observational reports, and they reported the prevalence of smoking amongst hospitalized COVID-19 patients [40].

As for the presence of cardiovascular diseases, the results of our study show that 50% of the participants had cardiovascular diseases, specifically 78% of them suffer from hypertension. Currently, the literature is controversial, also in the management of patients with hypertension since the SARS-CoV-2 uses ACE2 as a cell entry receptor [41]. It is unclear whether uncontrolled blood pressure is a risk factor for acquiring COVID-19, or whether controlled blood pressure among patients with hypertension is or is not less of a risk factor [42].

Although this observational study reports interesting data of 20 COVID-19 hospitalized patients, it has different limitations. Firstly, the small sample size, only 20 patients enrolled. This was given from different limitations on performing the study during the pandemic; the difficulty in enrolling patients with the abovementioned criteria during that period and the difficulty in having personnel available to administrate the questionnaire.

After the results raised, the questionnaires probably should have been done in a more specific way to better understand on which day of the disease the symptoms appear and if they had prior to the first symptom the symptoms they reported.

5. Conclusions

This study demonstrates the importance of the close link between SARS-CoV-2 and oral manifestations. There is no scientific evidence in the literature that certifies which oral symptoms SARS-CoV-2 can actually cause. In fact, from the analysis of our data, it is hard to notice that clinical conditions that patients manifest are due to the SARS-CoV-2. The presence of xerostomia in our patients suggests a symptom given by the virus, but it must always be correlated with the patient's therapy. In addition, it may be essential to carry out the measurement of the salivary flow before and after the COVID-19 diagnosis to demonstrate a close correlation of it with the virus. Furthermore, the dysgeusia present in only 25% of our study suggests that this symptom may be a warning signal for the patients. Finally, the reduction of oral hygiene conditions in the hospitalized patient (even if it was not the focus of this study) suggests how important it is to have a team specialized in dentistry within hospitals.

Further studies are necessary to better understand the symptoms of this new virus in order to faster detect its presence in humans; probably, a multidisciplinary team following the COVID-19 patients could be of key importance.

Author Contributions: Conceptualization, B.S., F.C., and S.C.; methodology, B.S., D.D., and M.S.; software, G.D. and I.R.; validation, B.S., S.C., and F.C.; formal analysis, P.D.C. and P.C.; investigation, F.C.; resources, B.S.; data curation, G.D. and I.R.; writing—original draft preparation, B.S., D.D., and M.S.; writing—review and editing, F.C. and S.C.; visualization, I.R. and G.D.; supervision, S.C. and F.C.; project administration, F.C.; funding acquisition, S.C. All authors have read and agreed to the published version of the manuscript.

Funding: This research received no external funding.

Acknowledgments: The authors received no financial support and declare no potential conflicts of interest with respect to the authorship and/or publication of this article.

Conflicts of Interest: The authors declare no conflict of interest.

Appendix A. Questionnaire

1. Age	
2. Sex	Male Female
3. Place of origin	
4. How many teeth do you have in your mouth?	>20 teeth 10–19 teeth 1–9 teeth totally edentulous patient
5. Are you a smoker?	Yes No
6. When did you last go to the dentist?	performed within 6 months performed within 1 year more than a year since the last visit
7. How many times did you brush your teeth in a day before being hospitalized?	times/after meals daily times daily 1 time daily Never
8. Did you use interdental brushes?	Yes No

9. If yes, how often weekly?	Yes, but it has been treated Yes, but I neglect the problem No, I wasn't told I don't know
10. When brushing your teeth, do your gums bleed?	Yes No
11. Did you clean your tongue before hospitalization?	Yes No
12. Did the dentist ever tell you that you have gum problems, gum infections or inflammation?	Yes, but it has been treated Yes, but I neglect the problem No, I wasn't told I don't know
13. Did the dentist extract your teeth because they had high mobility?	Yes No
14. Are you wearing a fixed prosthesis?	Yes
15. Are you wearing a removable prosthesis?	Yes, total Yes, partial Yes, both total and partial No
16. Has anyone in your family of origin (father, mother, siblings, uncles, ...) had gum problems such as periodontitis?	Yes No I don't know
17. Do you suffer from xerostomia (dry mouth)?	Yes No
18. Which home oral hygiene aids do you use now that you are hospitalized?	toothbrush + toothpaste + floss prosthesis brush + toothpaste + tablets toothbrush + toothpaste nothing
19. How many times do you brush your teeth a day, now that you are hospitalized?	1230
20. Do you still clean your tongue now?	Yes No
21. Do you currently bleed from your gums while cleaning your teeth?	Yes No
22. Did you have any chewing problems during the period of illness (COVID-19)?	Yes No
23. Did you have any swallowing problems during the period of illness (COVID-19)?	Yes No
24. Did you experience a burning sensation in your mouth during the period of your illness (COVID-19)?	Yes No
25. Did you experience halitosis during the period of your illness (COVID-19)?	Yes No
26. During the period of your illness (COVID-19) did you have tooth problems/pain?	Yes No
27. During the period of the disease (COVID-19) did you have any taste alterations?	Yes No

28. Did you suffer from xerostomia during the period of your illness (COVID-19)?	Yes No
29. Do you suffer from diabetes?	Yes No
30. Do you suffer from cardiovascular disease?	Yes No
31. Do you suffer from senile dementia?	Yes No
32. Did you experience any other oral problems during hospitalization?	Yes No

Appendix B. Statistical Results

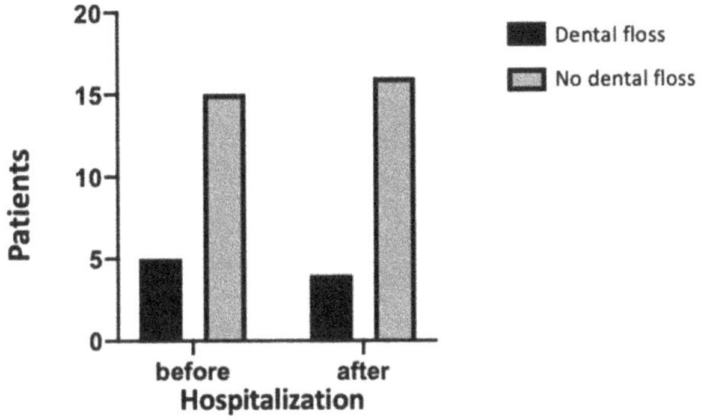

Figure A1. Use of dental floss before and after hospitalization of the patients. No statistical difference was shown between the study time points ($p > 0.99$).

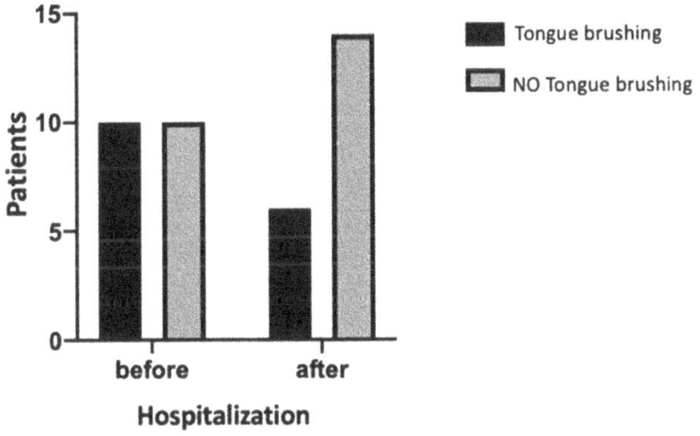

Figure A2. Habit of tongue-brushing before and after hospitalization of the patients. No statistical difference was shown between the study time points ($p = 0.333$).

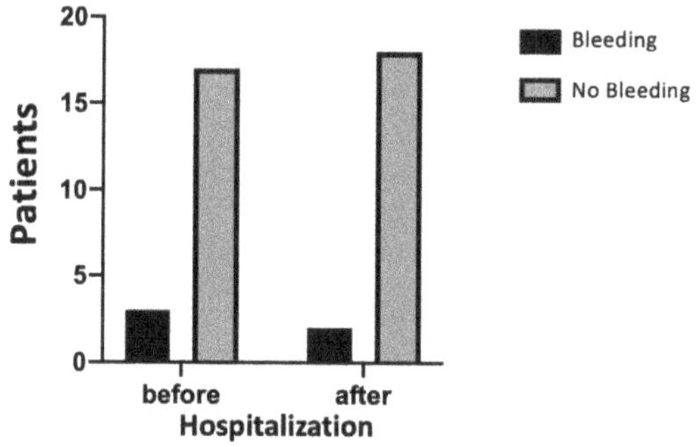

Figure A3. Bleeding of gums before and after hospitalization of the patients. No statistical difference was shown between the study time points ($p > 0.99$).

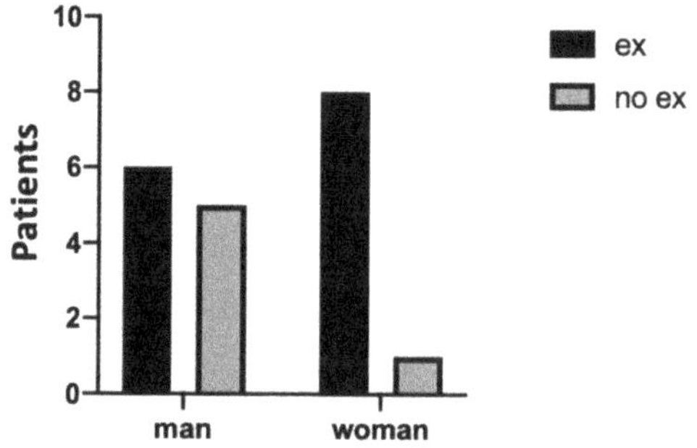

Figure A4. Tooth extraction (EX) carried out between males and females. No statistical significance ($p = 0.15$) was shown between the sexes on the tooth extraction performed.

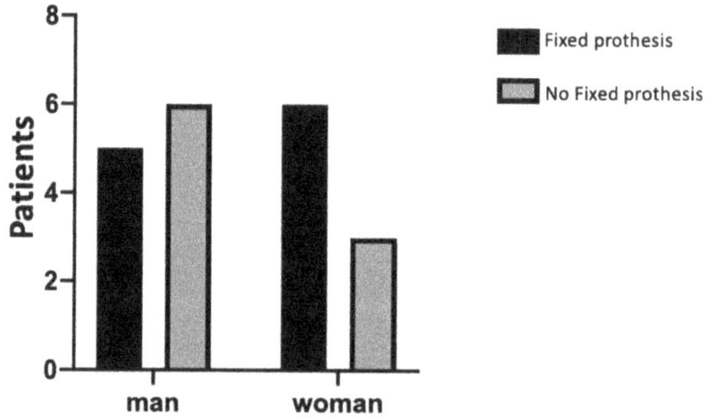

Figure A5. Difference between fixed-prosthesis wearers between males and females. No statistical significance ($p = 0.40$) was shown between the sexes.

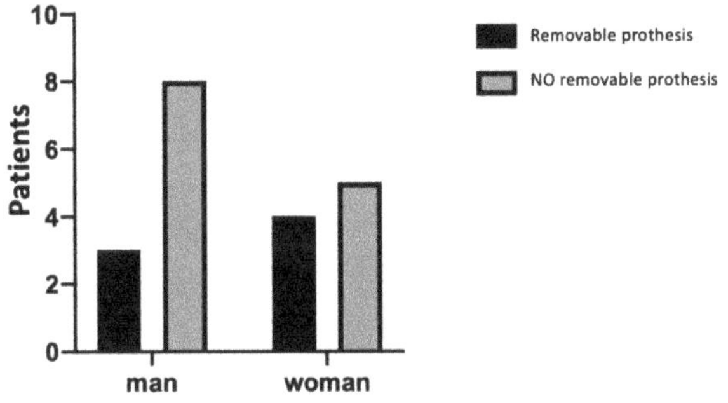

Figure A6. Difference between removable-prosthesis wearers between males and females. No statistical significance ($p = 0.64$) was shown between the sexes.

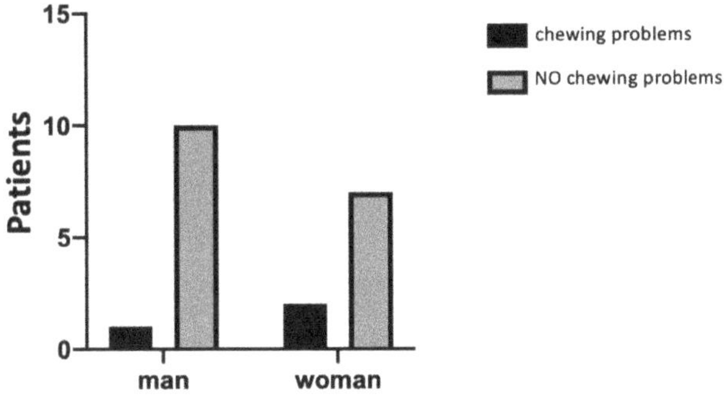

Figure A7. Difference between chewing problems between males and females. No statistical significance ($p = 0.56$) was shown between the sexes.

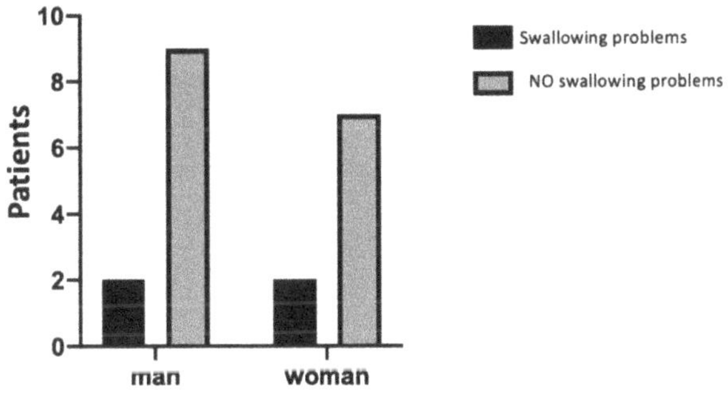

Figure A8. Difference between swallowing problems between males and females. No statistical significance ($p > 0.99$) was shown between the sexes.

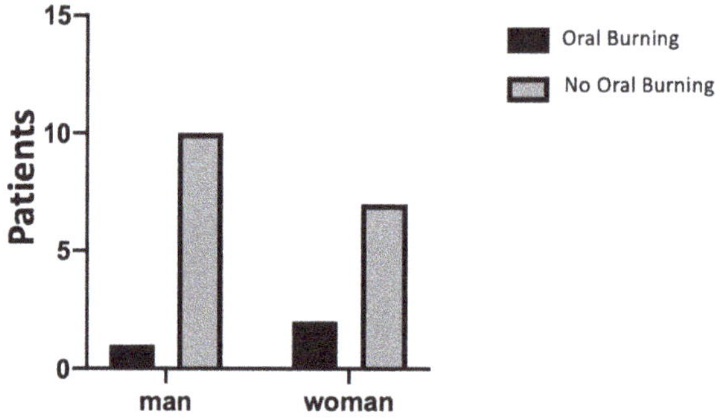

Figure A9. Difference between oral burning sensation between males and females. No statistical significance ($p = 0.56$) was shown between the sexes.

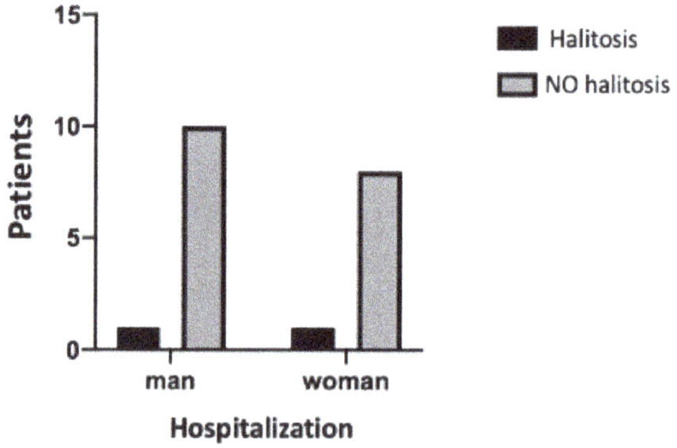

Figure A10. Difference of halitosis perception between males and females. No statistical significance ($p > 0.99$) was shown between the sexes.

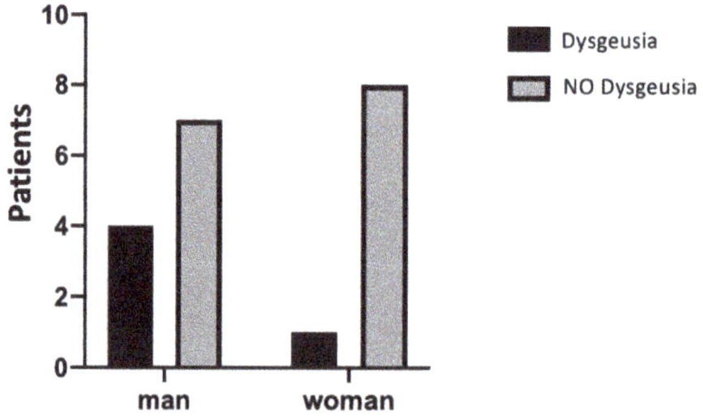

Figure A11. Difference of dysgeusia perception between males and females. No statistical significance ($p = 0.31$) was shown between the sexes.

References

1. Andersen, K.G.; Rambaut, A.; Lipkin, W.I.; Holmes, E.C.; Garry, R.F. The proximal origin of SARS-CoV-2. *Nat. Med.* **2020**, *26*, 450–452. [CrossRef] [PubMed]
2. Corman, V.M.; Muth, D.; Niemeyer, D.; Drosten, C. Hosts and Sources of Endemic Human Coronaviruses. *Adv. Virus Res.* **2018**, *100*, 163–188. [PubMed]

3. Wu, F.; Zhao, S.; Yu, B.; Chen, Y.-M.; Wang, W.; Song, Z.-G.; Hu, Y.; Tao, Z.-W.; Tian, J.-H.; Pei, Y.-Y.; et al. A new coronavirus associated with human respiratory disease in China. *Nature* **2020**, *579*, 265–269. [CrossRef] [PubMed]
4. Wang, Y.; Grunewald, M.; Perlman, S. Coronaviruses: An Updated Overview of Their Replication and Pathogenesis. *Methods Mol. Biol. Clifton NJ* **2020**, *2203*, 1–29.
5. Decaro, N.; Lorusso, A. Novel human coronavirus (SARS-CoV-2): A lesson from animal coronaviruses. *Vet. Microbiol.* **2020**, *244*, 108693. [CrossRef] [PubMed]
6. Yin, Y.; Wunderink, R.G. MERS, SARS and other coronaviruses as causes of pneumonia. *Respirol. Carlton VIC* **2018**, *23*, 130–137. [CrossRef] [PubMed]
7. Lu, R.; Zhao, X.; Li, J.; Niu, P.; Yang, B.; Wu, H.; Wang, W.; Song, H.; Huang, B.; Zhu, N.; et al. Genomic characterisation and epidemiology of 2019 novel coronavirus: Implications for virus origins and receptor binding. *Lancet Lond. Engl.* **2020**, *395*, 565–574. [CrossRef]
8. Chen, N.; Zhou, M.; Dong, X.; Qu, J.; Gong, F.; Han, Y.; Qiu, Y.; Wang, J.; Liu, Y.; Wei, Y.; et al. Epidemiological and clinical characteristics of 99 cases of 2019 novel coronavirus pneumonia in Wuhan, China: A descriptive study. *Lancet Lond. Engl.* **2020**, *395*, 507–513. [CrossRef]
9. Epidemiology Working Group for NCIP Epidemic Response, Chinese Center for Disease Control and Prevention. The epidemiological characteristics of an outbreak of 2019 novel coronavirus diseases (COVID-19) in China. *Zhonghua Liu Xing Bing Xue Za Zhi Zhonghua Liuxingbingxue Zazhi* **2020**, *41*, 145–151.
10. To, K.K.-W.; Tsang, O.T.-Y.; Yip, C.C.-Y.; Chan, K.-H.; Wu, T.-C.; Chan, J.M.-C.; Leung, W.-S.; Chik, T.S.-H.; Choi, C.Y.-C.; Kandamby, D.H.; et al. Consistent Detection of 2019 Novel Coronavirus in Saliva. *Clin. Infect. Dis. Off. Publ. Infect. Dis. Soc. Am.* **2020**, *71*, 841–843. [CrossRef]
11. ADA Council on Scientific Affairs; ADA Council on Dental Practice. Infection control recommendations for the dental office and the dental laboratory. *J. Am. Dent. Assoc.* **1996**, *127*, 672–680. [CrossRef] [PubMed]
12. Leung, R.L.; Schonfeld, S.E. Gypsum casts as a potential source of microbial cross-contamination. *J. Prosthet. Dent.* **1983**, *49*, 210–211. [CrossRef]
13. Sinjari, B.; Rexhepi, I.; Santilli, M.; D'Addazio, G.; Chiacchiaretta, P.; Di Carlo, P.; Caputi, S. The Impact of COVID-19 Related Lockdown on Dental Practice in Central Italy-Outcomes of A Survey. *Int. J. Environ. Res. Public. Health* **2020**, *17*, 5780. [CrossRef] [PubMed]
14. Yu, J.; Zhang, T.; Zhao, D.; Haapasalo, M.; Shen, Y. Characteristics of Endodontic Emergencies during Coronavirus Disease 2019 Outbreak in Wuhan. *J. Endod.* **2020**, *46*, 730–735. [CrossRef]
15. Wang, D.; Yin, Y.; Hu, C.; Liu, X.; Zhang, X.; Zhou, S.; Jian, M.; Xu, H.; Prowle, J.; Hu, B.; et al. Clinical course and outcome of 107 patients infected with the novel coronavirus, SARS-CoV-2, discharged from two hospitals in Wuhan, China. *Crit. Care Lond. Engl.* **2020**, *24*, 188. [CrossRef]
16. Vinayachandran, D.; Balasubramanian, S. Is gustatory impairment the first report of an oral manifestation in COVID-19? *Oral Dis.* **2020**. [CrossRef]
17. Freni, F.; Meduri, A.; Gazia, F.; Nicastro, V.; Galletti, C.; Aragona, P.; Galletti, C.; Galletti, B.; Galletti, F. Symptomatology in head and neck district in coronavirus disease (COVID-19): A possible neuroinvasive action of SARS-CoV-2. *Am. J. Otolaryngol.* **2020**, *41*, 102612. [CrossRef]
18. Saniasiaya, J. Xerostomia and COVID-19: Unleashing Pandora's Box. *Ear Nose Throat J.* **2020**. [CrossRef]
19. Martín Carreras-Presas, C.; Amaro Sánchez, J.; López-Sánchez, A.F.; Jané-Salas, E.; Somacarrera Pérez, M.L. Oral vesiculobullous lesions associated with SARS-CoV-2 infection. *Oral Dis.* **2020**. [CrossRef]
20. Chaux-Bodard, A.-G.; Deneuve, S.; Desoutter, A. Oral manifestation of Covid-19 as an inaugural symptom? *J. Oral Med. Oral Surg.* **2020**, *26*, 18. [CrossRef]
21. Soares, C.-D.; Carvalho, R.-A.; Carvalho, K.-A.; Carvalho, M.-G.; Almeida, O.-P. Letter to Editor: Oral lesions in a patient with Covid-19. *Med. Oral Patol. Oral Cirugia Bucal* **2020**, *25*, e563–e564.
22. Badran, Z.; Gaudin, A.; Struillou, X.; Amador, G.; Soueidan, A. Periodontal pockets: A potential reservoir for SARS-CoV-2? *Med. Hypotheses* **2020**, *143*, 109907. [CrossRef] [PubMed]
23. Metagenome of SARS-Cov2 Patients in Shenzhen with Travel to Wuhan Shows a Wide Range of Species—Lautropia, Cutibacterium, Haemophilus Being Most Abundant—and Campylobacter Explaining Diarrhea. Available online: https://www.researchgate.net/publication/340152514_Metagenome_of_SARS-Cov2_patients_in_Shenzhen_with_travel_to_Wuhan_shows_a_wide_range_of_species_-_Lautropia_Cutibacterium_Haemophilus_being_most_abundant_-_and_Campylobacter_explaining_diarrhea (accessed on 15 September 2020).

24. Zou, X.; Chen, K.; Zou, J.; Han, P.; Hao, J.; Han, Z. Single-cell RNA-seq data analysis on the receptor ACE2 expression reveals the potential risk of different human organs vulnerable to 2019-nCoV infection. *Front. Med.* **2020**, *14*, 185–192. [CrossRef] [PubMed]
25. Xu, H.; Zhong, L.; Deng, J.; Peng, J.; Dan, H.; Zeng, X.; Li, T.; Chen, Q. High expression of ACE2 receptor of 2019-nCoV on the epithelial cells of oral mucosa. *Int. J. Oral Sci.* **2020**, *12*, 8. [CrossRef]
26. Dziedzic, A.; Wojtyczka, R. The impact of coronavirus infectious disease 19 (COVID-19) on oral health. *Oral Dis.* **2020**. [CrossRef]
27. Amorim Dos Santos, J.; Normando, A.G.C.; Carvalho da Silva, R.L.; De Paula, R.M.; Cembranel, A.C.; Santos-Silva, A.R.; Guerra, E.N.S. Oral mucosal lesions in a COVID-19 patient: New signs or secondary manifestations? *Int. J. Infect. Dis. IJID Off. Publ. Int. Soc. Infect. Dis.* **2020**, *97*, 326–328.
28. Pedrosa, M.; Sipert, C.R.; Nogueira, F.N. Salivary Glands, Saliva and Oral Presentations in COVID-19 infection. *SciELO* **2020**. [CrossRef]
29. Gupta, A.; Madhavan, M.V.; Sehgal, K.; Nair, N.; Mahajan, S.; Sehrawat, T.S.; Bikdeli, B.; Ahluwalia, N.; Ausiello, J.C.; Wan, E.Y.; et al. Extrapulmonary manifestations of COVID-19. *Nat. Med.* **2020**, *26*, 1017–1032. [CrossRef]
30. Lenti, M.V.; Borrelli de Andreis, F.; Pellegrino, I.; Klersy, C.; Merli, S.; Miceli, E.; Aronico, N.; Mengoli, C.; Di Stefano, M.; Cococcia, S.; et al. Impact of COVID-19 on liver function: Results from an internal medicine unit in Northern Italy. *Intern. Emerg. Med.* **2020**. [CrossRef]
31. Herrera, D.; Serrano, J.; Roldán, S.; Sanz, M. Is the oral cavity relevant in SARS-CoV-2 pandemic? *Clin. Oral Investig.* **2020**, *24*, 2925–2930. [CrossRef]
32. Fu, L.; Wang, B.; Yuan, T.; Chen, X.; Ao, Y.; Fitzpatrick, T.; Li, P.; Zhou, Y.; Lin, Y.-F.; Duan, Q.; et al. Clinical characteristics of coronavirus disease 2019 (COVID-19) in China: A systematic review and meta-analysis. *J. Infect.* **2020**, *80*, 656–665. [CrossRef] [PubMed]
33. Tan, E.C.K.; Lexomboon, D.; Sandborgh-Englund, G.; Haasum, Y.; Johnell, K. Medications That Cause Dry Mouth as an Adverse Effect in Older People: A Systematic Review and Metaanalysis. *J. Am. Geriatr. Soc.* **2018**, *66*, 76–84. [CrossRef] [PubMed]
34. López-Pintor, R.M.; Casañas, E.; González-Serrano, J.; Serrano, J.; Ramírez, L.; de Arriba, L.; Hernández, G. Xerostomia, Hyposalivation, and Salivary Flow in Diabetes Patients. *J. Diabetes Res.* **2016**, *2016*, 4372852. [CrossRef] [PubMed]
35. Sinjari, B.; Feragalli, B.; Cornelli, U.; Belcaro, G.; Vitacolonna, E.; Santilli, M.; Rexhepi, I.; D'Addazio, G.; Zuccari, F.; Caputi, S. Artificial Saliva in Diabetic Xerostomia (ASDIX): Double Blind Trial of Aldiamed® Versus Placebo. *J. Clin. Med.* **2020**, *9*, 2196. [CrossRef]
36. Xu, J.; Li, Y.; Gan, F.; Du, Y.; Yao, Y. Salivary Glands: Potential Reservoirs for COVID-19 Asymptomatic Infection. *J. Dent. Res.* **2020**, *99*, 989. [CrossRef]
37. Carrillo-Larco, R.M.; Altez-Fernandez, C. Anosmia and dysgeusia in COVID-19: A systematic review. *Wellcome Open Res.* **2020**, *5*, 94. [CrossRef]
38. Lozada-Nur, F.; Chainani-Wu, N.; Fortuna, G.; Sroussi, H. Dysgeusia in COVID-19: Possible Mechanisms and Implications. *Oral Surg. Oral Med. Oral Pathol. Oral Radiol.* **2020**. [CrossRef]
39. Richardson, S.; Hirsch, J.S.; Narasimhan, M.; Crawford, J.M.; McGinn, T.; Davidson, K.W.; The Northwell COVID-19 Research Consortium; Barnaby, D.P.; Becker, L.B.; Chelico, J.D.; et al. Presenting Characteristics, Comorbidities, and Outcomes Among 5700 Patients Hospitalized With COVID-19 in the New York City Area. *JAMA* **2020**, *323*, 2052–2059. [CrossRef]
40. World Health Organization. *Smoking and COVID-19: Scientific Brief, 30 June 2020*; World Health Organization: Geneva, Switzerland, 2020.
41. Shibata, S.; Arima, H.; Asayama, K.; Hoshide, S.; Ichihara, A.; Ishimitsu, T.; Kario, K.; Kishi, T.; Mogi, M.; Nishiyama, A.; et al. Hypertension and related diseases in the era of COVID-19: A report from the Japanese Society of Hypertension Task Force on COVID-19. *Hypertens. Res.* **2020**, *43*, 1028–1046. [CrossRef]
42. Schiffrin, E.L.; Flack, J.M.; Ito, S.; Muntner, P.; Webb, R.C. Hypertension and COVID-19. *Am. J. Hypertens.* **2020**, *33*, 373–374. [CrossRef]

Journal of
Clinical Medicine

MDPI

Article

Managing the Oral Health of Cancer Patients during the COVID-19 Pandemic: Perspective of a Dental Clinic in a Cancer Center

Sunita Manuballa [1], Marym Abdelmaseh [1], Nirmala Tasgaonkar [1], Vladimir Frias [1], Michael Hess [1], Heidi Crow [1,2], Sebastiano Andreana [1,3], Vishal Gupta [4], Kimberly E. Wooten [4], Michael R. Markiewicz [4,5], Anurag K. Singh [6], Wesley L. Hicks Jr. [4] and Mukund Seshadri [1,7,*]

1 Department of Oral Oncology/Dentistry and Maxillofacial Prosthetics, Roswell Park Comprehensive Cancer Center, Buffalo, NY 14263, USA; Sunita.Manuballa@RoswellPark.org (S.M.); a.maryml@gmail.com (M.A.); Nirmala.Tasgaonkar@RoswellPark.org (N.T.); Vladimir.Frias@RoswellPark.org (V.F.); Michael.Hess@RoswellPark.org (M.H.); Heidi.Crow@RoswellPark.org (H.C.); Sebastiano.Andreana@RoswellPark.org (S.A.)

2 Department of Oral Diagnostic Sciences, University at Buffalo School of Dental Medicine, Buffalo, NY 14214, USA

3 Department of Restorative Dentistry, University at Buffalo School of Dental Medicine, Buffalo, NY 14214, USA

4 Department of Head and Neck/Plastic Surgery, Roswell Park Comprehensive Cancer Center, Buffalo, NY 14263, USA; Vishal.Gupta@RoswellPark.org (V.G.); Kimberly.Wooten@RoswellPark.org (K.E.W.); Michael.Markiewicz@RoswellPark.org (M.R.M.); Wesley.Hicks@RoswellPark.org (W.L.H.J.)

5 Department of Oral and Maxillofacial Surgery, University at Buffalo School of Dental Medicine, Buffalo, NY 14214, USA

6 Department of Radiation Medicine, Roswell Park Comprehensive Cancer Center, Buffalo, NY 14263, USA; Anurag.Singh@RoswellPark.org

7 Center for Oral Oncology, Roswell Park Comprehensive Cancer Center, Buffalo, NY 14263, USA

* Correspondence: Mukund.Seshadri@RoswellPark.org; Tel.: +1-716-845-1552

Received: 11 August 2020; Accepted: 24 September 2020; Published: 28 September 2020

Abstract: The practice of dentistry has been dramatically altered by the coronavirus disease 2019 (COVID-19) pandemic. Given the close person-to-person contact involved in delivering dental care and treatment procedures that produce aerosols, dental healthcare professionals including dentists, dental assistants and dental hygienists are at high risk of exposure. As a dental clinic in a comprehensive cancer center, we have continued to safely provide medically necessary and urgent/emergent dental care to ensure that patients can adhere to their planned cancer treatment. This was accomplished through timely adaptation of clinical workflows and implementation of practice modification measures in compliance with state, national and federal guidelines to ensure that risk of transmission remained low and the health of both immunocompromised cancer patients and clinical staff remained protected. In this narrative review, we share our experience and measures that were implemented in our clinic to ensure that the oral health needs of cancer patients were met in a timely manner and in a safe environment. Given that the pandemic is still on-going, the impact of our modified oral healthcare delivery model in cancer patients warrants continued monitoring and assessment.

Keywords: COVID-19; oral oncology; dental; oral surgery; head and neck cancer; cancer patients

1. Introduction

The outbreak of coronavirus disease 2019 (COVID-19) [1] has dramatically changed the practice of dentistry worldwide, given the close "person-to-person" contact involved in delivering dental care and treatment procedures that produce aerosols, often resulting in dental providers being exposed to blood, saliva and respiratory droplets [2,3]. Given the mode of transmission of COVID-19, dental healthcare professionals including dentists, dental assistants and dental hygienists are at high risk of exposure among all healthcare personnel [4,5]. In this regard, studies from multiple groups around the globe have reported on critical infection control measures [5–7] and guidelines for modifications to dental clinic workflows that were implemented during the pandemic [8,9]. Reports have also described the impact of COVID-19 on the practice of dental specialties, including oral medicine [10] oral and maxillofacial surgery [11–13], orthodontics [14] and endodontics [4,15].

Oral oncology (sometimes referred to as "Dental Oncology") is a branch of dentistry/oral medicine that provides specialized care to address the complex dental and oral health needs of cancer patients [16,17]. The division of Dentistry and Maxillofacial Prosthetics (DMFP) is a clinical service within the Department of Oral Oncology at Roswell Park, a National Cancer Institute (NCI)-designated Comprehensive Cancer Center located in Buffalo, New York. The center provides comprehensive cancer care to patients in the Buffalo–Niagara metropolitan area, surrounding counties in Western New York (WNY) and patients from New York State (NYS). The center also provides cancer care for patients from other states within the U.S. and Canada. The mission of DMFP is to provide high-quality oral healthcare to cancer patients. Specialized services provided by DMFP include management of existing dental conditions prior to the start of cancer therapy, prevention and management of oral complications from cancer treatment (radiation, chemotherapy and hematopoietic stem cell transplantation) and functional rehabilitation of patients after invasive cancer surgery [18–20]. Cancer patients are immunocompromised and, as a result, susceptible to oral and respiratory infections, including COVID-19 [21]. Given this "double whammy" (increased risk for cancer patients and dental providers), the pandemic has necessitated rapid implementation of changes to our oral healthcare delivery model, including adaptation of clinical workflows and diagnostic and treatment paradigms. Kochhar et al. have recently described recommendations for provision of dental care to cancer patients during the pandemic [22]. As a dental clinic in a comprehensive cancer center, we have continued to safely deliver dental care to cancer patients during this pandemic. This was accomplished through adaptation of clinical workflows to ensure that cancer patients can adhere to their planned cancer treatment. Timely implementation of practice modification measures was critical to ensure that patients and dental clinic staff remained protected and the risk of transmission remained minimal.

2. Overview of DMFP Clinic Responsiveness to COVID-19

The overview of the DMFP clinic response to COVID-19 is shown schematically in Figure 1. In response to the pandemic, a DMFP clinic task force was created in early March 2020 to implement clinic-centric measures that were in compliance with Centers for Disease Control and Prevention (CDC), the American Dental Association (ADA), NYS and institutional guidelines and develop protocols for safely providing dental care for cancer patients. The taskforce included the department chair, the clinical chief, a general dentist, the lead dental assistant and the clinic administrator. Such a composition of the task force ensured that all administrative and operational needs of the clinic and staff concerns were addressed. Given the relatively fluid nature of the situation, daily virtual meetings of the taskforce were conducted (via WebEx) to monitor the regional situation and to appraise team members of any updates to institutional policies regarding patient care and staff. The goals of the task force and the strategic approach undertaken to implement clinic-centric measures that complemented institutional measures are summarized in Figure 1.

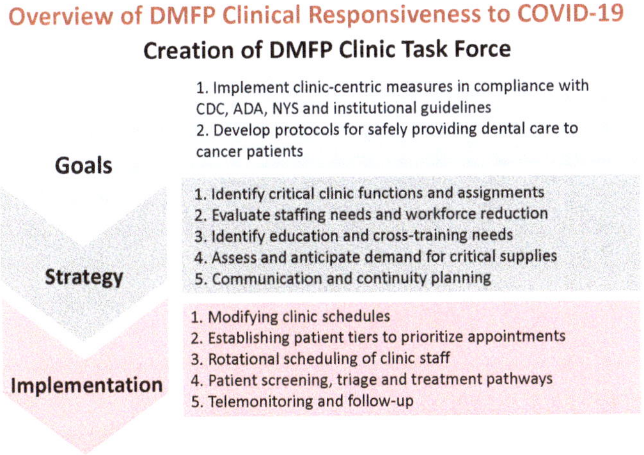

Overview of DMFP Clinical Responsiveness to COVID-19
Creation of DMFP Clinic Task Force
Goals
1. Implement clinic-centric measures in compliance with CDC, ADA, NYS and institutional guidelines
2. Develop protocols for safely providing dental care to cancer patients
Strategy
1. Identify critical clinic functions and assignments
2. Evaluate staffing needs and workforce reduction
3. Identify education and cross-training needs
4. Assess and anticipate demand for critical supplies
5. Communication and continuity planning
Implementation
1. Modifying clinic schedules
2. Establishing patient tiers to prioritize appointments
3. Rotational scheduling of clinic staff
4. Patient screening, triage and treatment pathways
5. Telemonitoring and follow-up

Figure 1. Schematic overview of the responsiveness of the Dentistry and Maxillofacial Prosthetics (DMFP) clinic at Roswell Park Comprehensive Center to the pandemic. (CDC—Centers for Disease Control and Prevention; ADA—American Dental Association; NYS—New York State).

The following measures were implemented in our clinic to limit traffic in clinical areas and ensure that the oral health needs of cancer patients were met in a timely manner and in a safe environment.

2.1. Identifying Critical Services Provided by the Dental Clinic

With the evolution of the pandemic in NYS and around the United States, the ADA, CDC and the New York State Dental Association (NYSDA) issued guidance on March 16, 2020, that all dental offices provide only emergency dental care for patients. A minimum of 3 weeks of postponement was recommended for all elective and non-emergent services. By mid-March 2020, the dental clinic taskforce had decided to scale down clinical operations to essential critical functions. In compliance with NYS, ADA and CDC guidelines, clinic visits were restricted to management of active cancer patients that needed medically necessary oral health evaluations (e.g., patients requiring dental clearance prior to start of radiation therapy, bone marrow transplant patients, patients scheduled for surgery) and urgent/emergent dental treatment.

2.2. Modifying Clinic Schedules

All clinic providers were asked to review their schedules for the months of March and April. Consistent with the framework [23] suggested by the Centers for Medicare and Medicaid Services (CMS), a three-tiered classification of patients was developed to modify clinic schedules as shown in Figure 2. Patients with scheduled appointments were immediately contacted and their health status assessed over the phone to determine the urgency of their treatment. The immune status of patients (undergoing active chemo/RT or immunotherapy, recent organ transplant; on immunosuppressive therapy) was also taken into consideration while determining the tier and type of appointment. Patients with appointments for elective dental procedures (e.g., routine follow-up appointments, prosthetic or routine oral hygiene maintenance patients that could wait) that could be safely deferred were rescheduled (on an average of 4–6 weeks from the initial appointment date). Patients were notified of their rescheduled appointments by the clinic receptionist along with the communication regarding the availability of all dentists and specialists for telephone consults.

Tier 1 (High acuity/risk)	**Lack of in-person oral health evaluation/timely care would result in harm.** • Active cancer patients including radiation/bone marrow transplant patients requiring dental clearance.
Tier 2 (Med acuity/risk)	**Lack of in-person oral health evaluation/care has the potential to result in harm/increase morbidity.** Existing dental/oral health issues may escalate into emergencies if treatment is delayed. • Cancer patients or survivors without any dental emergencies or urgent dental needs. Tele-monitoring and follow-up of these patients was implemented.
Tier 3 (Low acuity/risk)	**Oral health evaluation or care can be safely postponed for a short-term (3 months) without increased risk to the patient.** • Patients scheduled for regular, periodic follow-ups, hygiene appointments and maxillofacial prosthetics. Tele-monitoring and follow-up of these patients was implemented.

Figure 2. Three-tiered classification of patients based on their oral health needs for optimal scheduling of appointments during the pandemic.

2.3. Rotational Scheduling of Clinic Faculty and Staff

In alignment with the institutional "directed to leave campus" (DLC) policy, non-critical clinic staff, including personnel in administrative and research arms of the department, were scheduled to work remotely. Secure remote access (email, virtual desktop) was provided to staff members, which allowed them to continue their daily tasks from home. For essential clinic staff, a rotational schedule was implemented wherein one dentist and two dental assistants were assigned on a weekly basis. The providers and the assistants were on-site two days of the week to attend to patients requiring medically necessary dental procedures, but all providers were available for teleconsultation during the week. Additional emergent/urgent appointments were also handled by the same dentist /dental assistant team scheduled to be "on call" for the week. This arrangement also ensured a two-week window before the same provider/assistant team was scheduled to be back on-site (i.e., Week 1: Team A; Week 2: Team B; Week 3: Team C; Week 4: Team A). This temporal spacing of provider/staff schedules minimized overlap between faculty and staff from individual teams and allowed for a potential 14-day period of isolation or quarantine in the unfortunate event that one of the team members became symptomatic. All staff were instructed to continue self-monitoring and advised to stay home if they experienced flu-like symptoms.

2.4. Transitioning to a 'Virtual' Tumor Board

Another COVID-related modification in our clinical workflow involved a change in the conduct of a multidisciplinary head and neck conference ("tumor board"). The multidisciplinary conference serves as a valuable forum for discussions among team members regarding diagnosis and treatment planning of head and neck cancer patients. Roswell Park conducts a weekly head and neck tumor board meeting that is attended by faculty from the above-mentioned specialties along with nurse practitioners, physician assistants, physical therapists, palliative care and social workers. These weekly meetings are quintessential to ensure adequate work up for correct diagnosis, staging, discuss treatment strategies (surgery versus radiation), surgical reconstruction approaches for best quality of life and survivorship issues. In a pre-COVID-19 world, this involved an in-person meeting of about 25–30 specialists in a packed conference room. With the onset of the pandemic and the restrictions that followed, such a gathering was no longer possible. Given the large number of participants at these weekly meetings, a decision was made in March 2020 to move the tumor board to an online platform ("virtual" tumor board). We transitioned to weekly virtual tumor board meetings utilizing the WebEx platform developed by Citrix systems. The WebEx platform allowed both video and audio presentation, including a screen sharing ability. The platform was approved by Roswell IT and was compliant with the Health Insurance Portability and Accountability Act (HIPAA) regulations. Email invitations for these sessions were sent out to participants along with the pertinent WebEx information. Participation required a valid attendee name and a Roswell Park email login. The virtual format allowed for efficient participation of a large number of attendees with case presentations made in Microsoft Power Point format by the head and neck fellow, along with review of histology slides by a pathologist and imaging by the radiologist. Although not a new concept, we had no previous experience with virtual multidisciplinary conferences. Our experience to date with the virtual tumor board format has been positive, and the format has encouraged greater and timely participation from a large group of participants. In addition, since most of the attendees participated in the virtual meeting from their workstations, it provided them with the ability to instantly access not just patient records, but also published literature to clarify any points if needed. The biggest limitation of the virtual format is the lack of personal interaction and interactive conversations between multiple speakers. Despite a few initial technical glitches, this approach continues to be effective, allowing the entire team to engage in thoughtful discussions regarding treatment plans for individual patients without increasing the risk of exposure and potential members between clinic staff.

2.5. Screening of Patients Prior to Visits

Multiple measures were put in place for screening patients with scheduled appointments at our clinic. These included inquiry of symptoms over the phone ("tele-triage") 24 h prior to their appointment. Patients were screened (symptom checks, temperature measurements) at the main entrance to our cancer center and then at the clinic front desk at check-in. The duration of appointments for patients requiring medically necessary or emergency dental procedures was also lengthened (approximately 90 min) with adequate time (30–45 min) between appointments to allow clinic staff to perform all infection control procedures according to CDC guidelines.

2.6. Infection Control Training and Operatory Preparation

Recognizing the need for stringent infection control protocols, several institutional and clinic-centric training measures were implemented to train all clinical faculty and staff. In addition to the mandatory annual in-services routinely completed by all hospital staff, refresher training on infection control procedures was provided in the form of training videos, instruction sheets, flyers as well as presentations and group discussions (via WebEx). Topics covered in these training sessions included but were not limited to the basics of COVID-19, hand hygiene, respiratory etiquette, personal protective equipment (PPE), donning and doffing, sterilization and disinfection procedures, protection of all equipment (e.g., computer screens, monitors), proper disposal of single-use instruments and minimizing clutter (e.g., leaving all paperwork outside the operatory; removal of any potential sources of contamination, such as pictures from the walls) within the operatories. All providers, including assistants, wore full surgical garb (shoe covers, head covers, surgical gowns, gloves, N95 masks and face shields) while examining patients.

2.7. Clinical Care Guidelines for Dental Management of Cancer Patients

Given the unprecedented nature of events, guidelines for managing oral care of cancer patients were developed. Due to the known risk of COVID-19 transmission via respiratory droplets, a decision was made to avoid high aerosol-generating procedures including the use of high-speed hand pieces, ultrasonic scalers and air-water syringe. A prophylactic hydrogen peroxide mouth rinse was provided to all patients prior to their clinical examination. Aerosol-generating procedures were avoided in severely immunocompromised patients, and clinical evaluation of these patients was performed in dedicated operatories. Consideration was given and plans put in place for performing low aerosol-generating procedures in the operating room (OR) to these patients if clinically warranted. Conservative treatment for asymptomatic carious restorations and minimal debridement were provided without the use of ultrasonic equipment to reduce the microbial load prior to their treatments. Restorative procedures were performed following the principles of atraumatic restorative therapy [24]. Based on the depth of invasion and the presence/absence of symptoms, caries excavation and temporary restorations were placed. Alternatively, caries arresting measures, through the use of silver diamine fluoride (SDF 38% Advantage Arrest), were performed. Hand scaling was performed, and no ultrasonic scaling or polishing was done. Procedures were performed under rubber dam isolation, and radiography was limited to extra-oral radiographs. Extractions of non-restorable teeth were performed following the recommended PPE protocols. Extractions of teeth were only done when the teeth had significant mobility, poor bone support or a root morphology that was amenable to a simple extraction. For head and neck patients undergoing surgical procedures, dental extractions were performed in the operating room (OR) in close coordination with the head and neck surgeons. Contingency plans were also made for providing dental care in peri-operative surgical suites as alternatives to dental operatories, if needed. Emergency floor consultations were provided for in-patients and treatments provided as needed. During this time, the dental faculty maintained crucial communication with patients, their treating physicians (medical and radiation oncologists) and surgeons to maintain continuity of care.

2.8. Maxillofacial Rehabilitation of Cancer Patients during COVID-19

Maxillofacial prosthetics is the sub-specialty of prosthodontics that deals with the rehabilitation of head and neck defects beyond the immediate oral region. The most common procedures performed by a maxillofacial prosthodontist at a cancer center are the obturation or restoration of missing maxillary and mandibular structures and the replacement of missing orbital, nasal, auricular and cranial structures [16,17,25]. Other procedures performed include surgical placement of implants to support or retain prostheses or the creation of devices to aid the delivery of surgical or radiation treatment. The decision-making process during COVID-19 was complicated by the fact that, although many non-emergent prosthetic procedures could be postponed, the delay in adequate rehabilitation has major consequences, including deficient speech, swallowing as well as the psychosocial issues for patients due to a visibly missing body part. The treatment protocol at Roswell Park considered both the patient's medical status as well as the urgency of the procedure involved and attempted to provide treatment with the fewest number of visits and procedures to prevent exposure to the virus. Medically necessary surgical obturations that could be inserted with sutures or ligation were performed in the operating room. Removal of the surgical prosthetic and replacement with an interim prosthesis were evaluated on a case-by-case basis, and all adjustments were carried out under a laboratory hood. Since the creation of definitive prosthetics often requires multiple aerosol-generating procedures, these treatments were postponed. Conventional prosthodontic procedures and surgical implant placement also generate a large amount of aerosol and were delayed in order to limit the exposure of severely medically compromised patients. Fabrication of facial or somatic prostheses also requires multiple visits and would increase patient and provider risk of exposure (asymptomatic carriers) and was postponed.

2.9. Telemonitoring and Follow-Up

All phone consultations were documented in the electronic health record (EHR). The temporal scheduling of clinical faculty and staff enabled providers that were off-site to monitor requests for clinic appointments. Concerns and requests from patients seeking emergency appointments were reviewed by a dental provider to understand the nature of their emergency and the appropriate course of management. Phone consults were also performed for patients receiving radiation to follow up for dysphagia, mucositis or candidiasis. Individual prescription requests (e.g., fluoride toothpaste, chlorhexidine) were managed by the providers. Appropriate prescriptions were called into their pharmacies. All patient concerns were initially addressed with a phone call, and if a clinic visit was deemed necessary, the patient was scheduled for a visit.

2.10. Modifications to a General Practice Dental Residency Training Program

The DMFP department serves as a home to a 1-year General Practice Residency (GPR) program that is administered jointly with the State University of New York, University at Buffalo, School of Dental Medicine. The program has an annual intake of two residents who spend approximately 70 percent of their time in the clinical care of patients. The didactic portion consists of treatment-planning seminars and literature reviews, as well as lectures in diagnosis, prosthodontics, endodontics and practice management. When the directive to leave campus (DLC) for all non-essential staff was implemented at our cancer center, a distance education model based on an online learning curriculum and continuing education (CE) credits covering all areas of general dentistry was implemented. Subsequently, following the implementation of several risk reduction measures and enhanced infection controls, residents were allowed to return on a rotating basis and observe patient care, to minimize contact and exposure for an already vulnerable patient population. PPE donning/doffing procedures were extensively reviewed. Modifications to dental practice and clinical decision making in the context of a pandemic were thoroughly explained. Differences in risk–benefit considerations between ideal treatment plans versus minimally acceptable treatment to "clear" patients for oncologic care were discussed. Residents also participated in care by conducting assessment phone calls with patients calling the clinic with dental concerns. Residents learned to triage and classify dental emergencies and urgent care cases based on ADA interim guidelines. Emphasis was placed on gathering pertinent patient information to come up with working diagnoses before scheduling patients to minimize appointment times and overall exposure. Residents were tasked with leading virtual weekly case reviews. A thorough medical and dental history was presented for each patient that was seen in the clinic that week. Dental treatment that was proposed or completed to clear them to proceed with their cancer care was outlined and discussed with the faculty. Detailed discussions took place surrounding the modifications that had to be made in their oncologic and dental care as a result of COVID-19. Although not ideal, these modifications enabled the residents to effectively continue their dental and oral oncology training during the pandemic.

3. Conclusions

3.1. Teamwork Is Integral to Ensure Timely and Optimal Coordination of Care

Managing the oral health of cancer patients requires timely coordination of care between surgeons, radiation oncologists, medical oncologists, radiologists, pathologists, dentists and maxillofacial prosthodontists. For example, we have previously documented that stem cell transplant patients may have a narrow window of adequate disease control for successful transplantation [26]. Similarly, the time from a head and neck cancer diagnosis to the initiation of radiation therapy correlates with survival [27]. As a result, timely dental clearance of cancer patients is integral to their overall cancer care. While such coordination of care was routinely performed prior to the pandemic, the unprecedented outbreak of COVID-19 posed several logistical challenges and uncertainties in dental and oral healthcare delivery models. Therefore, the importance and the value of teamwork and communication between dentists and medical professionals cannot be understated.

3.2. The Road Ahead

We have recently begun resuming our clinical services in a phased manner with modified clinical workflow while maintaining social distancing guidelines in our clinic waiting rooms and continued incorporation of infection control procedures in our clinic areas. At the present time, clinical care is provided with staggered appointments while simultaneously managing unscheduled consultation requests and emergencies. Roswell Park currently offers COVID testing on-site by scheduled appointment, drive-up or in an expedited manner at point-of-care for cancer patients based on clinical need. As a result, we have routinely begun COVID testing our dental clinic patients. These modifications have enabled us to safely provide dental care to cancer patients while ensuring that they adhere to their planned cancer treatment. However, it is now being increasingly recognized that the impact of COVID-19 is likely to be long-standing (several months to years) with a possibility of a second wave of infections in the fall. As we gradually progress to a "new normal", evaluating the impact of these optimized practices and processes within the dental clinic will be important. Given the planned scale-down of our clinic operations, the number of patients seen by our clinic during this time was reduced. We are currently reviewing our clinic volume data (number of appointments, number and type of procedures performed) during March–September 2020 and comparing it to our "pre-COVID" (March–September 2019) metrics. Such a comparative assessment would have to take additional variables into consideration, including number of active providers (dentists and specialists) on staff, number of residents and so on., to recognize the true impact of COVID-19 on our practice. Equally important is measuring the impact of these practice modifications on patient outcomes and evaluating the overall impact of these changes to clinical workflows on patient experience. The impact of COVID-19 on healthcare economics for dentistry and oral medicine also warrants further investigation. In this regard, we have recently begun examining the financial consequences of COVID-19 on our clinical practice through a review of our billing records. We continue to closely monitor the impact of our clinic measures on treatment-related oral health complications and outcomes in cancer patients and hope to report our findings in the future.

Author Contributions: S.M., N.T., H.C. and M.S.: Contributed to conception or design, drafted and critically revised the manuscript. M.A., V.F., M.H., S.A., V.G., K.E.W., M.R.M., A.K.S. and W.L.H.J.: Contributed to conception or design and drafted the manuscript. All authors gave their final approval and agree to be accountable for all aspects of the work. All authors have read and agreed to the published version of the manuscript.

Funding: This research was funded by Roswell Park's Cancer Center Support Grant from the National Cancer Institute P30CA016056 and 3R01DE024595-05S1 from the National Institute of Dental and Craniofacial Research.

Conflicts of Interest: The authors declare no conflict of interest.

References

1. Guan, W.J.; Ni, Z.Y.; Hu, Y.; Liang, W.H.; Ou, C.Q.; He, J.X.; Liu, L.; Shan, H.; Lei, C.L.; Hui, D.S.C.; et al. Clinical Characteristics of Coronavirus Disease 2019 in China. *N. Engl. J. Med.* **2020**, *382*, 1708–1720. [CrossRef] [PubMed]
2. Meng, L.; Hua, F.; Bian, Z. Coronavirus Disease 2019 (COVID-19): Emerging and Future Challenges for Dental and Oral Medicine. *J. Dent. Res.* **2020**, *99*, 481–487. [CrossRef] [PubMed]
3. Odeh, N.D.; Babkair, H.; Abu-Hammad, S.; Borzangy, S.; Abu-Hammad, A.; Abu-Hammad, O. COVID-19: Present and Future Challenges for Dental Practice. *Int. J. Environ. Res. Public Health* **2020**, *17*, 3151. [CrossRef]
4. Ather, A.; Patel, B.; Ruparel, N.B.; Diogenes, A.; Hargreaves, K.M. Coronavirus Disease 19 (COVID-19): Implications for Clinical Dental Care. *J. Endod.* **2020**, *46*, 584–595. [CrossRef] [PubMed]
5. Izzetti, R.; Nisi, M.; Gabriele, M.; Graziani, F. COVID-19 Transmission in Dental Practice: Brief Review of Preventive Measures in Italy. *J. Dent. Res.* **2020**, *99*, 1030–1038. [CrossRef] [PubMed]
6. Abramovitz, I.; Palmon, A.; Levy, D.; Karabucak, B.; Kot-Limon, N.; Shay, B.; Kolokythas, A.; Almoznino, G. Dental care during the coronavirus disease 2019 (COVID-19) outbreak: Operatory considerations and clinical aspects. *Quintessence Int.* **2020**, *51*, 418–429. [CrossRef] [PubMed]
7. Jamal, M.; Shah, M.; Almarzooqi, S.H.; Aber, H.; Khawaja, S.; El Abed, R.; Alkhatib, Z.; Samaranayake, L.P. Overview of transnational recommendations for COVID-19 transmission control in dental care settings. *Oral Dis.* **2020**. [CrossRef]
8. Alharbi, A.; Alharbi, S.; Alqaidi, S. Guidelines for dental care provision during the COVID-19 pandemic. *Saudi Dent. J.* **2020**, *32*, 181–186. [CrossRef]
9. Peditto, M.; Scapellato, S.; Marciano, A.; Costa, P.; Oteri, G. Dentistry during the COVID-19 Epidemic: An Italian Workflow for the Management of Dental Practice. *Int. J. Environ. Res. Public Health* **2020**, *17*, 3325. [CrossRef]
10. Umansky Sommer, M.; Davidovitch, T.; Platner, O.; Inerman, A.; Yarom, N. The effect of COVID-19 pandemic on oral medicine services in a tertiary referral center. *Oral Dis.* **2020**. [CrossRef]

11. Barca, I.; Cordaro, R.; Kallaverja, E.; Ferragina, F.; Cristofaro, M.G. Management in oral and maxillofacial surgery during the COVID-19 pandemic: Our experience. *Br. J. Oral Maxillofac. Surg.* **2020**, *58*, 687–691. [CrossRef] [PubMed]
12. Yang, Y.; Soh, H.Y.; Cai, Z.G.; Peng, X.; Zhang, Y.; Guo, C.B. Experience of Diagnosing and Managing Patients in Oral Maxillofacial Surgery during the Prevention and Control Period of the New Coronavirus Pneumonia. *Chin. J. Dent. Res.* **2020**, *23*, 57–62. [CrossRef] [PubMed]
13. Zimmermann, M.; Nkenke, E. Approaches to the management of patients in oral and maxillofacial surgery during COVID-19 pandemic. *J. Craniomaxillofac. Surg.* **2020**, *48*, 521–526. [CrossRef] [PubMed]
14. Maspero, C.; Abate, A.; Cavagnetto, D.; El Morsi, M.; Fama, A.; Farronato, M. Available Technologies, Applications and Benefits of Teleorthodontics. A Literature Review and Possible Applications during the COVID-19 Pandemic. *J. Clin. Med.* **2020**, *9*, 1891. [CrossRef] [PubMed]
15. Yu, J.; Zhang, T.; Zhao, D.; Haapasalo, M.; Shen, Y. Characteristics of Endodontic Emergencies during Coronavirus Disease 2019 Outbreak in Wuhan. *J. Endod.* **2020**, *46*, 730–735. [CrossRef]
16. Petrovic, I.; Rosen, E.B.; Matros, E.; Huryn, J.M.; Shah, J.P. Oral rehabilitation of the cancer patient: A formidable challenge. *J. Surg. Oncol.* **2018**, *117*, 1729–1735. [CrossRef]
17. Sullivan, M. The expanding role of dental oncology in head and neck surgery. *Surg. Oncol. Clin. N. Am.* **2004**, *13*, 37–46. [CrossRef]
18. Sroussi, H.Y.; Epstein, J.B.; Bensadoun, R.J.; Saunders, D.P.; Lalla, R.V.; Migliorati, C.A.; Heaivilin, N.; Zumsteg, Z.S. Common oral complications of head and neck cancer radiation therapy: Mucositis, infections, saliva change, fibrosis, sensory dysfunctions, dental caries, periodontal disease, and osteoradionecrosis. *Cancer Med.* **2017**, *6*, 2918–2931. [CrossRef]
19. Epstein, J.B.; Barasch, A. Oral and Dental Health in Head and Neck Cancer Patients. *Cancer Treat. Res.* **2018**, *174*, 43–57. [CrossRef]
20. Levi, L.E.; Lalla, R.V. Dental Treatment Planning for the Patient with Oral Cancer. *Dent. Clin. N. Am.* **2018**, *62*, 121–130. [CrossRef]
21. Indini, A.; Rijavec, E.; Ghidini, M.; Cattaneo, M.; Grossi, F. Developing a risk assessment score for patients with cancer during the coronavirus disease 2019 pandemic. *Eur. J. Cancer* **2020**, *135*, 47–50. [CrossRef] [PubMed]
22. Kochhar, A.S.; Bhasin, R.; Kochhar, G.K.; Dadlani, H. Provision of continuous dental care for oral oncology patients during & after COVID-19 pandemic. *Oral Oncol.* **2020**, *106*, 104785. [CrossRef] [PubMed]
23. Non-Emergent, Elective Medical Services and Treatment Recommendations. Available online: https://www.cms.gov/files/document/cms-non-emergent-elective-medical-recommendations.pdf (accessed on 24 September 2020).
24. Schwendicke, F.; Frencken, J.E.; Bjorndal, L.; Maltz, M.; Manton, D.J.; Ricketts, D.; Van Landuyt, K.; Banerjee, A.; Campus, G.; Domejean, S.; et al. Managing Carious Lesions: Consensus Recommendations on Carious Tissue Removal. *Adv. Dent. Res.* **2016**, *28*, 58–67. [CrossRef]
25. Phasuk, K.; Haug, S.P. Maxillofacial Prosthetics. *Oral Maxillofac. Surg. Clin. North Am.* **2018**, *30*, 487–497. [CrossRef] [PubMed]
26. Chen, G.L.; Hahn, T.; Wilding, G.E.; Groman, A.; Hutson, A.; Zhang, Y.; Khan, U.; Liu, H.; Ross, M.; Bambach, B.; et al. Reduced-Intensity Conditioning with Fludarabine, Melphalan, and Total Body Irradiation for Allogeneic Hematopoietic Cell Transplantation: The Effect of Increasing Melphalan Dose on Underlying Disease and Toxicity. *Biol. Blood Marrow Transplant.* **2019**, *25*, 689–698. [CrossRef] [PubMed]
27. DeGraaff, L.H.; Platek, A.J.; Iovoli, A.J.; Wooten, K.E.; Arshad, H.; Gupta, V.; McSpadden, R.P.; Kuriakose, M.A.; Hicks, W.L., Jr.; Platek, M.E.; et al. The effect of time between diagnosis and initiation of treatment on outcomes in patients with head and neck squamous cell carcinoma. *Oral Oncol.* **2019**, *96*, 148–152. [CrossRef]

Journal of
Clinical Medicine

MDPI

Article

Children's Dental Anxiety during the COVID-19 Pandemic: Polish Experience

Aneta Olszewska [1,*] and Piotr Rzymski [2,3,*]

1 Department of Facial Malformation, Poznan University of Medical Sciences, 60-812 Poznań, Poland
2 Department of Environmental Medicine, Poznan University of Medical Sciences, 60-806 Poznań, Poland
3 Integrated Science Association (ISA), Universal Scientific Education and Research Network (USERN), 60-806 Poznań, Poland
* Correspondence: anetaol@ump.edu.pl (A.O.); rzymskipiotr@ump.edu.pl (P.R.)

Received: 14 July 2020; Accepted: 25 August 2020; Published: 25 August 2020

Abstract: Dental fear and anxiety is a significant issue that affects pediatric patients and creates challenges in oral health management. Considering that the coronavirus disease 2019 (COVID-19) pandemic, along with its associated sanitary regime, social distancing measures and nationwide quarantines, could itself induce public fears, including in children, it is of great interest to explore whether this situation and the necessity of reorganizing dental care could potentially affect the emotional state of pediatric patients facing a need for urgent dental intervention. The present study assessed the emotional state of children ≤ seven years old ($n = 25$) requiring dental healthcare during a nationwide quarantine in Poland, as well as the anxiety levels of their caregivers. The Faces Anxiety Scale was adopted, and the evaluation was independently performed by the dentist, caregivers and children themselves. The level of anxiety in caregivers was also measured. As demonstrated, children requiring dental intervention during the nationwide quarantine did not reveal a significantly higher anxiety level as compared to the age- and indication-matched pre-pandemic control group ($n = 20$), regardless of whether their emotional state was evaluated by the dentist, caregivers, or by themselves. However, the share of children scoring the lowest anxiety level in all assessments was smaller in the pandemic group. Boys in the pandemic group had a higher anxiety level, as indicated by a caregiver assessment, and displayed a negative correlation with age in all three types of evaluation. Moreover, caregiver anxiety levels were higher in the pandemic group as compared to the pre-pandemic subset and revealed stronger correlations with the dental anxiety in children. The results suggest that the reorganization of oral healthcare under the pandemic scenario did not have a profound effect on children's dental anxiety. Nevertheless, findings in young boys highlight that they may be more vulnerable and require special care to mitigate their anxiety and decrease the risk of dentophobia in the future—these observations must be, however, treated with caution due to the small sample size and require further confirmation. Moreover, it is important to reassure caregivers of the safety of the dental visit during the pandemic to minimize the effect of their own anxiety on dental fears in children.

Keywords: COVID-19; SARS-CoV-2; dental care; children; dentist-patient relation; pandemic

1. Introduction

The outbreak of the novel coronavirus disease COVID-19 in December 2019 that spread across the Asian continent and eventually turned into a pandemic [1,2] created numerous challenges in health care sectors unrelated to the management of infectious diseases, including dentistry [3–7]. Following the confirmation of the first case in an increasing number of countries, the physical infrastructure, including entire hospitals, hospital wards, beds and technical equipment, had to be repurposed. The workforce resources in health care have also undergone reorganization and reallocation to support the response to the pandemic. This has led to the limitation or postponing of non-emergency health care appointments and treatments. In the meantime, the rapidly evolving epidemiological situation has forced numerous countries to implement strict sanitary regimes and social distancing measures, and eventually impose nationwide quarantines to decrease transmission rates. Under such circumstances, and particularly lockdown-associated isolation, significant public distress can be seen, further magnified by mass media coverage, often based on sensational, panic promoting headlines, as well as by online social media through which the spread of unsupported claims and fake news could be seen [8–10]. This stress is not only related to a fear of contracting the disease but also to significant and rapid changes to lifestyle and work [11]. As already demonstrated, all of these factors can be so profoundly affecting that a relevant percentage of individuals are put at risk of less or more severe mental health issues [12], including children and their parents [13–16]. Moreover, one study in adults has already reported that the introduction of the pandemic caused anxiety in 25% of dental patients [17]. However, no research has specifically addressed dental anxiety levels during COVID-19, including that in children.

During the COVID-19 pandemic, children suffer from not going to kindergartens and schools, not having real contact with their friends and some family members and having to live at home with decreased ability to practice physical activity and carry out some of their hobbies. As shown in an Italian survey, a significant percentage of children become nervous when hearing about the pandemic (e.g., on television) [18]. To protect them from distress, parents might often avoid discussing the pandemic, although the research supports that sensitive communication during the crisis has benefits for children's wellbeing [19,20]. In addition, their emotional state can closely reflect that of caregivers, further adding to anxiety level [21].

Providing children with dental care during the COVID-19 pandemic, and in particular during the increased social restrictions, can be a challenging task. It is known that appointments are often met with dental fear and anxiety, while 7–8% of children in pre- and early school age display it at a level which might interfere with dental procedures [22,23]. This primarily originates from fears of procedure and pain [24–27], but under pandemic-related lockdown these emotions and feelings can potentially be further exacerbated by the new stressors present in their environment as well as by the psychological tension resonating from the caregivers who need to take a decision to leave home and potentially risk contracting SARS-CoV-2. Moreover, in the regular setting, there is a possibility of the effective management of children's fear, anxiety and phobia with the support of caregivers and through desensitization, tell-show-do, positive reinforcement, and other behavioral techniques [26,28]. As the main route of SARS-CoV-2 transmission is via airborne droplets, dental staff are required to use personal protective equipment (PPE), i.e., suits, goggles, face visors, and face masks. The PPE affects the voice tone, makes it more difficult for children to understand what a dentist is communicating, does not allow children to read facial expressions which are important for building their trust with a dentist, adds to white coat syndrome, and overall hinders interaction with the patient [7]. Although some techniques to manage the anxiety level are still possible and still performed, the additional safety measures may effectively worsen the relationship between pediatric patients and personnel.

Survey studies reported that 50–70% of dental professionals admit to experiencing higher stress and anxiety levels as a result of the COVID-19 pandemic [29,30], an effect that may, in turn, alter their relationship with the pediatric patient. All of this, along with empty dental clinics and the smell of ozone disinfectant, can affect the children's trust in and perception of the oral healthcare provider, particularly in patients with a high fear level, and potentially aggravate the possibility of reassuring and de-stressing them in the waiting room and dental office, and eventually this may reinforce dental anxiety.

The present study aimed to explore the level of anxiety in children and their caregivers during dental visits at the time of the nationwide quarantine in Poland. The first COVID-19 case in the country was confirmed on 4 March 2020. Following this, schools and universities were closed on 11 March and a nationwide quarantine was imposed on 24 March. The lockdown lasted till 4 May when hotels and shopping centers were permitted to reopen while on 6 May daycare centers and kindergartens were allowed to resume their activities. Despite the easing of social distancing rules, dental care will continue to be provided with new sanitary regimes. Evaluation of the emotional state of young patients and their caregivers during the pandemic and related nationwide lockdown is important to understand whether the additional safety measures can affect dental fear and to discuss the strategies that could effectively decrease this.

2. Experimental Section

2.1. Study Design

The study was designed to explore the emotional state of 25 children aged four–seven who required intervention at the Pediatric Dentistry Clinic at Poznan University of Medical Sciences, Poznań, Poland, during the nationwide quarantine in Poland (pandemic group), and to compare it to an age- and an indication-matched group of pediatric patients before the COVID-19 pandemic (pre-pandemic group). The pre-pandemic group used for comparison consisted of 20 children aged four–seven requiring dental intervention between January and June 2018. The level of anxiety related to the dental visit was also assessed in caregivers in both groups, as they remain in a close emotional relationship with their children and can affect each other. The following medical indications for dental appointments were considered in both groups of pediatric patients: tooth extraction, abscess, dental trauma (traumatic injury to orofacial tissues), mucosal lesion, and necessity of performing pulp treatment. All children enrolled in the study had a dental history of no more than three appointments, no history of chronic disease and no mental disorder. The following descriptive variables of the studied children were collected: age, sex, and medical indication for dental intervention.

The anxiety levels in the pandemic group was evaluated between 24 March and 30 April 2020 (pandemic group). At the time the study was initiated, COVID-19 infections were active in 195 countries and territories, including Poland, with 425,675 cases and 19,195 deaths confirmed globally. During the time the study was conducted, the total number of confirmed infections and fatal cases in Poland increased from 901 to 12,877 and from 10 to 644, respectively. This period represents the strictest national lockdown, which was imposed from 24 March with some restrictions lifted at the beginning of May when hotels, shopping centers, daycare centers, and kindergartens were permitted to reopen. During this period, the following modifications to dental healthcare procedures were undertaken:

1. To limit the direct time of the visit, medical history was taken via phone or online call.
2. Children's caregivers were informed about new safety regulations and measures employed by the dental clinic, and about additional safety measures.
3. Before the appointment, all caregivers were advised to explain the safety measures to children and show them a picture of dental staff in PPE to make them more familiar with the situation.
4. The body temperature of each child and caregiver was measured at the entrance to the waiting room.
5. Each child and caregiver was instructed to disinfect hands in the waiting room.
6. Only one adult caregiver was allowed to accompany a child during the visit to the dental office.
7. In the case of all appointments, two professionals (a dentist and assistant) were maximally present in the dental office.

All caregivers and children in the pandemic group adhered to the above-mentioned rules.

The purpose and protocol of the study were explained to every child and their supervisor. Participation in the research was entirely voluntary. Prior to participation, all supervisors were asked to give their written informed consent. The supervisor accompanied the child during the emotional assessment. The study protocol was submitted to the Bioethical Committee at Poznan University of Medical Sciences - according to the performed evaluation, it lacked the characteristics of a medical experiment and, in line with Polish law and the Good Clinical Practice, it did not require specific approval by the Bioethics Committee.

2.2. Emotional State Evaluation

The emotional state of children was evaluated in the waiting room prior to dental procedures by a caregiver, dentist and by the child. The whole procedure took max. 15 min. Dentists and caregivers independently assessed the children's emotional state using the faces mood scale (Figure 1). The scale was prepared by a graphic artist according to the facial muscle changes involved in a fearful expression and based on photographs of faces showing increased fear [31]. The evaluating individual selected one of the six drawn faces that suited the child's emotional state. The drawings were numbered as follows: 1—calm; 2—uncertain; 3—reserved, closed and uncooperative; 4—avoiding; 5—loud; 6—crying. The pediatric patients, given the paper with a blank face (Figure 1), were asked to complete the drawing by adding the facial elements: eyes, nose and lips. Prior to this, all children were instructed that a drawing should express their own emotions before the dental appointment. The dentist then categorized the children's drawings to the corresponding faces 1–6, mostly by matching eye and lip expressions. Such a graphical approach in the evaluation of the emotional state of children appears to be advantageous compared to the numerical scale assessment - it only requires simplified verbal instructions and is more accessible for children to understand than a translation of their inner state to a particular numerical score [32]. It has also been demonstrated that children and their caregivers tend to prefer the faces scale over other evaluation methods [33,34]. The numbers associated with each drawing were operationalized by transforming them into 1–6 Likert scales, where 1 and 6 indicated the lowest and highest level of anxiety, respectively.

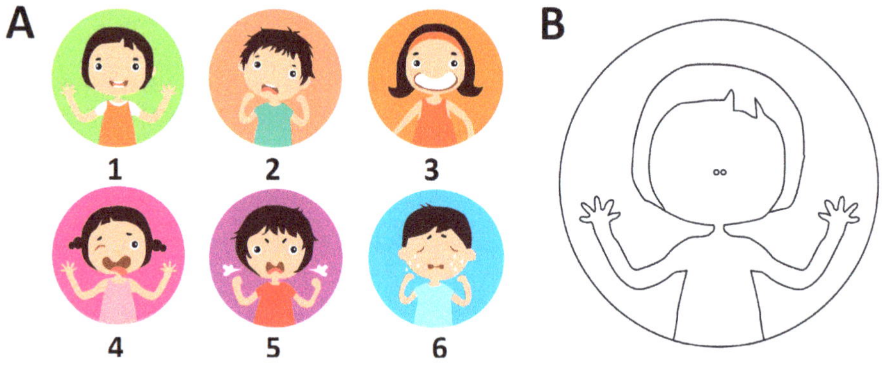

Figure 1. The graphical scale used to assess the emotional state of pediatric patients before the dental appointment (**A**) and a blank face (**B**) used by children to express their own emotional state by drawing missing elements: eyes, nose and lips.

Additionally, the caregivers were asked to assess their own level of anxiety related to the dental visit by using a Likert scale 0–10, where 0 corresponded to lack of fear, 5 indicated medium anxiety, while 10 represented a very high level of anxiety.

2.3. Statistical Analysis

The statistical analyses were performed using Statistica v.13.1 (StatSoft Inc., Tulsa, OK, USA). Because age did not meet the assumption of Gaussian distribution (Shapiro–Wilk test; $p < 0.05$) and the emotional state of children was measured in the ordinal scale, non-parametric methods were employed. The differences in the emotional state scores in pandemic and pre-pandemic groups, as well as between boys and girls, were assessed with the Mann-Whitney U test. The association between children's age and the scores were evaluated using Spearman's rank correlation coefficient (Rs). The differences in the prevalence of medical indications for dental intervention in the pandemic and the pre-pandemic group were assessed by Pearson's χ^2 test. A value of $p < 0.05$ was considered statistically significant.

3. Results

The pandemic group consisted of 25 children: 15 boys (mean ± SD age 5.1 ± 1.1 years) and 10 girls (mean ± SD age 5.3 ± 0.9 years). The pre-pandemic group consisted of 10 boys (mean ± SD age 4.5 ± 0.8 years) and 10 girls (mean ± SD age 5.6 ± 1.1 years). The comparative age of the two groups did not differ ($p > 0.05$, Mann-Whitney U test). The demographic breakdown of medical indications for a dental visit in both groups is summarized in Table 1. The prevalence of these indications did not differ between the studied groups ($p > 0.05$, χ^2 test in all cases); tooth extraction was the most frequent procedure (Table 2).

Table 1. Spearman's rank correlation coefficient calculated for the level of anxiety in the pre-pandemic ($n = 20$) and pandemic group of children ($n = 25$) before the dental appointment assessed by the dentist, caregivers and children themselves. All values are statistically significant.

	Group	Caregiver Evaluation	Children Evaluation
Dentist evaluation	pre-pandemic	0.88	0.59
	pandemic	0.86	0.75
Caregivers evaluation	pre-pandemic	-	0.79
	pandemic	-	0.82

Table 2. Medical indications for the dental visit in pediatric patients in the pandemic and pre-pandemic groups included in the present study.

Medical indication	Pandemic Group ($n = 25$)	Pre-pandemic Group ($n = 20$)
Tooth extraction (n/%)	14/56	10/50
Abscess treatment (n/%)	5/20	1/5
Mucosal lesion (n/%)	1/4	2/10
Pulp treatment (n/%)	2/8	5/25
Dental trauma (n/%)	3/12	2/10

The emotional state of children in the pandemic group did not differ from that in the pre-pandemic group, either when assessed by the dentist [median (interquartile range, IQR): 3 (2–5) vs. 2 (1–4)], caregiver [3 (2–5) vs. 3 (2–5)], or the children themselves [3 (2–4) vs. 2 (1–3)] ($p > 0.05$ in all cases, Mann-Whitney U test). However, the percentage of children for whom the highest anxiety score of 6 in the pre-pandemic and pandemic groups was 20.0 and 12.0% (dentist's evaluation), 20.0 and 16.0% (caregiver's evaluation) and 10.0 and 24.0% (self-evaluation by children), respectively In turn, the lowest anxiety score of 1 in these groups was 30.0 and 16% (dentist's evaluation), 15.0 and 12.0% (caregiver's evaluation) and 40.0 and 24.0% (self-evaluation by children), respectively The summary of scores in each group given by dentists, caregivers and children is presented in Figure 2. The scores given by the dentist, caregivers, and self-reported by the children were all highly correlated in both studied groups of children (Table 2).

Moreover, the gender of children did not differentiate the level of their anxiety in either pre- or pandemic groups ($p > 0.05$ in all cases, Mann-Whitney U test) (Figure 3). The only exception was the assessment of children's anxiety performed by parents in the pandemic group, with a higher score given for boys than girls [median (IQR): 4 (3–5) vs. 2 (2–3)] ($p < 0.05$, Mann-Whitney U test). The comparison of each gender across the two groups yielded no differences in anxiety level ($p > 0.05$ in both cases, Mann-Whitney U test).

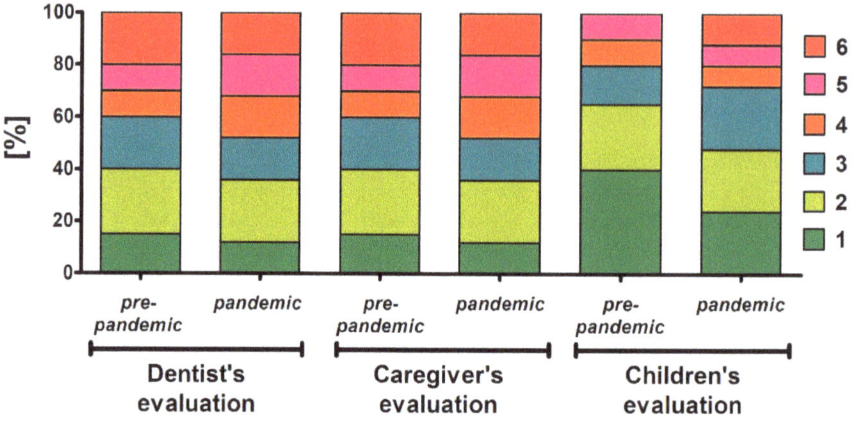

Figure 2. The emotional state of pediatric patients before the dental appointment in the pre-pandemic (n = 20) and pandemic group (n = 25) as assessed by dentists, caregivers and children themselves.

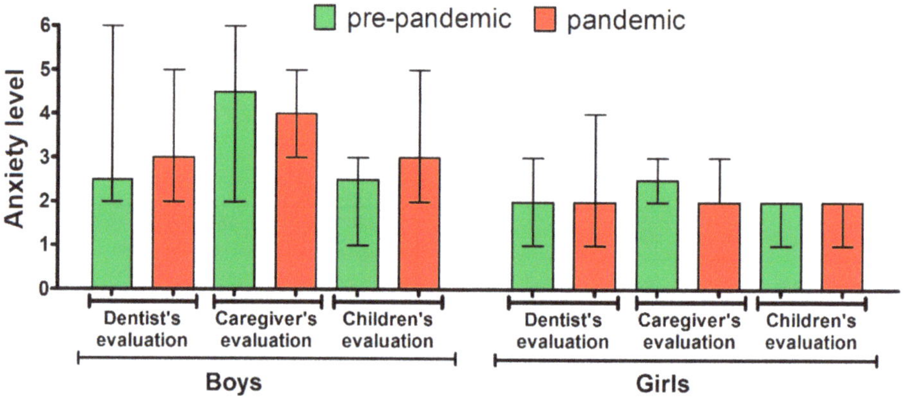

Figure 3. The emotional state of boys and girls before the dental appointment in the pre-pandemic (n = 20) and pandemic group (n = 25) as assessed by dentists, caregivers and children themselves. The bars represent median, the whiskers represent interquartile range.

However, as presented in Table 3, the percentage of boys in the pandemic group having the lowest and highest anxiety levels was respectively decreased and increased compared to the pre-pandemic subset in all three evaluations—such a phenomenon was not seen in the case of girls.

As shown in Table 4, a number of negative correlations were found between children's age in the pandemic group and the scores they were given, including their own assessment of emotional state. However, when differentiated by gender, these correlations were only significant for the subset of boys (Table 4). When evaluated by the dentist, caregivers and children themselves, the median (IQR) scores of anxiety in boys aged four from the pandemic group were 5 (5–6), 5 (5–6) and 4 (3–6), respectively, while for those aged seven, these scores were 1 (1–2), 2 (1–4) ad 2 (1–4), respectively.

A significant difference in the anxiety of caregivers accompanying children before and during the pandemic was observed with a median (IQR) level of 6 (4–8) and 3 (2–4), respectively ($p < 0.01$, Mann-Whitney U test). The number of caregivers indicating a score >5 (above the level of anxiety defined as 'medium') in pre-pandemic and pandemic groups was 1/20 (5%) and 13/25 (52%), respectively. The parental anxiety level in the pandemic group was positively correlated with children's dental anxiety as assessed by the dentist (Rs = 0.80, $p < 0.05$), the caregiver (Rs = 0.76, $p < 0.05$) and self-evaluated by the children (0.74, $p < 0.05$). In the pre-pandemic group, positive correlations with the children's anxiety evaluated by caregivers (Rs = 0.57, $p < 0.05$) and children themselves (Rs = 0.72 $p < 0.05$) were observed.

Table 3. The percentage of boys and girls with the lowest and highest anxiety levels before the dental appointment in the pre-pandemic (n = 20) and pandemic group (n = 25) as assessed by dentists, caregivers and children themselves.

Evaluation	Score	Boys		Girls	
		Pre-Pandemic (n = 10)	Pandemic (n = 15)	Pre-Pandemic (n = 10)	Pandemic (n = 10)
Dentist (%)	Lowest	20.0	6.7	40.0	30.0
	Highest	10.0	13.3	10.0	10.0
Caregiver (%)	Lowest	10.0	6.7	20.0	20.0
	Highest	10.0	20.0	10.0	10.0
Children (%)	Lowest	40.0	13.3	40.0	40.0
	Highest	10.0	13.3	10.0	10.0

Table 4. Relationship between the age of pediatric patients and their fear as evaluated by dentists, caregivers and self-reported by children (Spearman's rank correlation coefficient).

	Group	Dentist Evaluation	Caregiver Evaluation	Children Evaluation
Age	Pandemic	−0.67 *	−0.63 *	−0.44 *
	boys (n = 15)	−0.84 *	−0.69 *	−0.57 *
	girls (n = 10)	−0.34 ns	0.57 ns	−0.39 ns
	Pre-pandemic	−0.25 ns	−0.40 ns	−0.36 ns
	boys (n = 10)	−0.08 ns	−0.14 ns	−0.32 ns
	girls (n = 10)	−0.38 ns	−0.69 *	−0.52 ns

* $p < 0.05$; ns—not significant ($p > 0.05$).

4. Discussion

The present study is the first to report on the emotional state of children ≤ seven years during the COVID-19 pandemic. Its unique aspect is that it was specifically conducted during the strictest form of the nationwide quarantine. The previous research in adults has shown that dental patients reported feeling anxious about the pandemic, although this finding cannot be attributed directly to dental anxiety, and, contrary to our study, it did not investigate anxiety levels during the dental appointment [17]. In turn, dental fear and anxiety in children represent an important issue in dental management, and as hypothesized, fears related to the ongoing epidemiological situation and associated changes in the dental service organization could further potentiate them. This could be particularly expected given the fact that the emotional state of children is often influenced by that of their parents [35,36], and during the pandemic-related lockdown the fear of contracting SARS-CoV-2 during different activities, e.g., while shopping in the grocery store, were frequently reported [11]. On the other hand, the additional measures undertaken to shorten dental appointments via applying telemedicine, i.e., video/phone consultation to take medical history and talk through the proposed treatment, as well as efforts to make children as familiar as possible with the new sanitary regime during the dental visit, could possibly mitigate, at least to some extent, fear and anxiety in children. The observations of the present study indicate that children requiring dental intervention during the COVID-19 pandemic-related nationwide quarantine may not experience significant changes in their emotional state, as compared to the pre-pandemic, age- and indication-matched group. It should be however noted that the share of patients with the lowest anxiety level in all assessments was smaller in the pandemic group.

The emotional state of pediatric patients was evaluated in the present study by children themselves, but also by their caregiver and the dentist. Such an approach allows for a broader assessment of the child's inner state. As previously suggested by studies on pain intensity, self-reporting tools can be inaccurate for children younger than seven years due to poor understanding of the method and the skills needed to express their experiences not yet being fully developed [37,38]. Therefore, in such groups, complementary observational measures should be employed. In such a case, caregivers can be used as a proxy for patients' reports, especially in situations in which some communication barriers may exist. Finally, the assessment of the child by the dentist is also valuable as it is based on professional experience and not biased by the strong emotional relationship that exists between a child and a parent [39]. One should, however, note that a survey conducted in 30 countries reported increased levels of anxiety in dentists during the COVID-19 pandemic [29], and this may potentially alter their perception and assessment of the patient's emotional state. Importantly though, the present study demonstrated that the results on children's emotional state obtained using the face scale from the dentist, caregivers and self-reported by the pediatric patients generally agree with each other.

Previous research has related dental anxiety in children to various factors such as personality traits, increased general fears, a history of painful dental experiences, parental dental fears and other family-related factors [22,40,41]. Some studies have also found that it tends to be higher in girls than boys, and in younger children. These age and gender-related differences were, however, not always confirmed [42]. In the present study, gender-differences, with a higher level of anxiety in boys, were observed only in the group undergoing a dental procedure during the pandemic-related nationwide quarantine, and only when the assessment was performed by a caregiver. One should note that the percentage of boys in the pandemic group who displayed the highest and lowest level of anxiety increased and decreased, respectively, when compared to the pre-pandemic subset. Furthermore, the present study suggests that younger boys were the most vulnerable, as highlighted by the negative correlation of all anxiety assessments and their age, and the highest scores seen in patients aged 4. This is an interesting finding since general anxiety levels tend to be higher in girls during early childhood [43]. It can be hypothesized that under the pandemic scenario it may be more challenging to explain the nature of the situation to younger boys than girls, due to the difference in the development of their language skills [44–47]. As reported, four-year-old boys reveal a significantly lower expression of pivotal factors for human communication, such as FOXP2 protein [48]. Nevertheless, the present results highlight that special care may be needed for younger boys requiring a dental intervention during pandemic in order to mitigate their anxiety and decrease the induction of potential dentophobia in the future. One should however stress that implementation of any mitigation strategies in this regard should only be considered if the present results, based on small sample size, would find confirmation in future studies.

Importantly, the present study clearly shows that parental anxiety levels are correlated with the emotional state of children and that this association was stronger during the pandemic. The percentage of caregivers having anxiety above the medium level was over 10-fold higher in the pandemic group when compared to the pre-pandemic subset. Increased anxiety in adults during epidemiological events is not uncommon and has been observed previously, e.g., during the H1N1 pandemic in 2009–2010 [49–51]. Unsurprisingly, it has also been reported during the COVID-19 pandemic [52–54].

In turn, previous dental studies show that parents play a key role in children's anxiety and development [55–57]. Therefore, it is of high importance, particularly during the pandemic, to ensure that caregivers of pediatric patients are fully aware of these links and to educate them on how to make a dental visit a more comfortable event for children. Considering that parental anxiety levels in the pandemic group were higher than in the pre-pandemic group, it can be suggested that fears related to COVID-19 and contracting SARS-CoV-2 were responsible for this effect. It is, therefore, necessary for healthcare professionals to explain, prior to the appointment, all the measures undertaken to maximally limit the risk of infection in the dentist's surgery and to reassure patients of their safety. This can be achieved with a phone or video call preceding the dental visit during which medical history is also recorded.

Although the present study reports on the important issue of dental healthcare under a pandemic scenario, the study limitations must be emphasized. Firstly, the results represented a single-center experience and were obtained from a small population size. Moreover, dental anxiety in children is multifactorial, and this research did not explore the effect of personal traits and family-related issues, including socioeconomic status and level of education of caregivers [40,41,58–60]. Moreover, transforming the Faces Anxiety Scale into the Likert scale allowed for a more in-depth statistical elaboration of the results, although the study was not designed to delve into explaining the exact reasons for the observed anxiety levels in children. This would require additional questions, time spent in the dental clinic, and communication approaches that were challenging to apply during the dental clinical practice under the scenario of the most strict form of the COVID-19 related quarantine.

5. Conclusions

This is the first study to report on dental anxiety in children during the strictest form of the COVID-19 lockdown. In general, the present research indicates that, contrary to the concerns that pediatric children will be significantly more stressed due to dental appointments during a nationwide quarantine related to the COVID-19 pandemic, their anxiety levels, assessed by the dentist, caregivers and by themselves, did not differ from the pre-pandemic group of pediatric patients. Nevertheless, the percentage of children having the lowest level of anxiety in all employed assessments decreased in the pandemic group. The results suggest that younger boys may potentially be more vulnerable in this regard—this finding should be treated with caution and would require further confirmation in larger-scale studies. Moreover, parental anxiety levels were highly associated with the emotional state of children, particularly during the pandemic period. It seems reasonable to make parents aware of this association and, further, to reassure their safety by explaining that the risks of contracting an infectious agent during a dental visit are mitigated by appropriate measures.

Author Contributions: Conceptualization, A.O.; methodology, A.O.; validation, A.O. and P.R.; formal analysis, investigation, A.O. and P.R; writing—original draft preparation, A.O and P.R. All authors have read and agreed to the published version of the manuscript.

Funding: This research received no external funding.

Conflicts of Interest: The authors declare no conflict of interest.

References

1. Cucinotta, D.; Vanelli, M. WHO Declares COVID-19 a Pandemic. *Acta Bio-Med. Atenei Parm.* **2020**, *91*, 157–160. [CrossRef]
2. Bogoch, I.I.; Watts, A.; Thomas-Bachli, A.; Huber, C.; Kraemer, M.U.G.; Khan, K. Pneumonia of unknown aetiology in Wuhan, China: Potential for international spread via commercial air travel. *J. Travel Med.* **2020**, 27. [CrossRef]
3. Magro, F.; Perazzo, P.; Bottinelli, E.; Possenti, F.; Banfi, G. Managing a Tertiary Orthopedic Hospital during the COVID-19 Epidemic, Main Challenges and Solutions Adopted. *Int. J. Environ. Res. Public Health* **2020**, *17*, 4818. [CrossRef]
4. Wang, N.C.; Jain, S.K.; Estes, N.A.M., III; Barrington, W.W.; Bazaz, R.; Bhonsale, A.; Kancharla, K.; Shalaby, A.A.; Voigt, A.H.; Saba, S. Priority plan for invasive cardiac electrophysiology procedures during the coronavirus disease 2019 (COVID-19) pandemic. *J. Cardiovasc. Electrophysiol.* **2020**, *31*, 1255–1258. [CrossRef]
5. Pinheiro, R.N.; Coimbra, F.J.F.; Costa, W.L.D., Jr.; Ribeiro, H.S.D.C.; Ribeiro, R.; Wainstein, A.J.A.; Laporte, G.A.; Coelho, M.J.P., Jr.; Fernandes, P.H.D.S.; Cordeiro, E.Z.; et al. Surgical cancer care in the COVID-19 era: Front line views and consensus. *Rev. Colégio Bras. Cir.* **2020**, *47*. [CrossRef]
6. Coulthard, P. Dentistry and coronavirus (COVID-19)—Moral decision-making. *Br. Dent. J.* **2020**, *228*, 503–505. [CrossRef]

7. Bizzoca, M.E.; Campisi, G.; Lo Muzio, L. Covid-19 Pandemic: What Changes for Dentists and Oral Medicine Experts? A Narrative Review and Novel Approaches to Infection Containment. *Int. J. Environ. Res. Public Health* **2020**, *17*, 3793. [CrossRef]
8. Rzymski, P.; Nowicki, M. COVID-19-related prejudice toward Asian medical students: A consequence of SARS-CoV-2 fears in Poland. *J. Infect. Public Health* **2020**, *13*, 873–876. [CrossRef]
9. Shimizu, K. 2019-nCoV, fake news, and racism. *Lancet* **2020**, *395*, 685–686. [CrossRef]
10. Orso, D.; Federici, N.; Copetti, R.; Vetrugno, L.; Bove, T. Infodemic and the spread of fake news in the COVID-19-era. *Eur. J. Emerg. Med.* **2020**. [CrossRef]
11. Sidor, A.; Rzymski, P. Dietary Choices and Habits during COVID-19 Lockdown: Experience from Poland. *Nutrients* **2020**, *12*, 1657. [CrossRef]
12. Brooks, S.K.; Webster, R.K.; Smith, L.E.; Woodland, L.; Wessely, S.; Greenberg, N.; Rubin, G.J. The psychological impact of quarantine and how to reduce it: Rapid review of the evidence. *Lancet* **2020**, *395*, 912–920. [CrossRef]
13. Fontanesi, L.; Marchetti, D.; Mazza, C.; Di Giandomenico, S.; Roma, P.; Verrocchio, M.C. The effect of the COVID-19 lockdown on parents: A call to adopt urgent measures. *Psychol. Trauma Theory Res. Pract. Policy* **2020**. [CrossRef]
14. Thakur, K.; Kumar, N.; Sharma, N. Effect of the Pandemic and Lockdown on Mental Health of Children. *Indian J. Pediatr.* **2020**, *87*, 552. [CrossRef]
15. Clemens, V.; Deschamps, P.; Fegert, J.M.; Anagnostopoulos, D.; Bailey, S.; Doyle, M.; Eliez, S.; Hansen, A.S.; Hebebrand, J.; Hillegers, M.; et al. Potential effects of "social" distancing measures and school lockdown on child and adolescent mental health. *Eur. Child Adolesc. Psychiatry* **2020**, *29*, 739–742. [CrossRef]
16. Fegert, J.M.; Vitiello, B.; Plener, P.L.; Clemens, V. Challenges and burden of the Coronavirus 2019 (COVID-19) pandemic for child and adolescent mental health: A narrative review to highlight clinical and research needs in the acute phase and the long return to normality. *Child. Adolesc. Psychiatry Ment. Health* **2020**, *14*, 20. [CrossRef]
17. Peloso, R.M.; Pini, N.I.P.; Sunfeld Neto, D.; Mori, A.A.; Oliveira, R.C.G.d.; Valarelli, F.P.; Freitas, K.M.S. How does the quarantine resulting from COVID-19 impact dental appointments and patient anxiety levels? *Braz. Oral Res.* **2020**, *34*. [CrossRef]
18. Pisano, L.; Galimi, D.; Cerniglia, L. A qualitative report on exploratory data on the possible emotional/behavioral correlates of Covid-19 lockdown in 4-10 years children in Italy. *Psyarxiv* **2020**. [CrossRef]
19. Dalton, L.; Rapa, E.; Ziebland, S.; Rochat, T.; Kelly, B.; Hanington, L.; Bland, R.; Yousafzai, A.; Stein, A. Communication with children and adolescents about the diagnosis of a life-threatening condition in their parent. *Lancet* **2019**, *393*, 1164–1176. [CrossRef]
20. Dalton, L.; Rapa, E.; Stein, A. Protecting the psychological health of children through effective communication about COVID-19. *Lancet Child. Adolesc. Health* **2020**, *4*, 346–347. [CrossRef]
21. Spinelli, M.; Lionetti, F.; Pastore, M.; Fasolo, M. Parents' Stress and Children's Psychological Problems in Families Facing the COVID-19 Outbreak in Italy. *Front. Psychol.* **2020**, *11*. [CrossRef]
22. Dahlander, A.; Soares, F.; Grindefjord, M.; Dahllöf, G. Factors Associated with Dental Fear and Anxiety in Children Aged 7 to 9 Years. *Dent. J.* **2019**, *7*, 68. [CrossRef]
23. Wong, M.L.W.; Lai, S.H.F.; Wong, H.M.; Yang, Y.X.; Yiu, C.K.Y. Dental anxiety in Hong Kong preschool children: Prevalence and associated factors. *Adv. Pediatric Res.* **2017**, *4*, 1. [CrossRef]
24. Siegel, K.; Schrimshaw, E.W.; Kunzel, C.; Wolfson, N.H.; Moon-Howard, J.; Moats, H.L.; Mitchell, D.A. Types of dental fear as barriers to dental care among African American adults with oral health symptoms in Harlem. *J. Health Care Poor Underserved* **2012**, *23*, 1294–1309. [CrossRef]
25. Armfield, J.M.; Heaton, L.J. Management of fear and anxiety in the dental clinic: A review. *Aust. Dent. J.* **2013**, *58*, 390–407. [CrossRef]
26. Appukuttan, D.P. Strategies to manage patients with dental anxiety and dental phobia: Literature review. *Clin. Cosmet. Investig. Dent.* **2016**, *8*, 35–50. [CrossRef]
27. Dou, L.; Vanschaayk, M.M.; Zhang, Y.; Fu, X.; Ji, P.; Yang, D. The prevalence of dental anxiety and its association with pain and other variables among adult patients with irreversible pulpitis. *BMC Oral Health* **2018**, *18*, 101. [CrossRef]

28. Townsend, J.A.; Wells, M.H. 24—Behavior Guidance of the Pediatric Dental Patient. In *Pediatric Dentistry*, 6th ed.; Nowak, A.J., Christensen, J.R., Mabry, T.R., Townsend, J.A., Wells, M.H., Eds.; Content Repository: Philadelphia, PA, USA, 2019; pp. 352–370. [CrossRef]
29. Ahmed, M.A.; Jouhar, R.; Ahmed, N.; Adnan, S.; Aftab, M.; Zafar, M.S.; Khurshid, Z. Fear and Practice Modifications among Dentists to Combat Novel Coronavirus Disease (COVID-19) Outbreak. *Int. J. Environ. Res. Public Health* **2020**, *17*, 2821. [CrossRef]
30. Mahendran, K.; Patel, S.; Sproat, C. Psychosocial effects of the COVID-19 pandemic on staff in a dental teaching hospital. *Br. Dent. J.* **2020**, *229*, 127–132. [CrossRef]
31. Ekman, P.; Friesen, W.V. *Facial Action Coding System: A Technique for the Measurement of Facial Movement*; Consulting Psychologists Press: Palo Alto, CA, USA, 1978; Volume 3.
32. Sattler, J.M. *Assessment of Children: Behavioral and Clinical Applications*, 4th ed.; Jerome M. Sattler: La Mesa, CA, USA, 2002; p. 620.
33. Goodenough, B.; Piira, T.; Baeyer, C.L.V.; Chua, K.S.G.; Trieu, J.; Champion, G.D. Comparing six self-report measures of pain intensity in children. *Suff. Child.* **2005**, *8*, 1–25.
34. Keck, J.F.; Gerkensmeyer, J.E.; Joyce, B.A.; Schade, J.G. Reliability and validity of the faces and word descriptor scales to measure procedural pain. *J. Pediatric Nurs.* **1996**, *11*, 368–374. [CrossRef]
35. Ryan, R.; O'Farrelly, C.; Ramchandani, P. Parenting and child mental health. *Lond. J. Prim. Care* **2017**, *9*, 86–94. [CrossRef]
36. Power, T.G. Stress and Coping in Childhood: The Parents' Role. *Parenting* **2004**, *4*, 271–317. [CrossRef]
37. Von Baeyer, C.L.; Forsyth, S.J.; Stanford, E.A.; Watson, M.; Chambers, C.T. Response biases in preschool children's ratings of pain in hypothetical situations. *Eur. J. Pain* **2009**, *13*, 209–213. [CrossRef]
38. Von Baeyer, C.L. Children's self-report of pain intensity: What we know, where we are headed. *Pain Res. Manag.* **2009**, *14*, 39–45. [CrossRef]
39. Boutelle, K.; Eisenberg, M.E.; Gregory, M.L.; Neumark-Sztainer, D. The reciprocal relationship between parent–child connectedness and adolescent emotional functioning over 5 years. *J. Psychosom. Res.* **2009**, *66*, 309–316. [CrossRef]
40. Wu, L.; Gao, X. Children's dental fear and anxiety: Exploring family related factors. *BMC Oral Health* **2018**, *18*, 100. [CrossRef]
41. D'Alessandro, G.; Alkhamis, N.; Mattarozzi, K.; Mazzetti, M.; Piana, G. Fear of dental pain in Italian children: Child personality traits and parental dental fear. *J. Public Health Dent.* **2016**, *76*, 179–183. [CrossRef]
42. Raj, S.; Agarwal, M.; Aradhya, K.; Konde, S.; Nagakishore, V. Evaluation of Dental Fear in Children during Dental Visit using Children's Fear Survey Schedule-Dental Subscale. *Int. J. Clin. Pediatr. Dent.* **2013**, *6*, 12–15. [CrossRef]
43. Carter, A.S.; Godoy, L.; Wagmiller, R.L.; Veliz, P.; Marakovitz, S.; Briggs-Gowan, M.J. Internalizing Trajectories in Young Boys and Girls: The Whole is Not a Simple Sum of its Parts. *J. Abnorm. Child. Psychol.* **2010**, *38*, 19–31. [CrossRef]
44. Bleses, D.; Vach, W.; Slott, M.; Wehberg, S.; Thomsen, P.I.A.; Madsen, T.O.; BasbØLl, H. The Danish Communicative Developmental Inventories: Validity and main developmental trends. *J. Child. Lang.* **2008**, *35*, 651–669. [CrossRef]
45. Huttenlocher, J.; Haight, W.; Bryk, A.; Seltzer, M.; Lyons, T. Early vocabulary growth: Relation to language input and gender. *Dev. Psychol.* **1991**, *27*, 236–248. [CrossRef]
46. Maccoby, E.E. *The Development of Sex. Differences*; Stanford University Press: Palo Alto, CA, USA, 1966.
47. Ramer, A.L.H. Syntactic styles in emerging language. *J. Child. Lang.* **2008**, *3*, 49–62. [CrossRef]
48. Bowers, J.M.; Perez-Pouchoulen, M.; Edwards, N.S.; McCarthy, M.M. Foxp2 mediates sex differences in ultrasonic vocalization by rat pups and directs order of maternal retrieval. *J. Neurosci.* **2013**, *33*, 3276–3283. [CrossRef]
49. Wheaton, M.G.; Abramowitz, J.S.; Berman, N.C.; Fabricant, L.E.; Olatunji, B.O. Psychological Predictors of Anxiety in Response to the H1N1 (Swine Flu) Pandemic. *Cogn. Ther. Res.* **2012**, *36*, 210–218. [CrossRef]
50. Bults, M.; Beaujean, D.J.M.A.; de Zwart, O.; Kok, G.; van Empelen, P.; van Steenbergen, J.E.; Richardus, J.H.; Voeten, H.A.C.M. Perceived risk, anxiety, and behavioural responses of the general public during the early phase of the Influenza A (H1N1) pandemic in the Netherlands: Results of three consecutive online surveys. *BMC Public Health* **2011**, *11*, 2. [CrossRef]

51. Everts, J. Announcing Swine Flu and the Interpretation of Pandemic Anxiety. *Antipode* **2013**, *45*, 809–825. [CrossRef]
52. Fu, W.; Wang, C.; Zou, L.; Guo, Y.; Lu, Z.; Yan, S.; Mao, J. Psychological health, sleep quality, and coping styles to stress facing the COVID-19 in Wuhan, China. *Transl. Psychiatry* **2020**, *10*, 225. [CrossRef]
53. Petzold, M.B.; Bendau, A.; Plag, J.; Pyrkosch, L.; Mascarell Maricic, L.; Betzler, F.; Rogoll, J.; Große, J.; Ströhle, A. Risk, resilience, psychological distress, and anxiety at the beginning of the COVID-19 pandemic in Germany. *Brain Behav.* **2020**, e01745. [CrossRef]
54. Gualano, M.R.; Lo Moro, G.; Voglino, G.; Bert, F.; Siliquini, R. Effects of Covid-19 Lockdown on Mental Health and Sleep Disturbances in Italy. *Int. J. Environ. Res. Public Health* **2020**, *17*, 4779. [CrossRef]
55. Majstorovic, M.; Morse, D.; Do, D.; Lim, L.; Herman, N.; Moursi, A. Indicators of Dental Anxiety in Children Just Prior to Treatment. *J. Clin. Pediatric Dent.* **2014**, *39*, 12–17. [CrossRef]
56. Boynes, S.G.; Abdulwahab, M.; Kershner, E.; Mickens, F.; Riley, A. Analysis of parental factors and parent-child communication with pediatric patients referred for nitrous oxide administration in a rural community health center setting. *Oral Biol. Dent.* **2014**, *2*. [CrossRef]
57. Themessl-Huber, M.; Freeman, R.; Humphris, G.; Macgillivray, S.; Terzi, N. Empirical evidence of the relationship between parental and child dental fear: A structured review and meta-analysis. *Int. J. Paediatr. Dent.* **2010**, *20*, 83–101. [CrossRef]
58. Townend, E.; Dimigen, G.; Fung, D. A clinical study of child dental anxiety. *Behav. Res. Ther.* **2000**, *38*, 31–46. [CrossRef]
59. Eli, I.; Uziel, N.; Baht, R.; Kleinhauz, M. Antecedents of dental anxiety: Learned responses versus personality traits. *Community Dent. Oral Epidemiol.* **1997**, *25*, 233–237. [CrossRef]
60. Saheer, P.A.; Marriette, T.M.; Alappat, A.T.; Majid, S.A.; Hafiz, H.; Jamal, F.; Badar, N. Association of dental anxiety with personality traits among Al Azhar arts students in Thodupuzha, Kerala. *J. Glob. Oral Health* **2019**, *1*. [CrossRef]

Journal of
Clinical Medicine

MDPI

Review

Available Technologies, Applications and Benefits of Teleorthodontics. A Literature Review and Possible Applications during the COVID-19 Pandemic

Cinzia Maspero [1,2,*,†], Andrea Abate [1,2,†], Davide Cavagnetto [1,2,†], Mohamed El Morsi [1,2], Andrea Fama [1,2,‡] and Marco Farronato [1,2,‡]

1 Department of Biomedical, Surgical and Dental Sciences, School of Dentistry, University of Milan, 20100 Milan, Italy; andreabate93@gmail.com (A.A.); davide.cavagnetto@gmail.com (D.C.); moh.nagi90@gmail.com (M.E.M.); andreas.fama@hotmail.it (A.F.); marco.farronato@unimi.it (M.F.)

2 Fondazione IRCCS Cà Granda, Ospedale Maggiore Policlinico, 20100 Milan, Italy

* Correspondence: cinzia.maspero@unimi.it; Tel.: +39-338-334-4999

† These authors contributed equally to this work.

‡ These authors contributed equally to this work.

Received: 2 May 2020; Accepted: 15 June 2020; Published: 17 June 2020

Abstract: Background: COVID-2019 spread rapidly throughout the world from China. This infection is highly contagiousness, has a high morbidity, and is capable of evolving into a potentially lethal form of interstitial pneumonia. Numerous countries shut-down various activities that were considered "not essential." Dental treatment was in this category and, at the time of writing, only non-deferrable emergencies are still allowed in many countries. Therefore, follow-up visits of ongoing active therapies (e.g., orthodontic treatment) must be handled taking special precautions. This literature review aims at reducing in-office appointments by providing an overview of the technologies available and their reliability in the long-distance monitoring of patients, i.e., teledentistry. Methods: A literature review was made according to Preferred Reporting Items for Systematic Reviews and Meta-Analyses Protocols (PRISMA-P) guidelines. Randomized clinical trials, cross sectional, observational, and case-control studies were evaluated with the Mixed Methods Appraisal Tool for quality assessment and study limitations. Results: A primary search found 80 articles, 69/80 were excluded as non-relevant on the basis of: the abstract, title, study design, bias, and/or lack of relevance. Twelve articles were included in the qualitative analysis. Conclusions: Teleorthodontics can manage most emergencies, reassuring and following patients remotely. The aim set by dental teleassistance was met as it reduced patients' office visits whilst maintaining regular monitoring, without compromising the results. Although our preliminary findings should be further investigated to objectively evaluate the efficacy, cost-effectiveness, and long-term results, we are confident that teleassistance in orthodontics will have a role to play in the near future.

Keywords: COVID-19; dentistry; teleassistance; remote sensing technology; orthodontics; teledentistry; teleorthodontics

1. Introduction

A new type of coronavirus initially named Novel Coronavirus Pneumonia (NCP) and later renamed new Corona Virus 2019 (2019-nCoV or Covid-19) spread rapidly from China to the world from December 2019. It is the seventh coronavirus known to spillover to humans [1]. This viral infection is of great concern due to its high contagiousness and morbidity, as well as its ability to evolve into a potentially lethal form of interstitial pneumonia and its possible evolution into a potentially lethal form of interstitial pneumonia [2]. Preventive hygiene measures such as social distancing, quarantine, and isolation have been taken to limit its diffusion in most countries to different extent [3]. On 30 January 2020, the World Health Organization (WHO) stated that COVID-19 constituted a public health emergency of international relevance [4].

The National Health Committee keeps receiving an ever-increasing number of confirmed, suspected, and fatal cases reported from all over the world. To date, they are still carrying out world surveillance.

There was an estimated human-to-human healthcare-related transmission of about 41% at the beginning of the outbreak [5]. Many health care workers got and still are getting infected [5].

Government and healthcare services have put on their thinking hats to re-organize triage services in an attempt to reduce nosocomial infection by COVID 19 [5]. This task is particularly arduous as transmission is mainly through droplets and numerous subjects may be asymptomatic and/or in the incubation period. Dental clinics belong to a high-risk category as infection can be facilitated during dental maneuvers that generate droplets, including restorative procedures, professional hygiene sessions, etc., or whilst patients are in the waiting room [6]. Therefore, strict and effective hygiene protocols for infection control are urgently needed for dental practices to reduce dental practitioners' and patients' risk to get infected.

The use of appropriate personal protective equipment (PPE) is pivotal in avoiding cross infection during clinical practice between patients and healthcare workers and the adoption of adequate decontamination measures can help to reduce the risks. Although it has also currently been suggested that dental clinics limit their practice only to not deferrable emergencies, this is not always possible. Some ongoing treatment such as orthodontic therapies and/or critical situations, like conditions that must be identified in the early stages and treated immediately to avoid more serious outcomes, require timely follow-up appointments. Indeed, continuous monitoring by the orthodontist is a must in orthodontic treatment so as to evaluate the efficacy and/or any undesirable effects [7,8].

However, some periodic visits are not strictly necessary and others could be delayed by instructing the patient how to make simple changes to the appliance, for example by indicating which teeth to put the intraoral elastics on or how many activations to perform on the central screw of a rapid palatal expander.

At the time of writing, despite huge investments and research efforts, the current pandemic is still under investigation as are the best preventive measures to be adopted in individual fields. However, we are of the opinion that avoiding unnecessary follow-up appointments whilst maintaining the monitoring of treatment outcomes and current health status would be of great interest and importance for healthcare providers. Recently, an innovative approach has been proposed in the medical field. Although it was originally developed to provide healthcare services in remote areas, it may well be of use in managing healthcare services in this unprecedented emergency situation, i.e., telemedicine.

The World Health Organization (WHO) defines telemedicine as the use of telecommunications and virtual technologies to provide healthcare outside of traditional healthcare facilities [9]. In more detail, telemedicine is a set of technologies, especially Information and Communication Technologies (ICT), specifically aimed at providing healthcare services from a distance to lessen the need for contact between the patient and the healthcare provider [10,11] Secure communication of medical information, notes, sounds, pictures, or any other form of data necessary are required to prevent, or to diagnose pathologies, and therefore, to treat and to monitor patients [9].

Moreover, telemedicine is not only able to facilitate communication and interaction between the healthcare provider and the patient, but also between the providers themselves. Indeed, it can, to a certain extent, remove geographical and temporal barriers, bridging gaps in the dishomogeneous distribution of the healthcare offer. Therefore, it can provide care for more people, enabling them to benefit from healthcare services, especially those who live in remote areas and/or have poorly developed healthcare facilities. It can simplify online transmission of diagnostic tests and reduce waiting lists for consultations through an enhanced organization of appointments [12–14]. This makes these technologies a great resource in optimizing and reducing in-office visits and does not compromise necessary check-ups. Treatment progress and efficacy can be monitored in this time of social distancing, which will most likely be prolonged into the year to come as the international scientific community has declared that a definitive cure and/or vaccine is not yet available as research is still ongoing. Nowadays, telemedicine is becoming more and more widespread in the fields of oncology, cardiology, pediatrics, psychiatry, psychology, radiology, pneumology, dermatology, neurology, orthopedics, ophthalmology, and dentistry [15].

Although teleassistance in dentistry is far from new, it seems that its advantages in orthodontics have not yet been fully explored and is used on a limited scale.

Indeed, there are some reviews on teledentistry in general but none on teleorthodontics as most articles about teleorthodontics are relatively new.

As no reviews have yet been carried out on the efficacy of teleassistance in orthodontics as a way to manage patients at a distance, we would like to report on the evidence available as to the possibility of implementing new technologies in teleassistance, generally known by teleorthodontics to help during the COVID-19 pandemic to remotely monitor patients' conditions.

2. Experimental Section

2.1. Search Strategy

This topic is far from new, however, few studies have been reported, there is need for exploratory research for a better understanding. Given the above, a non-systematic literature review was performed [16]. The electronic literature was searched using the following databases: Medline, Pubmed, Embase, Cochrane Library, EBM Reviews, Web of Science, Ovid, and Google Scholar. The search was mainly based on five terms, i.e., teledentistry, teleorthodontics, virtual assistance, tele assistance, and telemedicine. Embase and PubMed were searched respectively using also the terms Embase subject headings (Emtree) and Medical Subject Heading (MeSH).

The EndNote software reference manager (Version X7 × 9.21, Thomson Reuters, released September 2014, Toronto, ON, Canada) was used/adopted to store/archive and view/analyze retrieved references studies. The research refers to the Preferred Reporting Items for Systematic Reviews and Meta-Analyses (PRISMA-P) 2015 [17,18]. Grey literature was also searched, but no data met the inclusion criteria. A hand search for relevant studies in the selected bibliography was also performed.

2.2. Inclusion Criteria

Studies involving new or already existing devices and software for teleassistance in orthodontics were included. Service provided, type of intervention, clinical outcomes, efficacy and efficiency of assessed methods, and possible time saving compared to traditional methods were evaluated. The following study designs were included: observational studies, longitudinal studies, prospective studies, case-control studies, systematic and narrative reviews, and clinical trials.

Given the state of technology and its rapid evolution, the search was limited to papers published over the previous 15 years.

2.3. Exclusion Criteria

Studies in a language other than English or on application areas unrelated to orthodontics were excluded.

Articles with a poor methodology description lacking at least two of the following were excluded: study design, sample size, hardware utilized, software installed. Letters to the editor, short communications, and all other publications not subjected to the peer review process were also excluded.

2.4. Data Extraction and Quality Assessment

Considering the variety of study designs in the articles included, Mixed Methods Appraisal Tool (MMAT) was used for quality assessment [17]. The score of each article was calculated by dividing the criteria that were considered satisfied by 4 (25% by 1 criterion, 100% if all 4 criteria were considered satisfied). The use of this system is compatible with a literature review that analyzes different research methodologies, as reported by Whittemore [18].

Two of the authors of this study (A.F and M.E.M) read the titles of the retrieved articles independently to ensure they met the eligibility criteria. If in doubt, the abstracts were read and the same method was applied. A final selection was then made by an independent evaluation of the full text of aforementioned papers before inclusion. Any disagreement between the assessors was resolved by their discussing the full texts. The studies selected according to eligibility criteria are reported in the evidence table (Table 1). One reviewer (A.F) extracted data from the full-texts and the other (M.E.M), independently verified the extracted data. Data extraction included: journal and year of publication, study design, clinical outcomes, and the conclusions of the research. The description of the included studies is reported in Table 1.

Table 1. Description of included studies and Mixed Methods Appraisal Tool (MMAT) score.

Author	Year	Study Design	Journal	Primary End Point	MMAT Score and Study Limitations
Morris R.S et al.	2019	Cross-sectional study	Am J Orthod Dentofacial Orthop	Digital models taken with Dental Monitoring software (DM) are precise enough for clinical application.	MMAT score 75%. The sample is too small to extend to the entire population.
Costa A.L.P. et al.	2011	Qualitative	Dental Press J. Orthod	Remote management of clinical cases was successfully carried out. Therefore, teleorthodontics is deemed a viable option. Available technologies, that are accessible and reduced in cost, suggest a quick development of teleassistance in orthodontics in the near future.	MMAT score 100%.
Bradley S.M et al.	2007	Survey	Primary dental care	Almost 50% of the responding dentists working in primary care in this area had a positive attitude towards a teledentistry-based referral scheme to the orthodontic consultants. These practitioners were more likely to be familiar with the use of digital camera and using removable appliances.	MMAT score 100%.
Estai M et al.	2018	Systematic review	J Telemed Telecare	There is emerging evidence as to the efficacy of the use of teledentistry technologies. However, there is some doubt about the price and the long-term efficacy. As the current evidence is inconclusive, further research is needed.	Not applicable
Favero L. et al.	2009	Survey	European Journal of Paediatric Dentistry	Teleassistance in dentistry is a new and powerful tool that makes for effective communication between the care provider and patient and between the providers themselves. The study stated that these technologies can be of significant help in treating orthodontic emergencies.	MMAT score 75%. The sample is not representative of the target population.

Table 1. *Cont.*

Author	Year	Study Design	Journal	Primary End Point	MMAT Score and Study Limitations
Dunbar A.C. et al.	2014	Prospective observational cross- sectional study	Health Eng.	Observations taken from this pilot study through the assessment of treatment planning and comparison between patients' opinion about traditional dental examinations (face to face) and teleorthodontics showed that the treatment planning was influenced by the diagnosis of the observer. However, the consultation system satisfied both the clinician and the patient.	MMAT score 50%. A bigger sample of patients should have been analyzed to evaluate the significance of differences in treatment planning because of the three diagnostic means. Most patients came from urban areas and only one center was considered. Concordance between operators in treatment planning was not possible to be assessed completely because not all the observers examined every subject clinically.
Hansa I. et al.	2018	Survey	Seminars in Orthodontics	This preliminary study assessed the possibility to reduce the number of in-office visits using teleorthodontics software. The patients' feedback on the use of the aforementioned software was positive.	MMAT score 100%.
Moylan H.B. et al.	2019	Cross-sectional study and survey	Angle Orthodontics	A comparison between measurements performed on models taken in-office or with Dental Monitoring software. Intercanine and intermolar distances showed little difference (below 0.5 mm). Therefore, this orthodontic teleassistence system is reliable to make clinical decisions.	MMAT score 100%.
Berndt J. et al.	2008	Case-Control Study	Am J Orthod Dentofacial Orthop	Children presenting malocclusions in remote areas with difficulties in accessing orthodontic care could get interceptive orthodontic treatment through cooperation between general dentists and orthodontists using teledentistry.	MMAT score 75%. It is unclear whether all the outcome data have been provided.
Mandall N.A. et al.	2005	Randomized Controlled Trial	Br Dent J	The authors deemed that teledentistry is an effective method to identify appropriate referrals. Moreover, they stated that teledentistry could increase treatment effectiveness.	MMAT score 100%. No limitations.

Table 1. *Cont.*

Author	Year	Study Design	Journal	Primary End Point	MMAT Score and Study Limitations
Kuriakose P. et al.	2019	Cross-sectional study and survey	Journal of the World Federation of Orthodontists	Dental Monitoring is a reliable tool to monitor rapid palatal expansion in the correction of the crossbite. Dental Monitoring, digital impression, and in-office examination showed no significant difference in assessing intermolar distances. The study concluded that in-office assessment of a rapid maxillary expander can be successfully substituted with teleorthodontics (DM software).	MMAT score 50%. This paper presents a small sample size due to several dropouts. The sample was selected from a pool of patients attending a single hospital and, therefore, the conclusions cannot be extended to a private setting.
Caprioglio A. et al.	2020	Qualitative	Progress in Orthodontics	Teleorthodontics is a useful tool to manage emergencies, and monitor patients at a distance using WhatsApp.	MMAT score 50%. The study is based on personal experience. No patients were analyzed, no results were evidenced

2.5. *Risk of Bias in Individual Studies*

Due to the differences in the design of the selected studies, understandable given the heterogeneity of what was taken into account, it was not deemed fit to apply common methods for evaluation of the risk of bias. There was a low or absent overall risk of bias as to data description but high risk of bias for the efficacy analysis of such a technology. All considered papers had high or unknown selection bias and reference standards. Moreover, as this is a novel topic, to the best of our knowledge, no validated protocol has yet been reported.

2.6. *Limitations of the Review*

Due to the heterogeneity of study designs and the technological tools assessed, it was not possible to carry out a meta-analysis of the data. Therefore, a thematic investigation was made, targeting the main topics that were analyzed in the selected papers. No other limitations appear to be present, as the review was carried out according to the PRISMA-P guidelines.

3. Results

Initially 129 articles were found. The primary search retrieved 80 articles, net of elimination of duplicates (n = 49). A total of 31 articles were then deemed irrelevant after screening the abstract, the title, or the study design and were therefore excluded. Twenty records were screened from the database and another 8 articles were excluded due to bias. Twelve studies were read in extenso and were included in the qualitative analysis. The summary of the studies that met the inclusion criteria is shown in Table 1. The PRISMA flow chart reports the search methodology (Figure 1).

Five studies assessed the benefits of teleassistance in orthodontics for the management of patients at a distance. They all stated that teleorthodontics has the potential to provide significant and determinant help even if further investigation is deemed necessary [19–23].

Five papers evaluated the efficacy and reliability of orthodontic teleassistance in the diagnosis treatment and follow-up of patients [24–28].

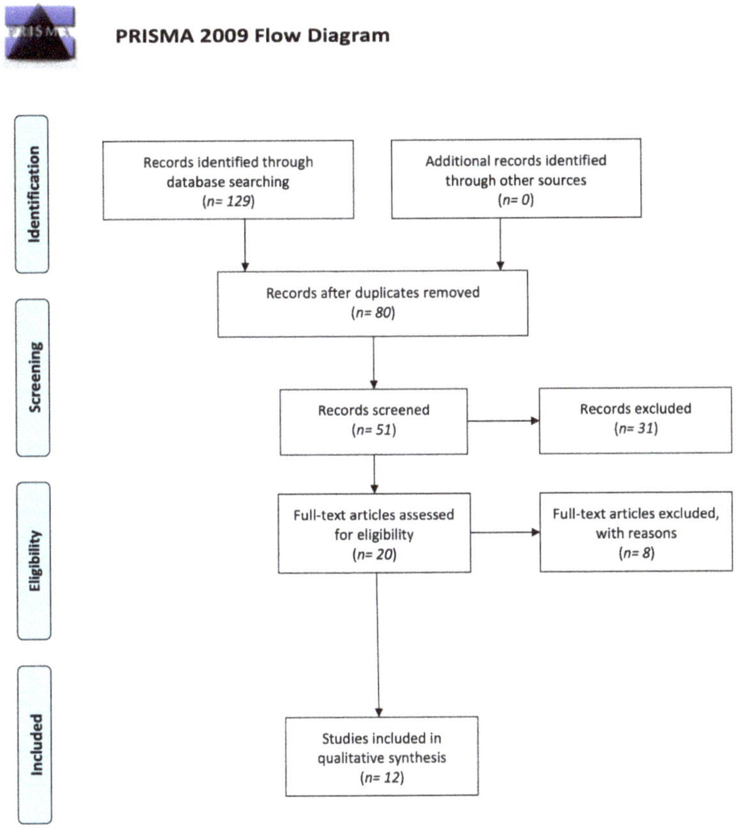

Figure 1. Preferred Reporting Items for Systematic Reviews and Meta-Analyses (PRISMA) flow chart.

One study endorsed the use of teleorthodontics for remote patient management [29].

One study evaluated which of the available IT technologies would allegedly be used in the near future for remote patient management [30]. All the included studies agreed on the advantages of introducing teleorthodontics into clinical practice. Taking into consideration the 11 included studies, one was not analyzed by MMAT, as this system is not suitable for non-empirical studies such as reviews and theoretical papers [20].

A total of 11 studies were analyzed by MMAT, nine of them were quantitative, two qualitative, and no studies used mixed methods. All the papers that were included were rated equal to or above 50% (average score 79.5%) according to the Mixed Method Assessment Tool and were therefore included. Table 1 presents a detailed summary of each of the 11 studies included.

3.1. Available Technologies

Currently, available technologies that can be used in teleorthodontics are: high-speed Internet connection, digital videos and photographs, smartphones, and websites. A review by Costa et al. [30]. emphasized that peer-to-peer communication services (MSN, Skype, etc.) can be helpful in patient management but that they are not sufficiently reliable by themselves, since they are products of big companies, they may be subjected to unpredictable changes. The authors of the aforementioned review thus recommend using websites instead, as they are easier to use and require no installation. In order to minimize problems involving safety, the same authors recommend using anti-virus and/or firewalls and adopt only sites with valid digital certification and end-to-end data encryption [31]. WhatsApp messenger seems to be the most widely used communication tool according to available literature [29]. Maintaining periodic virtual contacts, while it is impossible to do otherwise, is a valuable tool to build and maintain a positive patient–clinician relationship and a valuable therapeutic allegiance [29].

Digital technology in imaging and impression taking, that is now commonplace in most dental practices, is a powerful tool for the orthodontist to access, analyze and, if need be, communicate with patients, colleagues, and/or dental technicians. The widespread diffusion of smart phones among doctors and patients led to the development of a new option. [32,33] Indeed, an application for smartphones that allows remote monitoring of orthodontic patients using an algorithm of artificial intelligence, has recently been developed. This application is called Dental Monitoring™ (DM) [34]. Its purpose is to provide a precise record of the patient's occlusion with the integrated phone camera. DM was designed to carry out orthodontic follow-up at a distance. It tracks tooth movement through a 3D reconstruction of an intraoral movie taken with the smartphone camera and specific cheek retractors. The patients themselves make a video that is processed into a scan by DM™. Therefore, orthodontists can perform real-time monitoring of treatment outcomes anywhere and anytime.

This smartphone application (Android, iOS) was originally designed to provide access to orthodontic treatment for people living in places with limited access, to improve comfort and fruibility of the service for people who have busy schedules or travel frequently for work. Similarly, patients who are on orthodontic treatment during the COVID 19 pandemic period can benefit tremendously from remote monitoring, avoiding unnecessary follow-up appointments. Patient monitoring through this simple software may also improve treatment efficacy by avoiding late detections of problems such as debonded brackets, broken ligatures, non-tracking aligners, and are therefore able to solve the problem in the early stage [22].

3.2. *Benefits of Teleorthodontics*

A review on the benefits of teledentistry published in 2018, which considered only papers with high quality assessment scores, stated that not only is teledentistry potentially an effective tool for patient management, but it also has a positive economic impact on the dental profession. This review also pointed out that there is a rapid increase in the number of publications as to the efficacy of teledentistry, especially in oral medicine, periodontics, pediatric dentistry, and orthodontics [20].

However, due to the lack of conclusive evidence and the different methods (outcomes, assessment methods, main goal, etc.) they adopted, the findings cannot be generalized.

Other papers evaluate teleorthodontics as a means of performing initial examinations and report that there was no disagreement between in-office assessment and remote assessment through clinical photographs as to diagnosis and treatment planning [11,21]. They demonstrated that teleorthodontics reduced costs and provided treatment access to a wider range of persons able to benefit from specialist treatment at a distance, without compromising the quality of care [11,35,36].

A study by Favero et al. reported how new technologies applied to orthodontics allowed for remote management of several common orthodontic questions that would have otherwise necessitated in-office treatment: e.g., ligature displacement, discomfort from the appliance, cheek irritation [21].

A preliminary study by Hansa et al. [22]. evaluated whether the use of remote monitoring, carried out with DM™ software, is able to reduce the number of in-office visits compared to the traditional appointment management. The same study used a questionnaire to assessed patients' attitude towards the use of a remote monitoring software during treatment the patients who had remote monitoring had fewer in-office appointments: 1.68 in average during the 7-month follow-up taken into consideration. This means that over a 2-year treatment period, an average of 5.8 in-office appointments could be avoided by the use of DM software. Most patients classified the application as user-friendly (easy or very easy) (86%) and (84%) thought it was useful for their treatment. The questionnaire revealed that most patients using DM had the sensation of enhanced communication with their dentist and better convenience. However, this study [22] provides only preliminary results and, as do other studies, suggests that if the whole treatment period were to be considered instead of just 7 months, more precise information on the effects of teleorthodontics could be obtained.

Some studies analyzed the benefits of teleassistance in orthodontics and reported their utility in periodic check-ups for those in retention to make an early identification of problems and immediately book in-office appointments, thus maintaining a good doctor–patient relationship and a good level of surveillance over finished cases, without taking up the dentists' and patients' time unnecessarily [26].

3.3. *Effectiveness and Reliability of Proposed Methods*

Several studies have described teleorthodontics as an effective tool that allows the orthodontist to maintain treatment control in situations where the patient cannot go to the clinic [37]. These results are in agreement with data reported by Berndt et al. [19]. The authors provided evidence of the viability of teleorthodontics during interceptive treatment. Other studies have shown that the use of new patient monitoring technologies has enabled dental professionals to enhance the quality of treatment provided to their patients, as reported by Mandall and Stephens [23,38]. These authors stated that teledentistry is an effective way to identify appropriate referrals and that teledentistry may well increase treatment efficacy [20].

Dunbar et al. compared the reproducibility of treatment planning performed on digital records, clinical examinations, and standard records. The paper also considered patients' opinion of in-office visits and teleassistance [25]. It showed that that 50% of the observers were influenced by the type of records used to decide which treatment was more appropriate. The agreement between doctors was higher on standard records than on digital ones. The authors of this study concluded that it is possible to save money, time, and avoid the need to go to the dental office for a consultation [25]. Bradley et al. also made favorable comments about this system [28]. The attitudes toward teleassistance in orthodontics, and in general, dentistry by respective dental care professionals, was investigated in several studies which confirmed it was as an effective alternative to in-office visits for several routine procedures and to make consultations more accessible to dentists and patients [23,38]. Mandall concluded that teleassistance in dentistry is a reliable tool, enabling the screening of new patients and therefore, that it was of substantial help in lowering incorrect referral rates and reduced the waiting list for fist consultations [23].

Morris et al. [24] stated that three dimensional impressions taken with dental monitoring software do not differ greatly to those taken with an intraoral scanner (iTeroElement, Align Technology, Santa Clara, CA, USA). There was a clinically insignificant mean difference of 0.02 mm between the digital models generated with dental monitoring and intraoral scans, suggesting and therefore judging it clinically insignificant [24]. Heather et al. [26] evaluated the reliability and accuracy of DM. They assessed intercanine and intermolar distances during rapid maxillary expansion (RME) on DM scans and on digital models taken at in-office follow-up appointments. The paper reported a slightly higher margin of error for DM scans compared to digital model at the molar level. However, in-office and DM measurements differed by less than 0.5 mm. Therefore, the author of this study concluded that, as long as DM scans are of acceptable quality, they can be reliable in the formulation of clinical decisions. The reliability of DM in the evaluation of rapid palatal expansion treatment, compliance and satisfaction were also studied by Kuriakose et al. [27], who was in agreement with the aforementioned claims. That is, DM was able to make a remote assessment of the condition of posterior crossbite. No significant difference was noted in intermolar width between DM, digital model, or intraoral examination. On the basis of these data, it seems that in-office control of maxillary expansion can be substituted by teleassistance with DM software [27].

Bernd et al. [19] stated that facial orthopedic treatments can be delivered by sufficiently trained general dentists through remote supervision of an orthodontist using teleassistance technology. This may well make a significant improvement in conditions of malocclusion in children, who for various reasons, cannot be treated in-office by an orthodontist. Even if most patients treated with phase I orthodontics usually require a phase II treatment cycle, malocclusion is far less complex and is, therefore, easily managed.

4. Discussion

The ever more powerful capacity of modern computers has led to a continuous development of innovative technologies. Indeed, currently, various branches of medicine and dentistry are benefiting from the advances provided by new technologies for the diagnosis and treatment of several pathologies. Teledentistry is the part of telemedicine that deals with the application of ICT to dental care. Moreover, teledentistry and dental video phoning allow colleagues to readily exchange information. It can also become a cutting-edge screening system able to reduce patients' waiting time for specialist advice. As long as it is correctly set up, it is capable of improving service and working conditions and may even reduce costs [21]. Teleorthodontics generally refers to any orthodontic care delivered through information technology. A common and relevant example could be that of colleagues being able to discuss the digital records of clinical cases over the Internet and to exchange advice and share experience.

The first studies on teleorthodontics date back to the early 2000s [23,38]. A remarkable example that yielded promising results was a paper investigating the possibility to deliver orthodontic treatments through the remote real-time supervision of an orthodontic specialist for general dentists so as to reach patients with limited access to orthodontic care [19,38]. Another useful application is remote retention check-up by sending images rather than physically going to the dentist [22].

However, most likely, we shall have to wait for yet another decade before teleorthodontics becomes a viable option as technological and cultural obstacles still have to be overcome.

In recent years, the number of patients who wish to undergo orthodontic treatment requiring fewer in-office visits, while at the same time allowing the specialist to maintain control over the progress of their treatment, has grown. Teleorthodontics as a mean to further reduce unnecessary journeys to the orthodontic practice while maintaining control over treatment is allegedly one of the main reasons teleorthodontics has gained ground over the past few years. The development of clear aligners and lingual custom prescription brackets with robotic multi-wires has significantly reduced chair-side time and in-office visits [39,40]. As a rule, aligners or wires are changed during in-office visits at pre-established appointments that have been made on the basis of personal experience and common knowledge of an approximated time span for the wire to have exhausted its biological efficacy. However, a one size fits all approach is not always ideal, as average values do not take into account a patient's individual biological response. Teleorthodontics allows for tailor-made scheduled in-office visits though remote monitoring, promoting a more productive workflow.

These procedures are capable of reducing chair time and improving patient convenience.

As reported in the results of our review, it appears that the most promising technology for teleassistance in orthodontics is Dental Monitoring^{TM} (DM). This is based on three integrated platforms: a smartphone application that takes the patient through correct record taking; a software that adopts an algorithm that quantifies individual tooth movements (less than 0.5° for mesiodistal angulation and faciolingual inclination, and rotation) and an Internet-based interface where the dentist can check patients' updates as soon as they are uploaded and interact with the patient. Alerts can be set at certain thresholds to receive warnings should an emergency condition arise, e.g., debonded brackets, gingival issues depending on poor hygiene, non-tracking aligners, and so forth and/or for specific treatment objectives. All images recorded by the software are available on the clinician's platform. Physicians can take advantage of in-office photos (baseline and interim photos) as reference to better understand changes. The software allows four possible monitoring levels, i.e., the number of photos per period of time. Routine pre-treatment monitoring requires one picture every couple of months. The monitoring of active treatment requires one or two photos per week (for aligners and the other therapies respectively). The monitoring of the retaining phase has a more complex picture timing scheme: once weekly for a month, then once monthly for six months, followed by once every couple of months. The last possibility is known as DM Go Live, which is for use in aligner therapy, where pictures are taken once weekly and the patient is informed whether to keep the same aligner or to proceed to the next one. Although expectations are promising, teleassistance in orthodontics could have some limitations. Forwarding scans each 7 days may become a nuisance and frustrating for the patient as they may sometimes need to be taken again.

Moreover, the reduction in the time spent visiting the patient in person may deteriorate the patient–doctor relationship. Therefore, consent and education are needed for the patient to begin a similar path in order to build a positive and strong therapeutic allegiance [22]. During the pandemic outbreak, orthodontists had to significantly reduce, and in certain cases, suspend follow-up visits of patients currently under active treatments. We can therefore say that the use of applications for monitoring orthodontic therapy could be an effective solution to continue to keep deferrable orthodontic patients under control during the closure of dental practice due to COVID 19 and to reduce unnecessary in-office appointments.

The Italian Society of Orthodontics (SIDO) has recently published the recommended guidelines on the management of orthodontic patients during the COVID-19 outbreak. Orthodontic emergencies are unpredictable issues caused by orthodontic appliances that provoke pain or discomfort, thus requiring urgent dental care [29]. Orthodontic emergencies should be faced using a stepwise approach. The first recommended approach should be virtual assistance through photographic documentation or a video call. It is important to perform a preliminary triage to distinguish situations that require in-office treatment rather than those that are remotely manageable. Unlike other dental questions, orthodontic problems like traumatic injuries of teeth and periodontal structures, abscesses, etc., have a lower degree of severity and often do not necessitate in-office care to be solved. The most common orthodontic emergencies are related to the detachment of one or a few brackets and acute stinging of the lips and the oral mucosa caused by orthodontic wire or scraping brackets. Many of these problems can be readily solved at home with less stress for patients' families, saving time for both patients and dentists alike. Since they are not true emergencies, they can, more often than not, be easily resolved by providing the patient with simple instructions during a video call or with typed messages after photographic documentation of the problem, describing the intraoral condition. It has been suggested that dental caregivers become familiar with the potential social networks and modern web-based communication platforms have, thanks to the possibility of making a precise evaluation of indications and contraindications [41,42]. Patients should continue ongoing therapies, but should also be video checked periodically. Dental professionals and their team must select the number of eligible patients and organize this procedure [29]. In all other cases, it is advisable to contact each individual patient in therapy actively in order to give specific indications and it is recommended to make telephone appointments with patients 4–6 weeks apart to carry out a further check-up or fix an appointment in the studio, if strictly necessary [29]. Patients must be reassured and periodically checked, in particular if they have discomfort or problems related to their orthodontic appliance.

It is important to emphasize that not only must emergencies be managed by the orthodontist, but also all other patients with both mobile and fixed appliances. Teleorthodontics relies on information technology and telecommunications and allows for various types of orthodontic follow-up visits at a distance. Therefore, it is of fundamental importance to be able to avail oneself of teleorthodontics for the constant monitoring of all patients should the orthodontic practice be shut-down and/or visits significantly limited.

The professional, thanks to special devices, can check a patient's real situation remotely and compare it with the digital setups previously made, especially in the case of treatments with lingual orthodontics and aligners [26]. Based on the revised articles, new information technology improved the management of orthodontic patients, and in numerous cases, allowed for their remote management. Teleorthodontics has the potential to improve patient management and reduce treatment costs.

This review does have some limitations. One such limitation is the fact that the studies included had only a fair scoring in MMAT. Moreover, although most papers reported a positive attitude towards teleorthodontics, a publication bias may be present since all papers reported one or more positive outcomes for accuracy and/or efficacy and some papers are technical reports or pilot studies.

Only a limited number of papers made a controlled comparison of teleassistance in orthodontics with traditional methods. Many included studies focused on the evaluation of efficacy rather than the effectiveness of teleorthodontics. It would be of great importance to evaluate the appropriateness of teleassistance in orthodontics by assessing clinical outcomes and costs/template details the sections that can be used in a manuscript.

5. Conclusions

This review found a growing number of studies sustaining the efficacy of teleassistance in orthodontics. The advent of a large number of technological innovations over the past few years in dental and in orthodontic practices has allowed for substantial improvement. The COVID-19 pandemic will surely have long-term effects on patient management as it seems unlikely there will be any definitive treatment or vaccines available in the near future. This condition will require a different organization of dental appointments for several months to come and remote patient management could be efficiently carried out using instant messaging platforms to deliver healthcare consultancies. We believe that teleassistance in orthodontics should be considered a welcome resource, as it is able to successfully manage many dental emergencies, to reassure and follow patients at a distance without exposing them and/or dental practitioners to unnecessary risks. Moreover, most case issues can be promptly solved without the patients coming to the orthodontist office by communicating with photos and/or videos, saving both the patient's and clinician's valuable time.

The aim of teleorthodontics is fulfilled by reducing unnecessary follow-up visits while maintaining regular monitoring, thus not jeopardizing expected results. The potential of teleorthodontics is virtually endless; remote consultations could be carried out across the globe without the obstacles of distances or of scheduling appointments. This kind of approach could be of great help in the management of all dentofacial orthopedic removable appliances and of orthodontic treatments that need little in-office maintenance, such as some clear aligner therapies.

Even though in-office visits are still required for many dental and orthodontic procedures, teleorthodontics opens up open new horizons in the treatment and follow-up of many patients.

Nevertheless, currently, most studies report only pilot studies and evaluate short-term results of teleassistance in orthodontics. Therefore, there is limited evidence and the study designs differ, as do the interventions and endpoints assessed in the papers included, meaning that our findings cannot be strictly generalized. However, although we are of the opinion that further studies with higher levels of evidence are needed to objectively evaluate efficacy, cost-effectiveness, and long-term results, we are confident that teleassistance in orthodontics will have a role to play in the future.

6. Future Implications

Technological advances have substantially changed dentistry. In orthodontics, software like Dental Monitoring, which is capable of providing web-based platforms for sharing health data [43] between patients and doctors, may allow orthodontists to closely monitor their patients' status, reducing in-office visits and delivering more patient-centered treatment. The aim of teleassistance in orthodontics is to reduce unnecessary in-office visits and improving monitoring and early treatment of problems that may jeopardize the desired final outcome. Teleassistance in orthodontics may allow for remote consultations that can be carried out wherever without the need for the patient to be anywhere near the office. The downside of teleorthodontics is the reduced time to develop and maintain a positive relationship between doctor and patient [44,45].

Dunbar [25] reported in a feasibility study that 70% of patients thought that in-office consultation was extremely important, and most patients preferred it to teleorthodontics assistance.

Another important consideration are the points of law regarding patient confidentiality that may be in danger because of digital communication of sensible data over the Internet [46]. The quality of the doctor–patient relationship is particularly important should the treatment have complications or if outcomes are deemed unacceptable. Malpractice lawsuits may increase if patients feel they are not receiving treatment of a satisfying quality. Moreover, teleassistance in orthodontics and patients' confidentiality issues are more complicated in orthodontics because patients are often minors.

Therefore, the teleorthodontics we are implementing during the COVID 19 pandemic should not be seen in the future as a new treatment option for patients looking for cheaper and aesthetic alternatives to traditional orthodontics, as dental and orthodontic care should not be reduced to a simple question of "commodity" [47]. As already reported by Hansa et al. [22], orthodontists are still a little doubtful about treatment at a distance because of the possibility of limiting their patient base and due to the risk patients may face. It is the authors' opinion that, in the future, teleassistance in orthodontics will be helpful to maintain high standards of care while reducing unnecessary in-office visits in order to improve rather than reduce the quality of the service already provided by conventional orthodontics.

Author Contributions: Conceptualization, C.M., A.A. and D.C.; methodology, A.A., A.F., M.E.M. and D.C.; validation, A.A., D.C. and A.F.; data curation, A.A., D.C., M.E.M. and A.F.; writing—original draft preparation, A.A. A.F., D.C.; writing—review and editing, A.A., D.C. and C.M.; supervision, M.F.; project administration A.A., D.C. and C.M.; All authors have read and agreed to the published version of the manuscript.

Funding: This research received no external funding.

Acknowledgments: The authors thank Barbara Wade, contract professor at the University of Torino, for her linguistic advice.

Conflicts of Interest: The authors declare no conflict of interest.

References

1. Zhou, P.; Yang, X.L.; Wang, X.G.; Hu, B.; Zhang, L.; Zhang, W.; Si, H.R.; Zhu, Y.; Li, B.; Huang, C.L.; et al. A pneumonia outbreak associated with a new coronavirus of probable bat origin. *Nature* **2020**, *579*, 270–273. [CrossRef]
2. Zhu, N.; Zhang, D.; Wang, W.; Li, X.; Yang, B.; Song, J.; Zhao, X.; Huang, B.; Shi, W.; Lu, R.; et al. A novel coronavirus from patients with pneumonia in China, 2019. *N. Engl. J. Med.* **2020**. [CrossRef]
3. Phelan, A.L.; Katz, R.; Gostin, L.O. The Novel Coronavirus Originating in Wuhan, China: Challenges for Global Health Governance. *JAMA J. Am. Med. Assoc.* **2020**, *323*, 709–710. [CrossRef]
4. Mahase, E. China coronavirus: WHO declares international emergency as death toll exceeds 200. *BMJ* **2020**, *368*. [CrossRef] [PubMed]
5. Wang, D.; Hu, B.; Hu, C.; Zhu, F.; Liu, X.; Zhang, J.; Wang, B.; Xiang, H.; Cheng, Z.; Xiong, Y.; et al. Clinical Characteristics of 138 Hospitalized Patients with 2019 Novel Coronavirus-Infected Pneumonia in Wuhan, China. *JAMA J. Am. Med. Assoc.* **2020**, *323*, 1061–1069. [CrossRef]
6. Coulthard, P. Dentistry and coronavirus (COVID-19)-moral decision-making. *Br. Dent. J.* **2020**, *228*, 503–505. [CrossRef]
7. Maspero, C.; Fama, A.; Cavagnetto, D.; Abate, A.; Farronato, M. Treatment of dental dilacerations. *J. Biol. Regul. Homeost. Agents* **2019**, *33*, 1623–1627.
8. Farronato, G.; Giannini, L.; Galbiati, G.; Maspero, C. Comparison of the dental and skeletal effects of two different rapid palatal expansion appliances for the correction of the maxillary asymmetric transverse discrepancies. *Minerva Stomatol.* **2012**, *61*, 45–55.
9. Ryu, S. Telemedicine: Opportunities and Developments in Member States: Report on the Second Global Survey on eHealth 2009 (Global Observatory for eHealth Series, Volume 2). *Healthc. Inform. Res.* **2012**, *18*, 153–155. [CrossRef]
10. Dasgupta, A.; Deb, S. Telemedicine: A new horizon in public health in India. *Indian J. Community Med.* **2008**, *33*, 3. [CrossRef]
11. Nutalapati, R.; Boyapati, R.; Jampani, N.; Dontula, B.S.K. Applications of teledentistry: A literature review and update. *J. Int. Soc. Prev. Community Dent.* **2011**, *1*, 37. [CrossRef]

12. Ministero Della Salute. Telemedicina Linee di indirizzo nazionali. In *Conferenza Stato Regioni. Atti n*; 2012; Volume 16. Available online: https://scholar.google.com/scholar?hl=it&as_sdt=0%2C5&q=12.%09Della+Salute%2C+M.+Telemedicina+Linee+di+indirizzo+nazionali.+In+Conferenza+Stato+Regioni.+Atti+n%3B+2012%3B+Volume+16.&btnG= (accessed on 21 April 2020).
13. Marcin, J.P.; Shaikh, U.; Steinhorn, R.H. Addressing health disparities in rural communities using telehealth. *Pediatr. Res.* **2016**, *79*, 169–176. [CrossRef]
14. Field, M.J. (Ed.) *Telemedicine: A Guide to Assessing Telecommunications for Health Care*; National Academies Press: Washington, DC, USA, 1996.
15. Bashshur, R.L.; Mandil, S.H.; Shannon, G.W. Chapter 8: Executive Summary. *Telemed. J. E Health* **2002**, *8*, 95–107. [CrossRef]
16. Silva, A.A. *Prática Clínica Baseada em Evidências na Área da Saúde*, 1st ed.; Grupo Gen: São Paulo, Brazil, 2009.
17. Pluye, P.; Robert, E.; Cargo, M.; Bartlett, G. Proposal: A mixed methods appraisal tool for systematic mixed studies reviews. *Montréal McGill Univ.* **2011**, *47*, 1–8.
18. Whittemore, R.; Knafl, K. The integrative review: Updated methodology. *J. Adv. Nurs.* **2005**, *52*, 546–553. [CrossRef]
19. Berndt, J.; Leone, P.; King, G. Using teledentistry to provide interceptive orthodontic services to disadvantaged children. *Am. J. Orthod. Dentofac. Orthop.* **2008**, *134*, 700–706. [CrossRef]
20. Estai, M.; Kanagasingam, Y.; Tennant, M.; Bunt, S. A systematic review of the research evidence for the benefits of teledentistry. *J. Telemed. Telecare* **2018**, *24*, 147–156. [CrossRef] [PubMed]
21. Favero, L.; Pavan, L.; Arreghini, A. Communication through telemedicine: Home teleassistance in orthodontics. *Eur. J. Paediatr. Dent.* **2009**, *10*, 163–167.
22. Hansa, I.; Semaan, S.J.; Vaid, N.R.; Ferguson, D.J. Remote monitoring and "Tele-orthodontics": Concept, scope and applications. *Semin. Orthod.* **2018**, *24*, 470–481. [CrossRef]
23. Mandall, N.A.; O'Brien, K.D.; Brady, J.; Worthington, H.V.; Harvey, L. Teledentistry for screening new patient orthodontic referrals. Part 1: A randomised controlled trial. *Br. Dent. J.* **2005**, *199*, 659–662. [CrossRef] [PubMed]
24. Morris, R.S.; Hoye, L.N.; Elnagar, M.H.; Atsawasuwan, P.; Galang-Boquiren, M.T.; Caplin, J.; Viana, G.C.; Obrez, A.; Kusnoto, B. Accuracy of Dental Monitoring 3D digital dental models using photograph and video mode. *Am. J. Orthod. Dentofac. Orthop.* **2019**, *156*, 420–428. [CrossRef] [PubMed]
25. Dunbar, A.C.; Bearn, D.; McIntyre, G. The influence of using digital diagnostic information on orthodontic treatment planning—A pilot study. *J. Healthc. Eng.* **2014**, *5*, 411–428. [CrossRef] [PubMed]
26. Moylan, H.B.; Carrico, C.K.; Lindauer, S.J.; Tüfekçi, E. Accuracy of a smartphone-based orthodontic treatment–monitoring application: A pilot study. *Angle Orthod.* **2019**, *89*, 727–733. [CrossRef] [PubMed]
27. Kuriakose, P.; Greenlee, G.M.; Heaton, L.J.; Khosravi, R.; Tressel, W.; Bollen, A.-M. The assessment of rapid palatal expansion using a remote monitoring software. *J. World Fed. Orthod.* **2019**, *8*, 165–170. [CrossRef]
28. Bradley, S.M.; Williams, S.; D'Cruz, J.; Vania, A. Profiling the interest of general dental practitioners in West Yorkshire in using teledentistry to obtain advice from orthodontic consultants. *Prim. Dent. Care* **2007**, *14*, 117–122. [CrossRef]
29. Caprioglio, A.; Pizzetti, G.B.; Zecca, P.A.; Fastuca, R.; Maino, G.; Nanda, R. Management of orthodontic emergencies during 2019-NCOV. *Prog. Orthod.* **2020**, *21*, 10. [CrossRef]
30. da Costa, A.L.P.; Silva, A.A.; Pereira, C.B. Teleortodontia: Ferramenta de auxílio à prática clínica e à educação continuada. *Dental Press J. Orthod.* **2011**, *16*, 15–21. [CrossRef]
31. Cone, S.W.; Hummel, R.; León, J.; Merrell, R.C. Implementation and evaluation of a low-cost telemedicine station in the remote Ecuadorian rainforest. *J. Telemed. Telecare* **2007**, *13*, 31–34. [CrossRef]
32. Gupta, G.; Vaid, N.R.; Gupta, G.; Vaid, N.R. The World of Orthodontic apps. *APOS Trends Orthod.* **2017**, *7*, 73–79. [CrossRef]
33. Vaid, N. Up in the Air: Orthodontic technology unplugged! *APOS Trends Orthod.* **2017**, *7*, 1. [CrossRef]
34. Dental Care: Virtual Consultations and Remote Monitoring. Available online: https://dental-monitoring.com/ (accessed on 30 April 2020).
35. Daniel, S.J.; Wu, L.; Kumar, S. Teledentistry: A systematic review of clinical outcomes, utilization and costs. *J. Dent. Hyg.* **2013**, *87*, 345–352.
36. Vegesna, A.; Tran, M.; Angelaccio, M.; Arcona, S. Remote Patient Monitoring via Non-Invasive Digital Technologies: A Systematic Review. *Telemed. E-Health* **2017**, *23*, 3–17. [CrossRef] [PubMed]

37. Kravitz, N.D.; Burris, B.; Butler, D.; Dabney, C.W. Teledentistry, Do-It-Yourself Orthodontics, and Remote Treatment Monitoring. *J. Clin. Orthod.* **2016**, *50*, 718–726.
38. Stephens, C.D.; Cook, J. Attitudes of UK consultants to teledentistry as a means of providing orthodontic advice to dental practitioners and their patients. *J. Orthod.* **2002**, *29*, 137–142. [CrossRef] [PubMed]
39. Brown, M.W.; Koroluk, L.; Ko, C.-C.; Zhang, K.; Chen, M.; Nguyen, T. Effectiveness and efficiency of a CAD/CAM orthodontic bracket system. *Am. J. Orthod. Dentofac. Orthop.* **2015**, *148*, 1067–1074. [CrossRef] [PubMed]
40. Rossini, G.; Parrini, S.; Castroflorio, T.; Deregibus, A.; Debernardi, C.L. Efficacy of clear aligners in controlling orthodontic tooth movement: A systematic review. *Angle Orthod.* **2015**, *85*, 881–889. [CrossRef] [PubMed]
41. Veneroni, L.; Ferrari, A.; Acerra, S.; Massimino, M.; Clerici, C.A. Considerazioni sull'uso di WhatsApp nella comunicazione e relazione medico-paziente. *Recenti Prog. Med.* **2015**, *106*, 331–336.
42. Mars, M.; Escott, R. WhatsApp in clinical practice: A literature review. In *Studies in Health Technology and Informatics*; Santos: Amsterdam, The Netherlands, 2016; Volume 231, pp. 82–90.
43. Lindsten, R.; Ögaard, B.; Larsson, E.; Bjerklin, K. Transverse Dental and Dental Arch Depth Dimensions in the Mixed Dentition in a Skeletal Sample from the 14th to the 19th Century and Norwegian Children and Norwegian Sami Children of Today. *Angle Orthod.* **2002**, *72*, 439–448.
44. Vaid, N. A "Place for Everything," and "Everything in its Place! " *APOS Trends Orthod.* **2017**, *7*, 61. [CrossRef]
45. Lipp, M.J.; Riolo, C.; Riolo, M.; Farkas, J.; Liu, T.; Cisneros, G.J. Showing you care: An empathetic approach to doctor–patient communication. *Semin. Orthod.* **2016**, *22*, 88–94. [CrossRef]
46. Kotantoula, G.; Haisraeli-Shalish, M.; Jerrold, L. Teleorthodontics. *Am. J. Orthod. Dentofac. Orthop.* **2017**, *151*, 219–221. [CrossRef] [PubMed]
47. Vaid, N. Commoditizing orthodontics: "Being as good as your dumbest competitor? " *APOS Trends Orthod.* **2016**, *6*, 121. [CrossRef]